Oxford American Handbook of
Oncology

Second Edition

Published and forthcoming Oxford American Handbooks

Oxford American Handbook of Clinical Medicine
Oxford American Handbook of Anesthesiology
Oxford American Handbook of Clinical Dentistry
Oxford American Handbook of Critical Care
Oxford American Handbook of Emergency Medicine
Oxford American Handbook of Nephrology and Hypertension
Oxford American Handbook of Obstetrics and Gynecology
Oxford American Handbook of Oncology
Oxford American Handbook of Otolaryngology
Oxford American Handbook of Pediatrics
Oxford American Handbook of Psychiatry
Oxford American Handbook of Pulmonary Medicine
Oxford American Handbook of Rheumatology
Oxford American Handbook of Surgery
Oxford American Handbook of Clinical Diagnosis
Oxford American Handbook of Clinical Pharmacy
Oxford American Handbook of Sports Medicine
Oxford American Handbook of Physical Medicine and Rehabilitation
Oxford American Handbook of Geriatric Medicine
Oxford American Handbook of Neurology
Oxford American Handbook of Cardiology
Oxford American Handbook of Urology
Oxford American Handbook of Ophthalmology
Oxford American Handbook of Gastroenterology and Hepatology
Oxford American Handbook of Clinical Exam and Practice Skills
Oxford American Handbook of Endocrine and Diabetes
Oxford American Handbook of Hospice and Palliative Medicine
Oxford American Handbook of Infectious Diseases
Oxford American Handbook of Reproductive Medicine
Oxford American Handbook of Disaster Medicine
Oxford American Handbook of Radiology

Oxford American Handbook of Oncology

Second Edition

Edited by

Gary H. Lyman, M.D., M.P.H., F.R.C.P. (Edin)

Co-Director, Fred Hutchinson Institute for Cancer Outcomes Research
Divisions of Public Health Science and Clinical Research
Fred Hutchinson Cancer Research Center
Professor of Medicine, University of Washington School of Medicine
Adjunct Professor, Schools of Public Health and Pharmacy, University of Washington
Seattle, Washington

with

Jim Cassidy

Donald Bissett

Roy A.J. Spence

Miranda Payne

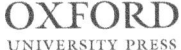

OXFORD
UNIVERSITY PRESS

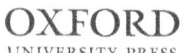

Oxford University Press is a department of the University of
Oxford. It furthers the University's objective of excellence in research,
scholarship, and education by publishing worldwide.

Oxford New York
Auckland Cape Town Dar es Salaam Hong Kong Karachi
Kuala Lumpur Madrid Melbourne Mexico City Nairobi
New Delhi Shanghai Taipei Toronto

With offices in
Argentina Austria Brazil Chile Czech Republic France Greece
Guatemala Hungary Italy Japan Poland Portugal Singapore
South Korea Switzerland Thailand Turkey Ukraine Vietnam

Oxford is a registered trademark of Oxford University Press
in the UK and certain other countries.

Published in the United States of America by
Oxford University Press
198 Madison Avenue, New York, NY 10016

Copyright © 2015 by Oxford University Press, Inc.

All rights reserved. No part of this publication may be reproduced, stored in
a retrieval system, or transmitted, in any form or by any means, without the prior
permission in writing of Oxford University Press, or as expressly permitted by law,
by license, or under terms agreed with the appropriate reproduction rights organization.
Inquiries concerning reproduction outside the scope of the above should be sent to the
Rights Department, Oxford University Press, at the address above.

You must not circulate this work in any other form
and you must impose this same condition on any acquirer.

Adapted from Oxford Handbook of Oncology, Second Edition by Jim Cassidy,
Donald Bissett, Roy AJ Spence, and Miranda Payne, 2006.

Library of Congress Cataloging-in-Publication Data
Oxford American handbook of oncology / edited by Gary H. Lyman ; with Jim
Cassidy, Donald Bissett, Roy A.J. Spence, Miranda Payne.—Second edition.
   p. ; cm.—(Oxford American handbooks)
Handbook of oncology
Based on (work): Oxford handbook of oncology / edited by Jim Cassidy ... [et al.].
3rd ed. 2010.
Includes bibliographical references and index.
ISBN 978–0–19–992278–9 (alk. paper)
I. Lyman, Gary H. (Gary Herbert), 1946–, editor.   II. Cassidy, Jim, 1958–, editor.
III. Bissett, Donald, editor.   IV. Spence, Roy A. J. (Roy Archibald Joseph), editor.
V. Payne, Miranda, editor.   VI. Oxford handbook of oncology. Based on (work):
VII. Title: Handbook of oncology.   VIII. Series: Oxford American handbooks.
[DNLM: 1. Neoplasms—Handbooks. QZ 39]
RC262.5
616.99´4—dc23
2014024777

This material is not intended to be, and should not be considered, a substitute for medical or other professional advice. Treatment for the conditions described in this material is highly dependent on the individual circumstances. Although this material is designed to offer accurate information with respect to the subject matter covered and to be current as of the time it was written, research and knowledge about medical and health issues are constantly evolving and dose schedules for medications are being revised continually, with new side effects recognized and accounted for regularly. Readers must, therefore, always check the product information and clinical procedures with the most up-to-date published product information and data sheets provided by the manufacturers and the most recent codes of conduct and safety regulation. Oxford University Press and the authors make no representations or warranties to readers, express or implied, about the accuracy or completeness of this material, including, without limitation, that they make no representation or warranties about the accuracy or efficacy of the drug dosages mentioned in the material. The authors and the publishers do not accept, and expressly disclaim, any responsibility for any liability, loss, or risk that may be claimed or incurred as a consequence of the use and/or application of any of the contents of this material.

The Editor and Authors dedicate this book to our patients, our families, and our colleagues

Preface

Welcome to the second edition of the *Oxford American Handbook of Oncology*. Based on the successful *Oxford Handbook of Oncology*, this volume has been updated and revised from the first edition by the multiple authors from the Fred Hutchinson Cancer Research Center and the University of Washington as well as Duke University and the Duke Cancer Institute. The updated version includes recently introduced diagnostic, prognostic, and therapeutic strategies emerging since the first edition. As before, the authors have particularly sought to approach each topic from a practical standpoint with pointers to effective diagnostic, staging, and management plans. It will serve as an information source for healthcare providers who come in contact with a broad range of oncology patients, as well as subspecialists who occasionally see cancer patients outside of their primary focus. It is also designed to be a resource for advanced residents and fellows, as well as others who are training or retraining in disciplines related to oncology. The editor and authors hope that this edition may also spark interest in others to pursue further training and focus both clinical and research interest on this fascinating and challenging group of diseases. I would like to thank all of the contributors for their outstanding efforts, and particularly Ms Andrea Parsek and Mrs. Nancy Thomasson, who have greatly assisted all of us in making this final volume one that we can all be proud of. And to our readers: you can thank us most by replying with comments and suggestions that can help us improve future volumes of this series, to make it more useful in your daily care of patients with cancer.

Gary Lyman
Fred Hutchinson Institute for
Cancer Outcomes Research Seattle, WA

Acknowledgments

The editor and authors would like to sincerely thank Ms. Andrea Parsek and Mrs. Nancy Thomasson for their outstanding support and assistance in the completion of this book.

Contents

List of contributors *xiii*
List of plates *xvii*

Part I Background
1 Molecular cancer biology ... 3
2 Etiology and epidemiology ... 15

Part II Cancer prevention and screening
3 Cancer prevention ... 29
4 Cancer screening ... 45
5 Genetic screening ... 51

Part III Principles of management
6 Principles of cancer treatment ... 61
7 Surgical oncology ... 65
8 Principles of radiation oncology ... 81
9 Principles of chemotherapy ... 101
10 Hematopoietic stem cell transplantation ... 151
11 Hormone therapy ... 165
12 Targeted therapies ... 175
13 Gene therapy and immunotherapy for cancer ... 185
14 Complementary and alternative medicine ... 195
15 Clinical trials ... 205

Part IV Complications and supportive care
16 Anemia and fatigue ... 215
17 Febrile neutropenia ... 229
18 Pain management ... 251

19 Venous thromboembolism	271
20 Metabolic emergencies	289
21 Paraneoplastic syndromes	303
22 Superior vena cava syndrome and raised intracranial pressure	321
23 Spinal cord compression	331
24 Other obstructive complications	337
25 Late effects of cancer treatment	351
26 End-of-life care	363

Part V Specific cancers

27 Thoracic cancers	395
28 Breast cancer	429
29 Gastrointestinal cancer I: esophagus, stomach, small intestine, carcinoid	465
30 Gastrointestinal cancer II: pancreas, biliary tract, hepatocellular	483
31 Gastrointestinal cancer III: colorectal, anus	499
32 Endocrine cancers	513
33 Genitourinary cancers I: renal, bladder, ureter, penile carcinomas	535
34 Genitourinary cancers II: prostate cancer	563
35 Genitourinary cancers III: testicular cancer	589
36 Gynecological cancer	605
37 Tumors of the central nervous system	625
38 Head and neck cancers	643
39 Cutaneous malignancies	667
40 Soft tissue and bone sarcomas	687
41 Acute leukemia	717
42 Chronic leukemias and myelodysplastic syndromes	729

43	Multiple myeloma	749
44	Malignant lymphoma	767
45	Cancer of unknown primary	789
	Appendix	801

Index *821*

List of contributors

Amy P. Abernethy, MD
Duke University
Medical Oncology

Ivy Altomare, MD
Duke University
Medical Oncology

Carrie Anders, MD
Duke University
Medical Center

Carey K. Anders, MD
Department of Medicine
University of North Carolina

Andrew J. Armstrong, MD
Duke University
Medical Oncology

Sally Barbour, MD
Duke University
Cancer Center Administration

Jason Cory Barnett, MD
Duke University
Medicine

Rhonda L. Bitting, MD
Duke University
Medical Center

Anne W. Beaven, MD
Duke University
Medical Oncology

Johanna C. Bendell, MD
Duke University
Medical Oncology

Andrew Berchuck, MD
Duke University
Ob/gyn Oncology

Gerard Blobe, MD, PhD
Duke University
Medical Oncology

Karen E. Bullock, MD
Duke University
Medicine

Jeffrey Crawford, MD
Duke University
Medical Oncology

Thomas A. D'Amico, MD
Duke University
Thoracic Surgery

Carlos M. deCastro, MD
Duke University
Medical Onclogy

Annick Desjardins, MD
Duke University
Medical Neurology

Louis F. Diehl, MD
Duke University
Medical Oncology

Phuong L. Doan, MD
Duke University
Medicine

Ashley Engemann, MD
Duke University
Cellular Therapy

Phillip Febbo, MD
Chief Medical Office
Genomic Health

Daphne Friedman, MD
Duke University
Medicine

Christina Gasparetto, MD
Duke University
Cellular Therapy

Daniel George, MD
Duke University
Medical Oncology

Jon Gockerman, MD
Duke University
Medical Oncology

Ranjit Goudar, MD
Duke University
Medical Center

Erika Hamilton, MD
Sarah Cannon Research Institute

Christina I. Herold, MD
Beth Israel Deaconess Medical Center
Instructor in Medicine Harvard Medical School

Bridget F. Koontz, MD
Duke University
Radiation Oncology

Nicole M. Kuderer, MD
Department of Medicine
University of Washington School of Medicine

Kathleen Lambert, MD
Duke University
Medicine

Mark C. Lanasa, MD
Associate Medical Director
MedImmune

Jacob Laubach, MD
Dana Farber Cancer Institute
Instructor in Medicine
Harvard Medical School

Thomas W. LeBlanc, MD
Duke University
Medicine

Matthew McKinney, MD
Duke University
Medical Center

Prateek Mendiratta, MD
Duke University
Medicine

Joseph Moore, MD
Duke University
Medical Oncology and Transplant SVC

Michael Morse, MD
Duke University
Medical Oncology

Jeanne Palmer, MD
Duke University
Medicine

Jeffrey Peppercorn, MD
Duke University
Medical Oncology

Arati V. Rao, MD
Duke University
Medical Oncology

Neal Ready, MD, PhD
Duke University
Medical Oncology

Richard Redman, MD
Duke University
Medical Center

Lindsay A. M. Rein, MD
Duke University
Medicine

Richard F. Riedel, MD
Duke University
Medical Oncology

David Rizzieri, MD
Duke University
Medical Oncology

April K. S. Salama, MD
Duke University
Medicine

Heather Shaw, MD
Duke University
Medical Oncology

Carling Ursem, MD
Duke University
Medicine

James Vredenburgh, MD
Duke University
Medical Oncology

J. Brice Weinberg, MD
Duke University
Medical Oncology

Christopher G. Willett, MD
Duke University
Radiation Oncology

S. Yousuf Zafar, MD
Duke University
Radiation Oncology

List of plates

Plate 1 IMRT plan for a left-sided oropharyngeal head and neck cancer
Plate 2 Benign pigmented lesion
Plate 3 Benign nevus close-up
Plate 4 Malignant melanoma close-up
Plate 5 Malignant melanoma close-up
Plate 6 Squamous cell carcinoma
Plate 7 Basal cell carcinoma

Part I
Background

1 Molecular cancer biology	3
2 Etiology and epidemiology	15

Chapter 1

Molecular cancer biology

Gerard Blobe
Phillip Febbo

Introduction to cancer *4*
Molecular alterations in cancer *6*
Cancer biology *10*

Introduction to cancer

Multistep carcinogenesis

The development of cancer is a multistep process characterized by accumulation of a number of genetic alterations. This process can be referred to as "oncogenesis." Genetic alterations can take the form of mutations (changes in the sequence of the DNA code), deletions (loss of sections of DNA), amplifications (multiple copies of the same DNA section), or epigenetic changes (altering the methylation status of DNA, resulting in activation or repression of genes in the region).

In the aggregate, multiple changes in the DNA of cancer cells alter normal cellular physiology so as to allow limitless proliferation, independence from external growth-promoting or growth-inhibiting influences, avoidance of programmed cell death (apoptosis), and recruitment of blood vessels (angiogenesis). Mutations in DNA repair genes appear to be a necessary feature of most cancers.

For cancer to spread beyond the site of origin, additional changes including loss of cellular polarity, decreased intracellular adhesion, and migratory or invasive characteristics are often required.

Most normal human cells can be transformed into tumor-forming cells by the introduction of four changes: the activation of telomerase (an enzyme that protects the ends of replicating chromosomes), the viral protein large T (which inhibits p53 and Rb proteins), the viral protein small t (which inactivates the signaling protein PP2A), and the expression of an activated *Ras* oncogene. Although this represents a minimal number of genetic changes required for human cells to acquire tumor-like characteristics, the development of a cancer in a person is likely to require additional changes.

Recent work suggests that colon cancers have, on average, nine mutations in cancer-related genes. Thus, although the genetic basis of cancer has been established, an understanding of the oncogenic process is far from complete.

Molecular alterations in cancer

Normal cellular function and homeostasis are regulated by a series of signal transduction pathways. All cancers result from disruption of these pathways, through germ-line, epigenetic, or somatic alterations. Whereas some cancers arise from a single genetic alteration (i.e., the BCR-ABL translocation resulting in chronic myelogenous leukemia), most human cancers arise from several to many sequential genetic alterations.

Functionally, these genetic alterations result in either the aberrant activation of an oncogene, whose protein product now promotes carcinogenesis, or inactivation of a tumor suppressor gene, whose protein product is now unable to mediate its homeostatic function (i.e., inhibiting cell growth or survival). In addition, an emerging number of microRNA genes, which do not encode proteins but instead regulate the expression of other genes, have been implicated in the pathogenesis of human cancers.

Types of molecular alterations
- Germ-line: although rare, result in hereditary (or familial) cancers
- Somatic: most common, result in sporadic cancers
- Genetic: result in changes in the primary DNA sequence
  - Point mutation (alteration of a base pair)
  - Deletion or insertion (loss or gain of genetic material)
  - Chromosomal rearrangements (inversions, translocations)
  - Gene amplification (increasing gene copy number) promoted by deficiency in DNA repair mechanisms
- Epigenetic: result in changes in gene expression that are not caused by changes in the primary DNA sequence, are thus potentially reversible
  - Promoter methylation
  - Histone deacetylation

Oncogenes
- Derived from normal cellular genes (see Table 1.1)
- Encode proteins that control cell growth and/or survival
- Usually gain of function or increased function relative to the normal cellular counterpart
- Protein products include
  - Transcription factors
  - Growth factors
  - Growth factor receptors
  - Signal transduction molecules
  - Regulators of apoptosis

Transcription factors
Often chromosomal translocations result in fusion proteins with aberrant activity.

Growth factors and growth factor receptors
Either overexpression of the growth factor or constitutive activation of the growth factor receptor occurs.

Signal transduction molecules
- Either nonreceptor protein kinases or guanosine-triphosphate binding proteins (G proteins)
- Nonreceptor protein kinases include both tyrosine kinases (ABL, SRC) and serine/threonine kinases (AKT, RAF)
- Usually activating mutations (constitutive or increased activity)

Regulators of apoptosis
- Two main pathways result in apoptosis, the death receptor or extrinsic pathway (ligands binding to death receptors) and the stress or intrinsic pathway (regulated by proteins with BCL-2 homology domains)
- Usually increased expression of inhibitors of these pathways

Table 1.1 Examples of oncogenes

Oncogene	Cancer	Alteration
Transcription Factor		
v-myc, N-MYC, L-MYC	Breast, lung, ovarian	Amplification, viral homolog
v-fos	Sarcoma	Viral homolog
Growth Factor		
v-sis	Glioma, fibrosarcoma	PDGF homolog, constitutive expression
Growth Factor Receptors		
EGFR	Colon, lung	Amplification, mutation
NEU	Breast, lung	Amplification, mutation
Signal Transduction Molecules		
SRC	Colon	Viral homolog, constitutive activation
H-RAS, K-RAS, N-RAS	Colon, lung, pancreas	Viral homolog, mutation
Regulators of Apoptosis		
BCL-2	Lymphoma	Chromosomal translocation
MDM2	Sarcomas	Amplification

CHAPTER 1 Molecular cancer biology

Tumor suppressor genes
- Encode proteins in pathways that normally control cellular homeostasis (growth, survival) (see Table 1.2)
- Usually loss of function or decreased function relative to normal
- Can require loss of both alleles to effect cell function
- Loss of function can be genetic (loss of heterozygosity, mutation), epigenetic, or both
- Can result in either familial cancer syndromes or sporadic cancers

microRNA genes
- Encode a single strand of RNA that anneals to mRNA to either degrade the mRNA or block translation of the mRNA (see Table 1.3).
- Many microRNA genes occur in chromosomal regions involved in translocations, deletions, and amplifications in human cancer, but with no known oncogenes or tumor suppressor genes.
- Can be upregulated (amplification, transcriptional, epigenetic) or downregulated (deletion, transcriptional, epigenetic silencing).
- Upregulated microRNA genes function as oncogenes by downregulating tumor suppressor genes.
- Downregulated microRNA genes function as tumor suppressor genes by downregulating oncogenes.

Table 1.2 Examples of tumor suppressor pathways and genes

Tumor suppressor pathway/genes	Familial cancer syndrome	Sporadic cancer
Hedgehog (PTC)	Gorlin syndrome	Breast, esophageal, gastric, medulloblastoma, pancreatic
HIF-1 (VHL)	von Hippel–Lindau syndrome	Renal cell carcinoma
PI3K/Akt (PTEN)	Cowden's disease	Breast, prostate, thyroid
Rb pathway (p14^{ARF}, p16^{INK4A}, p21^{CIP1}, p27^{KIP1})	Retinoblastoma, osteosarcoma	Most cancers
TP53 pathway	Li-Fraumeni syndrome	Breast, colon, lung, many others
Transforming growth factor-β (TGFBR2, SMAD4)	Hereditary non-polyposis colon cancer	Colorectal, gastric, pancreatic
Wnt (APC)	Familial adenomatous polyposis coli	Colorectal, gastric, pancreatic, prostate

Table 1.3 Examples of microRNA genes

MicroRNA	Target (effect)	Cancer
LET7	*RAS* (increased)	Lung
MiR15a	*BCL2* (increased)	CLL
MiR21	*PTEN* (deceased)	Breast, lung, prostate

Cancer biology

Deregulation of the cell cycle

One critical step in oncogenesis includes changes in genes that regulate cell growth and behavior so as to facilitate uncontrolled proliferation. The process of cell division is very similar in cancer and normal cells, but in many cases cancers exhibit loss of control of the cell cycle.

Cell cycle phases

The normal somatic cell cycle consists of two alternate phases.
- S phase
  - DNA is replicated
  - Duration is 78 hours
- Mitosis (M)
  - Cell division produces two daughter cells
  - Duration is one hour

Separating these are two phases where neither DNA synthesis nor cell division take place.
- G1
  - Between M and S
  - Variable duration
- G2
  - Between S and M

Cells may become quiescent and nondividing by leaving the cell cycle at G1 to enter a G0 phase. It is thought that cancer progenitor cells (also referred to commonly as cancer "stem cells") are often in the G0 phase.

Many of the molecules that drive and regulate the cell cycle have been identified. One important group consists of proteins called "cyclins" that can propel cells through the cycle by the activation of cyclin-dependent kinases (CDKs).

Regulation of the cell cycle normally ensures that cells have precise control of DNA duplication and subsequent cell division, protecting against a loss of genetic information. A number of checkpoints exist within the cell cycle and are crucial in this protection of the normal genome. Mechanisms to detect DNA damage due to incomplete or inaccurate replication often result initially in cell cycle arrest.

> Cell cycle control is essential to protect the integrity of normal genes.

G1–S transition

Exactly when a cell moves from G1 to S is tightly controlled to ensure survival, with factors such as cell size, metabolic state, growth factor availability, and DNA damage affecting whether a transition takes place. The most important checkpoint in the cell cycle is the restriction point, just before entry into S phase. Passage through this checkpoint is regulated by a number of growth factors and a number of critical genes, including *p53*.

p53 plays a key role in maintaining genomic stability. Normal cells with DNA damage become arrested in G1 and undergo programmed cell deaths (apoptosis) under the control of this gene. *p53* is the most commonly mutated gene in human cancer, which is not surprising because loss of control of genomic stability is a central feature of cancers.

- *p53* controls passage between M1 and S phase
- "Guardian of the genome"
- Most frequently mutated gene in human cancer

MYC is a transcription factor that regulates the expression of genes promoting proliferation. Burkitt's lymphoma is a type of cancer caused primarily by amplification of the *MYC* gene, but many more common types of cancers also have amplification of the *MYC* oncogene. Interestingly, if *MYC* is amplified in a normal cell, apoptosis often results.

A second change decreasing normal cell checkpoints is required in most cells in order for MYC to increase proliferation without causing apoptosis.

Cell cycle in cancer
Cancer cells characteristically demonstrate abnormalities in cell cycle and its control. Key features include the following:
- Uncontrolled proliferation with no physiological requirement
- Length of S and M phases is normal
- Short G1 phase
- Failure of checkpoints to arrest cell cycle
- Failure to trigger cell cycle arrest or programmed cell death in presence of damaged DNA
- Genomic instability with accumulation of multiple gene mutations

Independence from external growth-promoting and growth-inhibiting signals

Many normal cells enter the cell cycle (or delay entering the cell cycle) through growth signals from their environment. Through either endocrine (signals from distant cells) or paracrine (signals from adjacent cells) mechanisms, normal cells have a host of membrane-bound, cytoplasmic, and nuclear receptors that detect and relay growth signals to the cells either stimulating or inhibiting initiation of the cell cycle. Independence from these external growth signals is a common feature of cancer cells.

Receptor tyrosine kinases (RTKs) are membrane-bound proteins that relay growth signals. Members of this family of proteins commonly overexpressed in cancers include the following:
- Epidermal growth factor receptor 1 (EGFR/Her1)
- Her2/Neu
- Insulin-like growth factor receptor (IGFR)
- Vascular endothelial cell growth factor receptors (VEGFR)
- Platelet-derived growth factor receptors (PDGFR)
- Fibroblast growth factor receptors (FGFR)

Almost all cancers have constitutive activation of an RTK or downstream signaling member of an RTK pathway.

A paradigmatic example of how this mechanism is important in cancer oncogenesis includes small deletions of the *EGFR* gene encoding for the intracellular portion of the receptor. The subsequent change in the protein results in constitutive activation that is independent of any extracellular signals. These mutations have been found primarily in lung cancers, but similar activating mutations in other family members or other components of the pathways involved in sensing growth signals are found in most cancers.

Overall, changes in the sensing of external growth signals include
- Constitutive activation of progrowth RTKs
- Inactivating mutations, deletion, or epigenetic silencing of growth-inhibiting factors
- Self-production of growth-promoting factors (autocrine)
- Constitutive activation of downstream members of growth-promoting signaling pathways

A paradigm of the last point, constitutive activation of downstream members of growth-promoting signaling pathways, includes activating mutations of the *RAS* oncogene. In normal cells, *RAS* is activated by RTKs when they detect growth-promoting factors. In many types of cancers, most notably colon, pancreatic, and lung cancers, a specific mutation of the *RAS* gene results in constitutive activation.

Limitless replication

Most cells undergo a limited number of replications before becoming terminally differentiated and eventually experiencing programmed cell death (called "apoptosis"; see next page). If human cells are grown in tissue culture with supportive media that provide all their nutritional and metabolic requirements, they will grow and proliferate for approximately 10 to 15 population doublings and then stop dividing and experience senescence, characterized by a nonproliferative, metabolically inactive cell.

During DNA replication and cell division, the ends of each chromosome become shorter in the daughter cells. It is thought that this progressive shortening eventually results in the loss of critical DNA sequence and senescence.

A protein complex referred to as "telomerase" is now known to protect the ends of each chromosome during cell division by replacing the lost ends with repetitive DNA sequence. Cancers have been shown to routinely overexpress telomerase, thus protecting them from progressive shortening of the chromosomes and facilitating effectively limitless proliferation. Although telomerase is most commonly found to be activated in cancers, approximately 15% of tumors use an alternative mechanism that remains poorly understood.

- Telomerase protects the ends of the chromosome, replacing lost genetic material after each replication.
- Most cancers have increased telomerase activity.
- Alternative, as yet unknown, mechanisms exist to protect the ends of chromosomes.

Evasion of apoptosis

Apoptosis is the term that refers to programmed cell death and represents the natural end to most cells in the human body. Evasion from apoptosis is one mechanism by which normal cells can become transformed.

There are two basic apoptotic pathways. The intrinsic pathway generally results from cells sensing DNA damage or other internal stress and activating cytochrome c release from the cellular mitochondria with the subsequent activation of the apoptosome complex and a cascade of proteases called the "caspases."

The extrinsic pathway is triggered by external signals such as TRAIL or CD95 ligand but also eventually results in activation of the caspases. Inhibition of the intrinsic apoptotic pathway and/or insensitivity to the extrinsic apoptotic pathways is critical to the development and progression of cancer cells.

Follicular lymphoma is a cancer that results from the overexpression of bcl-2 through a genetic translocation—the aberrant juxtaposition of two pieces of DNA generally located on different chromosomes or parts of chromosomes. In follicular lymphoma, the *bcl-2* gene is placed adjacent to a gene that is generally expressed at much higher levels. As a result, *bcl-2* is expressed at much higher levels and significantly decreases intrinsic activation of apoptosis.

Establishing angiogenesis

Without recruiting new blood vessels, the size and extent of a tumor is severely limited. The recruitment and development of blood vessels (angiogenesis) is a universal characteristic of cancer cells. Often, cancer cells will express factors promoting blood vessel growth. This has been observed in different laboratory experiments; when cancer cells are compared with normal cells, they more rapidly and robustly establish blood vessels.

Growth factors that can be used to recruit blood vessels include
- Vascular endothelial growth factor (1 and 2)
- Platelet-derived growth factor (α and β)
- Fibroblast growth factor
- Angiogenin 1 and 2

Kidney cancer, specifically clear-cell carcinoma, has historically been known to be highly vascular. In patients with familial clear-cell carcinoma and in sporadic clear-cell carcinoma, mutations in the von Hipple-Lindau (*VHL*) gene are found approximately 85% of the time. *VHL* normally acts to suppress the activity of a gene called hypoxia-induced factor 1α (*HIF1α*). When cells experience hypoxia, *VHL* releases *HIF1α*, which acts as a transcription factor and increases the expression of genes that encourage new blood vessel formation (VEGF and others). The mutations of *VHL* found in familial and sporadic renal cell carcinoma also result in the release of *HIF1α* and the constitutive activation of signals encouraging new blood formation.

Invasion and metastasis

Most patients who die from cancer die from complications due to the metastatic spread of cancer cells throughout the body. Together with all the characteristics discussed above, cancer cells are frequently found to have the following characteristics:
- Anchorage-independent growth
- Decreased cell-to-cell adhesions
- Increased migration
- Increased invasion

The process of hematogenous metastasis (i.e., spread through the blood system) involves the sequential task of migrating through the stromal tissue present in most cancers, entering a blood vessel, traveling through the blood without getting stuck in the lungs or killed by immune cells, adhering to endothelial cells at a remote site, migrating through the endothelium to exit the vascular system, and growing and dividing in a foreign environment. The well established propensity for specific cancers to commonly spread to specific sites (i.e., prostate cancer to bone) is best modeled by a "seed and soil" hypothesis in which features of both the cancer cell and the environment of the metastatic site likely contribute to the observed predilections.

Some molecular changes associated with metastasis include
- Expression of matrix-metalloproteases
- Decreased expression of E-cadherin
- Alteration of specific integrin family member expression

Chapter 2

Etiology and epidemiology

Gary H. Lyman

Genetic factors 16
Smoking 18
Alcohol 19
Diet 19
Infections 20
Gender 22
Sun exposure 22
Other radiation exposure 23
Chemical exposures 24
Further reading 25

Genetic factors

Most cancers are monoclonal, i.e., a single cell accumulates sufficient mutations in key genes resulting in uncontrolled cell proliferation. Genes involved in the development of cancers fall into three categories.

Tumor suppressor genes—genes whose function is lost during carcinogenesis

Both allele copies must be inactivated before the tumor suppressor function is completely lost, resulting in the absence of normal protein product (recessive).
- *p53* gene produces a transcriptional regulator involved in cell cycle control and maintaining genomic integrity.
- Functional mutations result in loss of growth-inhibitory mechanisms.
- Mutations can be hereditary, i.e., germline mutations, or acquired.
- 50% of human cancers possess *p53* mutations, including carcinomas of breast, lung, pancreas, and colon, and brain tumors as well as malignancies seen in the inherited Li–Fraumeni syndrome.

Proto-oncogenes—genes whose function becomes enhanced in carcinogenesis

These usually play an essential role in controlling cell proliferation and encoding growth factors, growth factor receptors, and transcription factors. Mutations of oncogenes may impede normal regulation, resulting in uncontrolled cellular replication. Mutations in only one of the proto-oncogene alleles are needed for the mutant gene product to influence downstream events, i.e., mutations are dominant at the cellular level.
- *Ras* proto-oncogene encodes a membrane-associated G protein responsible for cellular signal transduction.
- Mutated *Ras* products remain activated even in the absence of the appropriate growth factor receptor signal.
- Mutations in *Ras* are implicated in 30% of all cancers including melanoma, lung, and pancreas.

DNA repair genes—genes whose usual function is to carry out DNA repair

Functional mutations of DNA repair genes accelerate accumulation of mutated tumor suppressor genes and proto-oncogenes.
- *ATM* gene (chromosome 11) encodes a protein involved in the detection of DNA damage, with an important role in cell cycle progression.
- Multiple double-stranded DNA breaks lead to high rates of chromosomal rearrangements producing the syndrome of ataxia–telangiectasia associated with progressive cerebellar ataxia, increased incidence of certain malignancies such as lymphomas and leukemias, and an enhanced response to treatment with ionizing radiation.

Specific genes that confer a high probability of susceptibility to specific cancer
- Usually highly penetrant
- Comprise 5% of total incidence of cancers

Examples of disorders (cancer), chromosome and gene relationships
- Retinoblastoma: 13q–*RB1*
- Wilms' tumor: 11p–*WT1*
- Familial adenomatous polyposis: 5q–*APC*
- Hereditary non-polyposis coli Lynch I (colon): 18q–*MSH2* Lynch II [gastrointestinal (GI), genitourinary (GU)]: 2p–*LCF2*
- Li–Fraumeni syndrome: 17p–*p53*
- Breast/ovary: 17p–*BRCA1*
- Dysplastic nevus syndrome: 1p–*CMM1*

Genes with modest effects that may interact with environmental factors
- Tumor viruses expressing genes that disrupt activity of tumor suppressor genes

Genetic (somatic) mutations caused by recognizable carcinogens causing sporadic cancers

Many exogenous carcinogens cause somatic mutations, e.g., aromatic hydrocarbons and ultraviolet (UV) radiation.

Smoking

- Tobacco smoking is the most important known carcinogen and the single greatest avoidable cause of premature death worldwide.
- It is associated most commonly with lung cancer but also has a causative role in many other cancers, such as cancers of the esophagus, head and neck, bladder, and pancreas.
- 15% of all cancer cases worldwide and >30% of cases in men from developed countries are attributable to smoking.
- Cigarette smoking has a synergistic (multiplicative) effect on the risk of developing cancer associated with other carcinogens, e.g., asbestos and radon.
- A substantial increase in the global burden of cancer can be expected unless measures to control tobacco distribution and use are strengthened. The growth in global cigarette consumption appears to be greatest among women and in developing countries.
- Smoking cessation reduces the risk of cancer, but programs promoting individual cessation have had only limited success.
- Passive exposure to tobacco smoke also contributes to the overall cancer risk.
- Active smoking is responsible for 85%–90% of cases of lung cancer, with radon exposure, passive smoking, and other environmental and occupational exposures accounting for the rest. The relative risk of lung cancer in a lifelong smoker compared with that of a lifelong nonsmoker is between 10- and 30-fold, depending on intensity and duration of exposure.

Alcohol

- Alcohol is implicated as a causal factor in several malignancies such as squamous cell carcinomas of the head and neck, and esophagus and hepatocellular carcinoma.
- Excess alcohol intake has a positive association with tobacco consumption.
- Alcohol and tobacco exposure may have a synergistic rather than additive effect on cancer incidence, but the association between the two can make assessment of the relative contribution of each difficult to elucidate.
- Alcoholic cirrhosis is a risk factor for hepatocellular carcinoma, although excessive alcohol intake in the absence of cirrhosis has a less clear role.

Diet

- Aflatoxin contamination in the developing world is associated with a very high rate of hepatocellular carcinoma.
- High intake of vegetables and fruit shows a consistent, inverse relationship with many cancers, including those of larynx, lung, and GI tract.
- High levels of vegetable consumption are associated with a reduced risk of colon cancer; alternatively, high levels of meat consumption appear to increase the risk.
- Obesity in adult life increases the risk of endometrial cancer as well as postmenopausal breast cancer and cancer of the kidney.
- Although difficult to prove, appropriate dietary modifications may significantly influence the incidence of certain cancers.
- The incidence of nasopharyngeal cancer in developing countries could be reduced by as much as 33%–50% by reducing intake of salt fish.
- Halving the median daily intake of aflatoxins produced by *Aspergillus* species may reduce the incidence of hepatocellular carcinoma in Africa and Asia by up to 40%.

Infections

It is estimated that 16% of the worldwide incidence of cancer is due to infection. For developed countries the proportion is 9%, and for developing countries the proportion is >20%.

Viral infections

Most tumor viruses are ubiquitous; prevalence of infection is much higher than the incidence of the respective form of tumor. Development of associated tumors requires many years of infection.

Viral infection plays a significant role in the initial phases of carcinogenesis. However, other cofactors are necessary for development of virally linked tumors, including genetic, immunological, and environmental factors. Examples of viruses directly linked to human tumors include the following.

Human papillomavirus

- Small, double-stranded DNA viruses (*Papovaviridae* family)
- They specifically infect squamous epithelial cells
- >100 different genotypes identified
- The strongest evidence for carcinogenicity is for HPV types 16 and 18 (cervical cancer).
- HPV infection accounts for >80% of cervical cancers worldwide

Hepatitis B and C virus

- 81% of cases of hepatocellular carcinoma (HCC) are attributable to chronic infection.
- 5% with primary hepatitis B virus (HBV) and upwards of 80% with acute hepatitis C virus (HCV) infection develop lifelong hepatic infection, hepatocellular injury, and chronic hepatitis.
- Chronic HBV infection is associated with a 100-fold risk of HCC.
- Prevalence of HBV carriers in Southeast Asia, China, and Sub-Saharan Africa may be >20%.

Epstein-Barr virus

- An endemic herpes virus.
- Epstein-Barr virus (EBV) may be associated with up to 60% of Hodgkin's disease in developed countries, and up to 80% in developing countries.
- EBV is thought to be causative in >90% of Burkitt's lymphoma in equatorial Africa, where Burkitt's is the most common childhood malignancy.
- EBV has a lesser role elsewhere, with <25% of cases outside Africa, the Middle East, and South America.
- Carcinogenic potential in EBV-endemic areas may be facilitated by coincidental infection with *Plasmodium falciparum* (malaria) depressing cytotoxic T-cell function. EBV infection escapes T-cell surveillance.
- There is greater uncertainty about its role in other types of non-Hodgkin's lymphoma.
- There is a highly consistent association with nasopharyngeal carcinoma.

RNA retroviruses associated with human malignancies
- Human T-cell lymphocytotrophic virus (HTLV)-1: adult T-cell leukemia
- HTLV-2: hairy cell leukemia variant
- Human immunodeficiency virus (HIV): Kaposi's sarcoma, lymphoma, and other cancers linked to the acquired immunodeficiency disorder (AIDS)

Bacterial infections

Helicobacter pylori
- May be associated with >60% of cases of gastric adenocarcinoma in developed countries
- Also likely to have a role in the development of gastric lymphoma
- Different strains of *Helicobacter pylori* may have different carcinogenic potential.

Parasitic infections

Schistosoma haematobium (Bilharzial bladder disease)
- Linked to hyperplasia, metaplasia, dysplasia, and invasive carcinoma of the bladder.
- 8% of cases of bladder cancer in the developing world, most commonly squamous cell carcinoma, may be attributable to infection.
- It is not associated with bladder cancer seen in the developed world.

Gender

- Many cancers occur more frequently in one gender or the other, e.g., stomach cancer is twice as frequent in men.
- It is difficult to distinguish innate differences in susceptibility from differences caused by other risk factors. For example, the greater incidence of carcinoma of the bladder in men was thought to represent an innate difference in susceptibility, but, when exposed to the same occupational carcinogens and tobacco smoke, women are at least as susceptible to the disease.

Sun exposure

- Epidemiological evidence suggests >90% of malignant melanoma is attributable to solar radiation.
- The most frequent primary sites are areas exposed intermittently but intensely, e.g., skin of the back.
- Australians who are mostly white and intensely exposed to UV radiation have the highest incidence of melanoma in the world, although recent declines have been reported.
- Rates of melanoma, however, continue to increase in the United States.
- Sun exposure, especially repeated burns in childhood, is a particular risk factor.
- Exposure to solar radiation is also associated with most nonmelanoma skin cancer.
- Basal cell and squamous cell carcinomas are associated with cumulative sun exposure, typically in maximally sun-exposed areas, e.g., the face and ears.

Other radiation exposure

Ionizing radiation includes both high-frequency, short-wavelength electromagnetic energy such as x-rays and gamma radiation, and high-energy subatomic particles such as electrons, protons, neutrons, and alpha particles.

Measures of ionizing radiation:
- Radiation release: 1 Curie (Ci) = 3.7×10^{10} decays/second
- 1 Becquerel (Bq) = 1 decay/second
- Roentgen: the amount of radiation, e.g., gamma, producing a charge of 2.58×10^{-4} coulomb in 1 kg dry air

Effects of radiation on tissue:
- Exposure to 1 Roentgen ~1 rad (radiation absorbed dose)
- 100 rads = 1 Joule/kg tissue = 1 Gray (Gy)
- 100 rem (radiation effect in man) = 1 Sievert (Sv)

- **High-dose exposure:** ionizing radiation at doses of 500–2000 mSv is known to be carcinogenic, potentially causing several malignancies, e.g., acute leukemia, thyroid cancer. Much of the data comes from the atomic bomb survivors of Hiroshima and Nagasaki.
- **Low-dose exposure:** much of the data comes from epidemiological studies of miners and studies of second malignancies in patients previously treated for cancer.
- The average per-capita dose from all sources of ionizing radiation is 3.6 mSv per year, with 82% from natural sources, of which two-thirds is from radon exposure. The remainder is primarily from medical exposures.
- Extrapolation from data on exposure to ≥500 mSv suggests that 1%–3% of all cancers may be attributable to radiation arising largely from natural sources.
- The initiating factor for radiogenic cancers is probably a mutation in a tumor suppressor or proto-oncogene and aberrant loss or gain of function.
- 3% of the population shows undue sensitivity to conventional doses of ionizing radiation without any obvious pretreatment phenotype apart from the presence of cancer. This group is at risk of excess toxicity from standard radiation therapy regimens. Greater understanding of underlying defects in DNA repair, cell cycling, and DNA damage signal transduction would allow appropriate tailoring of therapy.
- Rare radiosensitivity syndromes also exist, predisposing to early development of cancer, e.g., ataxia–telangiectasia and Bloom's syndrome. Susceptibility to DNA damage is enhanced, and both radiotherapy and chemotherapy regimens need adjustment accordingly.

Chemical exposures

Other exposures account for <5% of the cancer burden. Many chemical carcinogens have been identified.

Industrial exposure
- Dye and textile workers (naphythylamines): bladder cancers
- Chemical and rubber workers (benzene): hematological malignancies
- Vinyl chloride: angiosarcoma of liver
- Asbestos exposure: lung cancer, mesothelioma (notifiable)
- Beryllium, chromium, nickel: lung cancer

Pharmacological exposure
- Many chemotherapeutic agents used in the treatment of cancer are carcinogenic, e.g., alkylating agents.
- High-dose diethylstilbesterol during pregnancy, used in the 1960s to reduce the risk of miscarriage, in the development of clear cell carcinoma of the vagina at the time of menarche in a small percentage of the offspring of exposed women.
- Immunosuppressants have been associated with non-Hodgkin's lymphomas.

Environmental exposure
- Causal carcinogenic links with environmental pollutants have been difficult to establish.
- Estimates suggest 1% of U.S. lung cancer deaths are attributable to air pollution.
- Incidence of many cancers varies greatly between geographical areas: this includes variation between countries and between different regions within countries.
- Variations reflect complex interactions between genetic, environmental, socioeconomic, and behavioral factors.
- Migration between areas of contrasting incidence: a migrant population usually acquires the cancer pattern of their adopted country—i.e., environmental rather than genetic factors dominate, except in rare familial cases.
- Cancer incidence can vary between socioeconomic groups.
- Epidemiological studies continue to improve understanding of the etiology of different cancers and aid in development of strategies for disease prevention.

Further reading

Adami H, Hunter D, Trichopoulos D (2002). *Textbook of Cancer Epidemiology*. New York: Oxford University Press.

Jemal A, Siegel R, Ward E, et al (2008). Cancer statistics 2008. *CA Cancer J Clin* 58:71–96.

Lyman GH, Kuderer NM (1997). Basic population and cancer genetics and their use in the assessment of cancer risk. *Eur J Cancer* 33:2160–2166.

Stewart B, Coates A (2005). Cancer prevention: a global perspective. *J Clin Oncol* 23:392–403.

Part II
Cancer prevention and screening

3 Cancer prevention	29
4 Cancer screening	45
5 Genetic screening	51

Chapter 3

Cancer prevention

Gary H. Lyman

Prevention strategies: introduction 30
Cancer: genetic, environmental, and infectious risks 32
Smoking-related cancers 34
The role of surgery in cancer prevention 36
Cancer chemoprevention 38
Clinical trials of cancer prevention 40
Cancer prevention: diet 42
Further reading 44

Cancer prevention

Prevention strategies: introduction

Most cancer patients are diagnosed in late stage, and even those cancers that are diagnosed at an early clinical stage are the manifestation of a much longer preclinical carcinogenic process. These observations have prompted efforts to prevent cancers, particularly in those at highest risk.
- The World Health Organization (WHO) estimates that approximately one-third of all cancers are preventable through currently available strategies.

Overall cancer mortality rates have begun to decline in the United States, with an accelerated rate of decline observed in most recent years. This trend is thought to be due in part to more widespread adoption of primary and secondary (early detection) cancer prevention strategies.

The field of cancer prevention brings together the following disciplines:
- Epidemiology
- Carcinogenesis
- Experimental therapeutics
- Molecular biology
- Infectious diseases
- Genetics
- Public health

Approaches to cancer prevention include avoidance of chemical and physical carcinogens, excision of preinvasive lesions, prevention and eradication of cancer-associated infectious diseases, removal of organs at high risk for cancer, and chemoprevention.

Chemoprevention is the use of chemical agents or dietary compounds to reduce the incidence of cancer.

The chemical compounds could be trace elements, hormones, molecularly targeted agents, or other compounds; the dietary compounds could be fiber, nutrients, vitamins, or extracts of foodstuffs. A thorough understanding of the causes and mechanisms of carcinogenesis is the best guide to the designing of effective prevention strategies.

However, incomplete information for causation of a particular cancer type is the norm, thus the rationale for prevention strategies has often been based on epidemiological associations.
- For example, colorectal cancer is almost unknown in numerous tribes in Africa, possibly due to their high-fiber diet.
- Similarly, several studies have associated breast cancer with obesity and numerous studies have subsequently attempted to explore the relationship of fat in the diet and the onset of breast cancer.

Prevention strategies have appropriately been directed to individuals at highest risk for the target cancer.

Most current risk assessments are based on traditional clinical characteristics such as age, known exposure to carcinogens (e.g., tobacco), and presence of associated disease (e.g., ulcerative colitis).

Although some preventive approaches are now being applied more broadly to populations, such as vaccination against human papilloma virus, there is increasing emphasis on focusing prevention through use of genetic risk and more sophisticated biomarkers of cancer risk based on genomics and proteonomics. Having understood the cancer process and defined the population at greatest risk, it is easier to implement prevention approaches that are ultimately proven to decrease cancer incidence.

Cancer: genetic, environmental, and infectious risks

Genetic risks

Individuals with certain genetic defects are more likely to get cancer. Highly penetrant gene mutations have been associated with multiple familial cancer syndromes associated with a wide range of cancer types.

- These gene defects are transmitted as autosomal dominant traits, and individuals with these gene mutations usually have a very high risk of cancer during their lifetime.
- However, the prevalence of these gene mutations is low, thus the total population risk attributable to these genes is also low.

Table 3.1 lists examples of highly penetrant, low-prevalence, cancer-associated genes. There are more than 20 genes in this category. Population studies have also implicated genetic variants (polymorphisms) with a lower risk of cancer but much higher prevalence. To date, none of these studies has been sufficiently replicated to help guide clinical practice.

Environmental risks

- Several environmental factors are known to cause premalignant lesions; e.g., chewing tobacco frequently causes leukoplakia, which may progress to oral cancer.
- Smoking and lung cancer: cigarette smoking remains the most important avoidable environmental carcinogen worldwide (see Smoking-related cancers, p. 40).
- The association of ultraviolet (UV) light with skin cancer, including malignant melanoma, has been clearly demonstrated. The increasing incidence of malignant melanoma has been clearly linked to behaviors that increase the intensity and duration of sun exposure.

Table 3.1 Cancer types and associated genes

Cancer type	Gene
Breast	BRCA1, BRCA2
Colon	AFP, MSH2
Melanoma	CDKN2A, CDK4
Papillary renal cell	met
Thyroid	ret

Infectious causes of cancer

Viruses have been incriminated in the etiology of the following:
- Hepatocellular carcinoma (HCC; hepatitis B and C viruses)
- Cervical carcinoma (human papilloma virus [HPV] serotypes 16, 18, others)
- Anal carcinoma (HPV)
- Burkitt's lymphoma (Epstein-Barr viruses [EBV])
- Nasopharyngeal carcinoma (EBV)

Vaccines are available against some of these agents, but only hepatitis B and HPV vaccines have been tested long enough to show efficacy.

Helicobacter pylori has been linked to gastric carcinoma and early claims of eradication of the organism by antibiotics, and subsequent protection from cancer are being validated.

Smoking-related cancers

Tobacco smoke contains more than 4000 chemicals, of which more than 50 are known carcinogens. These agents cause DNA gene mutations.

Nicotine causes the addiction to tobacco and hence the exposure to the carcinogens, and it has recently been implicated as potentially contributing to carcinogenesis by activation of nicotinic acetylcholine receptors on bronchial epithelial cells.

- Tobacco use causes 30% of all deaths in the Western world.
- Smoking causes approximately 90% of lung cancers, with a clear dose-response relationship between the risk of developing cancer and cigarette consumption.
- Passive smoking is now well recognized as a danger and cause of smoking-related cancers.
- Male lung cancer deaths have been decreasing since approximately 1990, whereas in females, lung cancer deaths have only recently begun to decline, trends that reflect smoking patterns.
- Smoking is also the major cause of cancers of the larynx, mouth, tongue, pharynx, and esophagus, among others.
- Smoking is a factor in the development of cancer of the pancreas, kidney, stomach, colon, bladder, and cervix.

In an effort to stop exposure to passive smoking and discourage active smoking, some countries have banned smoking in workplaces, restaurants, bars, and other public areas.

Individual smoking cessation adjuncts include counseling (in person or by telephone, such as 1-800-QUIT-NOW) and pharmacological agents (buproprion, varenicline, nicotine replacement), but the most important factor remains patient readiness to quit.

The role of surgery in cancer prevention

Prophylactic surgery to prevent cancer in selected patients is of benefit in the following diseases.
- Multiple endocrine neoplasia (MEN) type II and familial medullary cell thyroid carcinoma, in particular the relatives of patients who have the MEN 2B and 2A syndrome. Prophylactic thyroidectomy is recommended under the age of five years.
- In patients with Barrett's esophagus, especially with high-grade dysplasia, there may be a role for prophylactic esophageal resection.
- Hereditary diffuse gastic cancer—there may be a role for preventative total gastrectomy.
- Ulcerative colitis of over 10 years in the patient with total colitis and who has dysplasia may warrant a total colectomy, although this is now less popular with the advent of regular surveillance colonosocopy.
- Hereditary colorectal cancer
  - **Familial adenomatous polyposis (FAP) coli.** After the diagnosis of this condition (with over 100 adenomas), total colectomy with a pouch procedure is now accepted practice to prevent the inevitable development of colorectal carcinoma.
  - **Hereditary non-polyposis colorectal cancer (HNPCC)** accounts for 5% of all colorectal cancers. There is currently no consensus regarding prophylactic subtotal colectomy in patients with HNPCC.

The 5%–10% of patients with hereditary breast carcinoma and who carry the *BRCA1* gene have a lifetime risk of 60%–85% of getting breast cancer.
- Some of these patients may opt for bilateral mastectomy and breast reconstruction.
- Women who carry a mutation in *BRCA1* and *BRCA2* genes are at a high risk of developing ovarian cancer.
- The lifetime risk lies between 60% and 85%, and after counseling, some of these women will opt for laparoscopic prophylactic oophorectomy.

Patients with an undescended testis have a higher chance of developing testicular cancer—more than 20 times that of the general population.
- 10% of testicular tumors arise from undescended testes.
- Orchidopexy is generally recommended within the first year or two of life; however, this does not abolish the risk of developing future testicular cancer.
- It is generally agreed that in the postpubertal boy, a nonpalpable undescended testicle should be excised.

The role of surgery in cancer prevention

Removal of preinvasive lesions

In addition to surgical removal of whole organs in high-risk individuals, a strategy to remove cancer precursor lesions has been widely adopted for two cancer types.
- Adenomatous colon polyps are now accepted as the morphological precursor of colorectal cancer. Colonoscopic removal of polyps reduces the incidence of invasive colorectal cancer.
- Women identified to have carcinoma in situ of the cervix (usually by biopsy prompted by an abnormal Paponicolou smear) can be prevented from developing invasive cervical cancer by surgical removal of part or all of the cervix.

Cancer chemoprevention

Principles of chemoprevention

Many human cancers are preventable because their causes have been identified in the human environment.

- Minimization of exposure of carcinogens in the environment (primary prevention) is an effective strategy in cancer prevention, e.g., smoking avoidance or cessation.

However, most environmental factors that initiate or promote cancer remain to be identified and, once identified, the avoidance of such factors may necessitate difficult lifestyle changes.

Epidemiological data suggesting that cancer is preventable by intervention with chemicals are based on the following:

- Time trends in cancer incidence and mortality
- Geographic variations and effect of migration
- Identification of specific causative factors
- Lack of simple patterns of genetic inheritance for the majority of human cancers

Chemopreventive agents

Epithelial carcinogenesis proceeds via multiple, discernible steps of molecular and cellular alterations, culminating in invasive neoplasms. These events can be separated into three distinct phases:

- **Initiation**, which is rapid, involves direct carcinogenic damage to DNA, and the resulting mutation is irreversible.
- **Promotion** follows initiation and is generally reversible; it involves the clonal expansion of initiated cells induced by agents acting as mitogens for the initiated cell.
- **Progression** results from promotion in the sense that cell proliferation caused by promoters allows cellular damage inflicted by initiation to be further propagated.

During tumor progression, genotypically and phenotypically altered cells gradually emerge. Both promotion and progression phases are prolonged. Depending on which phase of carcinogenesis they affect, chemopreventive agents can be divided into tumor "blocking" agents, which interfere with cancer initiation, and tumor "suppressing" agents, which inhibit promotion or progression (see Table 3.2).

Blocking agents such as oltipraz that prevent metabolic activation of carcinogens or their subsequent binding to DNA probably reduce the accumulation of initiating mutations.

Altered states of cell and tissue differentiation are characteristic of premalignant lesions long before they become invasive. It may be possible to reverse abnormal differentiation with a hormone-like nontoxic agent.

Two other approaches to controlling preneoplastic lesions are (1) to block their expansion with nontoxic agents that suppress cell replication or (2) to induce an apoptotic state in these cells.

Although in the past, cancer chemopreventive agents have been discovered serendipitously or developed empirically, recent advances in understanding of the molecular biology of carcinogenesis offers hope for more rational drug design.

Table 3.2 Mechanisms of tumor suppression and examples of cancer chemopreventive agents

Scavenging oxygen radicals	Polyphenols (curcumin, genistein), selenium, tocopherol (vitamin E)
Inhibition of arachidonic acid metabolism	N-acetylcysteine, NSAIDs (sulindac, aspirin), polyphenols, tamoxifen
Modulation of signal transduction	NSAIDs, retinoids, tamoxifen genistein, curcumin
Modulation of hormonal/growth factor activity	NSAIDs, retinoids, curcumin tamoxifen, finasteride
Inhibition of oncogene activity	Genistein, NSAIDs, monoterpenes (D-limonene, perillyl alcohol)
Inhibition of polyamine metabolism	2-Difluoromethylornithine, retinoids, tamoxifen
Induction of terminal differentiation	Calcium, retinoids, vitamin D_3
Induction of apoptosis	Genistein, curcumin, retinoids, tamoxifen

NSAIDs = nonsteroidal anti-inflammatory drugs.

Clinical trials of cancer prevention

The design of prevention trials in normal people is parallel to but significantly different from classical cancer therapeutic trials. For example, during the trials of tamoxifen given as an adjuvant therapy in early breast cancer, it was observed that the incidence of second primary breast cancer in the contralateral breast was lower in women treated with tamoxifen than in those with placebo. This led to the hypothesis that tamoxifen might be a cancer-preventive agent as well a cancer therapy.

There followed a series of trials leading to the landmark publication of the Breast Cancer Prevention Trial (BCPT) in 1998, which showed that tamoxifen could reduce by half the number of breast cancers observed in women at high risk. However, in two additional trials in different patient populations, no proven benefit was observed.

There remains controversy as to how effective this agent is, and in which healthy women it should be prescribed.

These trials have highlighted problems inherent in chemoprevention studies:
- Which healthy individuals should be invited to participate in such trials or be offered therapy off study?
- How should these individuals be identified and contacted?
- When should the drug be started and for how long should it be continued?
- Side effects that are quite acceptable in cancer patients may be unacceptable in healthy subjects.
- If chronic exposure can produce serious illness even rarely, the agent may be unsuitable for chemoprevention (e.g., tamoxifen rarely causes endometrial cancer).

Phase I/II clinical trials

The main objective of early clinical trials of chemopreventive agents is to establish tolerability and side effects of candidate compounds. One major difference from conventional cytotoxic agents is that the duration of administration of the preventive agent will be much longer than for a cytotoxic one, so chronic side effects are at least as important as acute side effects. For phase I studies:
- A major side effect would include either fatality or problems requiring intervention by a physician or long-term disability.
- Major side effects would automatically rule out any further development of chemopreventive agents.
- Minor side effects may preclude chronic dosing with the agent.
- The route of administration is usually oral, although inhalation and topical modalities are also of interest in some cancers.

A phase II trial will frequently be of longer duration and may have more than one dose level.
- It may be randomized with a placebo control to clarify toxicities and provide preliminary evidence of efficacy through measurement of an intermediate risk biomarker, if one has been validated for the disease under study.

- A crucial component in assessment of the agent at this stage is compliance, which may require pharmacokinetic confirmation.
- Duration may be six months to five years, and the sample size typically ranges from 50 to more than 1000 volunteers or potential patients.

The use of surrogate end points is extremely important for cost-efficient studies, although there are few biomarkers that are of proven value (e.g., development of carcinoma in situ or other precancerous lesion).

Ease of recruitment is important because "high risk" may be clear to a physician but not so clear to a normal individual.

Phase III clinical trials

Randomized placebo-controlled phase III studies of chemopreventive agents need to be large and lengthy because diagnosis of cancer is a relatively rare event. Because it is costly (in terms of time and resources) to test each new agent with the classical phase III design, two solutions are being tested:
- One is the concentration on high-risk groups of individuals.
- The other is the development of intermediate biomarkers.

Summary

Chemoprevention is in its infancy. New methodologies are being evaluated, and new surrogate end points and novel candidate interventions are emerging rapidly from the revolution in molecular biology and genetics. It is an extremely promising and exciting branch of oncology.

Cancer prevention: diet

This is a controversial area with conflicting data in the literature. Dietary modifications are difficult to promote in populations and compliance is often poor.

Dietary fat

Dietary fat promotes tumor growth in animal models and, conversely, energy restriction appears to reduce the incidence of tumors. Excess dietary fat is associated with cancer of the breast, colon, endometrium, and prostate.

Dietary studies are fraught with methodological problems:
- There are increasing case-control and cohort studies pointing towards an association of excess fat in the diet with breast and colon cancer in particular.
- However, conflicting data on these associations continue to appear.

Data on the relationship between a high-fat diet and prostate cancer are also conflicting.

Dietary fiber

Diets with increased fiber tend to reduce colonic transit time and bind some potentially carcinogenic chemicals. Randomized control trials of dietary manipulation are extremely difficult and are dogged by poor compliance.

Data from over a dozen case-control studies and a meta-analysis indicate an inverse relationship between fiber intake and colon cancer. However, prospective studies have yielded conflicting data, in particular the large Nurses' Health Study.

There is no evidence that increasing fiber in the diet inhibits the development of colorectal adenomas. Evidence that increased fiber in the diet inhibits the development of colorectal cancer is still uncertain, and data are conflicting. Similarly, although high-fiber diets may reduce the risk of breast cancer and stomach cancer, studies have revealed conflicting data.

Fruit and vegetable consumption

Data from the Nurses' Health Study have shown no association between the consumption of fruit and vegetables and subsequent cancer risk during over 1.5 million person-years of follow-up.

Some studies have found an inverse association between fruit and vegetable consumption and stomach cancer, although the data are conflicting.

There appears to be little association between fruit and vegetable consumption and the risk of breast cancer.

High consumption of fruit and vegetables may be protective for men and women who have never smoked in the development of lung cancer.

Folate

Folate may reduce carcinogenesis through DNA repair and DNA methylation. In animals, folate deficiency increases intestinal carcinogenesis.

A diet rich in folate may lower the risk of colorectal cancer and the precursor adenoma. Several studies have shown that folate supplementation can decrease colorectal cancer risk.

Carotenoids

These are antioxidants and promote cell differentiation.

β-carotene has been investigated and the data are conflicting. In smokers, β-carotene caused an increased risk of lung cancer in two large randomized studies and in other smaller studies.

Further reading

Chu DZ, Gibson G, David D, Yen Y (2007). The surgeon's role in cancer prevention. The model in colorectal carcinoma. *Ann Surg Oncol* 14:3054–3069.

Doll R, Peto R, Boreham J, Sutherland I (2004). Mortality in relation to smoking: 50 years observations on male British doctors. *BMJ* 328:1519–1528.

Fisher B, Constantino JP, Wickerham DL, et al (1998). Tamoxifen for prevention of breast cancer: report of NSABP-1 study. *J Int Cancer Inst* 90:1371–1388.

Fleshner N, Zlotta AR (2007). Prostate cancer prevention: past, present, and future [review]. *Cancer* 110:1889–1899.

Lindor NM, Petersen GM, Hadley DW, et al (2006). Recommendations for the care of individuals with an inherited predisposition to Lynch syndrome: a systematic review. *JAMA* 296:1507–1517.

Lucia MS, Epstein JI, Goodman PJ, et al (2007). Finasteride and high-grade prostate cancer in the Prostate Cancer Prevention Trial. *J Natl Cancer Inst* 99:1375–1383.

Willet WC, Stampfer MJ, Colditz GA, et al (1990). Relationship of meat, fat and fiber intake to the risk of colon cancer in a prospective study amongst women. *N Engl J Med* 323:1664–1672.

Chapter 4

Cancer screening

Gary H. Lyman

Principles 46
Limitations 47
Screening tests 48
Further reading 49

Principles

- The strongest evidence that early detection of cancer increases the chance of cure comes from randomized trials of cancer screening.
- This has led to public awareness campaigns to persuade individuals to seek advice regarding suspicious symptoms at an early stage.
- Unfortunately, most symptoms of cancer are symptoms of more advanced disease, and there is no evidence that encouraging early self-referral improves survival.
- The screening of asymptomatic individuals to detect a cancer that has yet to declare itself clearly holds more promise.
- For this to be effective in a population, there are certain criteria that should be met by the cancer in question, the screening test, and the screening program.

The cancer

- Its natural history should be well understood.
- It should be recognizable at an early stage.
- Treatment at an early stage of disease should be more effective and improve outcomes compared to that at a later stage.
- It should be sufficiently common in the target population to warrant screening.

The test

- It should be sensitive and specific.
  - **Sensitivity** is the proportion of individuals with the disease who have a positive test.
  - **Specificity** is the proportion of individuals without the disease who have a negative test.
- It should be reasonably acceptable.
- It must be safe.
- Ideally, it should be inexpensive.

The program

- There must be adequate facilities for diagnosis in those with a positive test.
- There should be effective treatment for screen-detected disease.
- Repeated screening should be feasible at intervals if the disease is of insidious onset.
- The benefit must outweigh the immediate and long-term physical and psychological harm.
- The benefit should justify the cost.

Limitations

It is crucial that treating the disease to be screened at an early stage is more effective than treating it at a later stage.

To justify a screening program, one should not compare the outcome of screen-detected disease with that of symptomatic disease, because three biases operate in favor of screen-detected disease.

- **Lead-time bias** arises from the fact that, if early diagnosis advances the time of diagnosis of a disease, then the period from diagnosis to death will lengthen irrespective of whether treatment has altered the natural history of the disease. If patients die of their cancer at the same age at which this event would have occurred without screening, no benefit has been afforded by screening. Screening will only be of value if it improves the survival curve of a screened population compared with that of an unscreened population.
- **Length bias** operates because slow-growing tumors are more likely to be detected by screening tests than fast-growing tumors, which are more likely to present with symptoms before a screening test can be applied or between tests. Thus, *screen-detected* tumors will tend to be less aggressive and associated with a relatively better prognosis than *interval-detected* tumors.
- **Selection bias** results from the characteristics of individuals who accept an invitation to be screened. Such a person is more likely to be health conscious than one who refuses or ignores screening and may therefore be more likely to survive longer, irrespective of the disease process.

Screening tests

In screening, it is also important to have a target population at increased risk to avoid applying the test without benefit in individuals at low risk of cancer. In screening for the common cancers, where the incidence is highly age-dependent, the age range should be that in which the disease is relatively more common and yet in which the patients are likely to be fit enough for curative treatment.

Several other predictors of risk may be important, including family history, particularly now that we can detect specific genetic mutations and to use these to screen close relatives. Examples of this include mutations in the APC gene in familial adenomatous polyposis, DNA mismatch repair genes in hereditary non-polyposis colorectal cancer (Lynch syndrome), and BRCA1 and -2 in familial breast and ovarian cancer.

A screening test should be acceptable, safe, and reasonably inexpensive, so that it will be adopted by the target population. It must also be remembered that screening may cause psychological harm as well as physical harm. The benefits gained through cancer screening must outweigh such morbidity, and society must decide whether the health gain justifies any risk and the associated costs.

When a screening program is established, it is important that the diagnostic facilities are adequate. Similarly, treatment of early disease must be associated with minimal morbidity and mortality.

Randomized trials of screening programs have been done in breast and colorectal cancer, and in both instances screening has been shown to significantly reduce cancer mortality.

Although guidelines vary from one agency to another, current screening recommendations for early detection of cancer in asymptomatic individuals of average risk from the American Cancer Society include:

- Breast cancer screening with breast self-exam and clinical breast exam in women starting at age 20 and annual mammography starting at age 40.
- Colorectal cancer screening stating at age 50 in both men and women with annual fecal occult blood testing or a fecal immunochemical test and either flexible sigmoidoscopy or double contrast barium enema every five years or colonoscopy every 10 years.
- Prostate cancer screening in men at age 50 with digital rectal examination and a prostate-specific antigen (PSA) annually.
- Cervical cancer screening in women starting within three years of the start sexual activity and no later than age 21.

Further reading

Berry DA (1998). Benefits and risks of screening mammography for women in their forties: a statistical appraisal. *J Natl Cancer Inst* **90**:1431–1439.

Elmore JG, Barton MB, Moceri VM, et al. (1998). Ten-year risk of false positive screening mammograms and clinical breast examinations. *N Engl J Med* **338**:1089–1096.

Harris R, Lohr KN (2002). Screening for prostate cancer: an update of the evidence for the US Preventative Services Task Force. *Ann Intern Med* **137**:917–929.

Peto J, Gilham C, Fletcher O, Matthews FE (2004). The cervical cancer epidemic that screening has prevented in the UK. *Lancet* **364**:249–256.

Shaheen NJ, Indomi JM, Overholt BF, Sharma P (2004). What is the best management strategy for high grade dysplasia in Barrett's oesophagus? A cost-effective analysis. *Gut* **53**:1736–1744.

Winawer S, Fletcher R, Rex D, et al (2003). Colorectal cancer screening and surveillance—clinical guidelines and rationale—update on new evidence. *Gastroenterology* **124**:544–560.

Chapter 5

Genetic screening

Christina I. Herold

Introduction 52
General Considerations 53
Specific Syndromes 54
   Hereditary "breast" syndromes 54
   Hereditary gastrointestinal syndromes 56
Developing issues 57
Further reading and resources 57

Introduction

Genetic screening for cancer predisposition has evolved from an investigational consideration to a standard part of clinical care in many oncologic conditions. Cancer specialists are the healthcare providers best positioned to initiate genetic screening, for several reasons:
- The results of genetic screening can influence management considerations in affected patients.
- Oncologists see the affected members of families with high rates of cancer.
- Affected individuals are most appropriately tested for genetic mutations, rather than unaffected family members.

General considerations

Genetic mutations that predispose to cancer are best considered as syndromes increasing the risk of cancer in many different organs, rather than just one organ. Although many syndromes have associated lists of criteria meant to guide referral for genetic evaluation, attention to a number of basic features can help in identifying appropriate patients:
- Cancer in two or more close relatives on the same side of the family
- Early age of onset (below 40 for most syndromes)
- Multiple primary tumors
- Bilateral disease in paired organs
- Multiple rare cancers in one family
- For most syndromes, evidence of autosomal dominant transmission

Patients and families demonstrating these characteristics are reasonable candidates for referral to a genetics specialist or genetic counselor. Critical in this process is collecting a reasonably detailed family history, including the following:
- At least three generations of family history information
- Some estimate of total number of individuals in each generation to determine how many potential at-risk members are present in the family
- Information on ethnic ancestry, because some populations have a higher prevalence of well defined "founder" mutations

Important elements of counseling for genetic testing are as follows:
- Determine whether testing is available for suspected syndrome
- Implications for screening and management with a positive or negative test
- Risk of passing mutation to children and risk to other family members, including siblings
- Assessment of psychological stress and family dynamics
- Discussion of discrimination considerations (health and life insurance, employment), although these concerns have not been strongly evident in clinical practice
- Discussion of testing accuracy: sensitivity, specificity, and possibility of genetic variation of unknown significance

Several useful models are available for evaluating family cancer histories.
- For example, the BRCAPRO model is a validated model using Baysian analysis of family histories to give pretest probabilities for carrying a *BRCA1/2* mutation.
- This model is part of the CAGene software, available free with registration at: www4.utsouthwestern.edu/breasthealth/cagene/default.asp.
- This software package will also give estimates for carrying genes causing other cancer syndromes.

Specific syndromes

Over 50 cancer predisposition syndromes have been identified, with a variety of classification systems proposed.
- These systems are based on features such as the organ(s) predominantly affected with cancer, or the molecular role of the gene mutated.
- No one system is uniformly accepted.

The following are noteworthy syndromes in adult oncology, listed by genes mutated in the syndrome with common name in parentheses; additional information is available in specific cancer chapters.

Hereditary "breast" syndromes

BRCA1/2 (breast/ovarian syndrome)
- Approximately 5%–10% of breast cancer cases (approximately 18,000/year); population carrier estimates are approximately 1 in 500 to 1000.
- 10% of ovarian cancer cases (approximately 2000/year).
- *BRCA1* penetrance is generally higher: breast risk to age 70 up to 70%; ovarian risk up to 40%. Breast cancers tend to happen at a younger age and are usually "triple-negative" in type.
- *BRCA2* penetrance is lower, with lifetime risks of breast cancer up to 50% and ovarian cancer up to 20%.
- *BRCA2* cancer risks also increased for pancreas, prostate, and melanoma; other cancer risks are less clear for *BRCA1*.
- Male carriers for mutations in both genes are at increased risk for breast cancer, although higher with *BRCA2*.
- Determination of mutation status in patients with breast cancer can guide local management and provide clear indication for oophorectomy as part of treatment.

P53 (Li-Fraumeni syndrome)
- Increased risk for breast, soft tissue sarcoma, osteosarcoma, leukemia, brain tumors, and adrenocortical tumors in classic syndrome.
- More recent studies suggest some increase in most adult epithelial cancers.
- Population carrier estimates are approximately 1 in 5000, making it rare.

PTEN (Cowden's syndrome)
- Benign and malignant tumors of the breast, thyroid (follicular more than papillary; not medullary), and endometrium
- Characteristic skin findings with lipomas, fibromas, and trichilemmomas

Checkpoint kinase 2 gene
- Mutations in the checkpoint kinase 2 gene (*CHEK2*) likely function as a low penetrance gene for breast cancer and may confer a two- to three-fold increased risk of breast cancer compared to the general population, particularly in white women of European ancestry.

- The clinical utility of testing for *CHEK2* mutation is unclear but may be considered for white women with breast cancer who have a family history of breast cancer and no evidence of a mutation in the *BRCA1/2* genes.

Serine Threonine Kinase (Peutz-Jeghers syndrome)

- Mutations in the serine threonine kinase gene (*STK11*) associated with characteristic hamartomatous polyps in the gastrointestinal tract as well as mucocutaneous melanin pigmentations in the lips and buccal mucosa.
- Autosomal dominant inheritance pattern associated with multiple cancers including those of the gastrointestinal system as well as cancers of the breast, ovary, uterus, and lung.
- Cumulative risks of breast cancer and ovarian cancer are estimated at 55% and 20%, respectively.
- Individuals with *STK11* mutation or familial characteristics of Peutz-Jeghers syndrome should undergo regular screening of the gastrointestinal system for polyp detection (including upper endoscopy, video capsule endoscopy, and colonoscopy) as well as enhanced screening for other associated cancers (including annual breast MRI).
- *CDH1* (hereditary diffuse gastric cancer syndrome)
- Autosomal dominant inheritance pattern. Mutations in the cadherin-1 gene (*CDH1*) are highly penetrant and associated with a lifetime risk of gastric cancer that exceeds 80%. These mutations are also strongly associated with increased lifetime risk, approximately 60%, of lobular breast cancer.
- Carriers of *CDH1* gene mutations may be counseled to consider prophylactic gastrectomy as well as enhanced screening for breast cancer (including annual breast MRI).

Hereditary gastrointestinal syndromes

Mismatch repair genes MLH1, MSH2, MSH6, PMS2 (Lynch syndrome or hereditary non-polyposis colon cancer)

- Approximately 5% of colon cancer cases (5000 cases/year)
- Predominance of right-sided colon cancers
- Colon cancers have "mutator" phenotype, microsatellite instability, and better prognosis
- Increased risk of endometrial, gastric, biliary tract, urinary tract, and ovarian cancers
- Mutations also account for other eponymous syndromes: Turcot's (glioblastomas plus colon cancer variant) and Muir-Torre (colon cancer plus sebaceous gland tumors)
- Observational studies have demonstrated survival benefit to more intensive colon cancer screening when mutation carriers are identified

APC and MYH (polyposis syndromes)

- Classic familial adenomatous polyposis (FAP) is usually clinically evident with the presence of thousands of colon polyps.
- Virtually all patients with classic FAP develop colon cancer eventually if the colon is left in place.
- Classic FAP is also associated with adenomas and carcinomas of the duodenum and rectum, desmoid tumors, osteomas, thyroid carcinoma, and hepatoblastomas (particularly in children).
- Some *APC* mutations give an attenuated clinical picture with many fewer polyps, but they still markedly increased risk of cancer.
- *MYH*-associated polyposis is a recessive disorder causing formation of fewer than 100 colon polyps, and associated colon cancer risk requiring more frequent screening.
- *MYH* carrier prevalence is approximately 2% of the population.

The resources listed under Further Reading and resources include useful Web sites for further information on other important syndromes such as multiple endocrine neoplasia (MEN), von Hippel-Lindau (VHL), and others.

Developing issues

With the mapping of the human genome and the generation of the HapMap (a catalog of polymorphic variation), whole genome association studies have become much more feasible. These studies are rapidly identifying genetic variants that have modest, but possibly clinically meaningful, effects on cancer predisposition.

Many private companies are beginning to offer whole genome "scans" in direct marketing to consumers. At present, obtaining such information should not be encouraged for guiding any cancer evaluation outside of a research context.

Further reading and resources

Online

- GeneTests: www.geneclinics.org. A National Institutes of Health (NIH)-supported Web site for information on medical genetics, including genetic testing laboratories.
- www.cancer-genetics.org: An educational resource on cancer genetics.
- Online Mendelian Inheritance in Man: www.ncbi.nlm.nih.gov/sites/entrez?db=OMIM. The definitive encyclopedia site for medical genetics.
- www4.utsouthwestern.edu/breasthealth/cagene/default.asp

Other

Garber JE, Offit K (2005). Hereditary cancer predisposition syndromes. *J Clin Oncol* 23:276–292.

Part III
Principles of management

6	Principles of cancer treatment	61
7	Surgical oncology	65
8	Principles of radiation oncology	81
9	Principles of chemotherapy	101
10	Hematopoietic stem cell transplantation	151
11	Hormone therapy	165
12	Targeted therapies	175
13	Gene therapy and immunotherapy for cancer	185
14	Complementary and alternative medicine	195
15	Clinical trials	205

Chapter 6

Principles of cancer treatment

Gary H. Lyman

CHAPTER 6 **Principles of cancer treatment**

The Modern management of patients with malignant disease generally involves several clinical disciplines

- Initial management includes establishing the diagnosis based on a definitive biopsy followed by appropriate staging procedures often including but not limited to various radiographic, radionuclide, magnetic resonance, or other imaging techniques.
- Management of patients with solid tumors generally involves primary surgical intervention frequently followed by systemic therapies and/or radiation therapy.
- The sequential orchestration of surgery, radiation therapy, chemotherapy, and hormonal therapy as well as newer target agents such as monoclonal antibodies and small molecule inhibitors have made the treatment of many malignancies very complex but increasingly effective at altering the course of disease, including the potential for survival or even cure.
- In addition, the rapid increase in knowledge from basic, clinical, and translational cancer research has led to an information explosion in the field of cancer that is beyond anyone's capability to stay abreast of.

Therefore, no single clinician has all the knowledge and all the skills necessary to effectively treat most cancers or even a single cancer in an optimal manner in today's world

- This has led to the development of multidisciplinary teams that deal with one or a limited class of specific types of cancer in a comprehensive manner.
- In addition to the assembly of pathologists, radiologists, and other imaging specialists, surgeons, radiation therapists, medical oncologists, and hematologists, such teams often include a broad array of essential allied healthcare specialists including but not limited to nurses, social workers, and pharmacists.
- Even as patients approach a point in their disease in which standard interventions are no longer reasonable or desired, a coordinated team of individuals is required to offer appropriate palliative or end-of-life care with optimal symptom control such as pain management, treatment of depression, etc.
- Thus, the makeup of the team may change over time to include individuals who are not directly involved in the initial treatment at presentation but have adjunctive roles at later stages in the course of the illness.

There should always be a sufficient range of expertise to allow for informed discussion of the best management policy for individual patients.

The team's various roles will include the following:
- Planning diagnostic and staging procedures
- Managing the primary treatment approach including any adjuvant therapy to be delivered pre- or postoperatively
- Preparing patients physically and psychologically for cancer treatment and subsequent follow-up
- Providing information on treatment, prognosis, side effects, and other pertinent questions that might arise
- Efficiently planning and delivering surgery, radiotherapy, and systemic therapy as appropriate
- Effectively managing treatment-associated toxicities with appropriate supportive care
- Aiding rehabilitation from the disease and its treatment
- Providing appropriate follow-up care
- Ensuring that the transition from curative to palliative care is appropriately and compassionately managed
- Facilitate the availability and possible recruitment to appropriate clinical trials

Patient management within such a multidisciplinary team structure results in better outcomes for patients.

Studies demonstrate survival advantages, and, equally important, patients experience less compromise of functional and psychological well being and better quality of life.

Further references

Lyman GH, Baker J, Geradts J, et al. (2013). Multidisciplinary care of patients with early-stage breast cancer. *Surg Oncol Clin N Am* 22:299–317.

Chapter 7

Surgical oncology

Thomas A. D'Amico

General principles 66
Tumor biology 67
Surgical techniques 68
Diagnosis and staging 70
Curative surgical resection 72
Palliative surgery 74
Surgery for metastatic disease 78

General principles

- Surgical resection is integral in the treatment of most patients with solid tumors.
- For some tumors (or certain stages of tumors), surgery alone is the treatment of choice; for others, surgery is a component of multidisciplinary care that may also include either induction or adjuvant therapy.
- Surgical approaches may be implemented with three goals in the management of cancer patients:
  - Diagnosis and staging
  - Curative intent
  - Palliation
- In general, the goals of surgical resection for curative intent include complete resection of the primary tumor (with negative margins) and adequate intraoperative staging, depending on the tumor type.
- There is also a role, in certain tumors, for prophylactic surgery.
- For example, this surgery might be used for familial polyposis coli colon cancer in the patient who is known to be a *BRCA1* gene carrier (breast cancer), and in some of the MEN syndromes (thyroid cancer).

Tumor biology

An understanding of tumor biology is essential in the planning of surgical treatment for cancer. The biology of solid tumors is diverse and often unpredictable. Even in patients where the primary tumor appears localized by radiographic evaluation, locally advanced disease or distant metastases may still be present, highlighting the need for rigorous preoperative staging. The three principal methods of spread are as follows:
- Direct extension
- Lymphatic involvement
- Hematogenous

Most cancers have the potential to disseminate by all three methods, although one method of spread may be predominant.

Breast and colorectal cancer exhibit both blood and lymphatic spread, whereas cancers arising in the upper gastrointestinal tract and the neck metastasize via the lymphatic system. Even cancers arising from the same cell type behave differently: papillary and follicular tumors of the thyroid give rise to lymphatic and hematogenous metastases, respectively.

Different surgical approaches will be required depending on tumor type.

Before performing surgery for curative intent, appropriate preoperative staging must be performed, including a complete history and physical examination, appropriate laboratory tests, and radiographic evaluation. The specific laboratory and radiographic tests used depend on the tumor type and clinical stage of the patient.

Recently, positron emission tomography (PET) has been demonstrated to improve the preoperative detection of distant metastatic disease, reducing the incidence of futile surgical exploration for patients with many (but not all) tumor types.

For many patients, multidisciplinary evaluation including (but not necessarily limited to) surgical, medical, and radiation oncologists will improve outcomes. In addition, appropriate knowledge and use of staging and treatment guidelines, such as those from the National Comprehensive Cancer Network (NCCN), have also been demonstrated to improve results.

Surgical techniques

For surgical procedures designed to achieve diagnosis and staging, the most minimally invasive technique possibly should be used. For surgical procedures performed for curative intent, the entire tumor must be resected with negative surgical margins.

The en bloc technique—removal of the primary tumor and an appropriate amount of adjacent soft tissue—is most often used in cancers with a predominantly lymphatic spread and to optimize the achievement of negative surgical margins. This technique is best developed in surgery of head and neck cancer, esophageal cancer, and soft tissue sarcomas.

Minimally invasive surgery

There has been an exponential growth in minimally invasive surgery (MIS) for cancer during the past decade. For some MIS procedures, proved advantages include decreased hospital stay, less postoperative pain and analgesia requirement, less inflammatory response, faster return to full activity, fewer overall complications, and more effective compliance with adjuvant therapy.

Conservative and radical surgery

There are increasing data to support conservative (less radical) resections for selected tumors. For example, thyroid lobectomy is the recommend surgical approach to treat minimally invasive follicular carcinoma of the thyroid gland, as opposed to total thyroidectomy; wide local excision (when followed by radiotherapy) is adequate treatment for selected breast cancer patients provided the resection margin is at least 0.5 cm.

Limb-conserving surgery, often with endoprosthetic bone and joint replacement, is suitable for young patients with bone tumors around the knee in highly specialized centers to avoid amputation.

Radical surgery still has its place in the patient with large hepatomas and mesothelioma, and total mastectomy is still required for some patients with breast cancer.

Occasionally, liver transplantation is performed for primary liver cancer or secondary endocrine tumors of the liver, but the benefits of such a transplant are debatable.

Reconstructive surgery

To return patients to an adequate and reasonable quality of life after cancer surgery, reconstruction should be offered, where possible (if the patient wishes). For example, after mastectomy the breast can be reconstructed using implant, tissue expander, transverse rectus abdominis muscle (TRAM), or latissimus dorsi flaps.

After major head and neck resections, oncological plastic surgeons use free vascularized flaps to replace skin, muscle, and bone. Examples include radial and fibular free flaps.

Although hand transplant is technically feasible, fewer than 10 have been performed worldwide because of poor functional results and considerable psychological morbidity.

Prophylactic cancer surgery

Surgical resection is used in the prevention of cancer in selected patients.

There are several conditions, either acquired or inherited, in which preventative surgery has a major role after careful counseling of the patient. These include the following:
- Orchidopexy or occasionally orchidectomy in the patient with a maldescended testis
- Total colectomy in patients with polyposis coli
- Total colectomy in patients with ulcerative colitis involving the entire colon (over 10 years) and who have changes of dysplasia
- Total thyroidectomy for patients at risk of medullary cell carcinoma of the thyroid gland, who have the MEN syndrome (type 2)
- Bilateral mastectomy in selected patients carrying the *BRCA1* gene

Further reading

Balch CM (2007). Prescribing patterns of surgical oncologists: are we surgeons, oncologists, or both? Results of a society of surgical oncology survey. *Ann Surg Oncol* 14:2685–2686.

Chan WM, Pang CP, Lam DSC, Gripp KW (2003). Genetics of colorectal cancer. *N Engl J Med* 348:2361–2362.

Chu DZJ, Gibson G, David D, Yen Y (2007). The surgeon's role in cancer prevention. The model in colorectal carcinoma. *Ann Surg Oncol* 14:3054–3069.

Croce CM (2008). Oncogenes and cancer. *N Engl J Med* 358:502–511.

Eubank WB, Mankoff DA (2005). Evolving role of positron emission tomography in breast cancer imaging. *Semin Nucl Med* 35:84–99.

Juweid ME, Cheson BD (2006). Positron-emission tomography and assessment of cancer therapy. *N Engl J Med* 354:496–507.

Lynch HT, de la Chapelle A (2003). Hereditary colorectal cancer. *N Engl J Med* 348:919–932.

Machens A, Niccoli-Sire P, Hoeel J, et al. (2003). Early malignant progression of hereditary medullary thyroid cancer. *N Engl J Med* 349:517–525.

Spechler SJ (2002). Barrett's esophagus. *N Engl J Med* 346:836–842.

Torigian DA, Huang SS, Houseni M, Alavi A (2007). Functional imaging of cancer with emphasis on molecular techniques. *CA Cancer J Clin* 57:206–224.

Yeatman TJ (2003). The future of cancer management: translating the genome, transcriptome, and proteome. *Ann Surg Oncol* 10:7–14.

Diagnosis and staging

Diagnosis and staging algorithms have been well described (NCCN Guidelines), and these should be followed closely in the majority of patients with known or suspected cancer.

The use of ultrasound, computerized tomography (CT), PET, and magnetic resonance imaging (MRI), as well as the performance of percutaneous (or transluminal) biopsy, allows the preoperative diagnosis of cancer to be made in most cases. These radiographic techniques may be interpreted to determine the clinical stage of a patient prior to surgical staging or therapy. Surgical procedures may be used for diagnostic and staging purposes, either before resection or to plan nonoperative therapy.

Although fine-needle aspiration and core biopsy often provide the diagnosis of cancer, it is important that the physician, pathologist, or radiologist performing these investigations direct their needle bearing in mind the possibility of tumor seeding.

Tumor seeding is not a problem with a fine-needle aspiration generally, but it may be more of a problem with core biopsy, especially with soft tissue sarcomas. Here, the needle track should be placed after discussion with the surgeon so that the needle track will be excised in the definitive surgery.

The surgeon may still be required to perform either an incisional or an excisional biopsy. In the former, compromise to the future definitive operation must not occur. The excisional biopsy should in many cases be carried out by the appropriate specialist who will be carrying out the definitive surgery. This applies particularly in melanoma where there is controversy over the excision margins (depending upon the depth of the melanoma).

When taking biopsies for diagnostic purposes, the surgeon should be aware of the quantity required for diagnosis and the appropriate conditions for storage of the biopsy. Tissue samples will need to be sent "fresh" if electron microscopy or other specialized stains or cytogenetics are required.

Some pathologic evaluations (such as receptor expression) require a certain minimum amount of tissue, and aspiration specimens for cytologic analysis may be inadequate. Diagnostic surgical procedures may provide specimens other than the primary tumor, including the adjacent lymph nodes, to stage the tumors most effectively.

A variety of surgical procedures may be used to effectively stage patients before resection or before induction therapy, or to plan definitive or palliative nonoperative therapy. For example, mediastinoscopy may be used to assess mediastinal lymph node involvement in patients with lung cancer, to determine whether resection (stages I or II), induction chemotherapy followed by resection (stage IIIA), or chemoradiotherapy (stage IIIB) should be used.

MIS procedures, such as laparoscopy or thoracoscopy, are also used in the diagnosis and staging of malignancy. Although image-directed biopsy can give a diagnosis in a large proportion of patients, some areas are not easily amenable.

MIS may be used for staging the following malignancies before definitive surgery: esophageal cancer, gastric cancer, pancreatic cancer, liver cancer, prostatic cancer, and ovarian cancer.

Sentinel node biopsy

Sentinel node biopsy is a minimally invasive technique that has been used for several years for patients with breast cancer or melanoma.

After injection of the primary tumor with a dye or a radioisotope, the "sentinel" lymph node (that which would be most likely to harbor metastatic disease) is identified and removed. Thereafter, if the gland is positive (on frozen section), the surgeon will proceed to complete resection of the regional nodes.

Further reading

Greene FL, Fritz AG, Balch CM, et al. (eds) (2002). *AJCC Cancer Staging Handbook* (6th edition). New York: Springer-Verlag.

Lyman GH, Giuliano AE, Somerfield MR, et al. (2005). American Society of Clinical Oncology Guideline recommendations for sentinel node biopsy in early-stage breast cancer. *J Clin Oncol* 23:7703–7720.

Posther K, McCall L, Blumecranz P, et al. (2005). Sentinel node skills verification and surgeon performance: data from multicenter clinical trial for early-stage breast cancer. *Ann Surg* 242: 538–549.

Redston M, Compton C, Miedea B, et al. (2006). Analysis of micro-metastatic disease in sentinel lymph nodes from resectable colon cancer: results of cancer and leukemia Group B Trial 80001. *J Clin Oncol* 24:878–883.

Sun Z, Wigle DA, Yang P (2008). Non-overlapping and non-cell-type-specific gene expression signatures predict lung cancer survival. *J Clin Oncol* 26:877–883.

Curative surgical resection

The long-term outcome after cancer surgery depends on tumor type and the stage of tumor at presentation.

- For some cancers, the outlook is favorable for the majority of patients. The five-year survival rate in breast cancer is over 80% and for colon cancer it is approximately 70%. Unfortunately, the cure rate for many tumors is much lower. The five-year survival rate for lung cancer is approximately 15%, and for pancreatic and esophageal cancer the five-year survival is less than 10%.
- Survival rates for some cancers have improved due to earlier presentation, improved public awareness, and screening programs (such as with breast and cervical cancer). Screening for colon cancer has also been successful, but screening is still under investigation for lung cancer.
- Improvement in surgical and anesthetic techniques has enabled the performance of extensive resections, with low risk (when performed by specialists) and excellent functional results, such as limb-preserving surgery for osteosarcoma, esophagogastrectomy, and pancreatectomy.

The concept of multidisciplinary evaluation and management of patients with cancer is extremely important

- Surgical resection may have an important role in the management of most solid tumors; however, pretreatment evaluation by medical oncologists or radiation oncologists may be necessary to optimize treatment planning.
- The use of either induction therapy (preoperative) or adjuvant therapy (postoperative) is well established for most tumor types, although the relative efficacy of each may evolve over time as new agents are developed and clinical trials are completed. For example, for patients with lung cancer, adjuvant chemotherapy has been shown to improve outcomes for patient with stage II disease, yet induction therapy is preferred for patients with stage IIIA disease.
- Similarly, preoperative chemotherapy may be used for locally advanced breast cancer, although most women will receive adjuvant chemotherapy only.

The tenets of complete surgical resection when possible are important for virtually every solid tumor

- **R0** resection refers to complete resection of all tumor. **R1** resection refers to resection of gross tumor, with microscopic disease remaining. **R2** resection denotes gross tumor unresected.
- The terminology for complete resection is important, but tumor margin may vary by tumor type, and close cooperation between the surgeon and the pathologist is essential. For example, wide local excision for breast cancer requires a margin of between 0.5 and 1 cm, whereas in colorectal cancer surgery a 5 cm margin proximally and a 2 cm margin distally should be achieved.

- The outcomes of many oncologic surgical procedures are superior in centers with higher volumes and when performed by surgeons with more experience, including pneumonectomy, esophagectomy, and pancreatectomy.
- Although colectomy is considered a relatively standard procedure, resection for rectal cancer is more complicated. Total mesorectal excision is essential to prevent local recurrence in the pelvis after rectal cancer, and this specialized technique is best done by surgeons who perform a considerable number of these procedures.

The use of MIS and robotic techniques in the definitive treatment of malignancy is evolving

- Currently, thoracoscopic lobectomy for lung cancer is an accepted option with numerous advantages, as is laparoscopic resection for colon cancer.
- Minimally invasive and robotic approaches to surgery of the kidney, thymus, esophagus, adrenal, and prostate are also performed.
- Through a collaborative process, the American Society of Clinical Oncology (ASCO), the NCCN, and the Commission on Cancer (CoC) have agreed on various quality measures in treatment of patients with breast cancer, colon cancer, and rectal cancer that surgeons should use. For example, at least 12 regional lymph nodes should be removed and pathologically examined for resected colon cancer.

Further reading

Baxter NN, Whitson BA, Tuttle TM (2007). Trends in the treatment and outcome of pancreatic cancer in the United States. *Ann Surg Oncol* 14:1320–1326

Begg CB, Cramer LD, Hoskins WJ, Brennan MF (1998). Impact of hospital volume on operative mortality for major cancer surgery. *JAMA* 280:1747–1751.

Farray D, Mirkovic N, Albain KS (2005). Multimodality therapy for stage III non-small-cell lung cancer. *J Clin Oncol* 23:3257–3269.

Guillem JG, Wood WC, Moley JF, Berchuck A, et al. (2006). ASCO/SSO review of current role of risk-reducing surgery in common hereditary cancer syndromes. *Ann Surg Oncol* 13:1296–1321.

Kaufmann M, von Minckwitz G, Smith R, et al. (2003). International expert panel on the use of primary (preoperative) systemic treatment of operable breast cancer: review and recommendations. *J Clin Oncol* 21:2600–2608.

Mulshine JL, Sullivan DC (2005). Lung cancer screening. *N Engl J Med* 352:2714–2720.

Pierce LJ, Levin AM, Rebbeck TR, et al. (2006). Ten-year multi-institutional results of breast-conserving surgery and radiotherapy in BRCA1/2-associated stage I/II breast cancer. *J Clin Oncol* 24:2437–2443.

Poplin EA, Benedetti JK, Estes NC, et al. (2005). Phase III Southwest Oncology Group 9415/Intergroup 0153 randomized trial of fluorouracil, leucovorin, and levamisole versus fluorouracil continuous infusion and levamisole for adjuvant treatment of stage III and high-risk stage II colon cancer. *J Clin Oncol* 23:1819–1825.

Punglia RS, Morrow M, Winer EP, Harris JR (2007). Local therapy and survival in breast cancer. *N Engl J Med* 356:2399–2405.

Thompson IM Jr, Tangen CM, Paradelo J, et al. (2006). Adjuvant radiotherapy for pathologically advanced prostate cancer: a randomized clinical trial. *JAMA* 296:2329–2335.

Palliative surgery

Surgical palliation falls into several different categories, requiring a broad range of expertise and knowledge.

A patient's life expectancy may vary from weeks to years, depending on their condition. The surgeon must know when not to operate and when to use palliative care teams and interventional radiology, as well as decide when and what operation is required.

Bowel obstruction

Patients with colon or ovarian cancer make up the bulk of those developing small- or large-bowel obstruction. In a colon cancer patient, confirmation of incurability will usually be made at laparotomy, after a decision to treat a large-bowel obstruction. Where possible, these patients should have the primary cancer excised and intestinal continuity restored by primary anastomosis.

Management of the obstructed ovarian cancer patient is usually more difficult, because the key decision is often whether the patient should have the operation. A multidisciplinary team discussion of these difficult patients, in consultation with the patients and their families, is essential. In general, a combined approach involving a colorectal surgeon and a cancer gynecologist is best.

Many patients will have multiple obstruction sites, with small and large bowel studded with tumors on the serosal surface. Such patients are not suitable for surgical palliation. Others will have one or two site obstructions. They can benefit from debulking, resection, and anastomosis or bypass surgery.

To differentiate these categories of patient, the following features and methods can be used: history of crampy abdominal pain, clinical examination revealing a distended tympanitic abdomen (as opposed to an abdomen with multiple sites of palpable tumor and ascites), plain x-rays revealing many loops of distended bowel with air-fluid levels, and CT evidence of pelvic or other single-site tumor deposit.

Laparoscopy will sometimes be helpful in the obstructed patient who has not had previous abdominal surgery. With modern techniques, laparoscopic bypass can be carried out by suitably trained surgeons in selected patients. This requires great care in the obstructed patient.

Fistulas

Fistulas caused by pelvic tumors or post-radiotherapy include the following:
- Rectovaginal
- Enterovaginal
- Colovesical
- Vesicovaginal
- Combination of above

Preoperative assessment to determine the exact type of fistula is important.
- A proximal end sigmoid colostomy, which can usually be performed without a formal laparotomy, is the treatment of choice for most rectovaginal fistulas if definitive surgery is not possible.
- Patients with combined rectovaginal and vesicovaginal fistulas may need an end colostomy and ileal conduit.
- A covered stent, delivered endoscopically or radiologically, should be considered for patients with a colovesical fistula.
- Patients with an enterovesical fistula will require laparotomy, resection of small bowel segment, and anastomosis.
- For low vaginal fistulas, coloanal sleeve procedures may be helpful. This should be done by an appropriate colorectal specialist.

Jaundice

Obstructive jaundice can be palliated surgically by choledochoenterostomy or cholecystenterostomy, although these procedures have been largely superseded by endoscopic and radiological placement of stents. Stents can become blocked, resulting in repeated cholangitis.

A trial has demonstrated a shorter overall hospital stay and decreased morbidity for surgical palliation of jaundice compared with endoscopic stenting and should be considered in medically fit patients.

Selected patients with inoperable hilar tumors will be best treated by segment III biliary enteric bypass. In those patients who require surgical bypass of obstructive jaundice, laparoscopic techniques have a role in selected patients by appropriately trained surgeons.

Ascites

Peritoneal-venous (Leveen) shunts can be inserted to relieve ascites in selected cases.

Careful preoperative assessment should be undertaken to ensure that ascites is not loculated and that the tumor is not mucinous; otherwise the shunt will become blocked. These are usually inserted using local anesthetic and sedation, with >50% of patients achieving good, long-term palliation. Postoperative coagulopathy may be a problem.

Pain

There are several options open to oncological surgeons to help patients with pain:
- Surgical debulking of large, slow-growing tumors (e.g., intra-abdominal, soft-tissue sarcomas in otherwise fit patients for whom expected morbidity of the procedure is low)
- Stabilization of pathological fractures and prophylactic pinning of bone metastases involving >50% of cortex
- Neurosurgical approaches for pain control, including cordotomy
- Thoracoscopic splanchnectomy for intractable pain secondary to pancreatic cancer

In general, with modern pain management and specialist pain clinics, the requirement for a surgical approach to the spinal cord or to peripheral nerves is now limited.

Gastrointestinal bleeding

A wide array of endoscopic and radiological techniques is available to stop bleeding from benign and malignant causes in patients with incurable cancer, including injection sclerotherapy (benign ulceration), laser coagulation (neoplastic ulcers), and radiological embolization (should other methods fail). Surgery should be reserved for those with a life expectancy of three months or more, for whom other methods fail.

Cytoreductive surgery

In some patients, extensive local disease may prevent removal of all disease by surgery, but partial resection is still appropriate. This applies particularly to ovarian cancer, for which subsequent chemotherapy can lead to good results, even in advanced disease.

Palliative resection of the primary tumor

Up to 10% of patients with breast cancer will present with metastatic disease; patients with visceral metastases have a poor prognosis, but patients with bone metastases have a median survival of over two years. Resection of the primary tumor to achieve locoregional control may improve patients' quality of life, preventing fungation or uncontrolled axillary metastases.

Patients with colorectal cancer are staged before surgery to determine the most appropriate therapy. In those in whom unresectable liver metastases are identified, primary tumor resection should still be considered to minimize the risk of bleeding, perforation, or obstruction, which may subsequently occur.

Laparoscopic surgery has a definite role in the palliation of malignancy, e.g., for gastric outlet obstruction, intestinal obstruction, and biliary bypass for obstructive jaundice (pancreatic cancer). Feeding tubes for nutrition can also be placed laparoscopically, the colon and small bowel can be decompressed, and stomata can be created using minimally invasive techniques.

Further reading

Randall TC, Rubin SC (2000). Management of intestinal obstruction in the patient with ovarian cancer. *Oncology* 14:1159–1163.

Rose PG, Nerenstone S, Brady MF (2004). Secondary surgical cytoreduction for advanced ovarian carcinoma. *N Engl J Med* 351:2489–2497.

Surgery for metastatic disease

For some tumor types (such as colorectal cancer, renal cell carcinoma, or sarcoma), patients with a single site or limited number of metastases may be considered for resection. Resection of the so-called oligometastatic disease is most commonly performed when the liver or lung are involved.

The diagnosis of metastatic disease may be recognized either synchronously or metachronously with the primary tumor. Some patients with limited secondary deposits in lung, liver, or brain may have prolonged survival, but the patients should be carefully assessed at a multidisciplinary team meeting to consider fitness for major surgery, likely benefit, potential complications, and patient and family wishes.

Indications for metastasectomy of the lung or liver include the following:
- The primary tumor is controlled (or controllable).
- There is no other evidence of metastatic disease.
- The metastases are completely resectable, allowing enough normal tissue for normal organ function.
- There is no medical therapy that would be superior to surgery.

For patients with liver metastases that are not surgical candidates, other therapies may be used:
- Cryotherapy
- Radiofrequency ablation
- Injection of alcohol
- Chemoembolization

Bone metastases

Presentation usually is that of a pathological fracture. Breast and prostate are the most common primary sites followed by lung, thyroid, and renal cancer. Mean survival is 3 months for lung cancer to over 2 years for breast cancer.
- **Investigations:** MRI and PET scanning are the most accurate investigations, followed by bone scanning.

Internal fixation is useful if:
- There is weight-bearing bone, especially if a lesion is >2.5 cm or involves circumference
- Painful secondary after radiotherapy
- It will improve mobilization and nursing care
- Patient is fit
- Bone quality will support fixation

Considerations in spinal secondary:
- Stability of spine
- Spinal cord compression

Treatment options
- Radiotherapy
- Hormone manipulation
- **Surgery:** stabilization preceded by bone tumor biopsy (occasionally it is possible to excise the secondary deposit)

- Internal fixation techniques include plates, intramedullary nails, and prosthetic replacement of metaphyseal lesions.
- Occasionally cast or brace immobilization or external fixation is used for patients with extensive localized disease that cannot be immobilized by internal methods. Rarely is amputation appropriate, except for fungating tumors, recurrent infections, and intractable pain.
- Minimally invasive treatment of metastatic bone lesions with radiographically guided percutaneous injection of bone cement is currently used in selected cases, for example, in the spine.

Brain metastases
- **Common:** Up to 10% of cancer patients have brain secondaries.
- The 5-year cumulative incidence of brain metastases is 16%, 10%, 7%, 5%, and 1% for patients with lung cancer, renal cell cancer, melanoma, breast cancer, and colorectal cancer, respectively. Lung and breast are the most common primary sites.
- **Blood-borne:** The distribution of brain metastases reflects blood flow—80% of lesions are found in the cerebrum, 15% in the cerebellum, and 5% in the brainstem.
- Presentations include headache, focal weakness, altered mental status, and epilepsy.
- Hemorrhage within brain metastases may cause an acute neurological state.
- Diagnosis is by CT or MRI (the latter picks up smaller secondaries).
- Mean survival without therapy is 2 months, 3 months with steroid therapy, and 6 months with radiotherapy.
- Surgery is useful to confirm diagnosis, relieve pressure effects, and improve local control and survival.
- Survival is poor in patients with systemic uncontrolled disease, poor general medical condition, tumors lying infratentorially, poor neurological status, and a short interval from the diagnosis of the primary tumor to the diagnosis of the brain metastases.
- Tumor deposits in the thalamus, brainstem, and basal ganglia are usually irresectable because of the associated morbidity and mortality.
- Resection of a single secondary can lead to prolonged survival (melanoma 7 months, lung cancer 12 months, renal cell cancer 10 months, breast cancer 1 year, and colon cancer 9 months).

Occasionally, resection of multiple metastases is worthwhile:
- Good palliation
- Underused
- Occasionally curative
- Postoperative radiotherapy helps
- Anatomical site is important

Malignant pleural effusion

Management may include thoracentesis, tube thoracostomy with or without pleurodesis, thoracoscopic drainage with pleurodesis, or placement of an indwelling pleural catheter.

Chemical pleurodesis may be performed with talc, bleomycin, or doxycycline. Talc is considered the most cost-effective agent, but side effects such as fever and malaise may limit its use in some patients. Rarely, talc may induce an adult respiratory distress syndrome (ARDS)-like syndrome.

Pleurectomy and decortication may be performed in selected patients with malignant mesothelioma.

Malignant pericardial effusion

In patients with a history of cancer, the development of a pericardial effusion is usually related to metastases, although it may be related to the treatment itself.

Except in patients in whom treatment of the primary tumor would be expected to improve the effusion, such as some patients with lymphoma, small cell lung cancer, and breast cancer, pericardial effusions are managed with surgical procedures.

Although pericardiocentesis may be effective, the recurrence rate is high and most patients with malignant pericardial effusion are managed with a pericardial window. A surgical pericardial window may be performed using a subxiphoid or thoracoscopic approach, with equivalent efficacy.

Malignant ascites

Although most patients with malignant ascites can be treated medically, peritoneal-venous shunting (Denver shunt) or the use of an indwelling catheter (Pleurx) may be useful in those with a reasonable life expectancy. Shunt occlusion and coagulopathy are limiting factors.

Further reading

Inoue M, Kotake Y, Nakagawa K, et al. (2000). Surgery for pulmonary metastases from colorectal carcinoma. *Ann Thorac Surg* 70:380–383.

Prasad D, Schiff D (2005). Malignant spinal cord compression. *Lancet Oncol* 6:15–24.

Putnam JB, Light RW, Rodriguez RM, et al. (1999). A randomized comparison of indwelling pleural catheter and doxycycline pleurodesis in the management of malignant pleural effusions. *Cancer* 86:1992–1999.

Thompson JF, Scolyer RA, Kefford RF (2005). Cutaneous melanoma. *Lancet* 365:687–701.

Vogelsang, H, Haas S, Hierholzer C, et al. (2005). Factors influencing survival after resection of pulmonary metastases from colorectal cancer. *Br J Surg* 91:1066–1071.

Chapter 8

Principles of radiation oncology

Bridget F. Koontz
Christopher G. Willett

Introduction *82*
Principles of radiobiology *84*
Principles of radiation physics *88*
External beam radiotherapy *92*
Specialized radiation therapy *96*
  Brachytherapy *96*
  Intraoperative radiotherapy *97*
  Stereotactic radiosurgery *98*
  Total body irradiation *98*
  Unsealed radionuclides *99*

CHAPTER 8 Principles of radiation oncology

Introduction

Radiation oncology is a medical specialty that uses ionizing radiation to treat malignancies and a few specific benign diseases. Radiation was first used to treat cancer only one year after the discovery of x-rays, and significant technologic advances have been made in the past century. It is now used in more than 50% of all patients with cancer.

Historical perspective

Important dates in the history of radiation oncology

1896	Discovery of x-rays by Wilhelm Roentgen
1898	Discovery of radium by Marie and Pierre Curie
1899	Treatment of skin cancer with x-rays
1915	Treatment of cervical cancer with radium implant
1934	Dose fractionation principles proposed by Regaud and Coutard
1950s	External radiotherapy using radioactive cobalt (1 MV)
1960s	Linear accelerators capable of megavoltage x-rays (4–25 MV)
1990s	Three-dimensional planning using CT imaging
2000s	Intensity-modulated radiotherapy and proton beam therapy

As a modality to treat cancer, radiation therapy can be used in several different ways:

- Definitive treatment with or without chemotherapy, e.g., head and neck cancer, lung cancer, prostate cancer
- Adjuvant treatment after completion of primary treatment, e.g., breast cancer, lymphoma
- Neoadjuvant treatment induces tumor regression prior to definitive therapy, e.g., rectal cancer, sarcoma
- Palliative treatment for symptom relief, e.g., brain or bone metastases, bronchial obstruction

In this chapter, we will discuss the guiding principles of radiobiology and radiation physics and the different strategies used to deliver radiation therapy.

Principles of radiobiology

Radiation dose is measured in Gray (Gy), which is the energy absorbed per mass of tissue (joules/kilogram). An older, non-SI unit of dose was the rad.

1 Gy = 100 rad

Fractionation is the division of a total prescribed radiation dose into small, often daily doses. Fractionation preferentially spares normal tissue injury, thereby allowing higher total doses and increased cancer cell kill. However, extending the treatment time of radiotherapy allows for tumor repopulation, negatively impacting the chance of cure.

Standard fractionation is 1.8 or 2 Gy per day.

Hyperfractionation uses smaller individual doses to reduce normal tissue injury.
- Administered multiple times per day to avoid increasing overall treatment time (e.g., 1.2 Gy bid).
- Treatments are given at least six hours apart to allow normal tissue time to complete repair of the previous fraction.
- Used most commonly in head and neck cancers, small cell lung cancer.

Hypofractionation uses fractions larger than 2 Gy/day.
- Reduces both repopulation and overall treatment time.
- Used most commonly for metastases.

Radiation-induced cell death

When x-rays pass through tissue, energy is absorbed, resulting in the ionization of molecules and generation of free radicals. The most biologically important target of these free radicals is DNA, causing double helix breaks. DNA damage can lead to cell death by two mechanisms:

1. Initiation of apoptosis through the p53-caspase pathway
2. Loss of cellular reproductive capacity through chromosome abnormalities

The biological effect of radiotherapy is related to the dose given and the timing of the treatment. This balances the DNA damage caused by radiation with repair processes of the cell.

The amount of DNA damage is dose-dependent, and so greater radiation doses cause more cell death. Therefore, the volume of disease before the start of radiotherapy can affect its success, with microscopic disease requiring less dose than visible tumor. Frequently, normal tissues in close proximity to the tumor limit the total doses of radiation therapy administered.

Repair processes act to inhibit cell kill. The cell-cycle phase during which the damage occurs affects the ability of repair, with mitosis and G2 having less repair capability than G1 and S phase. Treatment combining radiation with chemotherapy or hyperthermia may enhance tumor cell kill by attacking multiple pathways of DNA damage and repair.

Some tissues and organs are more sensitive to radiation than others. This is related in part to **repair** capabilities, ability to **repopulate**, and the relationship to other cells in the tissue.

An early-responding tissue will quickly respond to radiation but will also quickly recover through repopulation. These tissues typically have high cell turnover at baseline, and repopulation can be increased to meet radiation-induced cell loss. The degree of recovery relates to the total dose (number of stem cells remaining) and length of treatment (longer treatment allows for more repopulation).

- Early-responding tissues have high cell turnover.
- Toxicity presents during or within weeks of radiation and recovers quickly.
- e.g., GI mucosa and bone marrow

A late-responding tissue has dormant or slowly cycling cells that are better able to repair radiation-induced DNA damage. However, the tissue does not have a large reserve of stem cells able to regenerate the tissue after cell loss occurs. Thus, the effects of radiation arise after radiation is complete, but they are permanent. The degree of permanent injury relates to both fraction size and total dose (number of cells surviving).

- Late-responding tissues have minimal or slow cell turnover.
- Toxicity presents months to years after radiation and may be permanent.
- e.g., peripheral nerves, spinal cord, kidneys
- Skin is both an early- and a late-responding tissue, with the epidermis showing early effects and dermis showing late effects from radiation.

Organ structure can be visualized as functional units of cells either in parallel or in series, like an electrical circuit.

Parallel structures can tolerate high doses to small volumes because the untreated organ still functions, whereas relatively low doses to large volumes cause a significant decrease in organ function (e.g., lung, liver, kidney).

Serial structures require that all cells act in coordination, so that even small volumes receiving a high dose can cause significant injury (e.g., spinal cord, bowel).

Typical acute effects of radiation involve early-responding tissues and include mucositis, desquamation, and hematopoetic cytopenia. Late effects include fibrosis, ulceration, and organ dysfunction. Nonlethal DNA mutations caused by ionizing radiation can result in a radiation-induced malignancy. These typically occur after a long latent period of years and are related to the tissues irradiated and age of the patient at the time of treatment.

Strategies to improve radiosensitivity

Concurrent chemotherapy

Many chemotherapy agents also target DNA, and combination treatment can result in increased radiosensitivity, both of the tumor and normal tissues (Table 8.1). The most commonly used agents in combination with radiation are 5-fluorouracil and cisplatin. Anthracyclines and bleomycin are generally not used concurrently with radiation because of overlapping toxicities.

Reduce hypoxia

Because DNA damage is dependent on free radicals, hypoxic cells are relatively radioresistant compared with their nonhypoxic counterparts. Hypoxia can be combated by the following:
- Treating anemia to keep hemoglobin level above 10 g/dL
- Concurrent hyperthermia—heat improves blood flow and has direct cytotoxic effects
- Antiangiogenic drugs can normalize tumor vasculature to improve blood flow

Further reading

Hall E, Giacca A (2005). *Radiobiology for the Radiologist*, 6th ed. Philadelphia: Lippincott, Williams, and Wilkins.

Table 8.1 Radiosensitivity of different tumors and organs

Most sensitive	Lymphoma	Germ cells
	Small cell lung cancer	Bone marrow
Moderately sensitive	Rectal cancer	Lung
	Breast cancer	Kidney
	Lung cancer	Bowel
		Skin
Least sensitive	Melanoma	CNS
		Connective tissue

Principles of radiation physics

Types of radiation

Photons
- The most common type of therapeutic radiation
- Exponentially attenuated by tissue, due to absorption and scatter
- Higher energies have deeper penetration and less skin dose

Superficial x-rays	50–150 KV max dose at 1–2 mm
Orthovoltage	150–500 KV max dose at 0.5 cm
Megavoltage	>1000 KV max dose at 1–5 cm

- Beam travels through patient with substantial exit dose
- Photon energies between 6 and 20 MV are most common and used for deep or centrally located tumors.

Electrons
- Charged particles with limited penetration and full dose close to skin.
- The effective range (penetration depth of an electron beam) is approximately half the energy.
- The clinically useful range (depth at which dose falls to 80% of maximum) is one-third of the energy.

Range (cm) = E/2   80% isodose (cm) = E/3

e.g.: 12 MeV electron beam:
   Dose at 6 cm = 9.6%, at 4 cm = 80.0%

- Useful for superficial lesions while minimizing dose to deeper structures

Protons
- Charged particle that deposits most of its dose at the end of its path
- Can treat deep tumors with minimal exit dose
- Requires specialized accelerator, currently has limited availability

Neutrons
- Uncharged particle
- Used primarily for unresectable salivary tumors
- Requires specialized accelerator, currently has limited availability

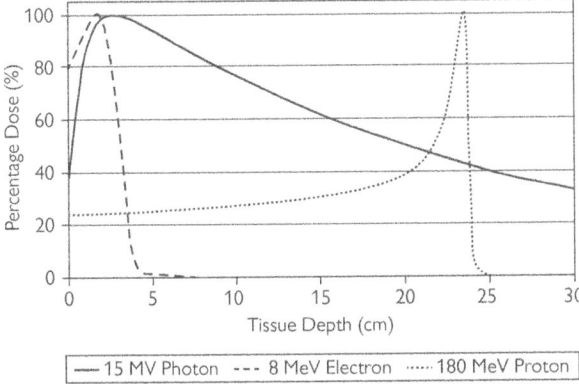

Figure 8.1 The percentage of dose based on tissue depth for representative electron (dash-dotted line), photon (solid line), and proton (dotted line) energies. The electron has a high skin dose but falls off quickly. The photon "spares" the skin and has a relatively shallow maximum dose, but it has a long tail. The proton deposits a small amount of dose initially with a sharp increase at the end of its range.

Sources of radiation

Ionizing radiation can be obtained from either a radioactive source or a linear accelerator, where electrons are accelerated to high kinetic energies before hitting a target, releasing x-rays.

Radioisotope
- Constant emission (radiation safety issue)
- Energy, half-life, and type of radiation depend on isotope (See Table 8.2)

Table 8.2 Characteristics of common isotopes

Isotope	Cobalt-60	Iodine-125	Iridium-192
Half-life	5 years	60 days	74 days
Energy	1.25 MV	0.027 MV	0.38 MV
Use	External beam irradiation	Permanent implants	Temporary implants

Linear accelerator
- Radiation is generated only when the machine is turned on.
- Energy can be manipulated based on electron acceleration.
- It can deliver photons and electrons.
- Specialized accelerators can deliver protons and neutrons.

Radiation safety

Radiation exposure of individuals is measured by *effective dose*, which considers dose, type of radiation, and tissue radiosensitivity (see Box 8.1). The SI unit is the Sievert (Sv). For most clinical therapeutic radiotherapy, 1 Gy = 1 Sv.

Regulations are in place to protect workers with potential radiation exposure (e.g., medical staff, nuclear power plant workers, airline staff). The annual occupational exposure limit is 50 mSv/year. The actual average effective dose received by a radiation worker is approximately 2 mSv/year.

> **Box 8.1 Annual effective dose in the U.S is 3.6 mSv, primarily due to radon exposure**
>
> *Natural sources*
> Radon   2 mSv
> Cosmic radiation   0.3 mSv
> Terrestial radioactivity 0.3 mSv
> Ingested radioactivity   0.4 mSv
>
> *Manmade sources*
> Medical imaging   0.5 mSv
> Consumer products   0.1 mSv
> Trans-Atlantic flight 0.05 mSv
>
> *Diagnostic tests*
> Chest X-ray   0.03 mSv
> Chest CT   8 mSv
> PET scan   4 mSv

External beam radiotherapy

Definitive radiotherapy
Many cancers can be cured using radiation as the primary modality, with or without concurrent chemotherapy (See Table 8.3). Concurrent chemotherapy is chosen to increase radiosensitivity when the tumor is large, radioresistant, or near critical structures. Use of definitive radiation allows for organ and tissue preservation, particularly for head and neck and skin cancers, by replacing potentially disfiguring surgeries.

Adjuvant radiotherapy
Radiation is given after primary surgery (e.g., breast cancer, prostate cancer) or chemotherapy (e.g., lymphoma) to eradicate microscopic residual disease. The dose required to treat adjuvantly is less than that required in the definitive setting because the tumor burden is less.

Neoadjuvant radiotherapy
Radiation PRIOR to primary treatment is most often used to reduce tumor size before surgery and improve the chance of a complete resection. In situations where adjuvant radiation would be generally recommended, radiation before surgery can often be performed with less toxicity, because smaller fields can be used and the tumor itself pushes normal tissue out of the radiation field.

Neoadjuvant radiation has been used with concurrent chemotherapy for GI malignancies and locally advanced breast cancers. Neoadjuvant radiotherapy is commonly used for sarcomas to reduce the need for amputation.

Palliative radiotherapy
Radiation is an excellent modality for relief of symptoms caused by metastatic or locally progressive disease. Brain metastases are commonly treated with radiation, which does not have the same blood-brain barrier limitations as chemotherapy. It is also commonly used for painful bone metastases or lesions impinging on vital organ functions, such as bronchial obstruction.

Treatment planning

Beam dosimetry
Before clinical use, the physical properties of the radiation beam must first be determined. Properties include output over time, dose at different depths, beam symmetry, and the penumbra (region of dose buildup beginning at the beam edge, typically 0.5–1 cm). These factors are used to calculate irradiation time required for a specific dose given.

Patient positioning, immobilization, and localization
Customizing radiation treatment to a particular tumor requires that the tumor position be reliably reproduced each day of treatment. During the planning process, immobilization devices are used to reduce daily "setup error." For treatment requiring very tight margins because of normal tissue constraints, stereotactic frames, implanted fiducial markers, or daily

pretreatment imaging of the target (by ultrasound or CT) can be used to determine the exact location of the tumor before treatment.

Target definition

For superficial tumors, the target can be defined clinically (i.e., skin cancers). For most cancers, however, imaging is used to ensure the tumor and areas at risk for microscopic spread are included in the radiation field. Imaging modalities can include:
- Fluoroscopy: bony anatomical markers used, e.g., bone metastases
- CT: structures "contoured" in planning system, e.g., lung, breast
- MRI: improved anatomical definition, e.g., CNS, prostate, sarcoma
- PET: improved staging, e.g., GI, lung

The radiation oncologist then defines organs to be avoided and several target volumes. This can be done in a planning software system or directly onto film:

- GTV: gross tumor volume, clinically apparent disease
- CTV: clinical target volume, GTV + expansion for microscopic disease based on known patterns of spread, often ~1 cm
- PTV: planning treatment volume, CTV + expansion allowing for daily target motion and setup uncertainty. This is 0.5–1 cm, depending on tumor location and immobilization techniques.

Field design

The direction and number of fields are chosen to optimize coverage of the target volume while ensuring that normal structures do not exceed dose tolerance limits. Multiple beam plans can be used to provide dose sculpting around the target and avoid normal structures. Increasing the number of fields increases the complexity of the calculation and can extend the daily treatment time. Field borders are chosen to include the PTV with additional consideration of the beam's penumbra. Blocks are used to shape the beam and protect normal tissues.

Dose calculation

The complexity of planning calculations depends on the type of plan selected by the radiation oncologist and is guided by location of the tumor, nearby normal tissue tolerances, and the goal of treatment. Image-based planning creates a topographical map of dose, called an isodose plan, which shows coverage of the target and normal structures.

Intensity-modulated radiation therapy

Intensity-modulated readiation therapy (IMRT) is a technology using non-uniform beam intensity within each field. Combined with multiple beam angles, the modulation of dose given within each field can sculpt dose around target and normal structures.

This technology increases the volume of tissue receiving a low dose, but it can dramatically reduce the volume of normal structures receiving a high dose of radiation. Treatment time is often increased because the beam is on for a longer period of time per field.

Quality assurance

If patient treatment is planned on a software system, fields are verified and marked on the patient before beginning treatment. Positioning is rechecked intermittently throughout the treatment to verify correct positioning (called "portal imaging"). IMRT and stereotactic treatment require additional quality assurance performed by medical physicists.

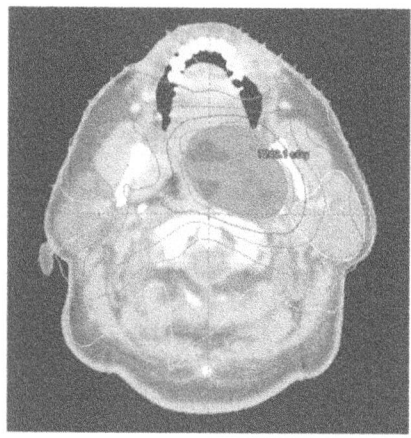

Figure 8.2 Example of an IMRT plan for a left-sided oropharyngeal head and neck cancer. The primary tumor (red) is covered by the 70 Gy isodose line (green). Nodal areas at risk (orange) receive at least 50 Gy (brown line). Note significant sparing of the right parotid (green), with the 60 (blue), 35 (pink), and 21 Gy (light green) isodose lines curving to avoid the structure. Right parotid is contoured in yellow. (see Plate 1 for a full color version.)

Table 8.3 Typical external beam radiation treatment for specific disease sites

Site	Stage	Treatment
Brain	High-grade astrocytoma	Surgery, then concurrent chemo-RT to 60 Gy
Head and neck	Early stage N0	Surgery or RT to 64–70 Gy
	Advanced stage	Chemo-RT to 70 Gy or Surgery, then chemo-RT to 60–66 Gy
Breast	Early stage (T1–2 N0)	Modified radical mastectomy or lumpectomy + 60 Gy to breast. Hormonal and/or chemotherapy
	Advanced stage (T3 or N+)	Surgery, Chemotherapy, RT 60 Gy to breast/chest wall and regional lymph nodes
Lung	Early stage (T1–2 N0)	Surgery or RT 60–70 Gy to tumor
	Advanced stage (N2+)	Preoperative chemotherapy ± 45–50 Gy or definitive chemo-RT to 60–70 Gy
Esophagus		Preoperative chemo-RT to 50 Gy
Stomach		Postoperative chemo-RT to 45 Gy
Pancreas		Preoperative or definitive chemo-RT to 50 Gy
Rectum		Preoperative chemo-RT to 50 Gy
Anus		Chemo-RT to 54 Gy
Hodgkin lymphoma	Stage I–II	Chemotherapy then involved field RT 20–30 Gy
Non-Hodgkin lymphoma	Stage I–II	Chemotherapy then involved field RT 30 Gy
Prostate		Prostatectomy or brachytherapy or definitive radiation 74–78 Gy ± androgen deprivation therapy

Specialized radiation therapy

Brachytherapy
Brachytherapy uses radioactive sources placed within or adjacent to a tumor. These sources typically deliver low-energy radiation with limited penetration, reducing the overall radiation dose to more distant normal structures.

Low-dose rate sources

These are used for permanent implants or temporary implants lasting 2–7 days. Sources can be placed in catheters implanted within a patient or implanted directly into tumor tissue.

Radiation staff receive exposure from preparing, placing, and removing low-dose rate (LDR) sources. To reduce this exposure, the radiation worker minimizes the **time** exposed, maximizes the **distance** from the source, and uses lead **shielding**. The most common sources for LDR implants are cesium-137, iridium-192 (Ir-192, for temporary implants), iodine-125, and palladium-103 (for permanent implants).

High-dose rate sources

The high-dose rate (HDR) source is guided through a catheter and delivers the prescribed radiation within minutes. HDR brachytherapy is often fractionated, giving a total of 3–5 fractions over 1–2 weeks.

The HDR source is housed in a remotely operated machine that prevents exposure to personnel during treatment. The source is located at the tip of a wire connected to a catheter placed at the desired treatment location. The most common source for HDR implants is Ir-192.

Typical brachytherapy treatment for specific disease sites
Intracavitary sources placed in a body cavity near the target tumor
Cervical cancer

Combined with external beam radiotherapy (EBRT), a brachytherapy implant is situated with a straight tandem catheter through the cervical os and two round ovoids (thus the implant is called T&O) on either side of the cervix. This results in a pear-shaped dose distribution overlying the cervix and medial parametrial tissue. This can be done in 1–2 LDR implants or 3–5 HDR implants.

Endometrial cancer

To reduce recurrence in the vaginal cuff after hysterectomy, a cylinder is placed in the vagina, and the cuff and proximal vagina are treated with 3–5 HDR treatments.

Lung cancer

Bronchial recurrence is treated by threading a catheter through and past the involved bronchial site by bronchoscopy. Radiation is typically given with 3–5 HDR treatments.

Bile duct cancer
HDR radiation is used to treat biliary stricture with the catheter placed by endoscopy into the biliary tree.

Ocular melanoma
A disc-shaped applicator containing the sources is surgically sewn onto the sclera at the site of the lesion and removed after five days of LDR radiation.

Interstitial sources placed in tissue

Prostate cancer
For early-stage prostate cancer, radioactive seeds can be permanently implanted into the prostate through the perineum using transrectal ultrasound guidance, or an HDR source is used over several fractions through catheters placed in the prostate.

Breast cancer
An HDR temporary implant is placed, using either catheters placed through the surgical lumpectomy site or a balloon placed into the lumpectomy cavity.

Sarcoma
Catheters are placed along the surgical bed. Either LDR or HDR sources can be used.

Penile cancer
For early shaft disease, catheters can be placed through the tumor. Both HDR and LDR sources can be used.

Intraoperative radiotherapy

Intraoperative radiotherapy is a subtype of brachytherapy in which lesions not otherwise accessible are given a single treatment with either low-penetration electrons or an HDR source during surgery. It is most commonly performed when resection is difficult and there is a high chance of microscopic or gross residual disease.

Once the tumor has been resected as much as possible, the surgical bed is prepared with lead shielding to protect nearby normal structures (i.e., bowel, kidney, nerves, blood vessels). Either a portable electron generator is placed over the target surgical bed or multiple HDR catheters embedded in a gel are placed against the surgical surface. The patient is kept under anesthesia and observed remotely while the treatment is delivered. Typically, it takes 10–45 minutes, depending on the size of the target field.

Because the dose is given in a single fraction, normal tissue injury is a concern, particularly for structures deep to the tumor bed that cannot be shielded. The dose given is usually between 10 and 20 Gy. The most common injury is neuropathy. Tumors treated in this fashion include abdominal or retroperitoneal tumors and recurrent rectal cancer.

Stereotactic radiosurgery

Intracranial stereotactic radiosurgery

Intracranial stereotactic radiosurgery (SRS) consists of a single large-dose but tightly focused radiation treatment. For intracranial SRS a stereotactic head frame is used that facilitates exact tumor positioning. The frame creates a three-dimensional coordinate system that is linked to the planning software and treatment equipment to allow for very tight margins on the target. Both CT and MR imaging are typically used.

SRS is offered to patients with a limited number of brain metastases and otherwise well controlled disease and for benign diseases such as acoustic neuromas and arteriovenous malformations. A single fraction of 12–24 Gy is prescribed, depending on the size of the lesion and its proximity to critical normal structures such as the brainstem and optic chiasm.

Stereotactic body radiotherapy (SBRT)

In extracranial stereotactic radiotherapy, typically 3–5 fractions are given to treat metastases or recurrent tumor. Tight margins are used to protect normal tissue when treating with high doses per fraction. Accuracy in positioning is essential. Instead of a head frame anchored to the skull, a body mold is used, often with hardware placed over the abdomen to reduce respiratory excursion.

For additional tumor targeting, use either pretreatment CT or radiographic matching to fiducial markers placed in or adjacent to the tumor.

Although SBRT is most commonly used for lung and liver metastases, it has also been used for recurrent disease previously treated by external radiation, such as spine lesions. Doses are 5–20 Gy in 3–5 fractions, taking into consideration size of the lesion and normal tissue tolerance. It is also becoming more common for curative treatment of early stage prostate and lung cancer.

Total body irradiation

Total body irradiation (TBI) is most typically used in conjunction with chemotherapy to prepare a patient for stem cell transplantation. The radiation serves several purposes:
- It eliminates residual disease, including sanctuary sites (CNS, testes).
- It suppresses the host immune system.
- It ablates native marrow to permit engraftment of donor marrow.

Ablative doses of radiation requiring either a full allogeneic or autologous transplant are in the range of 12–17 Gy. Low-dose TBI with a single 2 Gy fraction is used to suppress the immune system for non-myeloablative autologous transplants.

Acute side effects include nausea, mucositis, diarrhea, parotiditis, and fatigue. Possible late complications include cataracts, hypothyroidism, interstitial pneumonitis, veno-occlusive disease of the liver, sterility, and second malignancies. Children in particular are at risk for neurological deficits, growth deficits (both from impaired GH production and epiphyseal growth plate fusion), and second malignancies.

Treatment is given with opposed fields and low energies. Patients can be positioned lying, sitting, or standing, with either lateral or anterior-posterior (AP) and posterior-anterior (PA) beams that include the entire body.

Many dose schedules are in use, but they typically involve twice-daily treatment for 1 week. If sanctuary sites (areas with limited chemotherapy penetration, e.g., CNS, testes) are involved, additional radiation to boost these areas is used. The dose to the lung is reduced to 10 Gy in patients with normal lung function and to 7–8 Gy in those with reduced function. These calculations are made before treatment, and surface dosimeters are used to check the calculation on the first treatment.

Unsealed radionuclides

Unsealed radionuclides are most often used in diagnostic nuclear medicine imaging. They can also be used therapeutically for treatment of thyroid cancer, neural crest tumors, widespread bone metastases, or intraperitoneal malignancy. Targeted radionuclide therapy with radioisotopes attached to monoclonal antibodies is used to treat lymphoma.

Dosimetry calculations for unsealed nuclides must consider both the physical half-life of the isotope and the biological half-life, or length of time before the molecule is excreted. The radionuclide is typically secreted in bodily fluids, including saliva, sweat, and urine, which can pose a radiation exposure risk to other individuals.

Thyroid cancer

Thyroid cancer that absorbs iodine can be treated with radioactive iodine-131, which has a physical half-life of eight days. I-131 is selectively absorbed by differentiated thyroid cancer cells. After surgical resection of the thyroid, a low dose of I-131 is used to diagnose any residual disease. If present, a higher ablative dose can be used, with bone marrow being the limiting toxicity.

Neural crest tumors

Iodine-131 attached to metaiodobenzylguanidine (MIBG) is selectively absorbed by neuroendocrine tumors, including pheochromocytomas, neuroblastomas, and paragangliomas. This selective uptake can again be used both diagnostically and, at higher doses, therapeutically.

Bone metastases

Bone metastases can be treated with bone-selective radionuclides that concentrate in areas of bone turnover. Radium-223 has recently been approved by the U.S. FDA for treatment of bone metastases from prostate cancer. Myelosuppression can occur up to 6 weeks after treatment, and patients should be closely observed.

Peritoneal malignancies

Malignant ascites or metastatic peritoneal implants can be treated with an infusion of phosphorus-32, with a physical half-life of 14 days. The radionuclide emits electron radiation with very limited penetration, so the bowel tolerance is kept while treating superficial disease.

Lymphoma

Lymphomas expressing CD-20 can be targeted using anti-CD20 monoclonal antibodies. Two current agents, yttrium-90 conjugated to ibritumomab (Zevalin) and I-131 conjugated to tositumomab (Bexxar), have been effective in treating low-grade non-Hodgkin lymphoma. Bone marrow is again the dose-limiting toxicity.

Chapter 9

Principles of chemotherapy

Sally Barbour
Ashley Engemann

Rationale for combination therapy *102*
Alkylating agents *104*
Antitumor antibiotics *112*
Antimetabolites *118*
Cisplatin and derivatives *132*
Topoisomerase inhibitors *136*
Antimicrotubule agents *140*
Drug resistance *144*
Dose intensification *146*
Chemoradiation *148*

Rationale for combination therapy

Cytotoxic chemotherapy destroys cancer cells. Currently available drugs target
- Chemistry of nucleic acids
- DNA or RNA production
- Mechanics of cell division (e.g., spindle poisons)

The discovery and development of cytotoxics has paralleled the understanding of the chemical processes involved. The lack of selectivity inherent in this approach has limited the ability to kill cancer cells while leaving normal dividing cells unscathed.

Cytotoxic agents can be classified by the following:
- Chemical properties or mechanisms of action
- Source (e.g., natural products)
- Propensity to be cell cycle or phase specific

The following underlie the design of a potential combination therapy.
- Each drug should have single-agent activity in that tumor type.
- Each drug should have a different mechanism of activity.
- Drugs with non-overlapping toxicity patterns are preferable.
- Drugs that work in different parts of the cell cycle should be selected.
- Drugs should not all share the same resistance mechanisms.

Combination therapy aims to increase "fractional cell kill" leading to improved overall response of the tumor.

Higher doses of cytotoxic drugs tend to produce increased cell kill (at least within certain limits); thus, it is important not to compromise on the dose of each agent (hence, the need to select drugs with non-overlapping toxicity).
- Tumor mass is usually composed of cells that are asynchronously dividing, thus combinations of drugs that act at different points in the cell cycle will theoretically kill more cells.
- "Multidrug resistance" is displayed by some tumor types, resulting from, e.g., expression of an efflux pump on the cell surface that pumps the drug out of the cell.

Alkylating agents

Mechanism of action
Alkylating agents are among the oldest of anticancer agents used clinically. These cytotoxic agents exert their antiproliferative effects by covalently binding alkyl groups to cellular molecules.

Alkylation of DNA occurs through the formation of reactive intermediates that attack nucleophilic sites. The majority of clinically useful alkylating agents cause DNA cross-linking, which results in inhibition of DNA synthesis and cell death.

Some alkylating agents cause DNA strand breaks rather than cross-linking.

Resistance
Resistance to alkylating agents is multifactorial and may differ between classes of alkylating agents, e.g., resistance to nitrosoureas is probably mediated by increased expression of the enzyme O^6-alkyl transferase.

In addition to enhanced DNA repair, resistant cells may exhibit an increased ability to detoxify alkylating agents. Such mechanisms include increased
- Glutathione
- Metallothionein
- Glutathione-S-transferase

Nitrogen mustards
Chlorambucil
- **Clinical indications:** Chronic lymphocytic leukemia (CLL) and lymphomas.
- **Dosing:** CLL in adults: 0.1 mg/kg po daily for 3–6 months or until a remission is achieved. Maintenance is 2–4 mg po daily.

Adverse events
- Bone marrow suppression
- Nausea and vomiting
- Interstitial pneumonitis or pulmonary fibrosis (rare)
- Tumor lysis syndrome
- Infertility
- Secondary malignancies
- Rash (uncommon)
- Toxic epidermal necrolysis (rare)

Cyclophosphamide
Cyclophosphamide is a prodrug that requires hepatic activation in order to exert its cytotoxicity. In addition to cytotoxic effects, cyclophosphamide has significant immunosuppressant effects.
- **Clinical indications:** Acute and chronic leukemia, lymphoma, breast cancer, multiple myeloma, other solid tumors, autoimmune diseases, hematopoietic stem cell transplantation
- **Dosing:** 200–1000 mg/m^2 IV per cycle; oral regimens are also used

Adverse events
- Bone marrow suppression
- Nausea and vomiting (dose-related)
- Hemorrhagic cystitis
- Alopecia
- Pneumonitis or pulmonary fibrosis (rare)
- Tumor lysis syndrome
- Immunosuppression
- Syndrome of inappropriate antidiuretic hormone (SIADH)
- Infertility
- Secondary malignancies
- Cardiotoxicity (more likely in high-dose setting)
- Veno-occlusive disease of the liver (more likely in high-dose setting)
- Rash (uncommon)
- Toxic epidermal necrolysis or Stevens–Johnson syndrome (rare)

Additional comments
- Cyclophosphamide undergoes extensive hepatic P450 metabolism; caution is warranted when using inhibitors or inducers of these enzymes concurrently with cyclophosphamide.
- Patients should maintain adequate hydration to prevent hemorrhagic cystitis; mesna may be considered in the high-dose setting.

Ifosfamide
Ifosfamide is a synthetic analog of cyclophosphamide. It also requires hepatic activation to exert its cytotoxic effects.
- **Clinical indications**: Soft tissue sarcomas, osteogenic sarcomas, lung cancer, testicular cancer, lymphomas
- **Dosing**: Testicular cancer 1.2–2 g/m^2 per day IV for 5 days

Adverse events
- Bone marrow suppression
- Nausea and vomiting
- Hemorrhagic cystitis
- Neurotoxicity, encephalopathy
- Alopecia
- Renal insufficiency
- Infertility
- Secondary malignancies
- Cardiotoxicity

Additional comments
- Ifosfamide undergoes extensive hepatic P450 metabolism; caution is warranted when using inhibitors or inducers of these enzymes concurrently with ifosfamide.
- Patients should maintain adequate hydration to prevent hemorrhagic cystitis; mesna must always be given with ifosfamide.
- Neurotoxicity is thought to be caused by the metabolite chloroacetaldehyde; it is more common in patients with impaired renal function.

Mechlorethamine

Mechlorethamine is also known as nitrogen mustard.
- **Clinical indications**: Hodgkin's disease and lymphomas
- **Dosing**: 6 mg/m^2 IV on days 1 and 8 (MOPP regimen)

Adverse events
- Bone marrow suppression
- Nausea and vomiting (severe)
- Infertility
- Secondary malignancies
- Ototoxicity
- Alopecia
- Tumor lysis syndrome
- Thrombophlebitis
- Skin ulceration (vesicant)

Melphalan
- **Clinical indications**: Multiple myeloma, hematopoietic stem cell transplantation
- **Dosing**: Oral: 0.15 mg/kg per day for 7 days every 4 weeks or 0.25 mg/kg per day for 4 days every cycle or 6 mg daily; high-dose 140–200 mg/m^2 IV once

Dose should be reduced for impaired renal function.

Adverse events
- Bone marrow suppression
- Nausea and vomiting (with high doses)
- Vasculitis
- Alopecia
- Pruritis
- Rash
- SIADH
- Mucositis (with high doses)
- Hemorrhagic cystitis
- Interstitial pneumonitis or pulmonary fibrosis
- Hypersensitivity
- Infertility
- Secondary malignancies

Aziridine analogs

Thiotepa
- **Clinical indications**: Bladder cancer, breast cancer, ovarian cancer, lymphomas, sarcomas, intrathecal use for leukemia, lymphoma, and carcinoma, hematopoietic stem cell transplantation
- **Dosing**: 0.3–0.4 mg/kg IV once every 1–4 weeks

Adverse events
- Bone marrow suppression
- Nausea and vomiting (with high doses)
- Dizziness, fever, headache
- Confusion, somnolence (with high doses)

- Rash, pruritis
- Hyperpigmentation (with high doses)
  - Mucositis (with high doses)
  - Transaminitis, hyperbilirubinemia (with high doses)
  - Hemorrhagic cystitis
  - Infertility
  - Secondary malignancies

Alkane sulfonates

Busulfan

- **Clinical indications**: Oral therapy for CML (not commonly used today); oral and IV formulations used in hematopoietic stem cell transplantation
- **Dosing**: CML chronic phase: 4–8 mg po daily (or 1.8–4 mg/m^2 po daily); maintenance therapy: 1–3 mg/day po; stem cell transplantation: 1 mg/kg po q6h x 16 doses or 0.8 mg/kg IV q6h x 16 doses or 130 mg/m2 IV daily x 4 days

Adverse events

- Bone marrow suppression
- Nausea and vomiting (with high doses)
- Seizures (with high doses)
- Hyperbilirubinemia
- Veno-occlusive disease of the liver (sinusoidal obstruction syndrome)
- Mucositis (with high doses)
- Tumor lysis syndrome
- Cataracts
- Rash
- Alopecia
- Infertility
- Secondary malignancies
- Erythema multiforme (rare)
- Fever
- Headache
- Nail discoloration
- Skin hyperpigmentation
- Pulmonary fibrosis

Additional comments

- Phenytoin (or another antiepileptic medication) should be given to prevent seizures in patients receiving high-dose therapy.
- Therapeutic drug monitoring is commonly performed in the high-dose setting; maintaining drug concentrations within a given range has been shown to reduce the complication of veno-occlusive disease of the liver (sinusoidal obstruction syndrome).
- Busulfan is a substrate of cytochrome P450 3A4; caution should be used when inducers or inhibitors of this enzyme are used concurrently.

Nitrosoureas

Nitrosoureas are highly lipophilic and therefore cross the blood-brain barrier.

Carmustine
- **Clinical indications**: Brain tumors (IV and implantable wafers), multiple myeloma, Hodgkin's disease, non-Hodgkin's lymphoma, hematopoietic stem cell transplantation
- **Dosing**: 150–200 mg/m^2 IV every 6 weeks

Adverse events
- Bone marrow suppression (delayed, cumulative)
- Nausea and vomiting (severe, dose-related)
- Alopecia
- Infertility
- Secondary malignancies
- Elevated hepatic enzymes
- Encephalopathy
- Flushing
- Hypotension (with high doses)
- Headache
- Pneumonitis or pulmonary fibrosis (cumulative, dose-related)
- Rash
- Renal failure
- Seizures (primarily with implanted wafers or high doses)
- Skin hyperpigmentation
- Mucositis
- Injection site reactions
- Hypothyroidism
- Veno-occlusive disease of the liver (sinusoidal obstruction syndrome)

Additional comments
- Cycles of carmustine (BCNU) should only be given every 6–8 weeks to allow for bone marrow recovery.
- Diluent contains absolute alcohol, which is responsible for flushing and hypotension in the high-dose setting.

Lomustine
- **Clinical indications**: Brain tumors, Hodgkin's disease, non-Hodgkin's lymphoma, melanoma, renal carcinoma, lung cancer, colon cancer
- **Dosing**: 100–130 mg/m^2 po once every 6 weeks on an empty stomach as a single agent; consider dosage reduction with renal impairment

Adverse events
- Bone marrow suppression (delayed, cumulative)
- Nausea and vomiting (severe, dose-related)
- Alopecia
- Infertility
- Secondary malignancies
- Neurotoxicity
- Mucositis
- Diarrhea
- Renal failure, interstitial nephritis
  - Hepatotoxicity
  - Pulmonary fibrosis (cumulative)
  - Elevated hepatic enzymes

Additional comments
- Cycles of lomustine (CCNU) should only be given every 6–8 weeks to allow for bone marrow recovery.
- Lomustine is a substrate of cytochrome P450 2D6 and an inhibitor of 2D6 and 3A4; use caution when concurrently administering with substrates, inhibitors, or inducers of these enzymes.

Streptozocin
- **Clinical indications**: Carcinoid, colorectal cancer, pancreatic cancer
- **Dosing**: 500 mg/m^2 per day IV as a short or continuous infusion for 5 days every 4–6 weeks or 1000 mg/m^2 IV once weekly up to 1500 mg/m^2
  - Dosage reduction is recommended with renal impairment.

Adverse events
- Bone marrow suppression (delayed, cumulative)
- Nausea and vomiting (severe, dose-related)
- Nephrotoxicity (dose-related, cumulative)
- Injection site reactions (irritant)
- Hypoglycemia or hyperglycemia
- Lethargy, confusion, depression
- Infertility
- Secondary malignancies
- Diarrhea
- Elevated hepatic enzymes
- Hyperbilirubinemia

Hydration may reduce the incidence and severity of nephrotoxicity.

Nonclassical alkylating agents

Dacarbazine
- **Clinical indications**: Metastatic malignant melanoma, osteogeneic sarcoma, soft-tissue sarcoma, Hodgkin's disease

Dosing
- **Melanoma**: 100–250 mg/m^2 IV once daily for 5 days every 3–4 weeks or 850–1000 mg/m^2 IV once on day 1 repeated every 3–4 weeks
- **Hodgkin's disease**: 375 mg/m^2 IV days 1 and 15 every 28 days (ABVD regimen)

Adverse events
- Bone marrow suppression
- Nausea and vomiting (dose-related, severe)
- Facial flushing
- Headache
- Rash
- Alopecia
- Hepatotoxicity
- Myalgia
- Fever
- Hypotension (with high doses)

- Photosensitivity
- Vein irritation
- Infertility
- Secondary malignancies

Additional comments
- Dacarbazine (DTIC) requires activation by the liver to its active form, monomethyl triazenoimidazole carboxamide (MTIC)

Procarbazine
- **Clinical indications**: Hodgkin's disease, non-Hodgkin's lymphoma, brain tumors, melanoma, lung cancer, multiple myeloma
- **Dosing**: 100 mg/m^2 per day orally on days 1–14 every 28 days (MOPP regimen); consider dose adjustment with renal or hepatic dysfunction

Adverse events
- Bone marrow suppression
- Nausea and vomiting (severe)
- Mental depression
- Hallucinations
- Dizziness, ataxia
- Headache
- Confusion
- Seizures
- Weakness
- Paresthesias
- Neuropathy
- Tremors
- Pleural effusion
- Cough
- Alopecia
- Hyperpigmentation
- Mucositis
- Nystagmus
- Infertility
- Secondary malignancies
- Disulfiram-like reactions
- Hypertensive crisis
- Orthostatic hypotension
- Pneumonitis

Additional comments
- Procarbazine has monoamine oxidase inhibitor (MAOI) activity. Foods high in tyramine must be avoided.

Temozolomide
Temozolomide is an oral prodrug that undergoes rapid nonenzymatic conversion to form the same active metabolite as dacarbazine (MTIC); activation by the liver is not required.
- **Clinical indications**: Brain tumors, malignant melanoma
- **Dosing**: 150–200 mg/m^2 per day orally for 5 days every 28 days (reduce dose if giving concurrently with radiation). Consider dose reduction with severe renal or hepatic impairment; food reduces the rate and extent of absorption.

Adverse events
- Bone marrow suppression
- Nausea and vomiting
- Peripheral edema
- Headache
- Fatigue
- Dizziness
- Neurotoxicity
- Visual disturbances
- Rash
- Allergic reactions
- Infertility
- Secondary malignancies

Additional comments
- Administer *Pneumocystis carinii* pneumonia (PCP) prophylaxis if patient is receiving temozolomide in combination with radiation therapy.

Antitumor antibiotics

Anthracyclines

Anthracyclines (doxorubicin, daunorubicin, epirubicin, and idarubicin) are closely structurally related and have similar mechanisms of action and resistance, but they have different patterns of clinical activity and toxicity.

Pharmacology

The anthracyclines have several effects, and their specific mode of action is unclear.

- Complexes with DNA by intercalating between DNA base pairs, which interferes with strand elongation; results in inhibition of DNA and RNA synthesis.
- There are direct effects at the cell surface and also on signal transduction, specifically, activation of protein kinase C-mediated cell signaling pathways. The role of these actions in mediating anthracycline cytotoxicity is undefined.
- Their ability to undergo reduction to highly reactive compounds and to generate free radicals has clinically important implications. Characteristic cardiotoxicity of anthracyclines appears to be due to generation of free radicals in the heart, where defense systems are less active.
- The major target of anthracyclines is the enzyme topoisomerase II. During cell division, topoisomerase II binds to DNA, forming a "cleavable complex" that makes transient "nicks" in DNA, allowing torsional strain in DNA to be released, after which strands rejoin. Anthracyclines bind to the cleavable complex, disrupting this process, leading to DNA strand breaks and cell death.

Drug resistance

- Some tumors are inherently resistant to anthracyclines, whereas others initially respond but later become resistant.
- The *MDR1* gene codes for a P-170 glycoprotein (Pgp) that is a naturally occurring cell-surface pump. Its physiological function appears to be a protective mechanism, expelling toxic substances from the cell. Although expression is increased in some human cancers before treatment or at relapse, attempts to manipulate Pgp have had limited success.
- A second efflux pump associated with expression of multidrug resistance-associated protein (*MRP*) gene has been implicated in anthracycline resistance in the laboratory.

Toxicity

The dose-limiting acute toxicities are as follows:

- Myelosuppression and mucositis, both occurring 5–10 days after treatment.
- Alopecia occurs but is reversible.
- Extravasation injury can be severe; dexarazoxane may result in effective treatment.

Cumulative cardiotoxicity is specific to anthracyclines and appears to be caused by accumulation of free radicals in the heart. It typically presents with heart failure, the risk of which is dose related.

At doxorubicin doses below 450 mg/m², the risk is less than 5% but increases substantially at higher doses. In most cases, this threshold allows a full course of anthracycline to be given without risk. Irradiation of the heart increases risk of cardiotoxicity, as does preexisting cardiac disease. Liposomal encapsulation of doxorubicin reduces cardiotoxicity.

Epirubicin, daunorubicin, and idarubicin have less effect on the myocardium than doxorubicin.

Doxorubicin

- **Clinical use**: Doxorubicin plays a strong role in the management of breast, lung, gastric, and ovarian cancers, Hodgkin's disease, non-Hodgkin's lymphoma, sarcoma, myeloma, acute lymphocytic leukemia, and Kaposi's sarcoma.

Dosing

- Conventional: 15–75 mg/m² per dose
- Liposomal: 20–50 mg/m² every 3–4 weeks

Adverse events

- Bone marrow suppression
- Nausea and vomiting
- Tissue necrosis (conventional formulation is a vesicant; liposomal formulation is an irritant)
- Cardiotoxicity: heart failure (cumulative); arrhythmias
- Mucositis
- Alopecia
- Radiation recall
- Nail and skin discoloration
- Urine discoloration
- Palmar-plantar erythrodysesthesia (hand–foot syndrome) (with liposomal formulation)
- Anaphylactoid reactions
- Bronchospasm (with liposomal formulation)
- Secondary malignancies
- Impaired fertility

Additional comments

- The dose should be reduced in patients with hyperbilirubinemia.
- The incidence of cardiotoxicity increases significantly once a cumulative dose of 450 mg/m² is reached (for conventional formulation). Risk factors include previous cardiovascular disease, radiation to chest, bolus administration, and age; risk is lower with liposomal formulation.
- Dexrazoxane may be given to reduce incidence of cardiotoxicity.
- Substrate of CYP2D6 and 3A4.

Daunorubicin

- **Clinical use**: Acute leukemias, Kaposi's sarcoma

Dosing

- Conventional: 30–60 mg/m² IV daily for 2–3 days
- Liposomal: 40 mg/m² IV every 2 weeks or 100–140 mg/m² IV every 3 weeks

Adverse events
- Bone marrow suppression
- Nausea and vomiting
- Tissue necrosis (conventional formulation is a vesicant; liposomal formulation is an irritant)
- Cardiotoxicity: heart failure (cumulative); arrhythmias
- Mucositis
- Alopecia
- Radiation recall
- Nail and skin discoloration
- Urine discoloration
- Anaphylactoid reactions
- Secondary malignancies
- Impaired fertility

Additional comments
- The dose should be reduced in patients with hyperbilirubinemia or severe renal impairment.
- The incidence of cardiotoxicity increases significantly once a cumulative dose of 450 mg/m^2 is reached (for conventional formulation). Risk factors include previous cardiovascular disease, radiation to the chest, bolus administration, and age; risk is lower with liposomal formulation.
- Dexrazoxane may be given to reduce the incidence of cardiotoxicity.

Epirubicin
- **Clinical use**: Breast cancer, bladder cancer, gastric cancer, lung cancer, multiple myeloma, ovarian cancer, head and neck cancer, hepatocellular cancer, soft tissue sarcoma

Dosing
- 100 mg/m^2 IV on day 1 in combination with fluorouracil and cyclophosphamide every 21 days OR
- 60 mg/m^2 IV on days 1 and 8 in combination with oral cyclophosphamide and fluorouracil every 28 days for adjuvant treatment of breast cancer
- Adjust dose for hepatic impairment
- Maximum cumulative dose of 900 mg/m^2

Adverse event
- Bone marrow suppression
- Nausea and vomiting
- Tissue necrosis (vesicant)
- Cardiotoxicity: heart failure (cumulative); arrhythmias
- Mucositis
- Alopecia
- Radiation recall
- Nail and skin discoloration
- Urine discoloration
- Anaphylactoid reactions
- Secondary malignancies
- Impaired fertility

Additional comments
- The dose should be reduced in patients with hyperbilirubinemia or severe renal impairment.
- The incidence of cardiotoxicity increases significantly once a cumulative dose of 900 mg/m^2 is reached. Risk factors include previous cardiovascular disease, radiation to the chest, bolus administration, and age.
- Dexrazoxane may be given to reduce the incidence of cardiotoxicity.

Idarubicin
- **Clinical use**: Acute myelogenous leukemia (AML), acute lymphoblastic leukemia (ALL), chronic myelogenous leukemia (CML), myelodysplastic syndrome (MDS), breast cancer, non-Hodgkin's lymphoma (NHL)
- **Dosing**: 8–12 mg/m^2 IV once daily for 3 days in combination with cytarabine for AML

Adverse events
- Bone marrow suppression
- Nausea and vomiting
- Tissue necrosis (vesicant)
- Cardiotoxicity: heart failure (cumulative); arrhythmias
- Mucositis
- Alopecia
- Radiation recall
- Nail and skin discoloration
- Urine discoloration
- Secondary malignancies
- Impaired fertility

The dose should be reduced in patients with hyperbilirubinemia or severe renal impairment.

Mitoxantrone
Mitoxantrone is a synthetic anthracycline derivative called an anthracenedione. It exhibits less cardiotoxicity than that of classic anthracyclines and is not generally considered to be a vesicant. Mitoxantrone does not form oxygen free radicals, which is a feature that distinguishes this agent from traditional anthracyclines.
- **Clinical indications**: Acute myelogenous leukemia, prostate cancer, multiple sclerosis, other leukemias and lymphomas
- **Dosing**: 12 mg/m^2 IV daily for 3 days in combination with cytarabine (for AML); reduce dose for hyperbilirubinemia

Adverse events
- Bone marrow suppression
- Nausea and vomiting
- Cardiotoxicity: heart failure (cumulative); arrhythmias
- Mucositis
- Alopecia
- Radiation recall
- Nail and skin discoloration

- Injection site reactions, tissue necrosis
- Anaphylactoid reactions
- Urine discoloration
- Conjunctivitis
- Secondary malignancies
- Impaired fertility

Additional comments

- This agent binds to DNA and interacts with topoisomerase II but appears less potent in generating free radicals. It is also a substrate for Pgp.
- The main clinical use of mitoxantrone has been as an alternative to doxorubicin in advanced breast cancer, because it is substantially less cardiotoxic and less vesicant, and causes less alopecia.
- However, mitoxantrone is less effective than doxorubicin. It has some activity against other solid tumors, including non-Hodgkin's lymphoma and nonlymphocytic leukemia.

Dactinomycin (actinomycin D)

- **Clinical use**: Testicular cancer, melanoma, choriocarcinoma, Wilm's tumor, neuroblastoma, retinoblastoma, sarcomas
- **Dosing**: 500 µg IV daily for a maximum of 5 days (should not exceed 15 µg/kg per day or 400–600 µg/m^2 per day for 5 days in adults)

Adverse events

- Bone marrow suppression
- Nausea and vomiting (severe)
- Fatigue, malaise, fever
- Mucositis
- Hepatotoxicity
- Hypocalcemia
- Alopecia
- Radiation recall
- Tissue necrosis (vesicant)
- Anaphylactoid reactions
- Secondary malignancies
- Impaired fertility

Additional comments

- Actinomycin D binds strongly to DNA by intercalation and inhibits synthesis of RNA and proteins. It also appears to be a substrate for the Pgp pump. It is especially active against childhood tumors.

Mitomycin C

Mitomycin acts as an alkylating agent and has properties similar to other antitumor antibiotics

- **Clinical use**: Adenocarcinoma of the stomach or pancreas, bladder cancer, colorectal cancer, and as a radiation sensitizer
- **Dosing**: 10 mg/m^2 IV (combination therapy) or 20 mg/m^2 IV (single-agent therapy) every 6–8 weeks. Adjust dose in renal impairment; may be administered intravesicularly for bladder cancer

Adverse events
- Bone marrow suppression (delayed and cumulative)
- Nausea and vomiting
- Tissue necrosis (vesicant)
- Cardiotoxicity: heart failure (higher doses)
- Fever
- Mucositis
- Alopecia
- Radiation recall
- Nail banding and discoloration
- Paresthesias
- Interstitial pneumonitis
- Secondary malignancies
- Impaired fertility
- Hemolytic-uremic syndrome (rare)
- Renal failure (rare)

Additional comments
- Mitomycin C (MMC) is active against a range of solid tumors but is also used as a radiosensitizer in chemoirradiation.
- Mitomycin C is used in combination with other cytotoxics to treat breast cancer, non-small–cell lung cancer, and GI cancer.
- It is used as a radiosensitizer in the treatment of anal cancer.
- The most important toxicity of mitomycin C is myelosuppression, especially thrombocytopenia, which is delayed and can be cumulative. Accordingly, it is given systemically every 6 weeks, in contrast to the 3-weekly schedules usually used for other antitumor antibiotics.
- Hemolytic-uremic syndrome, pulmonary fibrosis, and cardiac complications are all uncommon side effects.

Antimetabolites

In general, antimetabolites mimic naturally occurring substrates and thus interfere with nucleic acid activity. Available antimetabolites vary in their specific mechanisms of action; however, classic antimetabolites are cell cycle phase-specific and inhibit DNA and/or RNA synthesis.

Some antimetabolites are incorporated into DNA and others may inhibit key enzymes important for DNA synthesis. Some examples are included in Figure 9.1. Fluorouracil and floxuridine inhibit thymidylate synthase whereas methotrexate inhibits dihydrofolate reductase. Pemetrexed is an inhibitor of both of these enzymes, in addition to other key enzymes involved in folate metabolism.

Antifolates

- Understanding antimetabolite action necessitates knowledge of folate biochemistry.
- The enzyme thymidylate synthase (TS) acts as rate-limiting step in the synthesis of thymidylate, converting dUMP into dTTP by transferring a methyl group from CH_2 to FH_4.
- The supply of reduced folate is maintained by the enzyme dihydrofolate reductase (DHFR).

Methotrexate (MTX)

Clinical indications

- Breast cancer, osteogenic sarcoma, GI cancers, choriocarcinoma, leukemias and lymphomas, and prevention of graft-versus-host disease, and for its immunosuppressive effects in various autoimmune disorders

Dosing

- The total dose per cycle ranges from a low dose (<100 mg/m^2) up to 10,000 mg/m^2 typically infused over 4–24 hours.
- The dose must be reduced for renal insufficiency.
- Consider dosage reduction for severe hepatic impairment.
- May be given intrathecally (usual adult dose 10–12 mg)

Adverse events

- Bone marrow suppression
- Mucositis
- Nausea and vomiting
- Nephrotoxicity
- Hepatotoxicity
- Encephalopathy (with high doses)
- Myelopathy
- Interstitial pneumonitis
- Pulmonary fibrosis
- Teratogenesis
- Impaired fertility
- Alopecia
- Dermatologic toxicity
- Ocular toxicity

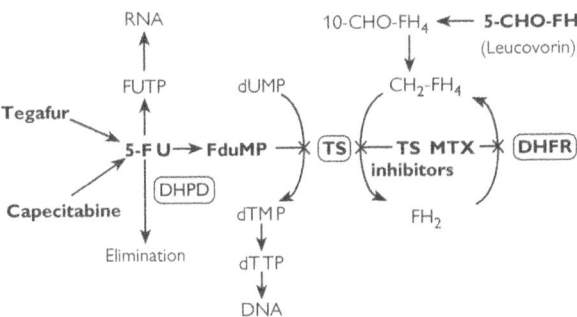

- MTX   Cytotoxics (MTX, methotrexate; 5, FU -5-fluorouracil; TS inhibitors include ralitrexed)
- dTTP   Normal metabolites
- ⟶✗   Indicates enzyme inhibition
- (DHPD) Enzyme (TS, thymidylate synthase; DHPD, dihydropyrimidine dehydrogenase; DHFR, dihydrofolate reductase)

Figure 9.1 Main sites of action of antimetabolites.

- Tumor lysis syndrome
- Rhythm disturbances
- Arachnoiditis (more likely with intrathecal administration)

Additional comments

- Methotrexate (MTX) distributes into third spaces; strong consideration should be given to draining identified effusions before the administration of methotrexate.
- Leucovorin must be given with "high-dose" methotrexate to effectively rescue normal cells from related toxicity.
- Toxicity of high-dose methotrexate can also be minimized by aggressively hydrating the patient and by alkalinizing the urine to promote excretion of the drug.
- Serum concentrations of methotrexate should be monitored until the drug has been cleared from the body.
- Widely used in many cancers, methotrexate is frequently used in breast cancer, osteogenic sarcoma, GI cancers, and choriocarcinoma.

Pharmacology

- MTX is well absorbed orally below 25 mg/m^2, but it is usually administered IV, except in maintenance regimens and treatment of benign connective tissue diseases.

- There is some hepatic metabolism to the active drug 7-OH-MTX, and approximately 10% of the drug is cleared by biliary excretion.
- Dose adjustments are not usually necessary with hepatic dysfunction.
- Significant third-space effects occur in the presence of fluid collections (e.g., ascites, pleural effusions) and can increase toxicity through reduced clearance.
- MTX excretion can also be inhibited by probenicid, penicillins (and cephalosporins), and nonsteroidal anti-inflammatory drugs (NSAIDs).
- Common toxicities include mucositis, myelosuppression, and nephrotoxicity.

Pemetrexed

Clinical indications
- Lung cancer and mesothelioma, bladder cancer, breast cancer, colorectal cancer, gastric cancer, head and neck cancer, pancreatic cancer, renal cell cancer

Dosing
- Mesothelioma: 500 mg/m^2 IV on day 1 of a 21-day cycle (in combination with cisplatin)
- Non-small–cell lung cancer: 500 mg/m^2 IV on day 1 of each 21-day cycle (single agent).
- Other regimens for lung cancer and other malignancies have been studied.
- Do not administer if CrCl <45 mL/min.

Adverse events
- Bone marrow suppression
- Nausea and vomiting
- Diarrhea
- Mucositis
- Elevated hepatic enzymes
- Nephrotoxicity
- Rash
- Neuropathy
- Dyspnea
- Anaphylactoid reactions

Additional comments
- Measures should be used to reduce toxicity associated with pemetrexed.
- Patients should receive folic acid 400 µg daily for at least 5 days before initiating pemetrexed and continuing for 21 days after completion of the final dose of pemetrexed.
- Vitamin B$_{12}$ 1000 µg IM should be given before initiating pemetrexed therapy and every three cycles thereafter.
- Dexamethasone 4 mg twice daily for three days should be considered beginning the day before each dose of pemetrexed to decrease skin reactions.
- Do not give pemetrexed if CrCl is <45 mL/min.
- Can give leucovorin rescue for severe or prolonged myelosuppression and/or mucositis.

Thymidylate synthase inhibitors
- New agents have been developed that directly inhibit thymidylate synthase (TS) (in contrast to indirect inhibitors, e.g., 5-fluorouracil [5-FU] and MTX) and interact with the folate-binding site of TS.
- Raltitrexed (Tomudex) causes prolonged inhibition of TS by enhanced retention in cells due to polyglutamation of the parent molecule.
- After IV administration it has triphasic elimination, with a rapid initial fall in concentration but very prolonged final phase.
- 50% of the drug is renally excreted unchanged. It is active in breast and colorectal cancer with toxicities including myelosuppression, diarrhea, and transaminitis.

Fluoropyrimidines
These prodrugs are intracellularly activated and their products inhibit pyrimidine synthesis.

5-Fluorouracil
- **Clinical indications**: Actinic keratosis, basal cell carcinoma, breast cancer, cervical cancer, colorectal cancer, gastric cancer, head and neck cancer, hepatocellular cancer, ovarian cancer, pancreatic cancer

Dosing
- 300–500 mg/m^2 IV bolus daily for 4–5 days every 28 days or 600–1500 mg/m^2 IV bolus once weekly or every other week
- 300–1000 mg/m^2 per day continuous IV infusion for 4–5 days every 28 days or 300 mg/m^2 per day continuous IV infusion indefinitely
- Numerous dosing schedules are used
- Consider dosage reduction with significant hepatic impairment

Adverse events
- Bone marrow suppression (dose-limiting with bolus injection or high-dose continuous infusion)
- Neurotoxicity or cerebellar toxicity (dose-limiting with high-dose continuous infusion)
- Diarrhea
- Mucositis
- Nausea and vomiting (mild)
- Palmar–plantar erythrodysesthesia
- Cardiotoxicity (angina, myocardial infarction)
- Ocular irritation
- Injection-site reactions
- Skin hyperpigmentation
- Photosensitivity
- Rash

Additional comments
- Do not use in patients with dihydropyrimidine dehydrogenase deficiency (severe toxicity will result from the inability to metabolize fluorouracil).
- Concurrent leucovorin administration may increase efficacy and toxicity.

- This is a widely prescribed agent with particular activity in breast cancer, GI cancers, and head and neck tumors.
- 5-FU is metabolized to FdUMP, which, in the presence of CH_2-FH_4, forms a stable complex inhibiting TS. It also inhibits RNA synthesis and pre-ribosomal RNA processing.

Pharmacology
- 5-FU is given IV both as a bolus and as a prolonged infusion. It has a short initial half-life, with significant hepatic, renal, and lung clearance. Active metabolites (e.g., 5dUMP and FUTP) have variable pharmacokinetics.
- Toxicities of 5-FU include myelosuppression and, particularly with longer administration schedules, stomatitis and diarrhea.
- Prolonged infusion overcomes the initial rapid clearance, resulting in differing toxicities with minimal bone marrow effects. Instead, cutaneous toxicity known as hand-foot syndrome occurs.
- Neurotoxicity and cardiotoxicity may also occur.

5-Fluorouracil prodrugs

Capecitabine
Capecitabine is an oral prodrug of fluorouracil. When administered twice daily, it somewhat mimics continuous IV infusion of fluorouracil.
- **Clinical indications**: Colorectal cancer and breast cancer
- **Dosing**: 2500 mg/m^2 per day in 2 divided doses with food for 14 days followed by 7 days of rest (repeat every 21 days)

The dose must be reduced for renal impairment (25% dose reduction for CrCl 30–50 mL/min; do not use if CrCl <30 mL/min).

Adverse events
- Myelosuppression including lymphopenia
- Diarrhea
- Mucositis
- Nausea and vomiting
- Palmar-plantar erythrodysesthesia
- Dermatitis
- Hyperbilirubinemia
- Paresthesia
- Eye irritation
- Dyspnea
- Venous thrombosis
- Headache
- Edema
- Fatigue
- Fever
- Angina
- Photosensitivity
- Radiation recall

Additional comments
- This is an orally active prodrug of 5-FU.
- It is preferentially activated in tumor and liver tissue and has the potential to replace prolonged or continuous-infusion 5-FU.
- It has been shown to be active in a wide range of cancers and is licensed for breast and colorectal cancer.

2-Fluoro-2'-deoxyuridine (floxuridine)

- **Clinical indications**: Used almost exclusively for hepatic artery infusion for colon cancer metastatic to the liver.
- **Dosing**: 0.1–0.6 mg/kg per day as a continuous intra-arterial infusion into the hepatic artery. Consider dose reduction with significant renal or hepatic impairment.

Adverse events
- Hepatotoxicity
- Cholangitis
- Bone marrow suppression
- Peptic ulcer disease
- Acute cerebellar syndrome
- Confusion, drowsiness
- Nystagmus, seizures, ataxia
- Alopecia
- Diarrhea
- Mucositis
- Rash
- Photosensitivity
- Skin hyperpigmentation
- Nausea and vomiting

Additional comments
- Given IV, this agent can be metabolized both into 5-FU and directly into FdUMP, theoretically giving increased efficacy.
- Its clinical use has largely been confined to hepatic artery infusion because it is less toxic than single-agent 5-FU used by this route for treating colon cancer.

Modulation of 5-Fluorouracil

- A number of agents have been combined with 5-FU to increase either its efficacy or therapeutic index.
- 5-FU and folinic acid combinations are the mainstay of treatment of colon cancer.
- Folinic acid is given by infusion, before or concomitant with 5-FU.
- By increasing the supply of CH_2-FH_4, folinic acid potentiates interaction between 5-FU and TS.
- Although more toxic, it has a higher response rate in advanced colorectal cancer with combined treatment than single-agent 5-FU.

Antipurines

Purine analogs

Purine analogs are widely used to treat leukemias and as immunosuppressives (azathioprine) and antivirals (acyclovir, gancyclovir).

6-Mercaptopurine (6-MP) and 6-thioguanine (6-TG) both inhibit de novo purine synthesis, and their nucleotide products are incorporated into DNA. Hypoxanthine guanine phosphoribosyl transferase (HGPRT) produces monophosphates that inhibit early stages of purine synthesis and then convert into triphosphates that are incorporated into DNA, causing strand breaks.

There are synergistic effects with MTX, due to 5-phosphoribosylpyrophosphate (PRPP) buildup, facilitating phosphorylation by HGPRT. Resistance develops due to HGPRT deficiency and reduced substrate affinity. Variable oral bioavailability may contribute to some treatment failures in childhood ALL.

Both drugs have a short half-life and are primarily metabolized. The important difference is that 6-MP is a substrate for xanthine oxidase, and dose alterations are necessary when coadministered with allopurinol. There is poor cerebrospinal fluid (CSF) penetration, but otherwise these agents are widely distributed.

The main toxicity is myelosuppression, but 6-MP can also cause hepatotoxicity. Nausea, vomiting, and mucositis can also occur, more commonly with 6-MP.

The most common indication is hematological malignancy: 6-MP is used for maintenance therapy of ALL, and 6-TG is used for both remission induction and maintenance in AML.

Cytarabine

Cytarabine is triphosphorylated and subsequently incorporated into DNA, which results in the inhibition of DNA synthesis.

Clinical indications

- Acute myelogenous leukemia, acute lymphocytic leukemia, carcinomatous meningitis, chronic myelogenous leukemia, Hodgkin's disease, non-Hodgkin's lymphoma

Dosing

- AML induction (usually in combination with daunorubicin or idarubicin): 100–200 mg/m^2 per day as a continuous infusion over 7 days
- AML induction (high-dose): 1000–3000 mg/m^2 IV twice daily for 8–12 doses
- Reduce dose for renal insufficiency
- Liposomal cytarabine (for intrathecal [IT] administration): 50 mg IT every 14 days on weeks 1, 3, 5, 7, 9 and then at week 13, then every 28 days on weeks 17, 21, 25, and 29
  - Administer dexamethasone 4 mg po/IV twice daily for 5 days beginning on the day of each administration.
  - If drug-induced neurotoxicity develops, decrease the dose to 25 mg.

Adverse events
- Bone marrow suppression
- Nausea and vomiting (dose-related)
- Mucositis
- Fever
- Hepatotoxicity
- Rash
- Palmar–plantar erythrodysesthesia
- Cerebellar toxicity (high doses)
- Chemical conjunctivitis (high doses)
- Respiratory distress
- Anaphylactoid reactions
- Peripheral neuropathy
- CNS toxicity (including arachnoiditis) with intrathecal therapy
- Tumor lysis syndrome

Additional comments
- Ara-C is actively transported, and its metabolite Ara-CTP is incorporated into DNA, inhibiting DNA polymerases and possibly phospholipid synthesis.
- Unlike gemcitabine, no further normal nucleotides are added, so that damaged DNA is susceptible to DNA repair.
- Ara-C is active in NHL and AML, but not in solid tumors.
- There is renal excretion of deaminated compound; because of rapid clearance, better activity is observed when Ara-C is given by continuous infusion.
- Side effects are emesis, alopecia, and myelosuppression.
- It can cause "Ara-C syndrome" with fevers, myalgias, rash, keratoconjunctivitis, and arthralgias. Rarely, lung and pancreatic damage occur.

Gemcitabine

Gemcitabine (difluorodeoxycytidine) is closely related to cytarabine; however, the spectrum of activity is significantly different. Gemcitabine is triphosphorylated and subsequently incorporated into DNA. An additional base pair is added after insertion of the analog into DNA, which inhibits DNA replication and repair. This is termed "masked termination." Ultimately, sensitive tumor cells exposed to gemcitabine undergo apoptosis.

Gemcitabine has self-potentiating effects, resulting in increased intracellular concentrations and prolonged intracellular retention.

Clinical indications
- Breast cancer, lung cancer, ovarian cancer, pancreatic cancer, bladder cancer, mesothelioma

Dosing
- Lung cancer (in combination with cisplatin): 1000 mg/m^2 IV on days 1, 8, 15 of a 28-day cycle, or 1250 mg/m^2 IV on days 1 and 8 of a 21-day cycle
- Lung cancer (in combination with paclitaxel): 1000 mg/m^2 IV on days 1 and 8 of a 21-day cycle

- Pancreatic cancer: 1000 mg/m² IV once weekly for up to 7 consecutive weeks followed by 1 week of rest then weekly for 3 weeks followed by 1 week of rest for subsequent cycles
- Additional regimens exist for breast and ovarian cancer

Adverse events
- Bone marrow suppression
- Fever
- Rash
- Alopecia
- Anaphylactoid reactions
- Injection-site reactions (irritant)
- Nausea and vomiting
- Diarrhea
- Mucositis
- Elevated hepatic enzymes
- Hyperbilirubinemia
- Hemolytic uremic syndrome
- Renal failure
- Dyspnea
- Pulmonary toxicity (rare)
- Radiation recall

Additional comments
- This fluorinated analog has better membrane permeation and affinity for deoxycytidine kinase than Ara-C.
- Intracellular retention is prolonged, partly due to a unique self-potentiation in which the bi- and triphosphates facilitate the phosphorylation of the parent compound, as well as inhibiting its catabolism.
- Active metabolite dF-CTP is incorporated into DNA, followed only by one more normal nucleotide, resulting in protection of the DNA from repair enzymes (masked termination).
- It is probably the saturable formation of dF-CTP that contributes to the clinical schedule dependency of gemcitabine, usually given IV, weekly for 3 weeks out of 4.
- Toxicities include flu-like symptoms, transaminitis, peripheral edema, myelosuppression, and possible nephrotoxicity.
- There is some evidence for synergy with cisplatin, the extent of which appears to be schedule-dependent. Gemcitabine is active in pancreatic cancer as well as in lung, breast, and bladder cancer.

Nelarabine

Nelarabine is a prodrug of 9-β-D-arabinofuranosyl guanine (Ara-G). Nelarabine undergoes intracellular phosphorylation to the active form Ara-GTP, which is toxic to T lymphocytes. The active form is incorporated into DNA, which results in inhibition of DNA synthesis and cell death. Ara-G also inhibits RNA synthesis and ribonucleotide reductase. Its mechanism of action is similar to that of other purine analogs such as cladribine, fludarabine, and pentostatin.

Clinical indications
- T-cell leukemia/lymphoma and chronic lymphocytic leukemia

Dosing
- **Adults**: 1500 mg/m^2 IV over 2 hours on days 1, 3, and 5 repeated every 21 days
- **Children**: 650 mg/m^2 IV over 1 hour daily for 5 days repeated every 21 days

Adverse events
- Neurotoxicity (dose-limiting, may be irreversible)
- Bone marrow suppression
- Nausea and vomiting
- Diarrhea
- Elevated hepatic enzymes
- Hyperbilirubinemia
- Tumor lysis syndrome
- Hypotension, sinus tachycardia, chest pain
- Cough, dyspnea, pleural effusion, wheezing
- Fatigue
- Fever
- Peripheral edema
- Mucositis

Additional comments
- Discontinue therapy in patients that develop grade 2 or higher neurotoxicity.
- Closely monitor patients with renal or hepatic impairment; dosage adjustments may be warranted with severe impairment, although specific recommendations are not available.

Adenosine analogs
- Three adenosine analogs have come into clinical practice, active in low-grade NHL, Waldenström's macroglobulinemia, and CLL.
- All have similar effects and interact with enzyme adenosine deaminase (ADA), a deficiency of which causes severe combined immunodeficiency.
- Toxicity includes myelosuppression with particular effects on lymphocytes, including depression of CD3 and CD4 levels, and reduced natural killer (NK) activity.

Cladribine
Cladribine (2-chlorodexocyadenosine; 2-CdA) is a synthetic purine analog that is resistant to the effects of ADA. It is phosphorylated intracellularly to its active form, which is toxic primarily against lymphocytes. It also has activity against myeloid malignancies.

Cladribine is incorporated into DNA and interferes with DNA synthesis. It also inhibits DNA polymerase, DNA ligase, and ribonucleotide reductase. Cladribine affects both resting and proliferating lymphocytes.

- **Clinical indications**: Hairy cell leukemia, other leukemias and lymphomas, hematopoietic stem cell transplantation
- **Dosing**: 0.09–0.1 mg/kg per day as a continuous IV infusion for 7 days; alternative bolus regimens also exist

Adverse events
- Bone marrow suppression
- Immunosuppression
- Fever
- Opportunistic infections
- Rash
- Nausea
- Neurotoxicity (dose-related)
- Nephrotoxicity (dose-related)
- Tumor lysis syndrome

Additional comments
- Consider prophylaxis against opportunistic infections.

Fludarabine

Fludarabine is a synthetic purine analog with a mechanism of action similar to that of cladribine. Its spectrum of activity is comparable.

Clinical indications
- Chronic lymphocytic leukemia, non-Hodgkin's lymphoma, other leukemias and lymphomas, hematopoietic stem cell transplantation

Dosing
- 25 mg/m^2 IV daily for 5 days repeated every 28 days as a single agent; alternative combination regimens exist

Dosage adjustments are recommended in patients with renal impairment:
- CrCl >70 mL/min: No adjustment required
- CrCl 30–70 mL/min: Reduce dose by 20%
- CrCl <30 mL/min: Do not administer

Adverse events
- Bone marrow suppression
- Immunosuppression
- Opportunistic infections
- Edema
- Nausea
- Neurotoxicity (dose-related)
- Nephrotoxicity (dose-related)
- Tumor lysis syndrome
- Autoimmune hemolytic leukemia
- Idiopathic thrombocytopenic purpura
- Interstitial pneumonitis

Additional comments
- Consider prophylaxis against opportunistic infections.
- Resistant to ADA, it is particularly useful in treating CLL.

- It is actively transported into the cells and its mode of action is a consequence of phosphorylation, following which it is incorporated into DNA and probably RNA, and may even cause topoisomerase II inhibition. It can cause hemolytic anemia.

Pentostatin

Pentostatin (2'-deoxycoformycin) is an inhibitor of adenosine deaminase. This inhibition results in the intracellular accumulation of deoxyadenosine triphosphate, which results in apoptosis of lymphocytes. The mechanism of action is similar to that of cladribine and fludarabine.

Clinical indications
- Hairy cell leukemia, other leukemias and lymphoma, hematopoietic stem cell transplantation, graft-versus-host disease

Dosing
- 4 mg/m^2 IV once every other week as a single agent; alternative regimens exist

The dose should be reduced for renal impairment:
- CrCl ≥60 mL/min: No dosage adjustment
- CrCl 30–60 mL/min: Reduce dose 50%
- CrCl <30 mL/min: Do not administer

Adverse events
- Bone marrow suppression
- Immunosuppression
- Opportunistic infections
- Nausea and vomiting
- Rash
- Neurotoxicity (dose-related)
- Nephrotoxicity (dose-related)
- Pulmonary toxicity
- Tumor lysis syndrome
- Anorexia and diarrhea
- Thrombotic thrombocytopenic purpura, hemolytic uremic syndrome

Additional comments
- Consider prophylaxis against opportunistic infections.
- It has a very high affinity for ADA, and the resultant complex is stable for over 24 hours, resulting in enzyme inhibition.
- Its major indication is treatment of hairy-cell leukemia.
- Actively transported into cells, it is phosphorylated and incorporated into DNA and also produces inhibitory dATP.
- It inhibits both DNA synthesis and DNA repair.

Clofarabine

Clofarabine is a purine analog with a mechanism of action similar to that of cladribine, fludarabine, and pentostatin.

Clinical indications
- Acute lymphocytic leukemia

Dosing
- Children: 52 mg/m^2 (up to 70 mg/m^2) IV over 2 hours daily for 5 days
- Adults: 40 mg/m^2 IV over 2 hours daily for 5 days

Adverse events
- Bone marrow suppression
- Immunosuppression
- Opportunistic infections
- Nausea and vomiting
- Dehydration
- Hypotension
- Diarrhea
- Elevated hepatic enzymes
- Hyperbilirubinemia
- Nephrotoxicity
- Edema
- Tachycardia
- Pericardial effusions
- Left ventricular systolic dysfunction
- Impaired fertility
- Capillary leak syndrome
- Respiratory distress
- Fever
- Mucositis

Additional comments
- Consider prophylaxis against opportunistic infections
- Consider prophylactic corticosteroids (hydrocortisone 100 mg/m^2 on days 1–3) to prevent signs and symptoms of systemic inflammatory response syndrome (SIRS) or capillary leak

Hydroxyurea

Clinical indications
- Myeloproliferative disorders, hyperleukocytosis with acute leukemias, use as a radiosensitizing agent, sickle cell anemia

Dosing
- 10–20 mg/kg per day initially by mouth; titrate to desired effect; consider dosage reductions in renal impairment

Adverse events
- Bone marrow suppression
- Edema
- CNS toxicity (dose-related)
- Erythema, rash, hyperpigmentation
- Tumor lysis syndrome
- Nausea and vomiting
- Mucositis
- Hepatotoxicity
- Weakness
- Peripheral neuropathy
- Pulmonary toxicity (rare)

Additional comments
- This oral agent inhibits ribonucleotide reductase, which reduces availability of all deoxynucleotides.
- It crosses the blood-brain barrier and is used in myeloproliferative disorders.
- Toxicities are myelosuppression, gastrointestinal toxicities, and sometimes hyperpigmentation of the skin.

Cisplatin and derivatives

Cisplatin is one of the most active anticancer drugs in clinical use with a very wide spectrum of antitumor activity. In view of its considerable toxicity profile, many attempts have been made to develop analogs with less toxicity, increased efficacy, or both.

Cisplatin

Mechanism of action
- Cisplatin binds directly to DNA, inhibiting synthesis by altering the DNA template via formation of intrastrand and interstrand cross-links.
- These cross-links are generated by an aquated complex that acts as a bifunctional alkylating agent.
- Cytotoxic effects of cisplatin are cell-cycle independent, and synergy between cisplatin and antimetabolites has been demonstrated both in vitro and in clinical trials.
- The mechanism behind this synergy has not been fully explained; the most commonly held hypothesis is that this is due to a malfunction in DNA repair processing.

Clinical indications
- Cisplatin was a major step forward in treatment of testicular cancer.
- In patients with metastatic disease, cisplatin-based combination therapy results in a complete clinical response in over 80% of patients, with the majority of these achieving long-term cure.
- Cisplatin is also a major component of treatment of ovarian cancer, genitourinary tumors, head and neck cancer, small-cell lung cancer, and non-small–cell lung cancer.
- Combinations of cisplatin with other cytotoxic agents are common and are used in a variety of human solid cancers and pediatric tumors.

Dosage
- Cisplatin is used in a variety of dosage schedules.
- The standard dose limit is 100 mg/m^2 as a single daily dose; higher doses have been explored in clinical trials, particularly in conjunction with neuroprotective agents.
- Alternate schedules such as five daily injections of 20 mg/m^2 are commonly used in the treatment of testicular and head and neck cancer.
- The initial clearance of cisplatin is rapid, followed by a much slower decline due to binding to plasma proteins.
- Clearance is prolonged in patients with renal insufficiency. Unlike carboplatin, there is no clear evidence of a pharmodyamic-pharmacokinetic relationship with cisplatin. Therefore, dosage is usually based on empirical body-surface calculations.

Side effects
- Nausea, vomiting: Doses ≥50 mg/m^2 cisplatin are highly emetogenic and cause significant delayed nausea and vomiting.

- Triple-drug regimens including steroids, serotonin antagonists, and NK-1 antagonists should be used; doses ≤50 mg/m^2 are considered moderately emetogenic with associated delayed nausea and vomiting.
- Antiemetic regimens for doses of moderate emetogenicty should include steroids and serotonin antagonists with NK-1 antagonists considered for patients with additional risk factors.
- Dose-dependent nephrotoxicity: All patients require adequate hydration before, during, and after administration.
- Electrolyte abnormalities: Hypokalemia and hypomagnesimia.
- Peripheral neuropathy is dose and duration dependent.
- Ototoxicity is manifested as tinnitus and high-tone deafness.
- Myelosuppression: Mild to moderate neutropenia and thrombocytopenia, greater propensity to cause anemia.
- Anaphylaxis rarely occurs.

Carboplatin

- Several analogs have been subject to clinical trials, but only carboplatin has emerged as a viable clinical candidate to use in patients instead of cisplatin.
- There is still a degree of controversy regarding the clinical equivalence of cisplatin and carboplatin. In limited situations such as with germ cell tumors, cisplatin still seems to be the agent of choice.
- However, in most other circumstances, carboplatin has supplanted the use of cisplatin.

Clinical indications

- Carboplatin can be regarded as a less toxic substitute for cisplatin and is used for similar indications.
- Patients resistant to cisplatin will also be resistant to carboplatin.
- However, the increased thrombocytopenia seen with carboplatin may be a disadvantage in some combinations, whereas reduced nonhematological toxicities may be an advantage in others.
- Furthermore, a low level of nonhematological toxicity makes carboplatin suitable for inclusion in high-dose regimens with bone marrow or stem cell rescue.

Dosage

- Initially, a dosage of carboplatin based on body-surface area resulted in a variable degree of thrombocytopenia, with several patients requiring platelet transfusion.
- Pharmacokinetically based dosing is now the adopted standard.
- The simple pharmacokinetics of carboplatin, with clearance being dependent almost exclusively on renal mechanisms, allows a dosing formula to be derived.
- The dose required to achieve a specific AUC (area under the curve) can be calculated for an individual patient.
- The most widely used formula is

    Dose = Desired AUC (GFR + 25)

where Dose is the total dose in milligrams to be given to the patient.

- Desired AUC is in mg/mL per mm. Typical AUCs are between 2 and 7, depending on the frequency of administration, previous treatment, and the drugs being used in combination.
- GFR is the glomerular filtration rate of the patient (mL/min), unadjusted for surface area (ideally measured by an isotope method such as $_{51}$CrEDTA clearance, but a carefully performed 24-hour urinary creatinine clearance is also acceptable).

Side effects
- Myelosuppression: dose limiting
- Thrombocytopenia: nadir at approximately day 14
- Leukopenia: nadir at approximately day 14
- Nausea and vomiting: moderate
- Nephrotoxicity: minimal to mild
- Neurotoxicity: minimal to mild
- Ototoxicity: mild
- Alopecia: absent to mild
- Anaphylaxis occurs rarely

Pharmacokinetic interactions with carboplatin
- Unlike cisplatin, carboplatin does not affect hepatic cytochrome P450 enzyme, and pharmacokinetic interactions with other drugs seem to be rare.

Summary
- Carboplatin has major advantages over cisplatin in terms of ease of administration and nonhematological toxicities, although the higher incidence of thrombocytopenia may be a problem in some circumstances.
- In treatment of many malignancies it can be regarded as an alternative to cisplatin, but current data suggest that cisplatin should still be used for treating testicular teratoma.
- Unlike cisplatin, carboplatin can be used in high-dose regimens. Carboplatin should generally be dosed on a pharmacokinetic basis.

Oxaliplatin
- Oxaliplatin is a platinum analog that differs from carboplatin and cisplatin in both chemical behavior and possibly its mechanism of action.
- In vitro oxaliplatin has a broad spectrum of activity, with marked differences from the spectrum seen with cisplatin or carboplatin.

Clinical indications
- It has become an established agent in the management of colorectal cancer following trials showing benefits in both the adjuvant and metastatic disease settings.
- Its wide utility is now being explored in the setting of many other solid tumor types.

Dosage

Two commonly used regimens exist:
- 85 mg/m^2 every 2 weeks as a 2- to 6-hour infusion
- 130 mg/m^2 over a similar length of time repeated every 3 weeks

However, a multitude of studies exist using a variety of different dosing regimens, including chronomodulated infusion together with 5-fluorouracil.

Side effects
- Neuropathy: dose limiting
- **Acute** effects are usually seen within the first 2 days, as paresthesias, dysesthesia, and hypoesthesia in the extremities, perioral area, or throat. They are exacerbated by cold temperatures and are usually reversible.
- **Chronic** effects are cumulative, persistent symptoms similar to those of acute effects but also include deficits in proprioception that interfere with activities of daily living.
  - Myelosuppression
  - Nausea and vomiting are moderate
  - Anaphylaxis rarely occurs

Topoisomerase inhibitors

Topoisomerase enzymes are a family of nuclear proteins with essential functions in regulating the topology of the DNA helix.

Eukaryotics have two forms of topoisomerase enzyme.
- Topoisomerase I (topo I) binds to double-stranded DNA and cleaves and relegates 1 strand of duplex DNA. Relaxation of supercoiled DNA is then used during processes of replication, transcription, and recombination.
- Topoisomerase II (topo II) creates transient double-stranded breakage of DNA, allowing subsequent passage of a second intact DNA duplex through the break.

Topoisomerase I inhibitors

Campothecin has been identified as the active constituent of an extract isolated from the Chinese tree, *Camptotheca acuminata*.

Currently, two CPT analogs have received regulatory approval for use in patients with solid tumors.

Irinotecan

Mechanism of action
- Mechanism-of-action studies demonstrated that irinotecan and its active metabolite, SN-38, stabilized covalent adducts between genomic DNA and topo I, resulting in single-strand DNA breaks.
- In addition, double-strand DNA breaks occur when a DNA replication fork encounters the irinotecan or SN-38–topoisomerase I complex.

Clinical indications
- Irinotecan is approved by the U.S. Food and Drug Administration (FDA) for the treatment of metastatic colorectal cancer.
- It is also used in treating small-cell lung cancer, malignant gliomas, and other solid tumors.

Dosage
- 125 mg/m^2 weekly for 4 out of 6 weeks
- 180 mg/m^2 weekly for 3 out of 4 weeks
- 350 mg/m^2 every 3 weeks
- Other dosing regimens have been studied.

Clinical pharmacology
- CPT-11 is in itself relatively inactive and must be converted by carboxylesterases to SN-38, which has potent topo I inhibitory activity.
- Glucuronidation and biliary excretion are the principal mechanisms of elimination for SN-38.
- Particular caution and dose reduction are recommended for patients with liver dysfunction or Gilbert's syndrome.

Side effects
- Diarrhea is common (early or late).
  - **Early**: It occurs during the first 24 hours of administration, with diaphoresis, abdominal pain, and cramping. It is usually transient and treated with low-dose atropine.
  - **Late**: It occurs more than 24 hours after administration, and it is treated with high-dose loperamide at the first sign of diarrhea.

- Myelosuppression
- Thrombocytopenia
- Neutropenia is common
- Anemia
- Alopecia
- Nausea and vomiting are moderate

Topotecan

Clinical indications
- Topotecan has FDA approved for the treatment of advanced ovarian cancer, cervical cancer, and small-cell lung cancers.

Dosage (available in both oral and IV dosage form)
- 1.5 mg/m^2 IV daily x 5 days every 3 weeks
- 2.3 mg/m^2 po daily x 5 days every 3 weeks

Refer to individual protocols for other dosing strategies and dosing in combination with other chemotherapy agents.

Side effects
- Myelosuppression is dose limiting
- Neutropenia is common
- Thrombocytopenia is common
- Anemia
- Diarrhea
- Alopecia
- Nausea/vomiting is low

Clinical pharmacology
- Topotecan has oral bioavailability of 30%–50%; both dosage forms are widely distributed throughout the body, with CSF topotecan concentrations 30%–50% of simultaneous plasma concentrations.
- Topotecan undergoes negligible metabolism and is primarily eliminated by the kidneys, with evidence for renal tubular secretion.
- A linear relationship between creatinine clearance and clearance of both total topotecan and lactone form has been demonstrated.

Topoisomerase II inhibitors

Etoposide and teniposide exert their action on topo II by
- Inhibiting the ability of the enzyme to relegate the cleaved DNA complex
- Generating high levels of DNA with potentially toxic double-stranded breaks
- Promoting mutation
- Permanent double-stranded breaks
- Illegitimate recombination
- Apoptosis

Etoposide and teniposide are poorly water-soluble and are formulated with a number of excipients including polysorbate (etoposide) or cremophor EL (teniposide).

Etoposide can be administered by either oral or intravenous routes; teniposide only by intravenous injection.

Clinical indications
- Teniposide and etoposide are widely used in treatment of adult and pediatric malignancies.
- Etoposide has been more broadly used in front-line therapy, particularly for small-cell lung cancer and germ-cell tumors.
- Teniposide is used in pediatric leukemias and other solid tumors.

Side effects
The pattern of toxicity is very similar between both agents and includes the following:
- Neutropenia
- Alopecia
- Mucositis
- Infusion-related blood pressure changes
- Hypersensitivity reactions
- Nausea/vomiting is low

Clinical pharmacology
- Etoposide absorption appears to be nonlinear with decreased bioavailability at doses above 200 mg.
- Both etoposide and teniposide are heavily protein bound; use in patients with low albumin concentrations will result in greater than expected systemic toxicity due to the larger free (unbound) drug concentrations.
- Both etoposide and teniposide are extensively metabolized. Etoposide is more rapidly eliminated than teniposide.
- Linear relationships between etoposide systemic clearance and creatinine clearance have been described for both adult and pediatric patients.

Antimicrotubule agents

Tubulin-interactive agents, commonly known as "spindle poisons," have a long history of use in cancer treatment. They act by binding to specific sites on tubulin, a protein that polymerizes to form cellular microtubules.

Table 9.1 focuses on important antimicrotubule agents in preclinical and clinical development.

Tubulin is an important target for anticancer drug development; several antitubulin agents have significant anticancer activity in the clinic. The taxanes (paclitaxel and docetaxel) were the most encouraging development in anticancer chemotherapy of the 1990s. Recent progress observed with taxanes has led to renewed interest in antimicrotubule analogs or drugs interacting with different sites on tubulin. In particular, agents with an improved pharmacological profile and/or activity in vinca/taxane-resistant cell lines are of interest.

Several new antitubulin agents are in preclinical development.
- Epothilones are a new class of antimicrotubule agent with a mechanism of action similar to that of the taxanes.
- Ixabepilone is the first drug in this class to be approved for commercial use.

Table 9.1 Antimicrotubule agents

Class of spindle poison (mechanism of action)	Useful indications	Drug administration (IV doses in mg/m²)	Main toxicities	Pharmacokinetics and metabolism	Comments of clinical interest
Vincristine (VCR) (destabilization of polymerized tubulin [β-tubulin])	Leukemias, lymphomas, pediatric tumors, small-cell lung cancer, multiple myeloma	0.5–1.4 q 1–4 weeks (total individual dose: 2 mg)	Neuropathy	Metabolized in the liver	VCR induces multidrug resistance (MDR) by P-glycoprotein (PgP). Mutations in α- and β-tubulin proteins enhance stability against depolymerization
Vinblastine (VBL) (same as VCR)	Lymphomas, germ cell tumors, Kaposi's sarcoma, breast cancer	6–10 q 2–4 weeks	Neutropenia, neuropathy	Metabolized in the liver	Neuropathy occurs less frequently than with VCR
Vindesine (VDS) (same as VCR)	Non-small-cell lung cancer (NSCLC), breast cancer, prostate cancer, lymphomas	2–4 q 1–3 weeks	Neutropenia, neuropathy	Metabolized in the liver	Randomized trials (breast, NSCLC, sarcomas, and melanoma) with VDS showed no advantage over treatments without VDS.
Vinorelbine (NVB) (same as VCR)	NSCLC, breast cancer	25–30 q 1–3 weeks combinations: cisplatin (NSCLC) and doxorubicin or 5-FU (breast). Oral form in clinical development	Neutropenia, constipation, neuropathy	Metabolized in the liver	Selective binding to the Taufamily of microtubule-associated proteins→tubulin aggregation into spirals and paracrystals.

Table 9.1 (Cont.)

Class of spindle poison (mechanism of action)	Useful indications	Drug administration (IV doses in mg/m^2)	Main toxicities	Pharmacokinetics and metabolism	Comments of clinical interest
					NVB not active and associated with severe neurotoxicity in paclitaxel-pretreated breast cancer patients
Paclitaxel (P) (microtubule stabilizer) (also anti-angiogenesis effect, disruption of Ki-Ras function, apoptosis induction by phosphorylation of bcl-2)	Ovarian, breast, and lung cancers (other tumors). Reproducible anti-tumor activity (response rate 15%–25%) in platinum-resistant ovarian cancer stimulated further clinical development	135 (24 h)–175 (3 h) q 3 weeks. 60–100 weekly Combinations: mainly with cisplatin or carboplatin (ovary) and doxorubicin (breast)	Neutropenia, neurotoxicity	Metabolized in the liver. Cisplatin→P: severe neutropenia; P→doxorubicin: more mucositis than the reverse sequence	Toxicities are sequence and schedule dependent. Steroids and H1 and H2 blockers are used to reduce hypersensitivity reactions. Water-soluble analogs and derivatives active in resistant cells of P are under development. Mutations in P53 cell lines confer sensitization to P. Resistance to P is due to PgP and/or alterations in the expression or structure of β-tubulin

Drug	Indication	Dose (mg/m²)	Toxicity	Pharmacokinetics	Comments
Docetaxel (D) (microtubule stabilizer)	Breast cancer, lung cancer (other tumors) Reproducible anti-tumor activity (response rate 35%–50%) in anthracycline-resistant breast cancer stimulated further clinical development	60–100 (1 h) q 3 weeks, 35 weekly	Neutropenia, retention syndrome (FRS)	Metabolized in the liver	Steroid premedication reduces and delays FRS. Tau and β4-tubulin expression correlate with D sensitivity in adenocarcinoma models
Ixabepilone (microtubule stabilizer)	Breast cancer	40 q 3 weeks	Peripheral neuropathy	Metabolized in the liver	H1 and H2 blockers are used to prevent hypersensitivity reactions. Steroids should be added in those patients who have experienced a previous reaction.
Estramustine phosphate (EP) (binds to the microtubule-associated proteins to promote microtubule disassembly)	Prostate cancer	560 mg × 2/day orally (with meal)	Gastrointestinal	75% of oral EP is absorbed. Terminal half-life: 20–40 h	Most responses observed in prostate cancer were subjective (objective response rate 710%). EP has been combined with other antimicrotubules (P, VBL) and etoposide with a clinical benefit in 30%–60% of patients. Overexpression of β (III & IVa)-tubulin and Tau may play a role in resistance to EP

Drug resistance

Most of the basic research into drug resistance has involved using pairs of sensitive and resistant tumor cells derived from the same parental cell line, usually by serial passage in increasing concentrations of the drug under investigation. This is an artificial situation, which often results in resistance that is really very substantial, with concentration variants in excess of 40- to 100-fold sometimes required to overcome such resistance. It is unclear whether this laboratory-derived resistance correlates with the types of clinical resistance outlined throughout this chapter.

Pharmacological resistance

The underlying concept of pharmacological resistance is that the dose of chemotherapy that can be safely given is insufficient to result in an effective concentration of the active drug at its target site. This may be due to the following:

- Toxicity in other organs
- Enhanced clearance of drugs
- Physical barrier between bloodstream and tumor cells (many tumors have avascular centers)
- De novo resistance—tumor does not respond despite full-dose chemotherapy
- Acquired resistance—initial response to chemotherapy, then tumor fails to respond and regrows
- Combination of de novo and acquired

Alteration of target or transport mechanisms

Tumor cells have the ability to mutate such that the drug is either not taken up by the cell or, having been taken up, is detoxified more rapidly than normal.

Alternatively, the actual target of the drug may change by mutation such that it becomes impervious to the form of attack. Or the normal repair mechanisms present in all mammalian cells may become more active and repair damage as produced by a cytotoxic agent in a more efficient manner, resulting in overall resistance to the agent.

Classical multidrug resistance

"Classical" drug resistance has been the most studied form of this phenomenon in the laboratory and results from overexpression of a 170 kDa glycoprotein known as P-glycoprotein. This spans the outer cell membrane and acts as an energy-dependent drug efflux pump. Thus, as the drug enters the tumor cell, by diffusion or transport, the drug in the interior of the cell is picked up and effluxed into the extracellular environment. This reduces the effective concentration of the drug within the cell and allows the cell to express resistance to the agent in question.

The development of this form of resistance is most commonly associated with exposure to the antitumor antibiotics, the anthracyclines, taxanes, and etoposide. In fact, resistance to one of this group of agents usually confers resistance to the other groups in addition, thereby leading to the phenomenon of multidrug resistance.

Multidrug resistance-associated protein

This protein is one member of a family of proteins that also act as energy-dependent pumps, in this case resulting in drug efflux or sequestration of the drug, within intracytoplasmic organelles or vacuoles.

The most studied member of this family of proteins is a 190 kDa protein that has a similar substrate specificity to P-glycoprotein but is usually associated with less resistance to the taxanes. The clinical relevance of this form of resistance is less clear than with the P-glycoprotein.

Glutathione

Glutathione is the predominant cellular thiol and participates in a complex biochemical pathway that interacts with the alkylating function of some agents (including cisplatin). Glutathione overexpression in cell lines results in relative resistance to alkylating agent attack. In addition, glutathione is able to detoxify free radicals, which may be an important pathway of action for some cytotoxics, including doxorubicin.

Clinical trials of glutathione depletion have been performed with somewhat equivocal results.

Failure to engage apoptosis

The common final pathway of cell death for many cytotoxics is apoptosis, an active process within cells somewhat akin to "cell suicide." The engagement of the apoptosis program is a complex interacting pathway.

At the center of this is p53, the so-called guardian of the genome. In cells that are unable to engage apoptosis, the damage done by cytotoxics can be "ignored" and cell division continues. This results in clinical drug resistance. Gene-therapy approaches to correct this apoptosis failure are being actively investigated.

Summary

- Clinical drug resistance is a major problem in oncology and the underlying mechanisms are multifactorial.
- In any one patient, it is unclear to what extent each mechanism contributes.
- Nevertheless, the potential clinical benefits of mechanisms to circumvent drug resistance are enormous.
- Undoubtedly, other mechanisms of drug resistance will be found as we come to understand more about the regulation of cell cycle, cell life, and cell death.

Dose intensification

Dose response

The strategy of therapeutic dose intensification in oncology has been largely driven by experimental evidence, suggesting that the drug resistance of cancer cells is often relative.

Results of studies indicate that arbitrary dose reduction should be avoided and suggest that clinicians consider use of prophylactic antibiotics, hematopoietic growth factors, etc. in situations in which neutropenia and its complications threaten to undermine timely delivery of potentially curative chemotherapy.

High-dose chemotherapy with hematopoietic support

In the clinic, dose escalation within a "conventional" range has an inconsistent effect on response rates and, with some exceptions, a negligible survival impact. Dose escalation is complicated by increased toxicity.

Substantial advances in hematopoietic support have allowed investigation of high doses of chemotherapy in the clinic. Autografting, using either autologous marrow or cytokine-mobilized peripheral blood progenitors, is seen to facilitate administration of high doses of those drugs dose-limited by myelosuppression.

An overview of hematopoietic stem cell transplantation is provided in Chapter 10.

Accelerated chemotherapy

An alternative approach to dose intensification is to shorten the interval between cycles of conventional chemotherapy, usually through granulocyte colony-stimulating factor (G-CSF) support. Preliminary results with this approach in adjuvant chemotherapy for high-risk breast cancer have been promising.

Chemoradiation

Chemotherapy and radiotherapy are complementary; integration of these treatment modalities underpins successful treatment of a number of tumors. Chemotherapy reduces the burden of local diseases and eradicates systemic micrometastases, but effective locoregional tumor control in some situations requires irradiation.

Sequential combined therapy

The traditional approach to combining chemotherapy and radiotherapy has been to attempt to predict whether eradication of systemic disease or local tumor control is of most immediate concern, then deliver the appropriate treatment first; the other type of treatment is delayed until after completion of the first. The main difficulties are the uncertain behavior of individual tumors and the inevitable delay in delivery of one form of treatment.

Chemotherapy as the first-line treatment has the added potential benefit that in downstaging the tumor, it may reduce both the volume of tissue that requires irradiation and the radiation dose required to control the tumor.

Concurrent combined therapy

Problems are avoided by delivering chemotherapy and radiotherapy together. This approach has advantages and some disadvantages (see Table 9.2).

Ideally, cytotoxics chosen for chemoirradiation regimens will have known activity against the tumor but will not have toxicities that overlap with the effects of irradiation of the relevant region. Agents such as cisplatin and 5-fluorouracil are particularly attractive because of their radiosensitizing effects.

At least in vitro, the interactions of chemotherapy and radiotherapy are complex and schedule dependent. An attempt must be made to minimize the normal tissue damage of radiation during combined therapy.

Table 9.2 Benefits and problems of concurrent combined therapy

Advantage	Disadvantage
No delay in either therapy	Increased toxicity
Additive cell kill by two therapies	Compromised dose of one or both treatments
Enhanced cell kill by radiosensitizing effects of chemotherapy	Large volume irradiated
Reduced likelihood of evolution of resistance to either therapy	Pharmacodynamic interactions (e.g., cell-cycle effects)

Anal and bladder carcinomas

For both of these pelvic malignancies, chemoirradiation offers the possibility of organ preservation and avoidance of a stoma.

There is good evidence that pelvic irradiation with concurrent 5-fluorouracil and mitomycin is the best-established therapy for anal carcinoma.

The combination of pelvic radiotherapy and cisplatin-based chemotherapy has proven successful in large phase II studies in muscle-invading transitional-cell carcinoma of the bladder.

Head and neck cancer and esophageal cancer

Chemoirradiation of intrathoracic tumors is hindered by risk of serious morbidity, in particular, pneumonitis and esophagitis. Chemoirradiation is superior to radiation therapy alone for esophageal cancer, but local failure rates remain high. Surgery after combined treatment may be the answer to this problem.

Primary chemoradiotherapy of head and neck cancers is widely used and can result in good response rates with some cures. This approach has some advantages over more radical surgical excision because of the possibility of organ and function preservation with resultant reduction of morbidity.

Surgical salvage can then be reserved for nonresponding or relapsing cases.

Rectal cancer

There is now clear evidence that combination of fluoropyrimidine-based chemotherapy with external beam radiotherapy leads to improved local control and enhanced survival.

Lung cancer

Concurrent chemoirradiation is considered the standard of care for limited-stage small-cell lung cancer and in some cases of non-small–cell lung cancer.

Chapter 10

Hematopoietic stem cell transplantation

Jeanne Palmer
David Rizzieri

Introduction 152
Donor selection 154
Pretransplant evaluation 156
Conditioning regimens 157
Post-transplant complications 158
Long-term complications of hematopoietic stem
 cell transplantation 164
Donor lymphocyte infusion 164

Introduction

Hematopoietic stem cell transplantation (HSCT) is a potentially curative therapy for many hematologic malignancies, errors of inborn metabolism, congenital immunodeficiency, and hemoglobinopathies. The specific indications for HSCT are covered elsewhere in this book. In this chapter, we will provide a brief overview of stem cell transplantation, including selection of donors, different types of transplantation, and short- and long-term complications.

Forms of transplantation

Autologous transplant

- Autologous HSCT uses the principle of "more is better."
- Very high doses of chemotherapy and/or radiation are used that would normally be lethal primarily due to overlapping toxicity to hematopoietic stem cells.
- To remedy this, the patient's own stem cells are collected before exposure to the high-dose therapy and reinfused subsequent to this exposure.
- This type of therapy has been shown to improve survival most commonly in relapsed Hodgkin's lymphoma, diffuse large B-cell lymphoma, and multiple myeloma.
- Autologous transplant has some similar risks to those of allogeneic transplant from the high-dose chemotherapy, but it does not carry the risk of graft-versus-host disease (GVHD; discussed in Post-transplant complications, pp. 156–160).
- Also, there was no significant long-term immunosuppression nor delayed immune reconstitution.
- The chemotherapy or radiation used is generally a regimen specific to the disease treated.
- Use of autologous HSCT in some solid tumors has been investigated but not routinely used, except in certain germ-cell and neural tumors.

Allogeneic hematopoietic stem cell transplantation

Allogeneic HSCT involves the infusion of donor cells into the patient. It is an intense process that involves preparing a patient to receive another hematopoietic system.

This preparation, or conditioning, involves use of immunosuppression typically through the use of chemotherapy and radiation. The goal is to both treat the disease and suppress or ablate the recipient immune system and allow the new immune system to engraft. The remainder of this chapter will cover this type of transplantation.

Donor selection

Human leukocyte antigens typing

Selection of a donor is based primarily on human leukocyte antigens (HLA), which are proteins expressed on cell surfaces on all cells in the body and involved in immune function.

These proteins are encoded on chromosome 6. There are two classes of major histocompatibility antigens that are important for transplant:
- *Class I* molecules are expressed on every cell in the body and allow recognition of self or non-self. They include HLA-A, B, and C.
- *Class II* molecules are expressed on antigen-presenting cells such as B cells and dendritic cells, and include HLA DQ, DP, and DR.

HLA typing is done by serologic and molecular methods.
- Serologic testing is indicated by the first two numbers, and done using sera that contains antibody to that specific HLA molecule, i.e., HLA-A02.
- Molecular typing uses a DNA allele-level analysis to be more specific, and it is indicated by the second two numbers—i.e., HLA-A0201.
- The matching done for HSCT evaluates at least HLA-A, B, and DR.
- There is emerging evidence that testing HLA-C, DQ, and other secondary loci may be important in unrelated or mismatched donor transplant as well.

Potential donors

Matched related donors are the preferred donors; however, with decreasing family sizes, only ~30% patients will have a matched related donor. In 1986, the National Marrow Donor Program was created,[1] which provides a registry of people throughout the country who are serologically typed for loci A and B.

When matched unrelated donors (MUD) were compared with matched related donors, outcomes were similar, although there were higher rates of severe side effects such as graft-versus-host disease (discussed in Post-transplant complications, pp. 156–160). To increase the donor pool for patients, alternative donors are currently being investigated. Alternative donors include both unrelated cord blood and haploidentical related donors.

Umbilical cord blood (UCB) transplantation has been used in children and is being tested in the adult patient population.[2]

---

1 Yakoub-Agha I, Mesnil F, Kuentz M, et al. (2006). Allogeneic marrow stem-cell transplantation from human leukocyte antigen-identical siblings versus human leukocyte antigen-allelic-matched unrelated donors (10/10) in patients with standard-risk hematologic malignancy: a prospective study from the French Society of Bone Marrow Transplantation and Cell Therapy. *J Clin Oncol* 24:5695–5702.

2 Laughlin MJ, Eapen M, Rubenstein P, et al. (2004). Outcomes after transplantation of cord blood or bone marrow from unrelated donors in adults with leukemia. *N Engl J Med* 351:2265–2275.

- **Benefits**: UCB allows a greater degree of mismatch to be tolerated without increasing GVHD. Also, when a matched cord exists, little wait time is required between the decision to transplant and availability of the cord.
- **Disadvantages**: UCB transplant results in slower engraftment, variability of the quality of the product between banks, and higher rates of infection and relapse. Part of the problem is due to the low number of nucleated cells per kilogram body weight. To overcome this, studies are being done using two or more cord blood units to increase the nucleated cell number per kilogram body weight.[3,4]

Another type of alternative donor transplant is haploidentical-related donor-matched transplant between 3 and 5/6.[5,6,7] When this type of transplant was initially tested using a myeloablative conditioning regimen, there were extremely high rates of GVHD. However, with nonmyeloablative approaches (with less toxic conditioning; see p. 155) and stringent T-cell depletion, treatment-related mortality and rates of severe GVHD are at acceptable levels.

- **Benefits**: Use of a haploidentical donor ensures that nearly everyone has an available donor.
- **Disadvantages**: This type of transplant results in higher rates of GVHD, longer times to engraftment, delay in immune reconstitution, and increased infection risks.

3 Barker JN, Weisdorf DJ, DeFor TE, et al. (2005). Transplantation of 2 partially HLA-matched umbilical cord blood units to enhance engraftment in adults with hematologic malignancy. *Blood* 105:1343–1347.

4 Ballen K, Spitzer TR, Yeap BY, et al. (2007). Double unrelated reduced-intensity umbilical cord blood transplantation in adults. *Biol Blood Marrow Transplant* 13:82–89.

5 Aversa F, Terenzi A, Tabilio A, et al. (2005). Full haplotype-mismatched hematopoietic stem-cell transplantation: a phase II study in patients with acute leukemia at high risk of relapse. *J Clin Oncol* 23:3447–3454.

6 Rizzieri DA, Kohl, LP, Long, GD, et al. (2007). Partially matched, nonmyeloablative allogeneic transplantation: clinical outcomes and immune reconstitution. *J Clin Oncol* 25:690–697.

7 Ogawa H, Ikegame K, Yoshihara S, et al. (2006). Unmanipulated HLA 2-3 antigen-mismatched (haploidentical) stem cell transplantation using nonmyeloablative conditioning. *Biol Blood Marrow Transplant* 12:1073–1084.

Pretransplant evaluation

Typically, one assesses disease status before transplant begins and assures adequate organ function with complete blood counts, comprehensive metabolic panel, HIV test, hepatitis B and C, and pulmonary function testing, echocardiogram, or equivalent testing.

Conditioning regimens

Myeloablative
- Myeloablative conditioning uses a combination of chemotherapy, total body irradiation (TBI) to wipe out all hematopoietic stem cells, and presumably any minimal residual disease.
- The conditioning regimens are designed to give maximal tolerated doses of several types of chemotherapy with avoiding overlap in nonhematopoietic toxicity.
- Often combinations of one or two of the following are used: busulfan, cyclophosphamide, thiotepa, etoposide, fludarabine ± TBI.
- This type of conditioning has significant toxicity and is usually reserved for patients under 55 years of age.
- This allows for the benefit of high-dose chemotherapy in addition to graft-versus-tumor effects to help control disease.

Nonmyeloablative
- Nonmyeloablative, or reduced-intensity, conditioning relies on immunotherapy rather than the effects of high-dose chemotherapy.
- This type of transplant has far less toxicity with conditioning and can be used in patients who are older or have comorbidities.
- The conditioning uses similar agents to those used in myeloablative conditioning but in doses more readily tolerated, such that the innate hematopoietic system of the patient is not immediately ablated.
- Thus, this approach relies less on chemotherapy benefits than on graft-versus-tumor effects for disease control, and it is most effective when the patient has minimal residual disease at initiation.

Post-transplant complications

Acute graft-versus-host disease

Overview

Acute GVHD (aGVHD) occurs in 10%–80% of HSCT, largely dependent on conditioning regimen and donor type. Risk factors for aGVHD include increased age of recipient, intensity of conditioning, and degree of HLA mismatch. The symptoms often observed include erythematous, itchy skin rash with peeling, profuse watery diarrhea with abdominal cramping, and elevated liver function tests.

There have been several grading systems developed (see Tables 10.1 and 10.2).

Acute graft-versus-host disease prophylaxis

Pharmacological

Immunosuppressant drugs have been tried alone or in combination in many trials.

- Current typical recommendations for myeloablative: Cyclosporine 3.0 mg/kg per day IV or tacrolimus 0.03 mg/kg per day plus methotrexate 15 mg/m² days 1 and 10 mg/m² on days 3, 6, 9, 11.
- Current recommendations for nonmyeloablative: Cellcept 15 mg/kg po q12h + cyclosporine 6.25 mg/kg po q12h (or tacrolimus equivalent)[1]
- Triple therapies have been tried, typically adding in steroids for prophylaxis; however, outcomes were not improved.
- Future directions for GVHD prophylaxis include tacrolimus + sirolimus, which had encouraging results in phase II trials and is currently in a phase III trial.

T-cell depletion

- T-cell depletion can be done both ex vivo and in vivo using thymoglobulin, alemtuzumab, or similar means.
- Many conditioning regimens employ use of these antibodies, which may persist for up to 1 month and continue to deplete donor T cells during early allogeneic recovery.
- Another method of T-cell depletion is positive CD34⁺ selection.
- Many studies have evaluated T-cell depletion in the matched-sibling context, and this seems to result in overall reductions in rates of GVHD, but increased rates of infection and graft rejection, thus no difference in overall survival.
- Use of stringent T-depletion methods is typically reserved for transplant conditions that have extremely high rates of GVHD such as haploidentical transplant.[2,3]

---

1. Mielcarek M, Martin PJ, Leisenring W, et al. (2003). Graft-versus-host disease after non-myeloablative versus conventional hematopoietic stem cell transplantation. *Blood* 102:756–76.

2. Aversa F, Terenzi A, Tabilio A, et al. (2005). Full haplotype-mismatched hematopoietic stem-cell transplantation: a phase II study in patients with acute leukemia at high risk of relapse. *J Clin Oncol* 23:3447–3454.

3. Rizzieri DA, Kohl, LP, Long, GD, et al. (2007). Partially matched, nonmyeloablative allogeneic transplantation: clinical outcomes and immune reconstitution. *J Clin Oncol* 25:690–697.

Table 10.1 Stage of graft-versus-host-disease by organ system

Organ	Grade	Description
Skin	+1	Maculopapular rash over <25% of body area
	+2	Maculopapular rash over 25%–50% of body area
	+3	Generalized erythroderma
	+4	Generalized erythroderma with bullous formation and often with desquamation
Liver	+1	Bilirubin 2.0–3.0 mg/dL; SGOT 150–750 IU
	+2	Bilirubin 3.1–6.0 mg/dL
	+3	Bilirubin 6.1–15.0 mg/dL
	+4	Bilirubin >15.0 mg/dL
Gut	+1	Diarrhea >30 mL/kg or >500 mL/day
	+2	Diarrhea >60 mL/kg or >1000 mL/day
	+3	Diarrhea >90 mL/kg or >1500 mL/day
	+4	Diarrhea >90 mL/kg or abdominal pain with or without ileus >2000 mL/day; or severe

Table 10.2 Comparison of International Bone Marrow Transplant Registry (IBMTR) and Glucksberg grading systems*

IBMTR grade	Glucksberg grade	Skin	Intestine	Liver
A	I	1	0	0
B	I	2	0	0
B	II	0–2	1	0–1
B	II	0–2	0–1	1
C	II	3	1	0–1
C	II	3	0–1	1
C	II	3	0	0
B	III	0–2	2	0–2
B	III	0–2	0–2	2
C	III	0–3	0–3	2–3
C	III	3	2–3	0–3
D	III	0–3	0–3	4
D	IV	0–3	4	0–4
D	IV	4	0–4	0–4

*In the Glucksberg system, any patient with a Karnofsky scale score of less than 30 is grade IV.

Acute graft-versus-host disease treatment
- Treatment given when aGVHD is higher than grade II. First-line treatment for GVHD is usually methylprednisolone 1–2 mg/kg daily.
- This is given until resolution of symptoms occurs, then tapered.
- One study indicated that response at 5 days may predict outcome. Those who obtained a response at 5 days had 49% 1-year survival; however, if they had no response it was only 27%.
- If the aGVHD is refractory to steroids, there are a variety of experimental options available, including ATG, anti-interleukin-2 receptor antibody, antitumor necrosis factor (TNF) antibody, or pentostatin, which have response rates of 19%–73%. However, none of these agents improved overall survival.[1]

Chronic graft-versus-host disease

Overview

Chronic GVHD (cGVHD) is a complication that occurs in 40%–70% of HSCT. Historically, it has been diagnosed when GVHD occurs after day 100. However, particularly with the rise in nonmyeloablative therapies, it is now thought to represent more a constellation of symptoms to make the diagnosis rather than any time point alone.

Chronic GVHD presents with any number of the following symptoms: sclerodermatous skin changes, dry mucous membranes, bronchiolitis obliterans, liver dysfunction, diarrhea, fatigue, cytopenias, and myalgias or arthralgias.

Increased risk for cGVHD occurs with peripheral blood stem cells rather than bone marrow in CML, increasing age, occurrence of aGVHD, a multiparous female donor, and increasing mismatch in HLA systems.

There have been multiple scoring systems proposed; more recently, a comprehensive scoring system has been recommended.[2]

Prophylaxis and treatment

There are no current recommendations for prophylaxis for cGVHD, other than preventing aGVHD first.

Treatment generally employs steroids and any number of immunosuppressants. In severe cases, photopheresis is used, which involves removal of a patient's lymphocytes, incubation with 8-methoxypsoralen, exposure to UVA light, then reinfusion into the patient. It is thought to kill the patient's newly expanding T cells and antigen-presenting cells and has been shown to work in cGVHD.

More studies are underway to confirm this hypothesis and determine the duration of treatment.

---

1. Antin JH, Chen AR, Couriel DR, et al. (2004). Novel approaches to the therapy of steroid-resistant acute graft-versus-host disease. *Biol Blood Marrow Transplant* 10:655–668.

2. Filipovich AH, Weisdorf D, Pavletic S, et al. (2005). National Institutes of Health consensus development project on criteria for clinical trials in chronic graft-versus-host disease: I. Diagnosis and staging working group report. *Biol Blood Marrow Transplant* 11:945–956.

Infection

Overview

It can take from 12 to 24 months for sufficient immune recovery after HSCT. Although initial neutrophil engraftment is usually observed within 4 weeks after transplantation, there are still significant detriments to the humoral and cytotoxic immune system. Furthermore, if the patient has developed GVHD, this also results in significant immunosuppression, both as a result of the GVHD and the treatment for it.

The type of infection varies depending on the time point after transplant: pre-engraftment, immediately post-engraftment, and late post-engraftment.

Pre-engraftment
- **Risks:** Neutropenia, organ dysfunction from conditioning regimen, mucositis
- **Infections:** HSV, gram-positive or gram-negative aerobes from mouth or gut, molds can occur, especially if there is preexisting infection

Immediately post-engraftment
- **Risks:** Continued mucocutaneous damage, adaptive immune system defects, GVHD, and subsequent treatment
- **Infections:** CMV, mold (aspergillus), fungi (candida), bacterial (*Listeria monocytogenes*), parasitic (PCP, toxoplasmosis), other viral infections

Late post-transplant
- **Risks:** Mucocutaneous compromise, delayed immune recovery
- **Infections:** Bacterial (especially encapsulated), viral infections (VZV, HSV, EBV)

Prophylaxis

Bacterial
- Current recommendations for infection prophylaxis include ciprofloxacin 500–750 mg po bid.
- If the patient has difficulty taking oral antibiotics or has an allergy to ciprofloxacin, ceftriaxone 2 g IV daily can also be used.
- Newer fluoroquinolones may be tried, but they are not as active against certain organisms of concern and do not counter polyoma virus in the bladder as ciprofloxacin may.

Fungal
- Fungal prophylaxis usually includes fluconazole, which has resulted in decreased candida fungal infections.
- One drawback is that it does not cover aspergillosis.
- Studies have evaluated the cost-effectiveness of using a more broad-spectrum antifungal such as posaconazole or voriconazole.
- Posaconazole has been shown to be superior to fluconazole for immunosuppressed patients with GVHD in development of invasive fungal infections and overall survival.
- A large study is underway to evaluate the benefit of voriconazole prophylaxis as compared with fluconazole. Preliminary results show no significant benefit, although long-term results are still being evaluated.[1]

Viral
- Viral prophylaxis is largely institution-dependent. Acyclovir is often used, and it protects against HSV.
- However, one of the bigger threats to a recovering patient is CMV, and although acyclovir is superior to placebo in protection against CMV, it is unclear how to interpret these results given that acyclovir has no in vitro activity against CMV.
- Some studies look at use of prophylactic gancyclovir to prevent CMV; however, this results in higher rates of neutropenia and may delay reconstitution of immunity against CMV. Furthermore, no survival advantage to prophylactic gancyclovir has been shown.
- One frequently employed model involves close monitoring for CMV in the blood post-transplant (polymerase chain reaction [PCR] testing for CMV), and if positive, treat with gancyclovir, which can often treat the reactivation before it has clinical ramifications (CMV disease).[2]

Hepatic veno-occlusive disease

Hepatic veno-occlusive disease (VOD) is a devastating complication of any type of transplant that employs high doses of chemotherapy or radiation. It is seen in myeloablative allogeneic and autologous transplantation.

The diagnosis is based on the presence of two or more symptoms noted within the first 20 days of transplant: elevation of bilirubin >2 mg/dL, hepatomegaly or right upper quadrant pain, and weight gain of >2% of body weight in fluid.[3]

The incidence of this complication varies by report and the criteria used for diagnosis. In two large studies it has was 5% and 54%. Risk factors for VOD are allogeneic BMT, high doses of chemotherapy, preexisting liver disease, and pretransplant use of gemtuzumab ozogamicin.

Prophylaxis

A randomized trial of heparin versus observation reduced the risk of VOD from 13.7% to 2.5% without increasing bleeding or transfusion requirements. Currently, the recommendations for prophylaxis include use of low-dose heparin.

Treatment

Once the patient develops VOD, treatment options are limited. One drug currently used is defibrotide, a single-stranded polydeoxyribonucleotide with fibrinolytic, antithrombotic, and anti-ischemic properties shown to improve survival in patients with severe VOD.[4]

---

1. Wingard JR, Carter SL, Walsh TJ, et al. (2007). Results of a randomized, double-blind trial of fluconazole (FLU) vs. voriconazole (VORI) for the prevention of invasive fungal infections (IFI) in 600 allogeneic blood and marrow transplant (BMT) patients. *Blood* 110:63.

2. Boeckh M, Gooley TA, Myerson D, et al. (1996). Cytomegalovirus pp65 antigenemia-guided early treatment with ganciclovir versus ganciclovir at engraftment after allogeneic marrow transplantation: a randomized double-blind study. *Blood* 88:4063–4071.

3. McDonald GB, Sharma P, Matthews E, et al. (1984). Venocclusive disease of the liver after bone marrow transplantation: diagnosis, incidence, and predisposing factors. *Hepatology* 4:116–122.

4. Richardson PG, Murakami C, Jin Z, et al. (2002). Multi-institutional use of defibrotide in 88 patients after stem cell transplantation with severe veno-occlusive disease and multisystem organ failure: response without significant toxicity in a high-risk population and factors predictive of outcome. *Blood* 100:4337–4343.

Long-term complications of hematopoietic stem cell transplantation

If the patient survives the first 2 years after transplantation, there is an excellent prognosis. In one analysis, 89% of those alive at the 2-year point remained alive at 7 years.[1] This review has covered many of the complications that occur within the first 2 years. The patient remains at risk for the following disorders more than 2 years after HSCT:
- Cataract disease
- Sicca syndrome
- Accelerated coronary atherosclerosis
- Secondary cancers
- Hypothyroidism
- Osteoporosis

Donor lymphocyte infusion

Although ideally hematopoietic stem cell therapy is a curative therapy, approximately 30% of patients will eventually relapse. One potential therapy for such relapses is use of donor lymphocyte infusions (DLI). DLI employs boosts of donor lymphocytes as immunotherapy. The hypothesis is that by infusion of these lymphocytes, a graft-versus-tumor effect can be observed. Unfortunately, this can also be accompanied by significant GVHD. The risk of GVHD is higher with increased cell dose and greater HLA mismatch.

Response rates are dependent on disease type. In CML, complete response rates have been reported as high as 100%, although they usually range from 60% to 70%. In AML and ALL, the response rates are not nearly as high, usually 15%–25%.[2]

A current area of active research is using DLI that have been depleted of alloreactive T cells or specifically selected for subsets such as NK cells that may allow better tumor kill with less risk of GVHD.

---

1. Socié G, Stone JV, Wingard, JR, et al. (1999). Long-term survival and late deaths after allogeneic bone marrow transplantation. Late Effects Working Committee of the International Bone Marrow Transplant Registry. *N Engl J Med* 341:14–21.

2. Schmid C, Labopin M, Nagler A, et al. (2007). Donor lymphocyte infusion in the treatment of first hematological relapse after allogeneic stem-cell transplantation in adults with acute myeloid leukemia: a retrospective risk factors analysis and comparison with other strategies by the EBMT Acute Leukemia Working Party. *J Clin Oncol* 25:4938–4945.

Chapter 11

Hormone therapy

Gary H. Lyman

Introduction *166*
Types of endocrine therapy *168*
Predictors of response *171*
Resistance to hormone therapy *172*
Controversies *173*

CHAPTER 11 **Hormone therapy**

Introduction

Hormones have been implicated in the etiology and growth of many malignant tumors including those of breast, ovary, thyroid, and endometrium and certain gastrointestinal and genitourinary tumors, melanomas, and meningiomas. The best evidence that hormones promote the growth of cancers relates to sex steroid hormones and cancers of their target organs, namely estrogens and progestins in breast and endometrial cancer and androgens in prostate cancer.

In general, the aim of hormone therapy for cancer is to deplete the circulating level of the hormone promoting tumor growth or to block binding of the hormone to its receptors within the tumor cell (Box 11.1). Both can result in tumor regression in response to reduction of hormone-dependent tumor cell proliferation and induction of programmed cell death (apoptosis).

> **Box 11.1 Principles of hormone therapy for cancer**
> - Either remove or reduce hormone levels driving cell proliferation or block binding of hormone to cell receptor.
> - This therapy results in inhibition of cell proliferation and/or programmed cell death.

The effects of endocrine therapy are generally confined to normal target organs for the hormone (see Box 11.2), and there are few side effects outside these organs. This accounts for the tolerability of these treatments compared with that of cytotoxic chemotherapy. In addition, tumor responses to hormone therapy may be durable even in advanced disease.

However, some cancers arising in hormone-dependent organs are resistant to endocrine therapy either at presentation or at the time of recurrence, and they become increasingly unresponsive during the course of treatment and disease progression. Thus, most patients with breast and prostate cancers die with hormone-independent disease.

> **Box 11.2 Hormone-responsive cancers**
> - Sex hormones
>   - Breast, prostate, endometrial cancer
> - Renal cancer, meningioma
> - Peptide hormones
>   - Thyroid, neuroendocrine cancers, carcinoid tumors

INTRODUCTION

Types of endocrine therapy

Ablation of endocrine glands

In men and premenopausal women, the major sites of sex hormone synthesis are the gonads.

Castration decreases circulating testosterone in males by over 95% and estrogens in premenopausal women by 60% relative to follicular phase levels. These endocrine effects produce clinical benefits in approximately 80% of men with metastatic prostate cancer and in 30%–40% of unselected premenopausal women with advanced breast cancer.

Oophorectomy is not beneficial in postmenopausal women because the postmenopausal ovary produces relatively little estrogen.

Hypophysectomy and adrenalectomy have been used in postmenopausal women with advanced breast cancer, the adrenal being one source of postmenopausal estrogen. These treatments produce benefit in approximately one-third of cases, but the procedures have significant morbidity and lack specificity, removing other classes of hormones in addition to the sex steroids.

The irreversible nature of surgical ablation of endocrine organs, when all patients cannot be guaranteed benefit, has provided the impetus to develop alternative pharmacological therapies that are specific, reversible, and self-limiting.

Agonists and supraphysiological doses of hormone

The gonadotrophins luteinizing hormone (LH) and follicle-stimulating hormone (FSH) provide the stimulus for gonads to produce steroid hormones. Their synthesis and release from the pituitary is regulated by the hypothalamic factor gonadotrophin-releasing hormone (GnRH) (or luteinizing hormone–releasing hormone [LHRH]).

Highly potent agonist analogs of GnRH have been synthesized by altering the amino acid sequence of the native peptide. When administered for short periods they cause a rapid release of gonadotrophins. However, in the long term, these agonists downregulate and desensitize the pituitary receptors, leading to a fall in circulating gonadotrophins, and abolish the trophic drive to the gonads, reducing circulating sex hormones to castration levels.

Depot formulations of LHRH agonists are available so that a single injection can maintain effective medical castration over prolonged periods.

The use of GnRH analogs in premenopausal women with breast cancer and men with prostate cancer has produced antitumor effects equivalent to surgical castration.

A similar mechanism of action explains the response seen in hormone-dependent cancers after use of pharmacological doses of steroid hormones such as

- Estrogen (diethyl stilbestrol)
- Progestogens (medroxyprogesterone and megestrol)
- Androgens (testolactone and fluoxymesterone)

Lower physiological doses of the same hormones may accelerate tumor growth.

Although downregulation of steroid hormone receptors occurs in target organs, other nonspecific effects can occur, such as thromboembolic complications.

Although a tumor flare may occur at the start of treatment, they are often of clinical benefit, e.g., high-dose progestogens for endometrial and breast cancer.

Inhibition of steroid-producing enzymes

This approach is illustrated by inhibitors of aromatase activity. The aromatase enzyme converts androgens to estrogens and is the last step of the synthetic cascade. It is the main source of estrogen in postmenopausal women. Inhibition of aromatase represents the most specific method of blocking estrogen production.

Since estrogen biosynthesis can occur in nonendocrine tissue such as adipose tissue and malignant tumors themselves, aromatase inhibitors have the potential to suppress estrogen levels beyond that achievable by adrenalectomy.

Two major types of aromatase inhibitors have been developed.
- Steroidal or type I inhibitors interfere with the attachment of androgen substrate to the catalytic site.
- Nonsteroidal type II inhibitors interfere with the enzyme's cytochrome P450.

Early type II inhibitors such as aminoglutethimide were neither potent nor specific, inhibiting other steroid-metabolizing enzymes that had a similar cytochrome P450 prosthetic group, so that steroid replacement therapy was required.

The current generation of triazole drugs (anastrozole, letrozole, vorozole) is 2000-fold more potent than amino-glutethimide and has differential affinity toward aromatase cytochrome P450 with highly selective inhibition of estrogen biosynthesis.

These drugs can reduce circulating estrogens in postmenopausal women to undetectable levels without influencing other steroid hormones.

Among type I inhibitors, formestane and exemestane are thought to act as "suicide" inhibitors, blocking aromatase irreversibly through their own metabolism into active intermediates by the enzyme; estrogen biosynthesis can only be resumed when aromatase molecules are synthesized de novo.

Steroid hormone antagonists

Antagonists for estrogens, progestins, and androgens have been developed blocking hormone-mediated effects usually at the level of their receptors (see Box 11.3).

The most extensive experience relates to the use of the antiestrogen tamoxifen in the treatment of breast cancer. Tamoxifen binds to the estrogen receptor and blocks the effects of endogenous estrogens. Responses are more likely to occur in tumors that are estrogen receptor-positive.

Tamoxifen incompletely blocks the trophic actions of estrogen and can demonstrate partial agonist activity, especially when endogenous estrogen levels are low. This explains its positive effects protecting against osteoporosis, but also unwanted stimulation of endometrial proliferation, which can cause polyps and occasionally endometrial cancer.

More potent "pure" antiestrogens have been developed, such as fulvestrant, which completely blocks the transcriptional activity of the estrogen receptor producing clinical responses in some patients with breast cancer resistant to tamoxifen.

Antiandrogens such as flutamide and casodex have clinical efficacy in the treatment of prostatic cancer.

Antiprogestins such as RU-486 and onapristone have been used against breast and endometrial cancer.

Box 11.3 Steroid sex hormone therapy treatment options
- Castration (surgical or medical)
- Synthetic pathway blockade (e.g., aromatase inhibition)
- Steroid receptor blockade
- Combination therapy

Single-agent versus combination hormone therapy

In the same way that combination chemotherapy has proven superior to single-agent therapy in many cancers, combined hormone treatments might be predicted to produce improved response rates.

However, for most hormone combinations, toxicity is increased, with no improvement in treatment outcome. Exceptions to this rule include castration plus tamoxifen, which is superior to either one alone in advanced premenopausal disease.

The combination of tamoxifen plus an aromatase inhibitor shows no benefit over an aromatase inhibitor alone in advanced disease or over adjuvant therapy. Nevertheless, sequential substitution of one hormone treatment by another can result in second and third responses when the previous treatment has failed in advanced disease.

Likewise, whereas castration plus antiandrogen has failed to produce clear benefits compared with castration alone, sequential addition of antiandrogen to castration can result in second responses in disease progressing postcastration.

Predictors of response

Given that hormone therapy is not effective in all tumors, indiscriminate application of treatment exposes patients with resistant cancer to the side effects of endocrine deprivation therapy and delays potentially beneficial treatment such as chemotherapy.

In breast cancer, the most widely used predictor is the estrogen receptor (ER). Between 60% and 75% of breast cancers are ER-positive by biochemical assay or immunohistochemistry and two-thirds of ER-positive advanced breast cancers respond to hormone manipulation, compared with <10% of ER-negative tumors.

The highest response rates are in tumors expressing both ER and progesterone receptors (PR), and the majority of ER-negative responding cancers are PR-positive.

The value of other markers such as the PR in endometrial cancer is less clear, and measurement of the androgen receptor in prostate cancer has not proven useful.

Although a previous response to hormone manipulation and longer disease-free interval are useful clinical predictors for benefit from second-line endocrine therapy, response rates to second- and third-line therapy fall progressively. Alternatively, progression on one hormone regimen is indicative of relative resistance to further endocrine manipulation.

Resistance to hormone therapy

Resistance to hormone therapy may be primary, i.e., no response to initial hormone therapy, or secondary (acquired), in which disease progresses during treatment after an initial response. Several possible mechanisms are known.

Primary resistance

- Mutations have resulted in hormone-independent proliferation in the tumor with or without loss of the hormone receptor.
- A hormone-dependent pathway is present but unresponsive to treatment, e.g., mutated receptor.
- Hormone-independent stimulation of pathway occurs, e.g., "cross-talk" from other growth factor receptors. There is good laboratory evidence for epidermal growth factor receptor (EGFR) and ER cross-talk in breast cancer.

Secondary (acquired) resistance

- Clonal selection of the above pathways may develop.
- Increased production of hormone receptor or hormone may occur.
- Increased affinity of receptor for hormone develops.
- Altered hormone-receptor interaction may occur in which hormone antagonists behave as agonists.
- Clinical evidence for this comes from observed responses to withdrawal of hormonal treatment in advanced breast cancer and withdrawal of antiandrogens in advanced prostate cancer.
- Induction of metabolic enzymes may occur, reducing intracellular levels of hormone antagonist.

Controversies

Duration of adjuvant therapy

If hormone deprivation therapy were not cytotoxic but cytostatic, therapy would need to be given indefinitely. The counterargument is that resistance may be accompanied by a change in tumor phenotype induced by the continued presence of the drug.

Discontinuation of the first adjuvant treatment followed by another non-cross-resistant regime might be more effective, e.g., ER-positive early breast cancer treated initially with tamoxifen and subsequently by an aromatase inhibitor.

Chemoendocrine therapy

If endocrine therapy is an effective systemic treatment and combination chemotherapy is beneficial, there is good reason to use chemoendocrine therapy. However, by suppressing tumor cell growth, hormonal therapy in theory may protect malignant cells from chemotherapeutic agents that are most effective against replicating cells. Likewise, toxicities may overlap between agents, leading to dose and schedule modifications that compromise long-term benefit.

In general, these treatment modalities are best given sequentially rather than concurrently with endocrine therapy started after completion of chemotherapy and radiation therapy, if indicated.

Chapter 12

Targeted therapies

Daphne Friedman
Ranjit Goudar

Introduction *176*
Small-molecule inhibitors *178*
Antibodies *180*
Conjugated agents *182*
Proteasome inhibitors *183*
Demethylation agents *183*
Histone deacetylase inhibitors *184*

Introduction

Targeted agents are designed to inhibit a specific cell-signaling pathway, cell-surface receptor, or intracellular process, making them fundamentally different from traditionally cytotoxic chemotherapy, which often interferes with cell division and may not be specific to malignant cells. The number of these targeted agents has increased rapidly, and many more such agents are currently under development.

Recent studies suggest that many of these targeted agents are more effective when combined with cytotoxic chemotherapy.

Categories of targeted agents
- Small-molecule inhibitors
- Antibodies
- Conjugated agents
- Proteasome inhibitors
- Demethylation agents
- Histone deacetylase inhibitors

Small-molecule inhibitors

BCR-ABL kinase inhibitors

A specific translocation between chromosomes 9 and 22 [Philadelphia chromosome, t(9;22)] fuses the *BCR* and *ABL* genes, producing a constitutively active tyrosine kinase that drives the uncontrolled proliferation of mature cells in chronic myeloid leukemia. Effective BCR-ABL kinase inhibitors include the following.

Imatinib (Gleevec)
- **Mechanism**: binds and inhibits the tyrosine kinase activity of BCR-ABL kinase, the platelet-derived growth factor receptor, and c-kit
- **Route**: oral
- **Uses**: chronic myeloid leukemia, Philadelphia chromosome-positive acute lymphocytic leukemia, gastrointestinal stromal tumor, dermatofibrosarcoma protuberans

Dasatinib (Sprycel)
- **Mechanism**: binds to the BCR-ABL kinase at a separate location than imatinib and inhibits kinase activity, inhibits SRC kinase
- **Route**: oral
- **Uses**: chronic myeloid leukemia (especially imatinib-resistant disease), Philadelphia chromosome-positive acute lymphocytic leukemia
- **Notes**: can cause pleural effusions and myelosuppression

Nilotinib (Tasigna)
- **Mechanism**: binds and inhibits BCR-ABL kinase
- **Route**: oral
- **Uses**: chronic myeloid leukemia
- **Notes**: can prolong the QT interval. Contraindicated in patients with long QT syndrome, hypokalemia, or hypomagnesemia

Epidermal growth factor receptor inhibitors

The epidermal growth factor receptors (EGFRs) are a family of receptor tyrosine kinases that include EGFR/ErbB1, HER-2/ErbB2, HER-3/ErbB3, and HER-4/ErbB4, and these EGFRs are commonly overexpressed or overactive in solid tumors. When activated by soluble extracellular ligands, EGFRs initiate intracellular signaling cascades that can control various cell functions, such as promoting cell division and inhibiting apoptosis.

Because of the similarity between the individual members of the EGFR family and their ability to form heterodimers, EGFR inhibitors are often able to target multiple different receptors. Available EGFR inhibitors include the following.

Erlotinib (Tarceva)
- **Mechanism**: binds and inhibits the tyrosine kinase activity of epidermal growth factor receptor (EGFR/ErbB1)
- **Route**: oral
- **Uses**: non-small-cell lung cancer (NSCLC), pancreatic cancer, squamous-cell head and neck cancer
- **Notes**: associated with acneiform rash and diarrhea

Lapatinib (Tykerb)
- **Mechanism**: reversible inhibitor of tyrosine kinase activity of the EFGR and the HER2/ErbB2 receptor
- **Route**: oral
- **Uses**: HER2-positive breast cancer
- **Notes**: common side effects include diarrhea and palmar-plantar erythrodysesthesia ([PPE] hand-and-foot syndrome)

Vascular endothelial growth factor receptor inhibitors

The vascular endothelial growth factor receptors (VEGFR-1, VEGFR-2, and VEGFR-3) are receptor tyrosine kinases. When stimulated by soluble VEGF, these receptors initiate a signal transduction pathway critical for angiogenesis, the development of new blood vessels. Since tumors are dependent on the formation of new blood vessels for growth and survival, the VEGF pathway is an important therapeutic target. Active VEGF receptor inhibitors include the following.

Sorafenib (Nexavar)
- **Mechanism**: inhibits vascular endothelial growth factor receptors (VEGFR-2, VEGFR-3), Raf kinase, platelet-derived growth factor receptor β (PDGFR-β), and the Kit receptor tyrosine kinase (KIT)
- **Route**: oral
- **Uses**: renal cell carcinoma, hepatocellular carcinoma
- **Notes**: common side effects include rash, diarrhea, and palmar-plantar erythrodysesthesia (hand-and-foot syndrome). It can lead to elevated PT-INR in patients on warfarin.

Sunitinib (Sutent)
- **Mechanism**: inhibits many receptor tyrosine kinases, including vascular endothelial growth factor receptors (VEGFR-1, VEGFR-2, VEGFR-3), PDGFR-β, KIT, and the glial cell-line derived neurotrophic factor receptor (RET)
- **Route**: oral
- **Uses**: renal cell carcinoma, gastrointestinal stromal tumor
- **Notes**: risk of decreased ejection fraction

Mammalian target of rapamycin inhibitors

Mammalian target of rapamycin (mTOR) is an intracellular protein kinase that serves as a nutrient sensor and can stimulate cell proliferation, and it may be overactive in malignant cells.

Temsirolimus (Torisel)
- **Mechanism**: temsirolimus is metabolized to rapamycin, and both molecules bind to FKBP12 to inhibit the mammalian target of rapamycin (mTOR)
- **Route**: intravenous
- **Uses**: renal cell carcinoma
- **Notes**: risk of hypersensitivity reaction, hyperglycemia, and rare risk of interstitial lung disease

Antibodies

Monoclonal antibody therapies are engineered proteins that bind specifically to soluble factors in the blood or to cell surface molecules. These antibodies may block normal function of target molecules and lead to clearance of targets by immune mechanisms.

Since antibody therapies are developed using humanized or chimeric versions of mouse antibodies, they carry a risk of infusion reactions including hives, hypotension, or, rarely, anaphylaxis. Clinically useful monoclonal antibodies include the following.

Alemtuzumab (Campath-1H)
- **Mechanism**: binds to CD52, a cell surface marker found on B and T cells
- **Route**: intravenous
- **Uses**: chronic lymphocytic leukemia, preparative regimens prior to transplantation
- **Notes**: can cause myelosuppression and increased risk of infections such as CMV

Bevacizumab (Avastin)
- **Mechanism**: binds to circulating VEGF, blocking its ability to bind to cells and thus inhibiting tumor neovascularization
- **Route**: intravenous
- **Uses**: metastatic colon cancer, metastatic non-small-cell lung cancer, renal cell carcinoma. Emerging uses include metastatic breast cancer, ovarian cancer, and pancreatic cancer.
- **Notes**: can cause hypertension and proteinuria, can impair wound healing, and low risk of thrombosis

Cetuximab (Erbitux)
- **Mechanism**: chimeric antibody that binds to the EGFR, blocking its kinase activity
- **Route**: intravenous
- **Uses**: metastatic colon cancer, squamous-cell head and neck cancer
- **Notes**: risk of severe or fatal infusion reactions. It may cause acneiform rash and hypomagnesemia.

Panitumumab (Vectibix)
- **Mechanism**: humanized antibody that binds to EGFR, blocking its kinase activity
- **Uses**: metastatic colon cancer
- **Notes**: low risk of infusion reaction. It may cause acneiform rash and hypomagnesemia.

Rituximab (Rituxan)
- **Mechanism**: binds to CD20, a cell surface marker found on B cells
- **Route**: intravenous
- **Uses**: B-cell malignancies, often in combination with cytotoxic chemotherapy
- **Notes**: low risk of infusion reaction

Trastuzumab (Herceptin)
- **Mechanism**: binds to HER-2, a cell surface molecule on HER-2-positive breast cancer
- **Route**: intravenous
- **Uses**: HER-2-positive breast cancer, both in the adjuvant and metastatic settings
- **Notes**: risk of decreased ejection fraction and congestive heart failure, particularly when combined with cardiotoxic chemotherapy

Conjugated agents

Conjugated agents consist of an antibody or protein linked to a toxin or radioisotope. This class of drugs confers specificity by localizing the cytotoxic insult to the malignant cell of interest. Available conjugated agents include the following.

Ibritumomab (Zevalin)
- Mechanism: CD20 antibody conjugated to the radioisotope Yttrium-90. Binds to B-cells, delivering local radiation
- Route: intravenous
- Uses: B-cell lymphomas, particularly follicular lymphoma
- Notes: can cause prolonged myelosuppression

Tositumomab (Bexxar)
- Mechanism: antibody to the B-cell marker CD20 that is conjugated to the radioisotope iodine-131, which binds and delivers local radiation to target cells
- Route: intravenous
- Uses: B-cell lymphomas, particularly follicular lymphoma
- Notes: can cause prolonged myelosuppression

Denileukin diftitox (Ontak)
- Mechanism: interleukin-2 conjugated to the diphtheria toxin, which binds to lymphocytes and inhibits protein synthesis
- Route: intravenous
- Uses: cutaneous T-cell lymphoma
- Notes: can cause hypersensitivity reactions, increased risk of infections, "vascular leak" syndrome, and risk of thrombosis

Proteasome inhibitors

When intracellular proteins are labeled by the addition of the ubiquitin protein, they are marked for degradation into smaller peptides by the intracellular proteasome complex.

Bortezomib (Velcade)
- **Mechanism**: binds and reversibly inhibits the 26S proteasome and inhibits nuclear factor (NF)-κB
- **Route**: intravenous
- **Uses**: multiple myeloma, mantle cell lymphoma, other non-Hodgkin's lymphomas
- **Notes**: can cause sensory neuropathy. Pulmonary complications including adult respiratory distress syndrome have been reported.

Demethylation agents

Methylation of DNA by DNA methyltransferase can suppress the transcription of tumor suppressor genes. By inhibiting DNA methyltransferase in a malignant cell, innate tumor suppressor activity can be restored. Active hypomethylating agents include the following.

Azacitidine (Vidaza)
- **Mechanism**: cytosine analog that is incorporated into DNA and RNA, irreversibly inhibiting DNA methyltransferase
- **Route**: intravenous
- **Uses**: myelodysplastic syndromes, acute myelogenous leukemia
- **Notes**: causes myelosuppression

Decitabine (Dacogen)
- **Mechanism**: deoxyribose form of azacitidine, a cytosine analog that incorporates into DNA only, irreversibly inhibits DNA methyltransferase
- **Route**: intravenous
- **Uses**: myelodysplastic syndromes, acute myelogenous leukemia
- **Notes**: causes myelosuppression

Histone deacetylase inhibitors

Histone deacetylase (HDAC) is a cellular enzyme that modifies histone proteins and regulates DNA transcription, and may lead to a survival advantage in cancer cells. HDAC inhibitors block this enzyme's activity and thus slow cancer cell growth.

Vorinostat (Zolinza)
- **Mechanism**: inhibits histone deacetylase
- **Route**: oral
- **Uses**: cutaneous T-cell lymphoma
- **Notes**: can cause fatigue, nausea, and myelosuppression. It can lead to elevated PT-INR in patients on warfarin.

Chapter 13

Gene therapy and immunotherapy for cancer

Matthew McKinney
Michael Morse

Introduction *186*
Manipulation of tumor suppressor
 genes and oncogenes *187*
Introduction of chemotherapy sensitization
 and resistance genes *188*
Immunotherapy for cancer *190*
Gene delivery *192*

Introduction

Limited progress has been made in extending survival of patients with many types of malignancies through use of conventional cytotoxic therapies. Specific cancer-targeted therapies have been devised as a way of attacking the tumor microenvironment while avoiding systemic toxicities.

Gene therapy for cancer represents the manipulation of genetic information in a way that affects the homeostasis of the tumor microenvironment for a therapeutic purpose. Such therapeutics may include the following:
- Introduction of therapeutic genes that alter cell differentiation or survival
- Genetic material that alters expression of genes or repairs somatic errors

The evolution of cancer gene therapy has evolved with expanding knowledge of the genetic changes associated with dysplastic and malignant transformation of normal tissues and with the development of improved technologies for genetic transfer.

In the United States, the FDA's Center for Biologics Evaluation and Research (CBER) regulates human gene therapies that are considered biologics through the investigational new drug (IND) approval process.
- A large number of phase I and II clinical trials have focused on gene therapy for cancer. However, there has not been an effective, safe therapy approved for commercial use in the United States.
- Recently, gencidine, a recombinant adenovirus encoding p53, was approved for use in China and represents the first commercially available gene therapy product worldwide.

Gene therapy approaches generally fall under the following categories:
- Correction of genetic error
- Tumor suppressor gene therapy
- Antisense, RNAi, or ribozyme correction of genetic error
- Suicide gene therapy
- Tumor microenvironment-targeted therapy (anti-angiogenesis, cytokine therapy)
- Immunomodulation

Somatic correction of deficits and suicide gene therapy directed at tumors are thought to be more useful in the setting of minimal residual disease states. Immunomodulatory strategies seem useful in similar settings and can be employed in systemic or adoptive strategies.

Gene therapy represents a powerful tool in the quest to define effective immunotherapies for malignancies and represents one of the more important uses in the field.

Manipulation of tumor suppressor genes and oncogenes

Expression of tumor suppressor genes

The most straightforward application of gene therapy involves introduction of genetic material that inhibits the progression of malignancies (tumor suppressor genes).

Tumor suppressor genes are genes lost during carcinogenesis and have the following qualities:
- They link the cell cycle to DNA damage and repair mechanisms.
- They stop cell division in the setting of irreparable DNA damage.
- They may affect tumor adhesion factors (metastasis-suppressive factors).

Tumor suppressor genes control the progression through cellular mitotic checkpoints and thus cell division and tumor growth. Approximately 50% of human cancers are noted to be deficient in the tumor suppressor gene *p53*, which encodes a transcription factor involved in cell progression; conversely, 100% of persons with Li-Fraumeni syndrome caused by *p53* mutations develop malignancies.

The *p53* tumor suppressor gene exerts exquisite control of the G1/S transition in the setting of DNA damage through bax and fas signaling. Introduction of *p53* into human malignancies has been studied as a way of inducing tumor regression.

The recently approved agent gendicin consists of a recombinant adenovirus-expressing p53 targeted to patients with head and neck cancers. Phase I and II trials have been carried out using retroviral vectors targeting lung malignancies.

Other examples of tumor suppressor genes include the following:
- E-cadherin
- Retinoblastoma (Rb) gene
- PTEN

Tumor suppressor gene therapy may also be used to increase responsiveness to radiotherapy or chemotherapeutic agents, regardless of tumor *p53* status. Trials of *p53* gene therapy involving radiation therapy (XRT) and cisplatin responsiveness are ongoing.

Correction of mutant oncogenes

Gene therapy may also prove useful by correcting mutations in human oncogenes. Mutations in the proto-oncogene k-RAS are common in a wide variety of human malignancies and may confer resistance to emerging therapies such as EGFR inhibitors such as cetuximab.

Knockdown of expression of oncogenes may be accomplished by antisense nucleotides as well as emerging therapies such as RNAi or ribozyme correction of mRNA templates. Antisense technology uses stable DNA molecules to bind complementary sequences of RNA or DNA and suppress transcription or translation of further gene products.

The anti-bcl-2 antisense agent G3139 (oblimersen) has been studied in prostate cancer patients.

Introduction of chemotherapy sensitization and resistance genes

One limitation of conventional chemotherapeutic approaches has traditionally been toxicity associated with administration of cytotoxic drugs, given the nonspecific nature of these agents. Gene therapy techniques can be used to either enhance prodrug concentration and effect within tumors or decrease toxic drug effects within normal tissues. Examples include genetic prodrug activating therapy (GPAT), genetic-directed enzyme prodrug therapy (GDEPT), or virus-directed enzyme prodrug therapy (VDEPT), which have the following mechanisms of action:
- Preferential insertion of genetic material into cancer cells that encodes prodrug modifying enzymes or cofactors
- GPAT uses tumor-specific transcription factors to up-regulate expression of gene products within tumor cells, whereas GDPT and VDEPT rely on vector targeting to deliver genetic information within the tumor environment
- Production of cytotoxic metabolites from administered prodrugs
- Preferential killer of cancer cells with reduced toxicity

Chemotherapy resistance genes
- Chemotherapy resistance genes are introduced into normal tissues (for example, multidrug resistance genes such as *MDR-1*).
- Gene products cause efflux or detoxification of chemotherapeutics in normal tissues, allowing increased dosages of cytotoxic agents with reduced toxicity profiles.
- Hematopoietic stem cells have been transduced with MDR-1 and then used adoptively with high-dose chemotherapy for relapsed leukemia or lymphoma.

For, example, direct injection of plasmid DNA expressing cytosine deaminase under the erB-2 gene promoter was used in a small trial of breast cancer patients. Production of 5-FU from 5-fluorocytosine was then used in a suicide gene approach to selectively target tumor cells to cytotoxic therapy.

Immunotherapy for cancer

Growing evidence suggests that loss of tumor immunosurveillance plays a major role in the progression of malignancy. The discovery of viruses involved in tumorigenesis (such as HPV in cervical cancer) and tumor-associated antigens (TAA) has led researchers to target malignancies through immunotherapeutic approaches. These may take the form of nonspecific or specific immunotherapy strategies.

The aim of nonspecific therapy is to boost immunity against malignancies through enhancement of the systemic immune response. Examples include interferon-γ (IFN-γ) injection or use of high-dose interleukin-2 (IL-2) in metastatic renal cell cancer.

Administration of gene therapies that boost cytokines may be a source of future investigation.

Specific immunotherapy targets TAA, which are present specifically in cancer cells, presented on major histocompatibility complex (MHC) molecules, and able to be recognized by immune effector cells. Examples of specific immunotherapies follow.

Peptide vaccines
- If MHC epitopes are known for a particular TAA, injections of peptides with appropriate adjuvant (IFN-γ, for example) may be used.
- Synthetic peptides are widely available and safe through intradermal or subcutaneous routes.
- Their use is limited by the need for known epitopes of TAA.

Tumor cell lysate preparation
- Extracts of a patient's own tumor cells are either reinjected, pulsed, or fused with antigen-presenting cells (APCs).
- Obviates need to specify TAA.
- Labor-intensive preparation and the requirement of prepared cancer tissue limit widespread use, although streamlined protocols for vaccination may make this modality more attractive in the future.
- One phase III randomized control trial (RCT) showed an increase in progression-free survival in a group of patients with stage III renal cell carcinoma; other trials have been reported.

DNA vaccines
Vaccination with recombinant DNA expressing genes known to be up-regulated in malignancies has been used as a targeted vaccination tool. Presentation of antigenic proteins then occurs after delivery of genetic information through a vector approach.

Recognition of antigenic material induces cytotoxic and humoral responses that slow progression of the tumor. Targets using this approach include the following:
- Carcinoembryonic antigen (CEA), a tumor marker expressed on most gastrointestinal malignancies. CEA-positive malignancies have been targeted in numerous clinic trials.

- Her2/neu, the epidermal growth factor receptor expressed on breast, stomach, and pancreatic cancers. Notably, humoral response to Her2 may be effective in slowing tumor progression.
- MAGE-1, which is an embryonic gene product associated with malignant melanoma.

DNA vaccines are useful because they afford a high degree of specific protein expression and MHC presentation without knowledge of epitope binding. Limitations of DNA vaccines include the requisite for TAA to be known for specific tumors and obstacles associated with vector delivery of DNA.

Dendritic cell vaccination

To optimize the immune response to TAA vaccination, investigations aiming to optimize antigen presentation are underway.

Dendritic cells (DCs) are potent antigen-presenting cells (APCs) due to their expression of high levels of costimulatory molecules and MHC complexes. Their role in TH_1 immunity and the direction of T-cell responses to tumor vaccines make them ideal targets for cancer immunotherapy. Cultured DCs take up exogenous antigen or can be transduced with DNA vaccines through a variety of methods including viral vectors.

Elucidation of techniques for large-scale storage and expansion of DCs has made clinical trials involving autologous DCs loaded with peptides or transduced with TAA possible.

Adoptive therapies

TAA-specific cytotoxic T cells may be isolated and expanded for infusion; this technique specifically targets TAA and produces a large number of TAA-specific T cells Alternatively, T cells may be transduced with specific T-cell receptors through DNA incorporation or viral vectors.

Small studies have suggested that these methods produce effective antitumor immunity, but the clinical impact of such an approach is not known.

Modulation of regulatory T-cell (T_{reg}) response in cancer immunotherapy

Evidence suggests that an inhibitory immune compartment consisting of $CD4^+CD25^+$ T cells suppresses immune responses, especially in the setting of self-vaccination (such as in TAA vaccines). Approaches to decrease this component of the immune response have undergone investigation. Denileukin diftitox (Ontak) has been used to eliminate $CD25^+$ cells in an effort to accomplish this. Further investigation and use of therapies targeting this will likely be important in guaranteeing effective immunization against TAA.

Gene delivery

One of the most important challenges in gene therapy involves gene delivery, i.e., efficient, reproducible delivery that avoids untoward side effects. Methods include physical means and biological vectors.

Physical means
- Injection or infusion of naked DNA particles
- Liposomal DNA delivery
- Electroporation or use of the DNA "gene gun"

Physical gene transfer is simple, because infusion of DNA or DNA-liposomal complexes is affordable and not associated with systemic side effects. Unfortunately, these methods result in ineffective gene transfer that only lasts transiently.

Biological vectors

Bacterial vectors
- Wide arrays of biological vectors have been introduced that are capable of efficient, stable gene expression.
- Disadvantages include neutralizing immune responses and systemic toxicities.
- The potential for propagation of infectious agents and the technological complexity of these methods further limit their use.

Viral vectors (see Table 13.1)
- Viral vectors are largely limited by cytolytic activity and cellular toxicity.
- Expression of genes by viral vectors may result in expressed protein accounting for up to 40% of total cellular protein.
- Since this is often cytotoxic, many viral vectors such as adenoviral vectors are only useful for immunotherapy in which vaccination requires high expression of cellular protein.
- Retroviral and lentiviral systems are now available but limited by insertional mutagenesis and difficulty in obtaining sufficient viral titers.

Gene delivery
- Ex vivo—transferred to cellular products that are infused adoptively
- In vivo—systemic delivery targeting specific tissues, i.e., tumor vaccines, or exploiting differences in transcriptional activity between malignant and normal tissues

Table 13.1 Viral vectors for gene therapy

	Retrovirus	Adenovirus	Adeno-associated virus	Herpes virus	Alphavirus	Lentivirus
Advantages						
	Small genome	High titers	Small genome	High viral titers	High viral titers	Small genome
	Carries 10 kb insert	Carries 30 kb insert	Carries 5 kb insert	Carries 15 kb insert		
		High gene transfer/expression	Can infect nondividing cells	High gene transfer/expression	High gene expression, few systemic effects (excellent for immunization)	Can infect nondividing cells
Disadvantages						
	Requires actively dividing cells	High existing immunity	Less clinical research experience with AAV vectors	Large genome	Robust gene expression toxic to infected cells	
	Low titer yield	Possibility for systemic toxicity				
	Random integration, mutagenesis					

GENE DELIVERY 193

Chapter 14

Complementary and alternative medicine

Heather Shaw

Overview of complementary and alternative medicine *196*
Issues in cancer complementary and alternative medicine *197*
Major categories of complementary and alternative
 medicine therapies *198*
 Alternative medical systems *198*
 Energy therapies *198*
 Exercise therapies *199*
 Manipulative and body-based methods *199*
 Mind-body interventions *200*
 Nutritional therapeutics *201*
 Pharmacologic and biologic treatments *202*
 Spiritual therapies *203*
Further reading *204*

Overview of complementary and alternative medicine

Complementary and alternative medicine (CAM) is often defined as any medical system, practice, or product that is not thought of as standard or conventional care. Some practitioners of CAM define it as any practice falling outside "Western" or allopathic medical training.

Complementary medicine
Complementary medicine is **used along with** standard medicine.

Alternative medicine
Alternative medicine is **used in place of** standard treatments.

Complementary and alternative medicine may include dietary supplements, complex herbal mixtures, dietary modifications, acupuncture, massage therapy, magnet therapy, spiritual healing, and meditation.

It is crucial that CAM therapies receive the same scientific evaluation used to assess standard healthcare approaches. Because CAM therapies are proven safe and effective, they may become part of standard healthcare, particularly in supportive care.

The National Cancer Institute (NCI) has established an Office of Cancer CAM (OCCAM) that specifically addresses the use of CAM in the treatment, palliation, and prevention of cancer.

Issues in cancer complementary and alternative medicine

Studies have reported that approximately 80% of cancer patients use some form of CAM, and more than 60% use supplements concurrent with their cancer treatment. Significant supplement-chemotherapy and supplement-radiotherapy interactions have been reported.

Multiple studies have shown that many patients (~50%) are reluctant to discuss CAM therapies with their standard healthcare teams. Few cancer CAM therapies have been tested in randomized controlled trials (RCTs).

Mass media and Internet sources for information on cancer CAM are unreliable. A recent review of breast cancer information Web sites revealed that those discussing CAM therapies were 15 times more likely to contain inaccurate information.

Major categories of complementary and alternative medicine therapies

Major categories of CAM have been defined by the OCCAM. Multiple CAM therapies can be classified under more than one category, such as yoga, which has both an exercise and meditation component.

Therapies have been assigned to one of the three following groups:
- Beneficial in cancer: Effective in RCTs. No significant adverse effects have been reported.
- Unproven benefit: Efficacy not shown in randomized clinical trials. No significant adverse effects have been reported.
- Potentially harmful: Significant adverse effects have been observed. This last category can be extended to all of the practices if used solely as alternative therapy, i.e., in lieu of standard therapy.

Alternative medical systems

Alternative medical systems are built upon complete systems of theory and practice. Often, these systems have evolved apart from and earlier than the conventional medical approach used in the United States.

Beneficial in cancer

Acupuncture
This is one of the key components of traditional Chinese medicine. Treatment typically involves stimulation of anatomical points by insertion of thin needles into the skin. Acupressure and electroacupuncture are also used.

Benefits:
- Reduction in cancer-related pain
- Reduction in chemotherapy-induced nausea

Unproven benefit
- **Ayurveda** is an ancient system of healthcare native to India. The majority of treatment is herbal, but metals and minerals may be added.
- **Homeopathy** is the use of medicine with similar side effects to the illness being treated, but at extremely high dilutions, such that less than one molecule remains.
- **Naturopathy** is the use of natural remedies for treatment. Individual components may be beneficial. Practitioners may vary widely in their training.
- **Traditional Chinese medicine** (TCM) is a very broad category, including the methods of diagnosis and treatment. Individual components have been tested and shown to be beneficial.
- **Tibetan medicine** is an ancient system of healthcare native to Tibet. The majority of treatment is herbal, but precious metals may be added.

Energy therapies

Energy therapies involve the use of energy fields. There are two types, biofield therapies and electromagnetic-based therapies.

Biofield therapies
These are intended to affect energy fields that purportedly surround and penetrate the human body. The existence of such fields has not yet been scientifically proven.

Unproven benefit
- Reiki
- Therapeutic touch
- Polarity therapy

Electromagnetic-based therapies

These involve the unconventional use of electromagnetic fields, such as pulsed fields, magnetic fields, or alternating-current or direct-current fields.

Unproven benefit
- Pulsed electromagnetic fields
- Magnet therapy

Exercise therapies

Exercise therapies are those that involve movement, such as t'ai chi, yoga asanas, and other aerobic exercise.

Beneficial in cancer
Physical activity
Many forms of physical activity involving aerobic exercise have shown benefit. The amount, frequency, and intensity of activity have varied in studies. Prospective observational studies have suggested a reduction in recurrence of multiple cancers.
Benefits:
- Reduction of therapy-related fatigue
- Improvement in quality of life indices

Unproven benefit
- T'ai chi chuan is a Chinese exercise form that includes relaxation, deep and regulated breathing techniques, and slow movements.
- Yoga asanas is the physical exercises of yoga practice.

Manipulative and body-based methods

Manipulative and body-based methods in CAM are based on manipulation and/or movement of one or more parts of the body.

Beneficial in cancer
Therapeutic massage
This involves the manipulation of soft tissue areas of the body. There are many different kinds of massage derived from both Western and Eastern traditions, including Swedish massage, trigger point therapy, lymphatic drainage, shiatsu, and Thai massage. Benefits include
- Reduction of chemotherapy-induced nauseas and vomiting (CINV)
- Reduction in anxiety

Unproven benefit
- Chiropractic methods focus on disorders of the musculoskeletal system and the nervous system, and the effects of these disorders on general health. The most common procedure is the manipulation of the spine; rarely, cervical spine manipulation may result in adverse events.
- Reflexology consists of firm pressure to specific points on the feet, hands, or ears. Reflexology is based on the principle that these regions contain links that correspond to every other part of the body.

Mind-body interventions

Mind-body medicine involves a variety of techniques designed to enhance the mind's capacity to affect bodily function and symptoms.

Beneficial in cancer

Meditation

Most trials have investigated mindfulness-based stress reduction (MBSR), which is a combination of mindfulness meditation—being "in the moment"—and yoga practices. There are numerous other forms of meditation, falling into either concentrative or mindfulness practices. Concentrative meditation focuses on clearing the mind and focusing on a single object, whereas mindfulness meditation involves close attention to physical and mental experiences.

Benefits:
- Reduction in mood disturbances
- Reduction in stress
- Improvement in sleep quality
- Reduction in fatigue
- Decreased blood pressure

Relaxation and guided imagery

This consists of progressive body relaxation and/or guided imagery. Typically, a tape will be used that gives direction on relaxation of parts of the body and/or imagination of being in a peaceful place.

Benefits:
- Reduction in anxiety and depression
- Reduction in CIMV
- Reduction in anticipatory nausea and vomiting
- Reduction in fatigue
- Decreased blood pressure

Yoga

Yoga is collection of spiritual techniques and practices aimed at integrating the mind, body, and spirit. There are many different yoga traditions. Those used in the West derive from the ancient Indian Hatha yoga, incorporating stretches and poses, breathing exercises, and meditation. Yoga tested in cancer clinical trials has generally been modified for use by cancer patients.

Benefits:
- Reduction in fatigue
- Reduction in mental distress
- Improvement in sleep

Art therapy

This is a form of expressive therapy using art materials. Benefits include
- Improvement in coping resources
- Improved health-related quality of life

Music therapy

This is a form of therapy using active music participation or passive listening. Benefits include
- Decreased mood disturbance
- Improved quality of life

Unproven benefit
- Aromatherapy is the use of aromatic essential oils in inhalation or massage settings.
- Support groups

Nutritional therapeutics

This involves an assortment of nutrients and non-nutrients, bioactive food components used as chemopreventive agents, and the use of specific foods or diets as cancer prevention or treatment strategies.

Beneficial in cancer
- Vitamin D plus calcium reduces the risk of breast cancer.
- Acetyl-L-carnitine reduces neuropathy due to taxanes and platinums.
- A low-fat diet reduces ovarian cancer risk and breast cancer recurrence.

Significant in prospective cohort studies
A number of dietary factors have been shown to influence the risk of cancer in prospective cohort studies. Some factors, such as alcohol consumption, cannot be tested in an RCT.
- Reduced alcohol intake
- Increased dietary lignan intake
- Reduced fat intake
- Decreased red meat intake
- Decreased processed meat intake

Unproven benefit
- Macrobiotic diet
- High fruit and vegetable diet
- Orthomolecular medicine
- Indole-3-carbinol (I3C)/3,3'-diindolylmethane (DIM)
- Selenium
- Coenzyme Q10
- Vitamin D
- Vitamin C
- Flaxseed

Potentially harmful
- **Gerson therapy** consists of a strict low-sodium diet, consumption of large amounts of juice from fruits, vegetables, and calf liver, and frequent coffee enemas. No credible cancer cures have resulted from this therapy, and deaths from the therapy have been reported.
- **Gonzalez regimen** combines prescribed diets, nutritional supplements, pig pancreatic enzymes, and twice-daily coffee enemas. Frequent enemas can cause significant electrolyte abnormalities.
- **Soy phytoestrogens**: Isoflavones in soy bind weakly to the estrogen receptor, potentially causing growth in estrogen-dependent cancers.
- **Vitamin E/α-tocopherol supplements** may increase risk of cancer development and impair efficacy of chemotherapy and radiation therapy.
- **Vitamin A/β-carotene supplements** may increase risk of cancer development and impair efficacy of chemotherapy and radiation therapy.

Pharmacologic and biologic treatments

Such treatments include off-label use of prescription drugs, hormones, complex natural products, vaccines, and other biological interventions not yet accepted in mainstream medicine.

Beneficial in cancer

- **Melatonin**: Prolonged survival after whole-brain radiation for brain metastases from solid tumors.

Unproven benefit

- **Immunoaugmentative therapy (IAT)** involves use of injections of unknown proteins derived from human blood. There is no scientific evidence that it treats or cures cancer. In the 1980s, patients were reported with serious infections; none have been publicly reported since then.
- **Low-dose naltrexone**: Use of naltrexone at approximately one-tenth the therapeutic dose to augment the immune system
- *714X* is an injected medication that contains nitrogen as its primary ingredient, camphor as its vehicle, mineral salts, and 18 trace elements. No evidence exists that it can treat or cure cancer. Importation to the United States is illegal.

Potentially harmful

- **Laetrile** is a purified form of the chemical amygdalin, found in many fruit pits. Side effects resemble those of cyanide poisoning.
- **Chelation therapy**: Disodium EDTA chelation therapy (oral or IV) has caused deaths from hypocalcemia. Renal failure and bone marrow toxicity have also resulted.
- **Hydrazine sulfate** has not proven effective in RCTs, and use may result in significant neurological side effects.
- **Dichloroacetic acid (DCA)** is a potent reducer of lactic acid but causes peripheral neuropathy and hepatotoxicity in adults.
- **Antineoplastons** are a mixture of amino acid derivatives, peptides, and amino acids found in human blood and urine. Severe neurotoxic side effects have been reported.

Subcategory: complex natural products

These remedies are derived from plants, fungi, other microorganisms, animal tissues, or marine organisms used for healing and treatment of disease. Products range from dried and pulverized material to crude, unfractionated organic extracts, and semipurified extract fractions. As the name implies, complex natural products contain dozens or hundreds of chemical compounds, in contrast to single-agent natural-product therapeutics such as paclitaxel or doxorubicin. Many of the products listed under "Unproven benefit" have shown promising results in preclinical cancer studies and are undergoing further investigation.

Beneficial in cancer

- *Lactobacillus* sp/**probiotic supplements** reduce 5-FU-induced diarrhea and radiation-induced diarrhea. Patients with immunosuppression are excluded from trials.

Unproven benefit (most commonly used, not a comprehensive list)
- Mistletoe (*Viscum album*) (Iscador, Helixor)
- Shark cartilage
- Noni juice (*Morinda citrifolia*)
- Milk thistle (*Silybum marianum*)
- Curcumin or turmeric (*Curcuma longa*)
- Fermented wheat germ (Avemar)
- MGN-3 is an extract of arabinoxylan from rice bran.
- Green tea or epigallocatechin-3-gallate (EGCG)
- Black cohosh (*Actea racemosa*)
- Garlic (*Allium sativum*)
- Ginger (*Zingiber officianale*)
- Ginkgo (*Ginko biloba*)

Potentially harmful
- **Red clover** (*Trifolium pratense*) is found in numerous herbal blends. It contains phytoestrogens that may increase growth of estrogen-dependent cancers.
- **Essiac** is a combination of several herbs, usually taken as a tea. One common component is red clover. There is no proven benefit in treating cancer.
- **Hoxsey therapy** is use of an herbal mixture internally and externally in combination with diet restrictions. Illegal in the United States, the internal tonic contains pokeweed, burdock root, licorice, barberry, buckthorn bark, stillingia root, red clover, prickly ash bark, potassium iodide, cascara, and sometimes other ingredients. Side effects include nausea, vomiting, and diarrhea.
- **St. John's wort** (*Hypericum perforatum*) is a potent inducer of CYP3A4, which is responsible for metabolizing 50% of prescription drugs. Its induction increases the drugs' clearance (and decreases their effectiveness). CYP3A4 metabolizes many chemotherapeutic drugs, including paclitaxel, etoposide, vinorelbine, imatinib, ifosfamide, and others.

Spiritual therapies

Such therapies have to do with deep, often religious, feelings and beliefs, including a person's sense of peace, purpose, connection to others, and beliefs about the meaning of life.

Unproven benefit
- Intercessory prayer
- Spiritual healing

Further reading

Deng G, Cassileth BR (2005). Integrative oncology: complementary therapies for pain, anxiety, and mood disturbance. *CA Cancer J Clin* 55:109–116.

Sparreboom A, Cox MC, Acharya MR, Figg WD (2004). Herbal remedies in the United States: potential adverse interactions with anticancer agents. *J Clin Oncol* 22:2489–2503.

Weiger WA, Smith M, Boon H, et al (2002). Advising patients who seek complementary and alternative medical therapies for cancer. *Ann Intern Med* 137:889–903.

Chapter 15

Clinical trials

Erika Hamilton
Jeffrey Peppercorn

Introduction 206
History of clinical trials 207
The ethics of clinical research 208
Safety and efficacy considerations 209
Phases of clinical trials 210
Additional information 212

CHAPTER 15 Clinical trials

Introduction

- Cancer still causes over 7.5 million deaths worldwide each year, and more effective interventions are needed in many settings.
- Clinical trials are research studies designed to evaluate new therapeutic options in human subjects and are often closely integrated with cancer care.
- Initial studies test the safety of novel interventions in small numbers of research subjects.
- Later studies evaluate efficacy and safety in larger numbers of subjects with specific types of cancer in specific settings.
- Most interventions will require testing in large randomized control trials (RCTs) to establish efficacy and safety compared with a standard treatment option.
- The design and conduct of cancer clinical trials thus carries special ethical responsibilities to safeguard the interests of research participants.
- These trials often require many years and millions of dollars to complete.
- Only a minority of compounds tested will successfully pass each successive phase of clinical testing.

History of clinical trials

- Medical practice was traditionally based on theory handed down from Hippocrates (460–361 B.C.) and Galen (129–200 A.D.).
- Several empirical studies challenged the dominance of theory over empiricism such as Cotton Mather's test of inoculation for smallpox in 1721 and James Linds trials at sea to test citrus to prevent and treat scurvy in 1747. Linds also used control groups for the first time.
- Pierre Louis pioneered the systematic evaluation of safety and efficacy of medical treatment through observational studies of blood letting and pneumonia, published in 1836.
- The first randomized trial was conducted by Johannes Fibiger who demonstrated the efficacy of diphtheria serum in 1896, but randomized comparison did not become standard for decades.
- The U.S. FDA was established by the Food, Drugs, and Cosmetics Act of 1938 in response to a scandal in which unsafe and insufficiently tested medication killed hundreds of patients.
- Modern randomized trial methodology began with the British Medical Research Council trial of streptomycin for pulmonary TB in 1946 and also featured blind assessment of the treatment groups.
- Cancer trials began in 1946 when Louis Goodman and Alfred Gilman demonstrated that nitrogen mustard could treat lymphoma.
- Multicenter cooperative groups were established by the National Cancer Institute in the 1950s to conduct cancer clinical trials.
- In 1962, the U.S. Congress required the FDA to evaluate efficacy, as well as safety, of medications.
- By the 1960s, the RCT was established as the gold standard for clinical research and adjuvant trials of chemotherapy, as well as trials for advanced disease.

The ethics of clinical research

- Concerns over the ethics of clinical trials, and the field of bioethics arose in response to scandals in human subjects research.
- In response to Nazi science, the Nuremburg Code of 1949 elaborated principles to guide medical research including requirement for voluntary informed consent by research subjects and the requirement to minimize harm to research subjects.
- Further definition of requirements for the ethical conduct of clinical trials continued in the Declaration of Helsinki (1964), the Belmont Report (1978), the establishment of the Common Rule (1981), and subsequent revisions of these documents and others.
- When testing novel cancer interventions among patients who actively need treatment, it is important to understand that by definition, we are subjecting the participants to unknown risks and benefits.
- Seven core principles of the ethical conduct of research common to most codes of ethics have been elaborated:
  1. The research must have social or scientific value
  2. The research methods must have scientific validity
  3. There must be fair selection of research subjects
  4. There must be a favorable ratio of risks to research subjects to the chance of benefit from the research
  5. The research must be independently reviewed
  6. Research subjects must provide informed consent to participate
  7. Respect for potential and enrolled subjects must be maintained at all times

Safety and efficacy considerations

Patient safety
- Protocols are designed to minimize harm to research subjects.
- "Clinical equipoise" is used to define a situation when based on available evidence that there is uncertainty within the medical community over whether an experimental intervention is likely to be superior, inferior, or equivalent to a standard therapy.
- If we can accurately claim that there is clinical equipoise among the arms of a given trial, it is considered ethical to randomly assign participants to any of the trial interventions.
- Studies are reviewed by independent Institutional Review Boards (IRB) at each study site to ensure that subjects' safety is protected.
- Data in large Phase III may be reviewed periodically by Data Safety Monitoring Board (DSMB), and trial may be stopped early if interim analysis suggests that one treatment is clearly superior or inferior to another.

Efficacy outcomes of interest
- Overall survival is the most clinically relevant endpoint, but it requires prolonged patient follow-up in many trials.
- Surrogate endpoints such as median time to progression or radiographic response rate are frequently used to shorten duration of clinical trials.
- For adjuvant trials, disease-free survival is often the primary endpoint.
- Quality of life is often an important secondary endpoint and can be assessed using validated surveys.
- Patient reported outcomes may better reflect the experience of toxicity and quality of life by trial participants.

Correlative science endpoints
- Increasingly, we want to understand not just whether a drug works, but also why or why not, and which patients are most likely to respond.
- Correlative science seeks to identify molecular features of a cancer that are associated with response or resistance to therapy.
- Such research often requires tissue, either from blood samples or tumor biopsies, and the consent of patients to obtain these samples.

Phases of clinical trials

Phase 0
- Novel concept of accelerated testing in humans using low doses of the investigational drug to measure pharmacokinetic and pharmacodynamic data.
- Designed to allow early elimination of compounds that do not perform as predicted in humans, and to save on expensive further testing.
- Less than 20 patients.

Phase I
- Standard initial study of novel interventions in humans, designed to evaluate safety.
- Standard design is dose-escalation study to determine the dose-limiting toxicities and maximal tolerated dose of the investigational agent.
- Alternative designs may evaluate biologically effective dose, in less toxic targeted agents.
- Single arm trials.
- Often <50 patients.
- Ensures the drug is safe and identifies the dose and delivery strategy to move to Phase II.

Phase II
- Studies to measure the efficacy and safety of the investigational agent in larger numbers of patients, and in a particular type of cancer.
- Typically single-arm trials.
- Randomized Phase II trials may be used to determine dose or regimen for further development in larger randomized trials.
- Often <100 patients.
- If the treatment shows sufficient efficacy in a specific cancer setting and further evidence of safety and tolerability, it may move to Phase III.

Phase III
- Comparison studies to evaluate efficacy and safety of novel interventions compared with standard therapy.
- Multiarm trials.
- Involve hundreds to thousands of patients.
- Patients are randomly assigned to one of the study arms to reduce potential for bias and confounding.
- Standard care arm may involve a placebo control in a setting where there is no proven benefit to therapy; this is rare in oncology clinical trials.
- Blinded trials, in which the subject or the subject and physician are unaware of the treatment assignment to reduce bias in interpretation of outcomes, are ideal, but they are rarely used in oncology due to the toxicity of many interventions and the reliance on hard outcomes such as survival.

Phase IV
- Postmarketing surveillance studies conducted after approval and sale of a new agent.
- Designed to evaluate for adverse effects that may not have been discovered in the smaller numbers of patients involved in initial clinical trials.
- Often involves thousands of patients.

Additional information

- Allison R, Baer RN, BSN, Mary Lou Smith JD, MBA, Deborah Collyar BS, Jeffrey Peppercorn, MD, MPH. (2010). Issues surrounding biospecimen collection and use in clinical trials. *J Oncol Pract* 6:206–209.
- Chabner BA, Roberts TG Jr. (2005) Timeline: Chemotherapy and the war on cancer. *Nat Rev Cancer* 5:65–72.
- Emanuel EJ, Wendler D, Grady C. What makes clinical research ethical? *JAMA* 283:2701–2711.
- Freedman B. (1987) Equipoise and the ethics of clinical research. *N Engl J Med* 317:141–145.
- Guideline for Good Clinical Practice, International Conference on Harmonization of Technical Requirements for Registration of Pharmaceuticals For Human Use. Federal Register Vol. 62, No. 90, May 9, 1997, pp. 25691–25709.
- Jemal A, Siegel R, Ward E, Hao Y, Xu J, Murray T, Thun MJ. (2008). *CA Cancer J Clin* 58:71–96. doi: 10.3322/CA.2007.0010. Epub 2008 Feb 20
- Vogel M, Rosenberg, C. *The Therapeutic Revolution*. Philadelphia; University of Pennsylvania Press, 1979.
- www.clinicaltrials.gov
  - database of ongoing clinical trials maintained by the U.S. National Institutes of Health
  - searchable by disease, therapy, and study locations

Part IV
Complications and supportive care

16 Anemia and fatigue	215
17 Febrile neutropenia	229
18 Pain management	251
19 Venous thromboembolism	271
20 Metabolic emergencies	289
21 Paraneoplastic syndromes	303
22 Superior vena cava syndrome and raised intracranial pressure	321
23 Spinal cord compression	331
24 Other obstructive complications	337
25 Late effects of cancer treatment	351
26 End-of-life care	363

Chapter 16

Anemia and fatigue

Gary H. Lyman

Introduction *216*
Overview of treatment of anemia *218*
Recommendations for the treatment of anemia *220*
Safety considerations *224*
Fatigue in patients with cancer *226*

Chapter 16: Anemia and fatigue

Introduction

Fatigue is common in patients with cancer. It is particularly common in those receiving chemotherapy. Causes of fatigue are multifactorial and include the following:
- Release of inflammatory cytokines
- Sleep disturbances
- Depression
- Malnutrition
- Hormone withdrawal (menopause and/or antiestrogen therapy in women, chemical castration in men)
- Pain and pain medications
- Systemic effects of chemotherapy
- Comorbidities including liver, heart, and kidney dysfunction

A significant proportion (15%–25%) of the fatigue experienced by cancer patients is due to moderate or even mild anemia.

Treatment of anemia in cancer patients is associated with improvements in energy levels and productivity. In managing fatigue in cancer patients, it is important to evaluate the hematologic status of the patient and address any anemia present.

Overview of treatment of anemia

Anemia is the most common hematologic abnormality encountered in cancer patients. Anemia in cancer patients is associated with considerable morbidity, mortality, and costs.[1]

Causes of anemia in cancer patients
- Nutritional anemia, including iron deficiency and vitamin B_{12} or folic acid deficiency, particularly in cancers of gastrointestinal origin
- Hemolysis, usually occurring in patients with lymphoid malignancies
- Anemia of chronic disease with suppression of endogenous erythropoietin production by circulating cytokines resulting in erythropoietin resistance or inadequate utilization of iron
- Myelosuppression due to chemotherapy or radiation therapy
- Rarely, bone marrow involvement with the malignancy

Treatment options

Red cell transfusions are usually limited to the treatment of severe anemia (hemoglobin level <8 g/dL) or in patients with active bleeding or other life-threatening complications.

Erythropoiesis-stimulating agents (ESAs) promote survival and proliferation of red cell precursors in the bone marrow, increasing red cell production. This leads to a decrease in transfusion requirements and fatigue and a decrease in fatigue in cancer patients receiving chemotherapy.[2]
- Epoetin-α is typically administered at a starting dose of 40,000 U/week by subcutaneous injection.
- Darbepoetin-α is usually administered at a starting dose of 200 μg subcutaneously every 2 weeks or 300 μg every 3 weeks in those with corresponding every 3-week chemotherapy regimens.[3]
- Epoetin-β is available in Europe but not in the United States.
- There is no convincing evidence that one ESA is more effective or less toxic than another when used in the treatment of anemia in cancer patients receiving chemotherapy.
- The ESAs are approved only for cancer patients who are receiving cancer chemotherapy and not for patients with anemia of cancer who are not receiving chemotherapy.
- Due to recent safety concerns and variation in reimbursement policies, the most current approved treatment setting and hemoglobin trigger along with the patients' insurance coverage for these agents may continue to change and should always be considered in the decision to support a cancer patient with an ESA.

---

1 Lyman GH, Berndt ER, Kallich JD, et al. (2005). The economic burden of anemia in cancer patients receiving chemotherapy. *Value in Health* 8:149–156.

2 Littlewood TJ, Bajetta E, Nortier JW, Vercammen E, Rapoport B (2001). Effects of epoetin-A on hematologic parameters and quality of life in cancer patients receiving nonplatinum chemotherapy: results of a randomized, double-blind, placebo-controlled trial. *J Clin Oncol* 19:2865–2874.

3 Vansteenkiste J, Pirker R, Massuti B, et al. (2002). Double-blind, placebo-controlled, randomized phase III trial of darbepoetin-α in lung cancer patients receiving chemotherapy. *J Natl Cancer Inst* 94:1211–1220.

- The safety and efficacy of ESAs in the treatment of patients with myeloid malignancies have not been established, so these agents should not be used outside of a clinical trial.
- A meta-analysis of randomized trials of ESAs found that the risk of transfusion is reduced by approximately 50% when ESAs are started early (e.g., hemoglobin 10 g/dL or higher) rather than late (e.g., hemoglobin 10 g/dL or less).[4]
  - Likewise, the greatest improvement in quality of life appears to be in the range of 10 g/dL to 12 g/dL hemoglobin.
  - There is often a delay between the initiation of ESAs and an increase in hemoglobin.
- Nevertheless, safety concerns have led to guideline recommendations from the American Society of Clinical Oncology (ASCO) and the National Comprehensive Cancer Network (NCCN) to recommend routine use of these agents only when hemoglobin levels fall to 10 g/dL or lower.[5]

---

4 Lyman G, Glaspy JA (2006). Are there clinical benefits with early erythropoietic intervention for chemotherapy-induced anemia? A systematic review. *Cancer* 106:223–233.

5 Rizzo JD, Sommerfield MR, Hagerty KL, et al. (2008). Use of epoetin and darbepoetin in patients with cancer: 2007 American Society of Hematology/American Society of Clinical Oncology clinical practice guidelines update. *J Clin Oncol* 26:132–149.

Recommendations for the treatment of anemia

Red blood cell transfusion
Patients with severe anemia (Hb <8 g/dL) should be considered for red blood cell transfusions, especially if they are experiencing cardiovascular symptoms.

Erythropoiesis-stimulating agents
The ESAs have been shown to reduce the frequency of severe anemia and the requirement for red blood cell transfusion and to improve the quality of life of anemic cancer patients receiving chemotherapy.
- ESAs may be considered in patients with solid tumors, chronic lymphocytic leukemia, or non-Hodgkin's lymphoma and in patients with multiple myeloma who are not receiving thalidomide and chemotherapy or corticosteroids.
- ESAs may be considered when the hemoglobin approaches or falls below 10 g/dL or, under special clinical circumstances, for hemoglobin levels in the range of 10–12 g/dL.
- Reassess at 4 weeks and adjust dose accordingly.

Initial treatment with epoetin-α may be dosed every 3 weeks or weekly, whereas darbepoetin can be dosed weekly or every 3 weeks.

Adjusting doses
- A target hemoglobin concentration of 12 g/dL is reasonable.
- If hemoglobin >12 g/dL and rising, ESA should be withheld and resumed at a reduced dose when hemoglobin falls below 11 g/dL.
- If the hemoglobin level is still beneath the target range, and a 1 g/dL increase in hemoglobin concentration is not observed within 4 to 6 weeks, increase the ESA dose. Rather than progressive dose escalation for the unresponsive or poorly responsive patient, give a therapeutic trial of parenteral iron.

Parenteral iron

Patients with cancer may have reduced iron reserves due to blood loss and decreased oral intake. Cancer patients may experience decreased iron absorption or develop functional iron deficiency from an inability to access storage iron because of increased hepcidin expression.

Randomized clinical trials have demonstrated greater increases in hemoglobin in chemotherapy-associated anemia when ESAs are accompanied by concurrent parenteral iron. Patients receiving a single infusion of the total calculated dose of dextran experience a greater ESA response.

Parenteral iron agents include the following:
- Iron destran: Total replacement dose as a single dose or 100 mg weekly. The rate should not exceed 50 mg/min.
- Ferric gluconate: 125 mg weekly for 8 weeks

Decision making may be difficult for cancer patients with anemia of chronic illness, because ferritin is often elevated and iron, iron-binding capacity, and saturation are decreased.

222 CHAPTER 16 **Anemia and fatigue**

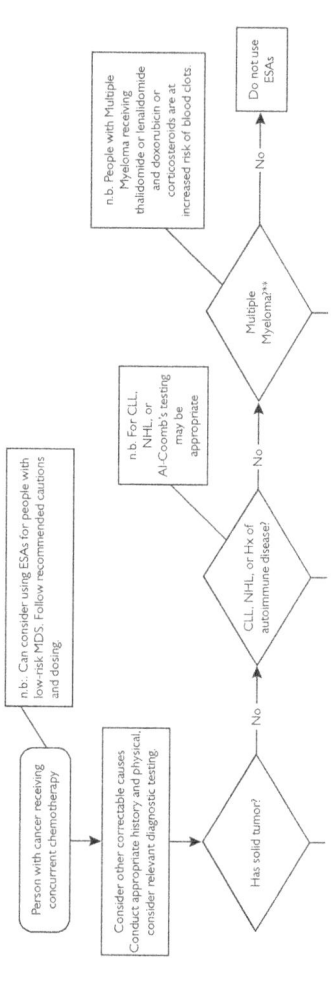

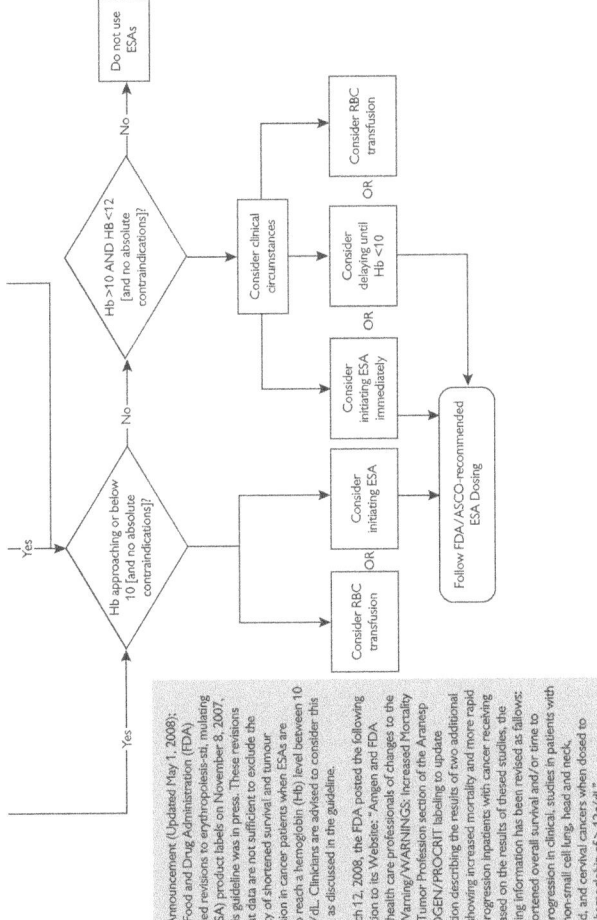

Safety considerations

Thrombosis

An increased risk of venous thromboembolism (VTE) has been found in a meta-analysis of randomized controlled trials of patients undergoing cancer chemotherapy and receiving ESAs.[1] The risk appears to be greatest in clinical trials targeting a hemoglobin level >12 g/dL.

However, the possible basis of any increased risk of VTE with the ESAs is unclear, because the cancer itself, cancer chemotherapy, and central lines are all recognized high-risk factors for the occurrence of VTE and similar levels of increased risk recently observed in cancer patients receiving red blood cell transfusions.

Nevertheless, ESAs should be used with caution in the following circumstances:
- A personal or family history of VTE
- Patients with an elevated platelet count (>350,000/mm^3)
- Symptoms or signs of infection, e.g., WBC >11,000/mm^3
- Obesity, e.g., body mass index >35 kg/m^2
- Certain high-risk cancers, e.g., gastric, pancreas

Until these safety issues are further addressed, a target hemoglobin level at or below 12 g/dL is recommended.

Other safety issues

A few recent randomized controlled trials in certain cancer populations have observed increased disease progression and even increased mortality.

A recent meta-analysis of randomized trials of ESAs in cancer patients receiving chemotherapy has shown a nonsignificant trend toward increased mortality (relative risk = 1.08 [95% CI: 0.99–1.19]).[1]

Increased risk was largely limited to studies in which hemoglobin was increased above recommended levels, e.g., 12 g/dL. An individual patient data meta-analysis is being conducted to further clarify any safety issues around disease progression and increased mortality. The safety of increasing hemoglobin levels above this range has not been demonstrated and should be avoided in this population

The safety of the ESAs has not been demonstrated in the following situations, and their use should be avoided until further safety data are available:
- Cancer of anemia in patients not receiving chemotherapy
- Patients receiving radiation therapy

---

1 Bohlius J, Wilson J, Seidenfeld J, et al. (2006). Recombinant human erythropoietins and cancer patients: updated meta-analysis of 57 studies including 9353 patients. *J Natl Cancer Inst* 98:708–714.

Fatigue in patients with cancer

Evaluation of the patient with fatigue
Fatigue represents a debilitating sense of a loss of energy that is often accompanied by depression, decreased appetite, cachexia, and general debilitation. Fatigue is arguably the most common symptom reported by cancer patients, including those who receive cancer chemotherapy.

Anemia may represent the most common treatable explanation for the high incidence of fatigue among cancer patients but explains less than half of the fatigue reported in this population. Fatigue may occur in the absence of significant anemia and have other explanations even among anemic cancer patients; it should generally be considered multifactorial.

Fatigue is a common complaint and may worsen during the period when cancer patients receive chemotherapy, hormonal therapy, immunotherapy, or radiation therapy.

Fatigue has been consistently reported in previously premenopausal women who experience premature, abrupt cessation of menstruation and symptoms of menopause during treatment with systemic chemotherapy and hormonal therapy.

Treatment of fatigue in the cancer patient
Treating accompanying causes of fatigue
In the patient with fatigue, it is important to address any treatable accompanying symptom of disease or treatment such as pain, fever or infection, insomnia, anorexia, depression, nausea, vomiting, and dehydration. Unfortunately, fatigue without other definable explanations may be an indicator of advanced or progressing cancer despite treatment.

The therapeutic options for cancer patients with severe fatigue without other definable symptoms or signs of disease or improvement after treatment of other symptoms remain limited and an area of active clinical investigation.

Treating unexplained fatigue

Traditional therapeutic efforts for unexplained or refractory fatigue in the patient with cancer have included the following:
- Nonsteroidal anti-inflammatory drugs (NSAIDs)
- Antidepressants
- Corticosteroids
- Central nervous system stimulants
  - Methylphenidate (Ritalin): 10 mg po bid or tid
  - Dexmethylphenidate (Focalin): 5 mg po bid initially (full therapeutic dose 25 mg po bid)
  - Modafinil (Provigil): 200 mg po qd

Regular exercise, when feasible, has been accompanied by measurable reductions in symptoms of fatigue among cancer patients.

Psychosocial support and counseling when indicated are components of the multidisciplinary care of patients with cancer.

Chapter 17

Febrile neutropenia

Gary H. Lyman
Nicole M. Kuderer

Introduction 230
Risk of febrile neutropenia 232
Complications of febrile neutropenia 234
Evaluation of the patient with febrile neutropenia 236
Empiric antibiotic therapy 242
Prophylaxis of febrile neutropenia 248
Key point summary 250

Introduction

Myelosuppression and febrile neutropenia

Myelosuppression remains the leading cause of dose-limiting toxicity associated with systemic cancer chemotherapy.

- Fever in the setting of neutropenia or febrile neutropenia (FN) is defined as a single temperature of ≥38.3°C (101.0°F) or a sustained temperature ≥38.0°C (100.4°F) for at least 1 hour in a patient with an absolute neutrophil count (ANC) <500 cells/mm^3 or <1000 cells/mm^3 and likely to fall below 500/mm^3.[1]

Early studies demonstrated that even in the absence of clinical signs or symptoms, most patients with FN have occult bacterial infections with a high risk of early mortality unless treated with immediate antibiotics.

FN is a **medical emergency** generally prompting immediate hospitalization for evaluation and the administration of empiric broad-spectrum antibiotics.

---

1 Hughes WT, Armstrong D, Bodey GP, et al. (2002). 2002 guidelines for the use of antimicrobial agents in neutropenic patients with cancer. *Clin Infect Dis* 34:730–751.

Risk of febrile neutropenia

The risk of FN increases in proportion to the severity and duration of neutropenia.

Patients with documented gram-negative bacteremia often experience a rapid and fatal outcome without antibiotic therapy while awaiting culture results.

Patients with FN should generally be hospitalized emergently for evaluation and administration of empiric, broad-spectrum antibiotics, which considerably reduce the mortality associated with FN.

Risk factors for febrile neutropenia

The risk of FN varies with the type and intensity of the treatment regimen, delivered dose intensity, and host-related factors such as age, the type of cancer, and various comorbid conditions. Risk factors for FN are summarized in Box 17.1.

The timing of febrile neutropenia

The risk of initial episode of FN appears to be greatest during the first cycle of chemotherapy, when the majority of patients receive full-dose intensity often without FN prophylaxis.[1]

Early neutropenic complications generally prompt chemotherapy dose reductions, treatment delays, or the addition of a myeloid growth factor in subsequent cycles.

---

1 Lyman GH, Morrison VA, Dale DC, et al. (2003). Risk of febrile neutropenia among patients with intermediate-grade non-Hodgkin's lymphoma receiving CHOP chemotherapy. *Leuk Lymphoma* 44:2069–2076.

Box 17.1 Risk factors for febrile neutropenia

Treatment-related
- Previous history of severe neutropenia with similar chemotherapy
- Type of chemotherapy (anthracyclines)
- Planned relative dose intensity >80%
- Preexisting neutropenia or lymphocytopenia
- Extensive prior chemotherapy
- Concurrent or prior radiation therapy to marrow containing bone

Patient-related
- Age
- Female gender
- Poor performance status
- Poor nutritional status, e.g., low albumin
- Decreased immune function

Cancer-related
- Bone marrow involvement with tumor
- Advanced cancer
- Elevated lactate dehydrogenase (lymphoma)

Conditions associated with risk of serious infection
- Open wounds
- Active tissue infection

Comorbidities
- Chronic obstructive pulmonary disease (COPD)
- Cardiovascular disease
- Liver disease (elevated bilirubin, alkaline phosphatase)
- Diabetes mellitus
- Low baseline hemoglobin

Complications of febrile neutropenia

Episodes of FN are associated with substantial morbidity, mortality, and cost as well as dose reductions and treatment delays that may compromise the delivery of full-dose intensity.[1]

Morbidity

FN compromises patient quality of life:
- Requirement for hospitalization
- Performance of multiple tests
- Delivery of intravenous antibiotics
- General sense of ill health associated with fever or other signs of infection

Mortality

The risk of mortality associated with FN ranges up to 20%, with higher mortality rates among patients with comorbid conditions and infectious complications including septic shock.

Documented sepsis may lead to septic shock with hypotension, oliguria, lactic acidosis, and ultimately multiorgan dysfunction.
- Sepsis in patients with FN occurs in the range of approximately 20%–40%.
- Mortality rates as high as 80% have been reported in patients with FN and septic shock.

Polymicrobial bacteremia in neutropenic patients is associated with high mortality rates.
- Mortality rates as high as 50% are reported when pseudomonas is a component of a polymicrobial bacteremia.

Cancer patients with FN and pneumonia experienced mortality rates in excess of 50% when associated with gram-negative or gram-positive bacteremia.

Costs

The costs associated with FN in the United States range from $5000 to $20,000 per episode depending on the type of malignancy and presence of comorbidities and infectious complications.

Reduced chemotherapy dose intensity

Substantially reduced chemotherapy dose intensity associated with FN has been observed in more than half of patients receiving chemotherapy for breast cancer or non-Hodgkin lymphoma.

---

1 Kuderer NM, Dale DC, Crawford J, et al. (2006). Mortality, morbidity, and cost associated with febrile neutropenia in adult cancer patients. *Cancer* 106:2258–2266.

Evaluation of the patient with febrile neutropenia

Initial evaluation

Patients with FN should be immediately admitted, evaluated, and started on broad-spectrum antibacterial therapy within 1 hour of presentation (see Table 17.1).

The initial evaluation should include a careful history, detailed physical examination, appropriate radiological and laboratory examinations, as well as blood, wound, and other cultures with Gram stains when indicated.

- Rectal and vaginal examinations and manipulations should generally be avoided unless absolutely necessary.
- The elderly or immunosuppressed patient may not manifest a fever and may actually be hypothermic.
- Infection in the patient with neutropenia may not manifest common signs and symptoms of infection related to leukocyte infiltration (redness, swelling, pain, warmth, pus, nuchal rigidity, CSF pleocytosis, pyuria, and pulmonary infiltrates on chest radiograph).

Cultures should be sampled from every possible site of infection including two sets of blood cultures, intravenous lines or other catheters, sputum, urine with urinalysis, and skin lesions. In patients with diarrhea, stool cultures are indicated and should undergo *Clostridium difficile* antigen assay.

Cultures will remain negative in more than half of patients with FN, despite the likely infectious etiology of the fever.

Common sites of infection

- Central nervous system
- Head and neck: mucositis, gingivitis, sinusitis,
- Chest: pneumonia (bacterial, fungal, viral, parasitic)
- Gastrointestinal (GI): esophagitis, typhlitis, *C. difficile*, perirectal abscess, perianal cellulitis
- Genitourinary (GU): urinary tract infection
- Skin: cellulitis, vascular-access device, tunnel infection (erythema or tenderness >2 cm from catheter exit site)

Infectious agents

Bacterial organisms

- The most common offending bacterial organisms are gram-positive cocci, including both coagulase-positive and -negative *Staphylococcus*, *Streptococcus pneumoniae*, and other streptococci.
- The most common gram-negative bacteria are *Escherichia coli*, *Klebsiella*, *Pseudomonas*, and *Enterobacter*.
- Less common bacterial organisms include *Proteus*, *Haemophilus*, *Listeria*, *Serratia*, and various anaerobic bacteria.

Fungal organisms
- Common fungal organisms in patients with FN include *Aspergillus*, *Candida albicans*, and other *Candida* species. Less common fungi include *Cryptococcus*, *Histoplasma*, and *Coccidiomycosis*.
- Fungal infections are more likely to occur later in the treatment course after repeated episodes of FN and extensive exposure to antibiotics.

Viral organisms
Common viral etiologies include the herpes complex, cytomegalovirus (CMV), and the enteroviruses.

Parasitic infections
The most common parasitic infection is due to *Pneumocystis carinii*.

Antibiotic-resistant organisms
The increasing emergence of antibiotic-resistant organisms has been of considerable concern:
- Methicillin- or oxacillin-resistant *Staphylococcus aureas* (MRSA/ORSA)
- Vancomycin-resistant enterococcus (VRE)
- Vancomycin-resistant coagulase-negative staphylococci

Changing patterns of antibiotic sensitivity and the greater frequency of gram-positive organisms in patients with FN relate to the frequent use of venous access devices and prophylactic antibiotics.

Table 17.1 Febrile neutropenia management check List

I Initial evaluation (<1 hour)

1. History
  - Careful history with focus on new symptoms and sites that are commonly infected (especially symptoms of upper and lower respiratory tract, upper and lower GI tract, GU tract, skin and soft tissue changes, neurologic changes and pain, symptoms of hypotension, dehydration, and bleeding)
  - Timing and type of chemotherapy, recent antibiotics or growth factor usage
  - Recent infections, procedures, catheter placements, or surgeries
  - History of MRSA, VRE, HIV, or fungal infections; sick contacts or other infectious exposures (TB, pets) and travel history
  - Allergies and recent changes in medications; comorbid conditions

2. Physical exam
  - Complete and detailed physical examination should be performed, including vital signs, oropharynx, sinuses, ears, ocular fundi, mental status changes and meningismus, lungs, abdomen, new or change in cardiac murmur, skin changes, especially the perianal and genitourinary area, recent surgical and other procedure sites including indwelling catheter sites.

3. Radiological imaging
  - Additional imaging such as ultrasound or CT when symptoms or signs of local infection justify it.
  - CT scanning will often reveal pulmonary nodules or infiltration in patients with persistent fever despite a normal chest X-ray

4. Therapy and management
  - Additional antibiotics if indicated
  - Consider colony-stimulating growth factors
  - Supportive care as indicated, low threshold for more intensive care
  - Monitor vital signs closely

III. Follow-up (<24 hours)

1. History
  - Monitor chief complaints and perform detailed review of system
  - Red flags: Altered mental status and new neurological symptoms, respiratory compromise and increased oxygen need, acute pain, bleeding, hypotension

2. Physical exam
  - Detailed physical exam

- Digital rectal and vaginal examination should generally be avoided as well as taking rectal temperature. It is generally understood that infection in the patient with neutropenia may not manifest common symptoms and signs associated with infections, i.e., leukocyte infiltration (e.g., redness, swelling, pain, warmth, pus, nuchal rigidity).

3. *Laboratory evaluation*
   - Complete blood count and differential
   - Two sets of blood cultures from at least two separate sites; isolator systems cultures as indicated
   - Cultures and Gram stains from other possible sites of infection, including: urine, sputum, skin, and catheters
   - Evaluate for need of lumbar puncture and viral culture
4. *Radiologic imaging*
   - Chest radiograph in most patients
5. *Therapy and management*
   - Appropriate empiric broad-spectrum antibiotics (see IDSA guidelines) should be given after blood cultures are obtained but within 1 hour of assessment.
   - Removal of clearly infected catheter
   - Intravenous fluid if no contraindications
   - Initiate neutropenic precautions (depending on institutional guidelines)

3. *Laboratory evaluation*
   - Follow-up blood counts and renal function and other abnormal laboratory results
   - Follow-up culture data
4. *Imaging*
   - Reassess need for further imaging
5. *Therapy and management*
   - Supportive care as indicated, low threshold for more intensive care
   - Monitor vitals signs closely

IV. **Further evaluation (>24 hours)**
1. *History*
   - Monitor closely any changes in symptoms.
2. *Physical exam*
   - Daily detailed physical exam, especially vital signs, oropharynx, lungs, abdomen, skin, and catheters
3. *Laboratory evaluation*
   - Daily complete blood counts and differential (to monitor neutropenia)
   - Follow renal function, hepatic function, and other abnormal laboratory values at least twice per week.
   - Follow-up culture data, repeat blood cultures every 24 hours if continued fever, other cultures as clinically indicated

Table 17.1 (Cont.)

II. Additional evaluation (1–6 hours)

1. *History and physical exam*
   - Finalize if not yet finished
2. *Laboratory evaluation*
   - Complete metabolic profile including renal and liver function
   - Coagulation studies if bleeding, low platelets, or concern for bleeding diathesis
   - Urine analysis and rest of cultures if not already done, if diarrhea is present get stool cultures for *C. difficile* toxin immunoassay
4. *Imaging*
   - Reassess need for further imaging, especially if fever persists for several days despite appropriate therapy.
5. *Therapy and management*
   - Reassess appropriateness and length of antibiotic therapy.
   - Reassess need for colony-stimulating factors.
   - Supportive care as indicated, low threshold for more intensive care if patient remains neutropenic
   - Monitor vital signs closely.

Empiric antibiotic therapy

Empiric broad-spectrum antibiotics should be started within 1 hour of presentation, following acquisition of cultures, without awaiting the results of testing.

Empiric antibiotic regimens

Multiple empiric antibiotic regimens have been demonstrated to be effective, with no single regimen shown to be clearly superior to others (see Box 17.2).[1]

Because of the high risk for mortality associated with untreated gram-negative septicemia, empiric regimens always provide coverage for gram-negative bacilli, especially *Pseudomonas aeruginosa*.

Initial therapy

Initial therapy in the uncomplicated patient may involve the following:
- **Monotherapy**, e.g., cefepime, ceftazidime, imipenem-cilastatin, and meropenem. Although controversial, ceftazidime has been associated with suboptimal treatment of resistant streptococci compared with that of other monotherapy options.
- **Combination therapy** is preferred in more complicated cases, generally including an aminoglycoside combined with either a semisynthetic antipseudomonal penicillin (piperacillin-tazobactam or ticarcillin-clavulanate) or an antipseudomonal cephalosporin (cefepime or ceftazidim) or a carbapenem (imipenem-cilastatin or meropenem).
- When a specific organism has been identified or is suspected, the antibiotic regimen should include optimal coverage for that organism while maintaining broad coverage for other unknown but potentially serious organisms.

Vancomycin usage

Vancomycin should be avoided in the initial empirical therapy because of the emergence of vancomycin-resistant organisms, except for patients at high risk of serious gram-positive infections:
- Clinically suspected, serious catheter-related infection
- Blood culture positive for gram-positive bacterium
- Mucosal damage and high risk for infection with penicillin-resistant *Streptococcus viridans*, especially patients with preceding prophylaxis with quinolone antibiotics or trimethoprim/sulfamethoxazole
- Known colonization with penicillin/cephalosporin-resistant pneumococci or methicillin-resistant *Staphylococcus aureus*
- Hypotension or other cardiovascular impairment without identified pathogen

Antifungal therapy

Empiric antifungal therapy should be considered in the persistently febrile patient despite adequate empiric antibacterial therapy for 5–7 days.

Newer and less toxic antifungals such as voriconazole, caspofungin, and itraconazole have largely replaced amphotericin as the empiric antifungal agents of choice.

---

1 Hughes WT, Armstrong D, Bodey GP, et al. (2002). 2002 guidelines for the use of antimicrobial agents in neutropenic patients with cancer. *Clin Infect Dis* 34:730–751.

Box 17.2 IDSA (2002) guidelines for use of antimicrobial agents in neutropenic patients with cancer: executive summary[1]

Initial antibiotic therapy

1. Monotherapy
   - Cefepime or ceftazidime or imipenem or meropenem
2. Dual therapy
   - Aminoglycoside plus antipseudomonal beta-lactam, cephalosporin (cefepime or ceftazidime), or carbapenem
3. Vancomycin should be added to either monotherapy or dual therapy only if criteria are met[2]
4. Oral therapy (only for low-risk adults)
   - Ciprofloxacin plus amoxicillin-clavulanate

Afebrile within first 3–5 days of treatment

1. If etiology identified: Adjust to most appropriate treatment
2. If no etiology identified:
   - Low risk: Change after 48 hours to oral antibiotics (ciprofloxacin/amoxicillin-clavulanate {adults}, cefixime {children})
   - High risk: Continue same antibiotics

Persistent fever during first 3–5 days of treatment

1. Reassess on day 3
   - If no change: continue antibiotics; stop vancomycin if cultures are negative
   - If progressive disease: Change antibiotics
   - If febrile after day 5: Consider adding an antifungal drug with or without antibiotic changes

---

Fluconazole should generally not be used for empiric antifungal coverage due to emerging resistance and its ineffectiveness against several organisms, including *Aspergillus* and various *Candida* species.

Duration of antibiotic therapy

Afebrile within 3–5 days

- Patients who defervesce rapidly without an identified organism should be continued on antibiotics through neutrophil recovery.
- With an identified organism, directed therapy is essential for a standard period of time, e.g., 7–14 days, while maintaining broad coverage during the neutropenic period (see Box 17.3).
- Treatment may generally be stopped after 7 days in patients with negative cultures who become afebrile and recover counts.

Persistent fever for 3–5 days

- In neutropenic patients with persistent fever after 3–5 days, the antibiotic coverage should be modified, e.g., addition of vancomycin when appropriate.
- Persistent fever beyond any alteration of antibacterial therapy should prompt consideration of antifungal coverage.

Box 17.3 Specific suggested duration of therapy
- Skin/soft tissue: 7–14 days
- Bloodstream infection (uncomplicated)
  - Gram-negative: 10–14 days
  - Gram-positive: 7–14 days
  - *Staphylococcus aureus*: 2 weeks
  - Yeast: ≥2 weeks
- Sinusitis: 14–21 days
- Pneumonia: 14–21 days

Fungal (mold and yeast)
- Continue therapy until there is clinical, microbiologic, and radiologic resolution of infection and resolution of neutropenia.

Viral
- Herpes simplex virus: 7–10 days
  - Acyclovir, valacyclovir, or famciclovir
- Varicella-zoster virus: 7–10 days
  - Acyclovir, valacyclovir, or famciclovir
- Cytomegalovirus: 21 days
  - Ganciclovir (pneumonia: add IV immunoglobulin)
  - Foscarnet
  - Consider suppressive antiviral therapy for 2–4 weeks following completion of cytomegalovirus infection treatment.
- For seasonal respiratory viruses use pathogen-specific regimens.

Persistent neutropenia
- Continue antibiotics for 7–14 days with early disappearance of fever.
- Persistently febrile patients should be evaluated for fungal infection.
- Consideration of a trial off antibiotics after 14 days if no infectious site has been identified with close monitoring for reoccurrence.

Catheter infection
Tunnel infection or persistent positive cultures should prompt catheter removal. Other catheter site infections may be treated with intravenous antibiotics without line removal.

Outpatient management of FN
- Early discharge and treatment of FN as outpatients should be limited to low-risk patients.
- Such patients should be monitored closely for clinical deterioration, because available risk models, although useful, have limited accuracy.

Risk assessment in patients with febrile neutropenia

High-risk febrile neutropenic patients
A variety of risk factors for serious medical complications including death in patients with established FN have been reported. These include the development of FN as an inpatient, hypotension, sepsis, various comorbidities such as cardiovascular and pulmonary disease, leukemia, or lymphoma diagnosis, age >65, the severity and duration of neutropenia, prior fungal infection, visceral organ involvement, organ dysfunction, and uncontrolled malignancy.

Low-risk febrile neutropenic patients
In an effort to identify low-risk individuals for possible outpatient management, the Multinational Association of Supportive Care of Cancer (MASCC) identified independent factors at the time of presentation with FN among 756 cancer patients. A risk score was designed on the basis of multivariate analysis (see Table 17.2).[2]

Table 17.2 MASCC scoring index: Identifying low-risk febrile neutropenic patients*

Characteristics	Score
Burden of illness	
No/mild symptoms	5
Moderate symptoms	3
No hypotension	5
No chronic obstructive pulmonary disease	4
Solid tumor or no previous fungal infection	4
No dehydration	3
Outpatient at onset of fever	3
Age <60 years	2

* Score range 0–26: A risk score ≥21 indicates a low-risk patient for medical complications and mortality. Adapted from Klastersky et al. (2000).[2]

In the validation population, a risk score ≥21 identified low-risk patients for serious medical complications including death. Although the MASCC Index is used to identify low-risk patients, the limited test performance (sensitivity 71%; specificity 68%; positive predictive value 91%) and ability to identify low-risk patients should be kept in mind.

2 Klastersky J, Paesmans M, Rubenstein EB, et al. (2000). The Multinational Association for Supportive Care in Cancer risk index: a multinational scoring system for identifying low-risk febrile neutropenic cancer patients. *J Clin Oncol* 18:3038–3051.

Therapeutic use of myeloid growth factors

The myeloid growth factors are not recommended for routine use in the treatment of established FN. They may be considered in addition to antibiotics in critically ill patients especially with sepsis, pneumonia, or organ dysfunction.

A recent Cochrane meta-analysis of colony-stimulating factors (CSFs) as an adjunct to empiric antibiotics in patients with established FN indicated significant reductions in the length of hospitalization and infection-related mortality.[3]

The use of the CSFs should be considered in higher-risk patients hospitalized with FN, including the elderly, those with significant comorbidities (lung, heart, renal, liver disease), infectious complications such as hypotension, documented sepsis, and pneumonia, and those with very severe (absolute neutrophil count [ANC] <100/mm^3) or prolonged neutropenia (>7 days).

---

3 Clark OA, Lyman GH, Castro AA, et al. (2005). Colony-stimulating factors for chemotherapy-induced febrile neutropenia: a meta-analysis of randomized controlled trials. *J Clin Oncol* 23:4198–4214.

Prophylaxis of febrile neutropenia

Prophylactic antibiotics
Prophylactic antibiotics reduce the risk of FN and documented infections but are also associated with toxicity, the emergence of antibiotic-resistant bacteria, and fungal overgrowth.[1]

Trimethoprim-sulfamethoxazol (TMP-SMZ)
- Reduces the risk of *Pneumocystis carinii* pneumonia and may reduce the risk of bacterial infections.
- Adverse reactions include allergies to the sulfonamide, myelosuppression, development of drug-resistant bacteria, as well as more frequent candidiasis.
- The Infectious Disease Society of America (IDSA) recommends against routine prophylaxis with TMP-SMZ in neutropenic chemotherapy patients.

Quinolones
- Quinolone antibiotics are capable of preventing FN and infection and reducing infection-related mortality in hematologic cancer patients.
- A significant reduction in all-cause and infection-related mortality, fever, clinically documented infections, and microbiologically documented infections has been reported with fluoroquinolone prophylaxis in a meta-analysis mainly of patients with hematologic malignancies.
- Recent double-blind, placebo-controlled RCTs of levofloxacin prophylaxis demonstrated significant reductions in the risk of fever and hospitalization but not severe infection or infection-related mortality.
- Significant increases in resistant gram-negative and gram-positive isolates were observed in high-risk patients.
- The IDSA recommends against routine FN prophylaxis with the fluoroquinolones.
- They should not be used in institutions where parenteral quinolones are routinely used as a part of empiric therapy.

Vancomycin
Evidence for antibiotic resistance and limited clinical benefit argue against the use of prophylactic vancomycin in neutropenic patients.

Antifungal prophylaxis
- Antifungal prophylaxis has been shown to significantly reduce superficial and invasive fungal infection as well as fungal-related mortality.
- The risk of invasive *Aspergillus* is not affected.
- The most benefit is seen in studies of stem cell transplantation and patients with hematologic malignancy.

---

1 Hughes WT, Armstrong D, Bodey GP, et al. (2002). 2002 guidelines for the use of antimicrobial agents in neutropenic patients with cancer. *Clin Infect Dis* 34:730–751.

Prophylactic colony-stimulating factors

Prophylactic G-CSF in adult cancer patients reduces the risk of FN and documented infection and risk of infection-related mortality while sustaining chemotherapy dose intensity.[2] A significant increase in bone pain is reported in approximately 20% of patients.

Prophylactic CSFs in childhood cancer reduce the risk of FN, documented infection, length of hospitalization, and use of amphotericin.

Pegylated G-CSF reduced the risk of FN from 17% to 1% in breast cancer patients who received chemotherapy, consistent with previous studies, suggesting a further reduction in risk of FN compared with that of filgrastim.

Clinical practice guidelines from the American Society of Clinical Oncology (ASCO), the National Comprehensive Cancer Network (NCCN), and the European Organization for Research and Treatment of Cancer (EORTC) recommend primary prophylaxis with CSF in patients receiving chemotherapy regimens associated with a risk of FN above 20% and with less intensive regimens in certain high-risk settings, based on age or comorbidities (see Figure 17.1).[3]

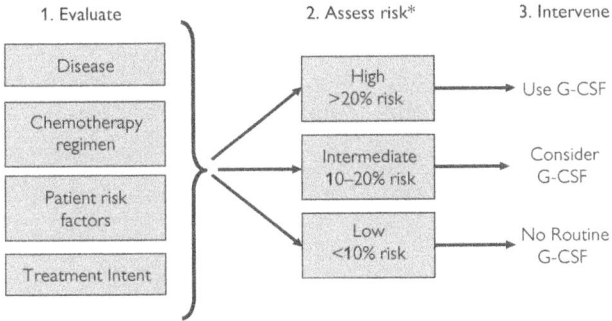

* Risk of FN or neutropenic event compromising treatment

Figure 17.1 Algorithm for primary G-CSF prophylaxis. Lyman GH: Guidelines of the National comprehensive cancer network on the use of myeloid growth factors with cancer chemotherapy: A review of the evidence. *J Natl Compr Canc Netw* 2005; 3:557–571.

2 Kuderer NM, Dale DC, Crawford J, Lyman GH (2007). Impact of primary prophylaxis with granulocyte colony-stimulating factor on febrile neutropenia and mortality in adult cancer patients receiving chemotherapy: a systematic review. *J Clin Oncol* 25:3158–3167.

3 Smith TJ, Khatcheressian J, Lyman GH, et al. (2006). 2006 update of recommendations for the use of white blood cell growth factors: an evidence-based clinical practice guideline. *J Clin Oncol* 24:3187–3205.

Key point summary

- Myelosuppression and its complications including FN represent the major dose-limiting toxicity of systemic cancer chemotherapy, often compromising dose intensity in potentially curable malignancies.
- FN is associated with substantial morbidity, mortality, and cost.
- FN represents a medical emergency requiring immediate evaluation and prompt administration of empiric broad-spectrum antibiotics.
- FN often occurs early in the course of chemotherapy.
- Risk factors for serious medical complications may influence the choice of therapy including empiric antibiotics and myeloid growth factors.
- The role of prophylactic antibiotics continues to be defined in the context of drug toxicity and emerging antibiotic resistance.
- The myeloid growth factors are indicated for dose-dense chemotherapy and for prophylaxis of FN and sustaining chemotherapy dose intensity in the curative setting.

Chapter 18

Pain management

Amy P. Abernethy
Thomas W. LeBlanc

Introduction 252
Assessment 253
Causes of cancer pain 254
Understanding the patient's cancer pain 255
Management of cancer pain 256
Management of breakthrough pain 262
Other pain management interventions 266
Further reading 269

Introduction

Incidence
Pain is one of the most dreaded and most prevalent cancer-related symptoms. Estimates derived from World Health Organization (WHO) data and from numerous national and international surveys report that one-third of cancer patients receiving active therapy experience cancer pain. This proportion increases to 60%–90% among patients with advanced disease. Over 80% of cancer patients with pain have two or more sites of pain.[1]

General management
In most cases, cancer pain is a manageable concern. Approximately 80%–90% of cancer-related pain can be relieved relatively simply with oral analgesics and adjuvant drugs.

Inadequate pain control may exacerbate many other problems:
- Fatigue
- Anorexia and nausea
- Constipation
- Depression
- Hopelessness

It is also more difficult for a patient in pain to continue with demanding cytotoxic treatment and hospital visits.

Relief of pain at the expense of side effects is unacceptable to most patients; therefore, a variety of treatment modalities is required.

---

1 Agency for Health Care Policy and Research (1994). *Management of Cancer Pain. Clinical Practice Guidelines*, Vol. 9. Washington, DC: U.S. Department of Health and Human Services.

Assessment

Pain scales

The Joint Commission for the Accreditation of Healthcare Organizations has mandated that pain scales be used in routine clinical care to measure pain intensity.[1]

A number of validated pain assessment instruments exist. Some of the most common choices are the following:
- Numerical Rating Scale or Visual Analog Scale
- Brief Pain Inventory
- Memorial Pain Assessment Card
- McGill Pain Questionnaire
- Faces Rating Scale
- Pain Thermometer

Choice of pain scale should take into account characteristics of the individual patient, e.g.,
- Numerical rating scale or visual analog scale for the cognitively intact adult
- Faces rating scale for children
- Pain thermometer or faces rating scale for the elderly

After selecting one scale for a particular patient, the clinician should use that same scale for initial evaluation and all follow-up; the scale used, as well as pain intensity, should be documented.

---

1 Berry PH, Dahl JL (2000). The new JCAHO pain schedule: implications for pain management nurses. *Pain Manag News* **1**(1):3.

Causes of cancer pain

Primary causes
At the outset of cancer pain management, a careful history should be taken to identify any reversible or remediable causes of the patient's pain and to better understand potential prognosis of the pain itself.

Cancer pain may derive from the following:
- Tumor progression and related pathology
- Procedural intervention
- Treatment toxicity
- Infection
- Musculoskeletal issues

The most common causes of pain in cancer patients include
- Peripheral neuropathies secondary to chemotherapy or tumor invasion
- Tissue injury secondary to radiotherapy
- Chronic postsurgical incisional pain
- Bone metastases
- Visceral pain

Exacerbating factors
Cancer pain can be exacerbated by the following:
- Other physical symptoms, including insomnia, loss of appetite, fatigue
- Psychological symptoms, including distress, anxiety, and depression
- Social factors (e.g., family distress)
- Spiritual or existential suffering
- Medical crisis

Undertreatment of cancer pain
Although cancer pain is manageable, it is often undertreated. The most common reasons for uncontrolled cancer pain are
- Inadequate assessment resulting in misdiagnosis of the cause and type of pain and failure to detect general distress, which in turn lowers the pain threshold. Psychological distress can contribute significantly to the pain experience, and it must be managed appropriately.
- Lack of a systematic approach to analgesia. "Panic prescribing" is more likely to result in unacceptable side effects.
- Lack of knowledge of opioid pharmacology, including failure to anticipate and prevent side effects

Understanding the patient's cancer pain

Because treatment must be tailored for the individual according to the nature, likely mechanisms, and subjective component of pain, thorough inquiry is the starting point of cancer pain management.

Is the pain acute or chronic?
- A diagnosis of cancer itself should not be taken as sufficient reason for a patient to experience or endure pain.
- Pain of sudden onset may suggest an acute complication of the malignancy, the treatment, or an unrelated cause, e.g., a new pathological fracture or mucositis due to radiotherapy.
- Chronic escalating pain may represent underlying disease progression, e.g., soft tissue or nerve root infiltration, but the etiology of that pain must also be assessed.

What is the nature of the pain?
- **Somatic**: Typically localized and persistent, e.g., bone metastases, localized inflammation such as cellulitis
- **Visceral**: Usually poorly localized, of variable intensity, and often occurring with associated symptoms such as nausea, e.g., hepatic metastases, malignant abdominal lymphadenopathy
- **Neuropathic**: Classically described as a "shooting pain" or "burning," usually following a nerve distribution, and typically less responsive to opioid therapy, e.g., compression of a spinal nerve root

How does the patient interpret the pain?
- Pain has a strong affective component and is greatly influenced by mood and morale.
- An understanding of the patient's perception of their pain will help formulate an effective management plan.
- The clinician should discuss the issue of pain with the patient, to determine whether he or she has specific anxieties related to this pain, such as fear that it will adversely affect functionality or that it heralds the final stages of illness.
- Addressing any anger, fear, or distress will increase the likelihood of achieving satisfactory pain control.

Management of cancer pain

The approach to cancer pain management entails a foundation of pharmacologic management, which is tailored with individualized care.

The basic pillars of cancer pain management are the following:
- WHO analgesic ladder as foundation of care
- Individualized therapy
- Around-the-clock dosing
- Breakthrough dosing
- Oral formulation, whenever possible
- Proactive treatment and/or prophylaxis of side effects
- Discussion of therapeutic goals is essential. Complete relief may not be a reasonable expectation and it is important to set achievable goals

Pharmacological pain relief

Pharmacologic pain management follows the approach depicted in Figure 18.1 by the WHO analgesic ladder. In applying the WHO analgesic ladder, it is important to
- Determine the strength of analgesia based on the *severity of pain* rather than on the stage of disease.
- Prescribe regular medication to prevent pain from occurring or reoccurring.

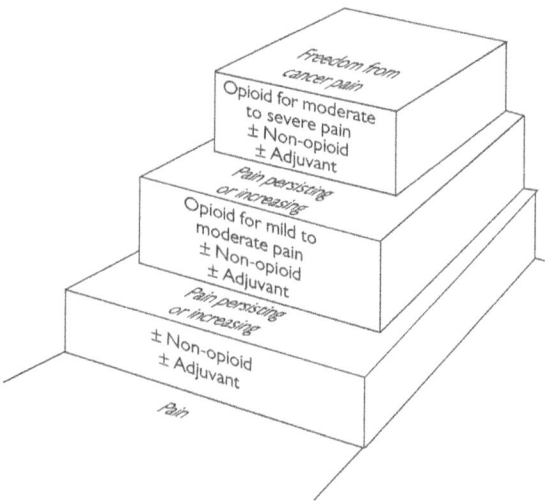

Figure 18.1 The WHO analgesic ladder. Reproduced with permission from the WHO. http://www.who.int/cancer/palliative/painladder/en/index.html

- Make appropriate "as needed" (prn) immediate-release medication available for pain escalation or breakthrough pain, in doses calculated on the basis of the regular prescribed dose.
- Recognize that monotherapy rarely suffices.
- Use opioids in combination with nonopioids, in most cases.
- Initiate treatment with immediate-release formulations; switch to sustained-release formulations when the dose is stable.
- Choose adjuvant analgesia according to the cause and type of pain. Adjuvants can be added at any step in the ladder.

Step 1. Initial treatment of mild-to-moderate pain: nonopioid analgesia

Begin with a nonopioid analgesic plus adjuvant(s) as appropriate for the individual. Good nonopioid analgesic options are the following:
- Acetaminophen, an antipyretic with no anti-inflammatory action. Adverse reactions are rare at prescribed doses (i.e., up to 1 g 4 times per day [qid] in the absence of liver disease).
- Nonsteroidal anti-inflammatory drugs (NSAIDs; e.g., ibuprofen 400–800 mg 3 times per day [tid], naprosyn 250–500 2 times per day [bid], choline magnesium trialicylate for patients when platelets are a concern). Be aware of issues regarding gastric protection and renal function as well as cardiac risks with long-term use.
- Acetaminophen in combination with an NSAID.
- Cox-2 inhibitors (e.g., celecoxib) are also anti-inflammatory and may result in lower incidence of gastric irritation and renal toxicity, but they have been associated with increased risk of myocardial infarction and stroke.

Nonopioid analgesics can be paired with adjuvants such as the following:
- Agents for neuropathic pain, including gabapentin, duloxetine, amitriptyline, and capsaicin. With gabapentin, start at low doses (100 mg daily to 100 mg tid) and increase by 100–300 mg every 1–3 days to effect. The usual effective total daily dose is 900–3600 mg, administered in three divided doses per day; some patients may need higher doses, but sedation is a common dose-limiting side effect.
- Bisphosphonates for bone pain, particularly effective in breast cancer and multiple myeloma but also in lung, gastrointestinal, and prostate cancer. Standard starting doses are zoledronic acid 4 mg IV over 15 minutes or pamidronate 90 mg IV administered over 2 hours.
- Corticosteroids for bone pain. Starting doses reported in the literature are as follows: oral methylprednisolone, 16 mg bid; dexamethasone, 4–8 mg 2 to 3 times per day; prednisone, 20–30 mg 2 to 3 times per day.

Step 2. Mild-to-moderate pain not responsive to Step 1 or initial treatment of severe pain: low-doses of opioid analgesia

If pain is not adequately controlled with nonopioid analgesia alone, then a low dose of an opioid analgesic is usually added.

Historically, this step has focused on "weak opioids." Contemporary approaches recognize that low doses of any opioid represent less potency, and that the classically defined "weak opioids" (e.g., codeine) can be "strong" when given in high enough doses. High doses of these agents are usually limited because of side effects.

Good options at this step of the ladder include the following:
- Codeine phosphate, 30–60 mg tid. Avoid subtherapeutic doses (<30 mg qid) of codeine, such as over-the-counter (OTC) preparations. This drug causes substantial nausea and vomiting in many patients, so consider adding an antiemetic when prescribing.
- Low dose of morphine, <40 mg total daily dose, or a similar dose of oxycodone.

The patient should continue regular nonopioid analgesics alongside weak opioids.
- Weak opioids are often prescribed in combination formulations with acetaminophen or aspirin (e.g., codeine plus acetaminophen, hydrocodone plus acetaminophen).
- Possible side effects of any opioid include nausea and constipation, and should be treated preventively.
- Step 2 agents can be combined with adjuvants to tailor the pain management plan to the individual patient's needs.

Step 3. Pain not responsive to Step 2: more potent doses of opioid analgesia

If pain continues despite the addition of low-dose opioid to nonopioid analgesia, substitute a more potent opioid agonist or increase the dose of the Step 2 opioid.

1. Choose an initial drug and dose.

Opioid agonists generally used for cancer pain include morphine, oxycodone, fentanyl, hydromorphone, and methadone.
- Avoid meperidine because of the risk of seizures.

Use sustained-release product (e.g., sustained-release morphine every 8–12 hours, sustained-release oxycodone every 12 hours, transdermal fentanyl patch every 48–72 hours), combined with an immediate-release formulation for breakthrough pain and inadequate analgesia.

For conversions between agents and comparing potency, work in terms of oral morphine equivalents (OMEs).
- Example: 30 mg OME daily = 15 mg sustained-release 2x/day = 10 mg sustained-release oxycodone 2x/day (see opioid-conversion Table 18.1)

Gauge potency of opioid and starting dose. Small doses of potent opioids can be considered in the same way as full doses of less potent opioids.
- Opioid-naïve patient: Start at 20–40 mg OME/day (this is really Step 2)
- Opioid-tolerant patient: Start at 40–80 mg OME/day (this is Step 3)
- Cut initial dosing by 50%–75% for elderly patients, and for individuals with liver or renal dysfunction

Morphine metabolites contribute to side effects including nausea, myoclonus, and sedation. These metabolites can accumulate, especially in patients with renal dysfunction.
- Oxycodone, fentanyl, hydromorphone, and methadone do not have the same metabolites and may have fewer side effects.

Methadone may be more effective for neuropathic pain and is very inexpensive. However, methadone has an unpredictable half-life and safety concerns raised by its effects on the QT interval; it should be prescribed by experienced clinicians only.

2. *Titrate drug to desired analgesic effect and tolerable side effects.*
- Titrate both long-acting and short-acting formulations. A long-acting formulation provides background analgesia, and a short-acting one provides relief of episodic breakthrough pain (see Box 18.1) and inadequate background analgesia.
- Increase by 30%–100% OME daily, or by adding in the previous day's prn dose.
- Do not increase the methadone dose any more frequently than every 5–7 days, unless in very controlled settings; monitor the QTc interval.
- In the outpatient setting, monitor the patient frequently (e.g., every 24–48 hours by phone, with an office or home visit every 3–5 days until pain subsides).

Box 18.1 Example: titration using short-acting morphine

A patient with severe pain of 7/10 on a 0–10 numerical rating scale did not get relief with low doses of opioid using Step 2 guidelines.
- Make sure the patient is receiving a nonopioid and any required adjuvants.
- Advance to Step 3.
- Start a regular dose of immediate-release morphine sulfate at 10 mg every 4 hours around the clock with 10 mg every 2 hours as needed for breakthrough pain. Total prescribed OME = 60 mg sustained-release per day.

If the patient requested 30 mg of immediate-release morphine during the preceding day, in addition to the 60 mg regularly prescribed (total OME = 90 mg), then
- Increase the regular dose to 15 mg every 4 hours. Total prescribed OME = 90 mg/day.
- Increase prn dose to 15 mg.
- Continue this titration every day until pain <2/10 and/or the patient reports that pain is adequately controlled.

When the required dose is stable, convert the total usage into a sustained-release formulation. For example:
- Current stable dose is 20 mg immediate-release morphine sulfate every 4 hours (total prescribed OME = 120 mg/day).
- Change to sustained-release morphine at 60 mg bid.
- Breakthrough morphine dose is 10–15 mg immediate-release morphine as needed.

3. *Manage side effects.*
- **Nausea**: Prescribe an antiemetic, e.g., metaclopramide 5–10 mg every 6 hours as needed.
- **Constipation**: Co-prescribe a laxative plus stool softener with the opioid, and start these therapies at the same time, e.g., docusate with senna.
- **Distress**: Use oral formulations when possible. Communicate with the patient and family to establish an expectation of pain relief.
- **Dry mouth**: Treat with access to fluids or mouth care.
- **Hallucinations**: Be aware of this possibility. If they occur, treat with haloperidol, 1.5–3 mg as needed.
- **Respiratory depression** is rare in cancer patients and usually only seen at doses above those required for analgesia or if the drug is accumulating (e.g., due to renal impairment, methadone titrated too quickly). Naloxone is an opioid antagonist for emergency use in such settings.
- **Pruritus**: Treat with antihistamines such as diphenhydramine or hydroxyzine, the latter of which may be less sedating. In some older patients, these medications can cause urinary retention, confusion, or both; switching to a different opioid may be more helpful.

Management of breakthrough pain

Breakthrough pain refers to intermittent flares of pain that occur even though the patient is properly taking around-the-clock analgesics and pain is generally well managed. One-half to two-thirds of patients with chronic cancer pain experience episodes of breakthrough cancer pain.[1]

Educate patients and caregivers about breakthrough pain and include them in discussion of the clinical plan for preventing or alleviating it.

Alongside each long-acting sustained-release opioid, prescribe an immediate-release opioid, at an appropriate dose relative to the long-acting product (see Table 18.1).

- The short-acting dose should be approximately 10% of the long-acting dose, adjusted for efficacy vs. side effects based on the patient's report of symptoms.
- Exception: The dose of short-acting transmucosal fentanyl products is determined by titration to the effective dose and not based on the relative dose of the long-acting product. Tailor dosing of short-acting fentanyl products to patient report only.
- Example: A patient taking 100 mg of long-acting oxycodone daily should have a breakthrough dose of 10 mg of short-acting oxycodone.

Increasing analgesic requirements and persistent pain

A slow increase in opiate requirement can be anticipated over time. Opioid responsiveness falls along a continuum, yet certain types of pain (e.g., neuropathic pain) require larger doses of opioids.

- Titration may be limited by unacceptable side effects such as sedation. In these situations, adjuvant analgesics become particularly important.

When a cancer patient has persistent pain despite the appropriate use of analgesics, one has to consider whether the patient has developed progressive disease, tolerance, withdrawal, or hyperalgesia.

Progressive disease
Most often, progressive disease is the cause of pain that is suddenly difficult to control in cancer patients.

Tolerance
- Leads to increasing doses of analgesics being required to maintain the same level of pain control
- Rare in cancer patients
- Usually responds to increasing the opioid dose or switching to a different opioid

Withdrawal
- Secondary to decreasing or stopping an opioid
- Can lead to worsening pain, but this should improve by adding back the opioid or increasing the opioid dose

---

[1] Portenoy RK, Hagen NA (1990). Breakthrough pain: definition, prevalence and characteristics. *Pain* 41(3):273–281

Hyperalgesia

- Opioid-induced hyperalgesia occurs when opioids lead to increasing pain as the opioid dose is increased.
- Hyperalgesia is often characterized by "allodynia," wherein nonpainful stimuli are perceived as painful (such as light touch).
- If standard adjustments to the patient's analgesic regimen do not lead to improved pain control, referral to a pain specialist should be considered.

Addiction

- Many patients and families harbor concern about the possibility of addiction to strong opioids.
- Dependency can be physical, psychological, and due to habituation. In most cases, when properly managed, addiction is not an issue.
- It should nonetheless be discussed with patients and families to allay anxiety and to reaffirm the goal of sufficient pain control.
- The risk of addiction in this setting is approximately 1 in 1000 cancer patients.

*These new products are only available under the U.S. FDA's Risk Evaluation and Mitigation Strategy (REMS) program for registered prescribers. Due to the possible risks of these thereapies, consult a pharmacist before attempting to use them; you must be a registered prescriber.

Table 18.1 Dose equivalents

Drug	IM/SC/IV (mg)	PO/PR/SL (mg)	Duration (hours)
Morphine	10	20–30	3–4
Codeine	120–130	200	3–4
Hydromorphone	2	4	3–4
Oxycodone		15–20	3–4
Fentanyl	100 µg (0.1)		2–3
Fentanyl (transdermal)	25 µg/h = 30–67 IV morphine/24 h	25 µg/h = 60–134 po morphine/24 h	3 days
Fentanyl, oral (lozenge or dissolving buccal film)	*	*	*
Methadone		Depends	>5 days

Adjuvant analgesics

The WHO guidelines indicate that adjuvant analgesics should be considered at every stage in pain management. Appropriate selection of therapy requires an understanding of the mechanism of pain.

Each selected medication should be given an appropriate trial of efficacy and withdrawn if it proves ineffective. Otherwise, the patient can easily accumulate a vast list of tablets, requiring a complex timetable of administration and without clear symptomatic benefit.

Useful adjuvants include the following:
- **Steroids** are helpful for pain due to increased intracranial pressure (ICP), nerve compression, distension of the liver capsule (due to metastases), or soft tissue infiltration.
  - Example: Dexamethasone, up to 16 mg/day acutely; review dose regularly and titrate down to a minimum as soon as practicable.

Potential side effects include fluid retention, gastric irritation, hypomania, hyperglycemia, and iatrogenic Cushing's syndrome. Dexamethasone has fewer mineralocorticoid-related effects; prednisone has less glucocorticoid activity.

- **Tricyclic antidepressants** (TCAs) are particularly effective in neuropathic pain (e.g., amitriptyline, 25 mg every evening titrated upward according to response). Side effects include sedation, dry mouth, constipation, dizziness, and urinary retention.
- **Anticonvulsants**. Gabapentin, carbamazepine, lamotrigine, sodium valproate, oxcarbazepine, and pregabalin can all be prescribed for neuropathic pain. Carbamazepine is generally indicated only if TCAs have failed, because it entails a high risk of drug interactions and side effects.
- **Anxiolytics**. Benzodiazepines are indicated for anxiety, agitation, restlessness, and insomnia, all of which may exacerbate pain. They are also sedative, antiemetic, and useful in managing anticipatory nausea.
- **Neuroleptics** are particularly useful for opioid-induced hallucinations. These (e.g., haloperidol) are antiemetic and sedative.
- **Bisphosphonates** reduce pain due to skeletal metastatic disease in breast, prostate, and lung cancer, reduce bone-related complications (e.g., pathological fractures), and they play a role in multiple myeloma. Their role in other malignancies remains to be established. Analgesic effect takes up to 2 weeks to develop. Treatment is currently IV (e.g., pamidronate or zolendronic acid, every 3 to 4 weeks). Monitor renal function and serum Ca^{2+} for risk of hypocalcemia.

Other pain management interventions

Anesthetic techniques
Various anesthetic approaches are available as alternatives, or adjuncts, to oral or parenteral drug therapies.

Nerve blocks
Nerve blocks interrupt the sympathetic nervous system. Blocks are usually used to control pain arising from malignancies of the abdominal and pelvic viscera.

Visceral pain manifests as constant, deep, and difficult to localize or describe. When visceral pain does not respond to drug and behavioral therapy, or if the patient cannot tolerate drug therapy, seek consultation to consider the potential benefits of a neurolytic block.

- **Celiac plexus block** is appropriate for upper abdominal pain (e.g., from pancreatic cancer) and pain involving the GI tract from the distal third of the esophagus to the transverse colon, liver and biliary tract, adrenals, and mesentery.
- **Superior hypogastric plexus block** is appropriate for lower abdominal pain, involving the GI tract from the descending colon to the rectum, as well as the urogenital system.
- **Brachial plexus block** may relieve pain due to malignant axillary disease infiltrating the brachial plexus.
- **Ganglion impar block** alleviates pain involving the rectum and perineum.

Neurolytic blocks have certain advantages over epidural anesthetic techniques. They are often less expensive and obviate the need for hardware (e.g., catheters, tubes, pump), which are distressing to patients and families, can be cumbersome, may malfunction, and pose an infection risk.

Epidural anesthesia
Epidural anesthesia can provide superior regional analgesia compared with conventional systemic routes (IV or oral). Drugs administered in the epidural space are extremely potent because the drug is delivered close to the site of action.

Hence, systemic side effects (e.g., nausea, sedation, constipation) are minimized. In palliative care, epidural analgesia may be appropriate for patients with regional pain (e.g., pelvic pain from cervical cancer) and/or patients who do not tolerate or obtain relief from other drug and nondrug therapies.

- Example: Pathological fractures in patients ineligible for surgical fixation may benefit from epidural anesthesia.

Intrathecal anesthesia
Intrathecal anesthesia, in which drug is delivered through a catheter placed within the neuraxis, is appropriate for management of severe pain when conventional drug therapy proves ineffective or produces intolerable side effects. It provides superior analgesia when pain is widespread or does not respond to high-dose epidural anesthesia.

- Continuous somatic pain and continuous visceral pain are the types of pain most responsive to intrathecal anesthesia; neuropathic pain is less responsive.

Palliative radiotherapy

External beam radiotherapy can be effective at reducing pain due to local tumor effects.

The maximum benefit of radiotherapy is achieved 3–6 weeks after delivery. Radiotherapy may acutely exacerbate pain, causing a "pain flare." Thus, pain control must be adequately addressed while the patient is undergoing treatment and in subsequent weeks.

- **Bone metastases**: Bone-targeted radioisotopes (e.g., strontium-89) can be considered for diffuse pain from osteoblastic metastases unresponsive to conventional analgesia. External beam radiation achieves pain relief in >75% of patients with bone metastases. Analgesia requires up to 3 months to take effect. Myelosuppression can be a significant toxicity.
- **Epidural metastases**: External beam radiation constitutes the primary definitive treatment, in conjunction with a short course of steroids.
- **Brain metastases**: Either whole-brain external beam radiation or stereotactic radiosurgery for small lesions can relieve symptoms including pain as well as potentially extend survival time.

Psychological and cognitive-behavioral approaches

Psychological and psychoeducational approaches should be integrally incorporated into cancer pain management. Pain has a profound effect on emotional distress, and, conversely, psychosocial factors such as depression, anxiety, and family strain intensify the pain experience.

Several psychological variables contribute to the suffering associated with cancer pain; these include perceived loss of control, the meaning of pain, fear of death, depressed mood, and hopelessness. The individual's personality, coping ability, social support, and medical factors influence the level of psychological distress they experience with cancer pain.

Potentially beneficial therapeutic approaches include the following:
- Psychoeducational strategies
- Cognitive-behavioral therapies (e.g., pain coping skills training)
- Partner-assisted pain coping
- Psychological counseling
- Support groups

Complementary and alternative medicine approaches

A host of complementary and alternative approaches, including mind-body modalities, energy medicine techniques, and relaxation therapies, may help alleviate the pain either directly or indirectly as mediated by reduction in distress and other psychological states.

Patients with cancer-related pain may experience benefit from the following:
- Acupuncture
- Aromatherapy
- Reflexology
- Hypnosis and guided imagery
- Massage
- Feldenkrais, and other mind-body modalities
- Healing touch, Reiki, and other energy-based modalities
- Yoga therapy, if specifically adapted for cancer pain
- Transcutaneous electrical nerve stimulation (TENS)
- Occupational therapy
- Physical therapy

Referrals should be made only to providers who are appropriately credentialed, who have had specialized training in the care of cancer patients, who work closely with oncologists to be alert to patient-specific considerations, and whom the referring clinician knows to be both competent and compassionate.

Further reading

Abernethy AP (2007). Older persons with cancer: A framework for managing cancer pain. In 2007 *American Society of Clinical Oncology (ASCO) Educational Book* from the 43rd Annual Meeting, Chicago, June 1–5, 2007, pp. 301–306.

Abernethy AP, Foley KM. Management of Cancer Pain. In: DeVita VT, Lawrence TS, Rosenberg SA, eds. Cancer: Principles & Practice of Oncology. 9th ed. Philadelphia: Wolters Kluwer/Lippincott Williams & Wilkins; 2011:2426-2446.

Guideline for the Management of Cancer Pain in Adults and Children. American Pain Society, ©2005.

Pain management. In Watson M, Lucas C, Hoy A, Back I (eds.). *Oxford Handbook of Palliative Medicine*. Oxford: Oxford University Press, 2005, pp. 169–236

NCCN Clinical Practice Guidelines in Oncology: Adult Cancer Pain. http://www.nccn.org.

Chapter 19

Venous thromboembolism

Nicole M. Kuderer

Risk of venous thromboembolism 272
Consequences of venous thromboembolism 275
Clinical presentation 276
Prevention and treatment of venous
  thromboembolism 278
Clinical practice guidelines for prophylactic
  anticoagulation 280
Key point summary 285
Thrombosis of central venous catheters 286

Risk of venous thromboembolism

The risk of venous thromboembolism (VTE) is *substantially* increased in cancer patients.

Risk factors for venous thromboembolism
(see Table 19.1)
- Virchow's triad
  - Venous stasis
  - Vascular trauma
  - Hypercoagulability of the blood

The risk of VTE in cancer patients is particularly increased in those hospitalized, especially those with
- Neutropenia and presumed infection
- Older age
- Immobility and comorbidities such as obesity, pulmonary disease, and renal failure

The risk of VTE in hospitalized cancer patients appears to be *increasing*. Additional risk factors for VTE in cancer patients include the following:
- Type of cancer, including cancers of the pancreas, stomach, brain, lung, and ovary
- Stage of disease
- Type of treatment, including chemotherapy, hormonal therapy, and surgery
- Central venous catheters

The risk of VTE also appears to be increased in ambulatory cancer patients on active systemic chemotherapy.

A number of new cancer therapies appear to be associated with an increased risk of VTE. The erythroid-stimulating agents (ESAs) and Bevacizumab also place patients at higher risk of VTE.

Time course of incident venous thromboembolism relative to date of cancer diagnosis

Most cancer-associated VTE events occur within a few months of the date of diagnosis.

The *extent or degree of spread* of a cancer is among the strongest predictors of VTE.

Risk factors associated with cancer treatment
The following treatment factors increase the risk of VTE:
- Chemotherapy: 2- to 6-fold increased risk
- Hormonal therapy: 1.5- to 7.1-fold increased risk
- Bevacizumab-containing regimens have been associated with high rates of VTE.
- Patients on erythropoiesis-stimulating agents have significantly greater VTE.
- Major surgery, e.g., laparotomy, laparoscopy, or thoracotomy lasting greater than 30 minutes

Thalidomide therapy and to a lesser degree lenalidomide in combination with chemotherapy or corticosteroids is associated with a high risk of venous thrombosis.
- Given as a single agent in the treatment of multiple myeloma, the reported incidence of VTE with thalidomide is 3%–4%.
- Thalidomide combined with dexamethasone alone or with other chemotherapeutic drugs for treatment of multiple myeloma has a reported incidence of VTE that ranges from 9% to 58%.

Lenolinamide, a potent analog of thalidomide, is also associated with an increased risk of VTE.
- The reported VTE incidence with lenolinamide and dexamethasone combination therapy is 19%, compared to 4% with lenolinamide alone.

A risk model for venous thromboembolism in cancer patients
Predictive factors in a tumor type and stage-adjusted multivariate model for VTE among adult cancer patients receiving chemotherapy in the ambulatory setting are as follows:
- Platelet count ≥350,000/mm^3
- Hemoglobin <10g/dL and/or use of erythropoietin
- Leukocyte count >11,000/mm^3
- Body mass index ≥35

This model distinguishes low-risk patients with VTE rates <1% from those having rates up to 7% in the high-risk category.

Biomarkers
Some of the following biomarkers are under active investigation:
- Platelet and leukocyte count
- Tissue factor
- D-dimer
- C-reactive protein
- P-selectin

Table 19.1 Selected risk factors for cancer-associated thrombosis

Patient-related factors

- Older age
- Female gender
- Race
  - Higher in African Americans
  - Lower in Asians or Pacific Islanders
- Comorbidities
  - Infection, renal disease, pulmonary disease, obesity
- Inherited prothrombotic mutations
  - Factor V Leiden, prothrombin gene mutation
- Prior history of VTE

Cancer-related factors

- Primary site of cancer
  - Brain, pancreas, kidney, stomach
  - Lung, gynecologic, lymphoma, myeloma
- Advanced stage of cancer
- Initial period (3–6 months) after diagnosis

Treatment-related factors

- Cancer therapy
  - Chemotherapy
  - Hormonal therapy
  - Anti-angiogenic agents: thalidomide, lenalidomide, bevacizumab (for arterial)
  - Erythropoiesis-stimulating agents
  - Major surgery
  - Hospitalization
  - Central venous catheter

Adapted from Rao MV, Francis CW, Khorana AA (2007). Who's at risk for thrombosis? Approaches to risk-stratifying cancer patients. In Khorana AA, Francis CW (eds.). *Cancer-Associated Thrombosis: New Findings in Translational Science, Prevention, and Treatment.* New York: Informa Healthcare.

Consequences of venous thromboembolism

Thromboembolism represents a leading cause of death in cancer patients.
- VTE is associated with a variety of adverse consequences including increased mortality.
- VTE remains a leading cause of death in cancer patients.
- Hospitalized cancer patients with documented thromboembolism have a greater in-hospital mortality.

Outcomes of interest in cancer patients at risk for venous thromboembolism
- VTE and its consequences
- The impact and complications of VTE treatment or prevention
- Mortality
- Delivery of cancer therapy
- Cancer-related outcomes
- Use of health-care resources

The impact of anticoagulation on the overall survival of patients with chemotherapy has been the focus of a number of prospective clinical trials.
VTE is associated with reduced survival after adjusting for age, race, sex, cancer type, stage, and comorbid conditions. The effect of VTE on survival may be greatest in patients with early-stage cancer.

Possible reasons for early deaths in patients with venous thromboembolism
- Pulmonary embolus
- Anticoagulant related bleeding
- Serious underlying comorbidity
- More aggressive cancer

Clinical presentation

Deep vein thrombosis
- Deep vein thrombosis (DVT) can be part of presentation of cancer or may predate diagnosis.
- Signs and symptoms are as for any DVT, but may be multiple or mixed with superficial clots, or "thrombophlebitis migrans."
- Use Wells clinical DVT model (see Table 19.2).
- Diagnosis of DVT is most often based on duplex ultrasound. If this is negative but suspicion remains high, CT venography may be considered.
- Therapy is with anticoagulants. It is preferable to use low-molecular-weight heparin (LMWH).

Pulmonary embolism
- This is a medical emergency.
- Symptoms can be tachycardia, chest pain, dyspnea, and hemoptysis, although often not all of these are present and can be very subtle.
- Have a high index of suspicion in all cancer patients.
- Treat with cardiovascular support and anticoagulation.
- Use Wells clinical pulmonary embolism (PE) model (see Table 19.3).
- Diagnosis of PE is often based on a CT angiogram. If it is negative but suspicion is high, a duplex ultrasound of the lower extremity or pulmonary scintigraphy can be considered. Pulmonary angiogram remains the "gold standard" diagnostic test, but can be avoided in most situations. Due to its chronic elevation in cancer patients, D-dimer only tends to be helpful in diagnostic decision making when it is not elevated in this patient population.

Table 19.2 Wells clinical deep thrombosis model

Clinical characteristic	Score
Active cancer (patient receiving treatment for cancer within 6 months or currently receiving palliative treatment)	1
Paralysis, paresis, or recent plaster cast immobilization of the lower extremities	1
Recently bedridden for 3 days or more, or major surgery within the previous 12 weeks requiring general or regional anesthesia	1
Localized tenderness along the distribution of the deep venous system	1
Entire leg swollen	1
Calf swelling at least 3 cm larger than the asymptomatic side (measured 10 cm below the tibial tuberosity)	1
Pitting edema confined to the symptomatic leg	1
Collateral superficial veins (nonvaricose)	1
Previously documented deep vein thrombosis	1
Alternative diagnosis at least as likely as deep vein thrombosis	−2

A score of <2 indicates that a deep vein thrombosis is unlikely. A score of 2 points or higher indicates that a deep vein thrombosis is likely.

Table 19.3 Wells clinical pulmonary embolism model

Clinical characteristic	Score
Active cancer (patient receiving treatment for cancer within 6 months or currently receiving palliative treatment)	1
Surgery or bedridden for 3 days or more during the past 4 weeks	1.5
History of deep venous thrombosis or pulmonary embolism	1.5
Hemoptysis	1
Heart rate >100 beats/minute	1.5
Pulmonary embolism judged to be the most likely diagnosis	3
Clinical signs and symptoms compatible with deep venous thrombosis	3

A score of ≤4 indicates that pulmonary embolism is unlikely. A score of >4 indicates that pulmonary embolism is likely.

Prevention and treatment of venous thromboembolism

Randomized clinical trials of prophylactic anticoagulation in cancer patients
Efforts to prevent VTE are premised on the following:
- Potential benefits and harms associated with treating established VTE and the associated life-threatening complications including pulmonary embolism
- Bleeding risk of full-dose anticoagulation

RCTs of anticoagulant treatment in cancer patients may be categorized on the basis of the following primary objectives:
- **Primary medical prophylaxis**: prevention of VTE and its complications without a prior occurrence in the medical setting
- **Primary surgical prophylaxis**: prevention of VTE and its complications in patients without a prior occurrence in the perioperative or postoperative setting
- **Secondary prophylaxis**: prevention of a recurrence of VTE or its complications in patients with a recent VTE
- **Improve overall survival**: attempt to reduce mortality or improve disease control in cancer patients without a history of VTE

Meta-analyses of anticoagulation in cancer patients
Methodological challenges
While the ideal for meta-analyses remains access to individual patient data, the vast majority of meta-analyses reported in oncology are based on aggregate patient data largely derived from the published literature.
Limitations of previous meta-analyses include the following:
- Incomplete search and selection strategies
- Post hoc subgroup analyses of the proportion of the study population with cancer

Primary prophylaxis
Only three studies of a primary prophylaxis strategy in ambulatory cancer patients have had VTE as a primary outcome, and no meta-analysis of this issue has been completed.

Secondary prophylaxis
The impact of LMWH versus vitamin K antagonists on recurrence of VTE in cancer patients has been addressed in four RCTs, all of which have shown a trend toward a lower risk of recurrent VTE for LMWH.

Surgical prophylaxis
A large number of RCTs of prophylactic anticoagulation have been performed in the perioperative and postoperative setting among cancer patients, which reveal efficacy in VTE prevention.

A variety of methods for VTE prophylaxis have been studied including compression stockings, intermittent compression devices, and various anticoagulants.

After major surgery, anticoagulation is the preferred method of prophylaxis. LMWH prophylaxis extended 4–5 weeks after surgery significantly further reduces the risk of venographically detected DVT.

Impact on overall survival

A number of RCTs of anticoagulation treatment in cancer patients without a diagnosis of VTE have suggested improvement in overall mortality in some cancer types.

Improvement in overall survival in cancer patients that is due to anticoagulation needs to be confirmed in ongoing prospective RCTs.

Clinical practice guidelines for prophylactic anticoagulation

American college of chest physicians
The American College of Chest Physicians (ACCP) guidelines recommend VTE prophylaxis with either low-dose unfractionated heparin (UFH) or LMW-heparin for both surgical patients and hospitalized medical patients.

Although these recommendations are based on studies with a limited number of cancer patients, given the high risk in these patients, extrapolation is considered acceptable.

These guidelines provide limited information concerning VTE prophylaxis specifically in cancer patients.

National comprehensive cancer network
The guidelines cover the diagnosis and evaluation of VTE in cancer patients, risks and contraindications of anticoagulation, available therapies for prophylaxis and treatment of VTE. The current version of the National Comprehensive Cancer Network Venous Thromboembolic Disease Guideline (version 2.2008) can be found at http://nccn.org.

Clinical practice guidelines from the American Society of Clinical Oncology
1. Hospitalized cancer patients should be considered for VTE prophylaxis in the absence of contraindications to anticoagulation.
    - Heparin, low-molecular-weight heparins, and fondaparinux all provide effective prophylaxis.
    - Nonmedical therapies such as ambulation, exercise, and graduated compression stockings offer only some protection.
    - Anticoagulant prophylaxis in hospitalized medical patients significantly reduces the risk of all PEs as well as fatal PE.
2. Routine prophylaxis with an antithrombotic agent is currently not recommended in ambulatory cancer patients during systemic chemotherapy except for high-risk situations, such as patients receiving thalidomide or a thalidomide analog in conjunction with chemotherapy or dexamethasone.
    - The rate of thrombosis in ambulatory cancer patients appears to vary widely with the type of cancer, treatment, and comorbid conditions.
    - There are very few data available on the primary prevention of thrombosis in ambulatory cancer patients.
    - In the solid-tumor setting, low-dose warfarin has been shown to reduce the risk of VTE in women with metastatic breast cancer receiving chemotherapy.
    - Data on prophylaxis in this setting with low-molecular-weight heparins have been conflicting.

3. Unless contraindicated, patients undergoing major surgical procedures for cancer should receive VTE prophylaxis, with a consideration of combined mechanical prophylaxis and anticoagulation in high-risk patients.
    - Cancer patients undergoing major surgical procedures are at increased risk for VTE and at greater risk of bleeding complications.
    - Risk factors include age over 60, previous history of VTE, operation time in excess of 2 hours, operation for advanced-stage disease, and prolonged bed rest postoperatively in excess of 4 days.
    - Mechanical devices include graduated compression stockings or intermittent pneumatic calf compression devices.

Pharmacologic agents for venous thromboembolism prophylaxis in surgical cancer patients
    - Vitamin K antagonists have not been fully evaluated and must be monitored. Drug interactions remain a problem and many cancer patients have poor oral intake and nutrition.
    - Low-dose unfractionated heparin reduces risk of fatal PE.
    - Low-molecular-weight heparins are equally effective and require minimal monitoring.
    - Extended prophylaxis for up to 4 weeks reduces the risk of venographically detected VTE in patients undergoing major abdominal and pelvic surgery with high-risk features such as residual malignancy, obesity, and those with a previous history of VTE.

4. Initial therapeutic options for treatment of cancer patients with established VTE to prevent recurrent VTE include the following:
    a. Unfractionated heparin (UFH)
    b. Low-molecular-weight heparin (LMWH)
    c. Fondaparinux

- LMWH therapy is the preferred agent for long-term therapy for cancer outpatients.
- If vitamin K antagonists are planned for long-term therapy, acute treatment with UFH, LMWH, or fondaparinux should be continued for at least 5 days and until INR ≥2.
- Cancer patients with continuing risk for VTE should be continued on anticoagulant prophylaxis following a VTE for a minimum of 3–6 months.
- Dalteparin is currently the only FDA-approved LMWH for the extended treatment of VTE in cancer patients.
- Longer durations of anticoagulation may be warranted if the cancer is clinically active and the patient is receiving cancer therapy.

Special circumstances need to be considered in the treatment and prevention of VTE:
- Severe bleeding and severe thrombocytopenia are contraindications to anticoagulation.
- Anticoagulation is contraindicated in patients with active risk or at high risk for bleeding.
- In patients with documented VTE and contraindication to anticoagulation, vena cava filters should be considered.

5. Cancer patients should be encouraged to participate in clinical trials designed to evaluate anticoagulant therapy as an adjunct to standard anticancer therapies.
   - Meta-analyses of trials that compared initial therapy of VTE with UFH versus LMWH demonstrated a survival benefit in cancer patients randomized to LMWH.
   - Several RCTs have studied whether anticoagulants administered to cancer patients without VTE improve overall survival and have reported mixed results.
   - Overall, these data are not sufficient to suggest that anticoagulation improves survival among cancer patients.

Regimens for prophylaxis and treatment of venous thromboembolism in cancer patients and estimated cost data

See Table 19.4.

Table 19.4 Regimens for prophylaxis/treatment of venous thromboembolism in cancer patients*

Management	Drug	Regimens	Estimated Weekly Cost	Estimated 6 month Cost
Prophylaxis				
Hospitalized medical or surgical cancer patients	Unfractionated heparin	5000 U q 8 h	$12.08	$313.95
	Dalteparin (Fragmin®)	5000 U daily	$152.40	$3,962.50
	Enoxaparin (Lovenox®)	40 mg daily	$154.59	$4,019.29
	Fondaparinux (Arixtra®)	2.5 mg daily	$199.92	$5,197.92
Treatment				
Initial[5]	Dalteparin (Fragmin®)	100 U/kg q 12 h	$426.73	n/a
		200 U/kg daily	$426.73	n/a
	Enoxaparin (Lovenox®)	1 mg/kg q 12 h	$541.06	n/a
		1.5 mg/kg daily	$405.79	n/a
	Heparin	80 U/kg IV bolus, then 18 U/kg/hr IV (adjust level based on PTT)	$24.99	n/a
	SQ heparin	333 u/kg SQ, followed by 250 u/kg SQ q12h		

Table 19.4 (Cont.)

Management	Drug	Regimens	Estimated Weekly Cost	Estimated 6 month Cost
	Fondaparinux (Arixtra®) (6)	<50 kg, 2.5 mg daily	$199.92	n/a
		50–100 kg, 5 mg daily	$399.84	n/a
		>100 kg, 7.5 mg daily	$599.76	n/a
	Tinzaparin (Innohep®)	175 U/kg daily	$198.17	n/a
Long term[a]	Dalteparin (Fragmin®) (3)	200 U/kg daily for 1 m; then 150 U/kg daily	$334.12	$8,687.04
	Warfarin	Daily dose; adjust dose to maintain INR between 2 and 3	$4.43	$115.15

Lyman G, Khorana A, Falanga A et al. (2007). American Society of Clinical Oncology Guideline: Recommendations for venous thromboembolism prophylaxis and treatment in patients with cancer. *J Clin Oncol* 25(34): S490–S505. Originally published by the American Society of Clinical Oncology. Reprinted with permission.

[a] Cost is estimated based on 70kg person and 2006 Medicare data. Warfarin cost estimates do not include cost for laboratory testing

Key point summary

- Patients with cancer, especially those who are hospitalized and those undergoing surgery or systemic treatment, are at significantly increased risk for VTE.
- The primary and secondary prevention of VTE in cancer patients represent a continuing clinical problem for the practicing oncologist.
- The possible adjunctive role of anticoagulants in improving survival remains an intriguing opportunity that will require further randomized controlled clinical trials.

Thrombosis of central venous catheters

Thrombus related to long-term venous catheterization of patients with cancer is relatively common; e.g., studies suggest a 3%–30% incidence of catheter-induced axillosubclavian vein thrombosis. This is a population already prone to thrombosis in which a thrombogenic focus has been introduced.

Presentation
- Commonly asymptomatic—high index of suspicion is needed
- Local symptoms, e.g., unilateral hand or arm edema, shoulder pain, prominent collateral veins visible on chest wall
- Pulmonary embolism

Investigation
- Usually by duplex ultrasound examination
- Occasionally with a venogram.

Management
- **Line removal**, if at all possible, i.e., removal of the thrombogenic stimulus. Commonly this is a decision that potentially complicates treatment of the underlying cancer and therefore needs to be addressed on an individual basis.
- **Anticoagulation** with low-molecular weight heparin or warfarin. The duration of anticoagulant therapy is dependent on past medical history, ongoing presence of the venous catheter, other risk factors, etc.
- **Catheter-directed thrombolysis**. There is no current evidence that this is superior to conservative management. However, it can be considered in selected patients, particularly those with a good prognosis from their cancer who have serious, acute thrombus-related symptoms.
- Thrombolytic therapy should be reserved for patients with massive limb-threatening central venous catheter (CVC)-associated thrombosis.

Thrombus of the catheter lumen
The inability to withdraw blood from or infuse into a venous catheter is common.
- A chest X-ray will help exclude kinking or line migration.
- Instillation of a fibrinolytic agent into the line, e.g., tissue plasminogen activator or an equivalent, may clear intraluminal thrombus.

Further reading

Ambrus JL, Ambrus CM, Mink IB, et al. (1975). Causes of death in cancer patients. *J Med* 6:61–64.

Khorana AA, Francis CW, Culakova E, et al. (2006). Thromboembolism in hospitalized neutropenic cancer patients. *J Clin Oncol* 24:484–490.

Khorana AA, Kuderer NM, Culakova E, et al. (2008). Development and validation of a predictive model for chemotherapy-associated thrombosis. *Blood* 111:4902–4907.

Kuderer NM, Khorana AA, Lyman GH, Francis CF (2007). A meta-analysis and systematic review of the efficacy and safety of anticoagulants as cancer treatment: impact on survival and bleeding complications. *Cancer* 110:1149–1160.

Lee AY, Levine MN, Baker RI, et al. (2003). Low-molecular-weight heparin versus a coumarin for the prevention of recurrent venous thromboembolism in patients with cancer. *N Engl J Med* 349:146–153.

Lyman GH, Khorana A, Kuderer NM, et al. (2013). Venous thromboembolism prophylaxis and treatment in patients with cancer: American Society of Clinical Oncology Clinical Practice Guideline Update. *J Clin Oncol* 31:2189–2204.

Chapter 20

Metabolic emergencies

Gary H. Lyman

Hypercalcemia 290
Hyponatremia 294
Hyperkalemia 296
Hyperglycemia and hypoglycemia 297
Acute renal failure in patients with malignant disease 298
Renal tubular dysfunction 299
Tumor lysis syndrome 300

Hypercalcemia

- Complicates 10%–20% of all cancers
- Commonly the presenting feature of malignancy
- Occurs in both solid tumors and hematologic malignancies

It is especially associated with
- Breast cancer
- Multiple myeloma
- Lung cancer, especially squamous cell carcinoma

Free Ca^{2+} ≥3.0 mmol/L leads to multisystem dysfunction.
- Free (ionic) Ca^{2+} is dependent on serum albumin and arterial pH.
- Free (ionic) Ca^{2+} = measured Ca^{2+} + [(40-albumin) × 0.02].

Pathophysiology

- Local increased bone resorption (osteolysis) induced by bone metastases is attributed to tumor cell production of cytokines, particularly interleukins and tumor necrosis factor (TNF) activating osteoclasts.
  - It is the dominant mechanism in certain malignancies, e.g., lymphoma, non-small–cell lung cancer. Serum PO_4^{3-} is usually normal.
- There is systemic release of humoral mediators activating osteoclasts, e.g., parathyroid hormone-related peptide (PTHrP).
  - In some tumors, humoral mechanisms causing hypercalcemia are believed to dominate particularly in the absence of bony metastases, e.g., squamous cell carcinoma of the lung.
- Often associated with low PO_4^{3-} from inhibition of PO_4^{3-} reabsorption

Dehydration exacerbates hypercalcemia.
- Ca^{2+} is a potent diuretic causing salt and water loss.
- As diuresis continues, Ca^{2+} levels increase, causing further volume depletion, etc.

Tumor-specific mechanisms include the following examples:
- Multiple myeloma—secretion of an osteoclast-activating factor with or without deposition of Bence-Jones proteins leads to renal impairment and decreased Ca^{2+} excretion.
- Some lymphomas (usually T cell) produce active metabolites of vitamin D, increasing intestinal absorption of Ca^{2+}.

In many cancers, more than one mechanism may contribute, e.g., osteolytic, and humoral mechanisms appear to be important in breast cancer.

Presentation

- Acute or insidious
- May be incidental finding in an asymptomatic patient
- Neurological features: malaise, fatigue, weakness, depression, cognitive dysfunction, coma
- Gastrointestinal features: nausea, vomiting, anorexia, abdominal pain, constipation, pancreatitis

- Renal signs: polydipsia, polyuria, dehydration, signs of uremia, renal calculi
- Cardiac disorders: arrhythmias, with increased or decreased BP

Investigations
- Urea and electrolytes (U & E), corrected serum Ca^{2+}, PO_4^{3-}, Mg^{2+}
- Full blood count (FBC): a normal Hb in the presence of significant hypercalcemia is likely to fall once the patient is rehydrated.
- Plasma PTH is appropriately undetectable in malignant hypercalcemia.

Nonmalignant causes of hypercalcemia are common and may coexist with a diagnosis of cancer, e.g., primary or tertiary hyperparathyroidism.

Management
- Establish intravenous access and monitor urine output.
- Rehydration is given to produce volume expansion, restore glomerular function, and increase urinary Ca^{2+} excretion.
  - Fluid deficit may be many liters.
  - Aim for 3–6 L/24 hours if cardiac function and urine output permit.
  - Reassess fluid status regularly.
- Monitor U & E: Renal impairment should improve with fluid resuscitation. K^+ and Mg^{2+} may fall with rehydration and require IV replacement (K^+ 20–40 mmol/L, Mg^{2+} up to 2 mmol/L of normal saline).
  - Check Ca^{2+} and albumin daily.
- Loop diuretics, e.g., furosemide po/IV, lower Ca^{2+} (inhibits reabsorption in the loop of Henle) and maintain diuresis once patient is rehydrated
- Bisphosphonates: Consider if free Ca^{2+} remains ≥3.0 mmol/L despite rehydration
  - They cause inhibition of osteoclast activity, leading to low Ca^{2+}.
  - Typical schedule is *pamidronate* 60–90 mg infused in 1 L normal saline over 2–4 hours, provided renal function is adequate following 24 hours of rehydration. Then continue fluids.
  - Onset of action is from 48 hours and patient is usually normocalcemic within 3–7 days.
  - Cannot repeat dose for 7 days, i.e., the *acute* management of hypercalcemia is fluid resuscitation. Optimal interval is ≥3 weeks.
  - Side effects include transient fever, hypocalcemia.
  - Zolendronic acid (4 mg IV over 15 minutes) is superseding pamidronate as the bisphosphonate of choice to treat malignant hypercalcemia because of shorter infusion time and greater potency.
- Steroids have little role. They may be helpful in treating multiple myeloma (prednisolone 30–60 mg qd).
- Avoid immobility: Lack of weight-bearing induces increased osteoclastic activity while reducing bone formation, which may precipitate hypercalcemia.

CHAPTER 20 Metabolic emergencies

- Dietary Ca^{2+} *restriction* is not appropriate in most patients, as gut Ca^{2+} absorption is usually appropriately reduced. Rare exceptions are some patients with lymphoma associated with raised levels of vitamin D metabolites.
- Treat the underlying malignancy if possible. Usually hypercalcemia is associated with advanced disease and treatment is palliative.
- Salmon calcitonin leads to increased renal Ca^{2+} excretion and decreased bone reabsorption. Use IM or SC administration. There is a rapid onset of action but efficacy is limited to the initial 48 hours of treatment (tachyphylaxis).

Hyponatremia

Etiology in malignant disease
With low plasma osmolality
There is excess antidiuretic hormone (ADH).
- Ectopic tumor production of ADH is most commonly associated with small cell lung cancer (SCLC) but also described in many other cancers including carcinoid tumors, lymphomas, leukemias, and pancreatic cancer.
- Syndrome of inappropriate ADH secretion (SIADH) exhibits reduced excretion of ingested H_2O with or without resetting of the osmostat (maintaining serum Na^+ at a stable, lower level). Multiple causes include major surgery, pulmonary disease (e.g., concurrent pneumonia), and raised intracranial pressure. Apparent idiopathic SIADH is often associated with occult malignancy, particularly SCLC.
- Stimulation of ADH secretion can be caused by cytotoxic drugs used in the treatment of cancer, e.g., ifosfamide, vincristine, high-dose IV cyclophosphamide.

Adrenal insufficiency, e.g., following rapid withdrawal of long-term exogenous steroid therapy, may be accompanied by increased K^+ with or without metabolic acidosis.
- Excess intravenous fluid replacement.

With normal or high plasma osmolality (pseudohyponatremia)
This may occur secondary to hyperglycemia or retention of hypertonic mannitol used in prehydration regimes for chemotherapy. High plasma osmolality is produced, drawing intracellular water out into the circulating volume and, hence, producing apparent hyponatremia.
- There is no hypo-osmolality and thus no risk of cerebral edema due to movement of water into the brain.
- Treatment directed at correcting the serum Na^+ is not indicated.

Presentation
Hyponatremia is often asymptomatic. Presence of symptoms is dependent on the following:
- Degree of hyponatremia
- Rapidity of onset
- Age and sex of patient, with premenopausal women being most at risk

Symptoms, when they occur, are primarily neurological:
- Nausea, malaise, and weakness
- Confusion, headache, and drowsiness
- Seizures, coma, and respiratory arrest

Investigation
- Plasma and urinary Na^+: Low serum Na^+ with inappropriately normal to high urinary Na^+ excretion
- Plasma and urinary osmolality: Urinary osmolality exceeds plasma osmolality.

Management

- Fluid restriction to approximately 0.5–1 L/day is often sufficient, i.e., to below the level of urine output.
- Inhibition of the action of ADH on the renal tubule, e.g., with demeclocycline
  - Only consider in occasional patients with persistent, significant hyponatremia who cannot tolerate water restriction.
  - Renal function needs to be monitored.

Infusion of hypertonic (3%) saline should be considered only if the hyponatremia is life threatening, and then only under careful supervision.

- Overly rapid correction must be avoided, particularly in chronic hyponatremia.
- It is not appropriate in treating most malignant causes of hyponatremia as Na^+ handling is intact in SIADH.
- Administered Na^+ will simply be excreted unless the osmolality of the administered fluid exceeds urine osmolality.

Hyperkalemia

Etiology in malignant disease
- Renal failure is probably the most frequent cause.
- Tumor lysis syndrome usually follows initiation of therapy for large-volume treatment of responsive disease.
- Concurrent septicemia
- Adrenal insufficiency is usually secondary to glucocorticoid withdrawal or, rarely, adrenal destruction by a tumor.
- Acute graft-versus-host disease following allogeneic bone marrow transplantation
- Drugs, e.g., diuretics such as spironolactone

Presentation
- Often asymptomatic
- Cardiac dysrhythmias and arrest
- Signs and symptoms of underlying cause

Management
- 12-lead ECG and continuous cardiac monitoring: Effects of increased K^+ on cardiac conducting tissue include tented T-waves, broadening of the QRS complex, and flattened P-waves.
- Establish IV access and give 10 mL 10% calcium gluconate IV, as this is cardioprotective. It can be repeated every 10 minutes until the ECG normalizes.
  - Up to 50 mL may be required.
- 50 mL 50% dextrose with 10 U insulin infused over 15–30 minutes
- Polystyrene sulfonate resin enema (calcium resonium) increases gut K^+ losses.
- If there is associated renal failure, consider intravenous rehydration; you will need central access and possibly intravenous sodium bicarbonate to correct acidosis
  - E.g., 50–100 mL 8.4% bicarbonate IV over 30 minutes via central line
- Hemodialysis is occasionally necessary.

Hyperglycemia and hypoglycemia

- Corticosteroid administration will increase insulin requirements in patients with diabetes mellitus and may precipitate the need for hypoglycemic medication in those with impaired glucose tolerance.
- Loss of appetite, nausea, and vomiting may complicate management of blood sugars in the diabetic patient.
- Inappropriate insulin production can result from islet cell tumors and pancreatic APUDomas.
- Large metastatic tumors, particularly in the liver, rarely can produce insulin-like growth factors (IGF) that are released into the circulation, especially in response to treatment.

Acute renal failure in patients with malignant disease

Diagnosis
Certain causes of acute renal failure may be seen more commonly in the patient with malignant disease. Identification of treatable causes is the priority.

Causes can be divided into the following categories.
- **Prerenal**: Hypovolemia, e.g., dehydration due to vomiting or hypercalcemia, concomitant sepsis
- **Renal**: Cytotoxic agents, e.g., platinum-based chemotherapy, and other nephrotoxic drugs, nonsteroidal anti-inflammatory analgesia, tumor lysis syndrome, multiple myeloma with production of Bence-Jones proteins
- *Postrenal*, e.g., obstruction secondary to a pelvic tumor or pathological lymphadenopathy, renal vein thrombosis

Appropriate management
- Correct life-threatening electrolyte derangement and achieve euvolemia if possible.
- Confirm the cause of renal failure. Use Doppler imaging to assess blood flow. CT of the abdomen or pelvis may identify filling defects consistent with inferior vena cava thrombus.
- Treat the underlying cause if possible.

Renal tubular dysfunction

Cytotoxic agents
Cisplatin and ifosfamide can disrupt normal renal tubule function.

The following electrolyte abnormalities commonly occur from increased urinary loss:
- ↓Ca^{2+}
- ↓Mg^{2+}
- ↓K^+
- ↓Na^+

Symptoms may include the following:
- Perioral and limb dysesthesia
- Tetany/carpopedal spasm
- Lethargy
- Constipation
- Hypotension and arrhythmias
- Seizures

Patients receiving these drugs require regular monitoring of electrolyte concentrations and replacement where necessary.
- Oral calcium and vitamin D may be required to maintain serum calcium levels.
- For chronic treatment of hypomagnasemia, oral magnesium glycerophosphate is preferred to other oral magnesium preparations, as diarrhea is less of a problem with this formulation.

Tumor lysis syndrome

This is a syndrome of metabolic abnormalities and renal impairment due to rapid lysis of tumor cells. Suspect the diagnosis in patients with large-volume malignant disease developing acute renal failure in the presence of hyperuricemia and/or hyperphosphatemia.

The syndrome is most commonly associated with bulky chemosensitive disease, e.g., aggressive lymphomas, high blast-count leukemias, and metastatic germ cell tumors. It has been described in many other cancers, e.g., breast cancer and multiple myeloma.

It usually follows treatment, with onset within hours or days of commencing chemotherapy. Steroid monotherapy can induce the syndrome in patients with lymphoma or acute lymphoblastic leukemia. It can follow radiotherapy for a similar spectrum of cancers.

Spontaneous tumor lysis of tumors with high cell turnover can occur, although is not usually associated with hyperphosphatemia.

Metabolic abnormalities

- Hyperuricemia: can be associated with urate nephropathy and oliguric renal failure.
- Hyperphosphatemia
- Hyperkalemia is exacerbated by deteriorating renal function.
  - It can cause cardiac arrhythmias
- Hypocalcemia/hypomagnesemia is secondary to increased PO_4^{3-} and precipitation of calcium phosphate.
  - Symptoms include muscle weakness with or without tetany.
  - Contributes to cardiac dysrhythmias
- Acute renal failure is due to acute uric acid nephropathy and/or hyperphosphatemia.
  - It may be exacerbated by deposition of calcium phosphate in the renal parenchyma.
- Metabolic acidosis

Prophylaxis

- Allopurinol, e.g., 300 mg po qd. Pretreatment for 48 hours prior to chemotherapy results in a marked decrease in the incidence of post-treatment hyperuricemia.
- Optimize renal function before and during treatment.
  - Relieve urinary tract obstruction if possible.
  - Correct electrolyte abnormalities, e.g., hypercalcemia.
  - Ensure adequate fluid replacement, e.g., intravenous hyperhydration to maintain high urine output.
  - The osmotic diuretic mannitol is sometimes used in pretreatment hydration regimes.
  - Loop diuretics (e.g., furosemide) can also help maintain appropriate diuresis during therapy.
- Leukophoresis, if peripheral blast count is high

Management

- Urgent correction of hyperkalemia
- Monitor fluid balance.
  - Urinary catheterization may be helpful.
  - Careful assessment of circulating volume and intravenous rehydration if patient is volume depleted
- Urinalysis may demonstrate uric acid crystals but may be normal due to oliguria from obstructed nephrons.
- Exclude postrenal causes of renal failure, e.g., ureteric obstruction.
  - Suspect this particularly if there is flank pain.
- Monitor electrolytes and urea twice daily until the patient is stable.
- Calcium supplementation is not usually necessary unless there is neuromuscular irritability.
- Consider alkalinizing the urine, e.g., with acetazolamide or sodium bicarbonate. This reduces uric acid precipitation by converting uric acid to the more soluble urate salt.
- Assess need for hemodialysis to remove excess circulating uric acid.

Chapter 21

Paraneoplastic syndromes

Jeffrey Peppercorn

Introduction 304
Endocrine paraneoplastic syndromes 306
Neurological paraneoplastic syndromes 310
Hematological paraneoplastic syndromes 316
Dermatologic and skeletal paraneoplastic syndromes 318
Further reading 320

Introduction

Paraneoplastic syndromes (PNS) are manifestations of disease arising from substances produced by cancer cells or in reaction to cancer cells, rather than as a direct consequence of cancer invasion or metastasis.

Fever and cachexia are the most common PNS by this definition, and they are frequently associated with many cancers and may precede diagnosis. Other PNS are rare, occurring in less than 1% of most cancers, but they can occur more frequently in association with some specific tumor types and may be underdiagnosed.

A PNS may be the presenting feature of an undiagnosed cancer, occurring months to years before cancer diagnosis.

Cancers commonly associated with paraneoplastic syndromes include the following:
- Small cell lung cancer (endocrine PNS, Lambert-Eaton syndrome)
- Non-small–cell lung cancer (clubbing, osteoarthopathy)
- Pancreatic neuroendocrine tumors (endocrine PNS)
- Pancreatic cancer (Trousseau syndrome)
- Lymphoma (Dermatologic PNS)
- Breast, ovarian cancer (neurologic PNS)
- Thymoma (red cell aplasia)
- AML (Sweets syndrome)
- Myeloma (POEMS syndrome [polyneuropathy, organomegaly, endocrinopathy, M protein, skin changes])

Although the mechanisms of many PNS are not fully understood, they have been associated with
- Inappropriate secretion of hormones and/or growth factors by cancer cells
- Production of anticancer antibodies that cross-react with normal tissue antigens

Endocrine paraneoplastic syndromes

Syndrome of inappropriate antidiuretic hormone
Production of antidiuretic hormone (ADH) by the tumor is most commonly associated with small cell lung cancer (SCLC).

Cancer types
- SCLC (11% of patients)
- Pancreatic
- Prostate
- Non-Hodgkin's lymphoma (NHL)
- Hodgkin's disease (HD)
- Non-small–cell lung cancer (NSCLC)
- Breast
- Gynecologic

Presentation
- Often asymptomatic
- CNS effects: fatigue, headaches; progressing to altered mental state, confusion, and seizures

Diagnosis
Exclude nonmalignant causes:
- CNS disease (infection, trauma, vascular)
- Pulmonary disease (infections, cystic lesions, asthma)
- Drug-induced (thiazides, cytotoxics, SSRI, narcotics)
- Hypovolemia

Management
- Fluid restriction (0.5–1.0 L/day)
- Democlocycline (150–300 mg 8 hourly)
- Avoid rapid correction
- Frequently responds to treatment of underlying malignancy

Laboratory criteria for diagnosis of syndrome of inappropriate antidiuretic hormone
- Hyponatraemia Na+ <130 mmol/L
- Normal serum albumin and glucose.
- Serum hypo-osmolarity <275 mmol/kg
- Urine osmolarity > serum osmolarity
- Urinary sodium >25 mmol/L
- Nonsuppressed ADH

Cushing's syndrome
This syndrome involves production of adenocorticotrophic hormone (ACTH) by tumor, and it is most commonly associated with lung cancer.

Cancer types
- SCLC (1%–5%)
- NSCLC
- Pancreatic
- Thymic
- Carcinoid

- Ovary
- Breast
- Cervix
- Colon

Presentation
- Weakness
- Hypertension
- Muscle wasting
- Hyperpigmentation
- Altered mental status
- Metabolic disturbances (e.g., hyperglycemia, hypokalemic alkalosis)

Diagnosis
- Clinical features: hyperpigmentation, muscle wasting
- Labs: hypokalemia, hypernatremia, metabolic alkalosis
- High 24-hour urinary cortisol
- High plasma ACTH/precursors
- Corticotropin-releasing hormone (CRH) stimulation test after low-dose dexamethasone administration (no response in plasma ACTH in Cushing's syndrome [CS])
- Desmopressin stimulation test (brisk response in plasma ACTH in CS)
- Exclude pseudo-Cushing's: depression, alcohol abuse, polycystic ovarian syndrome, excess body fat

Management
- Specific antitumor treatment
- Decrease cortisol secretion either surgically (bilateral adrenalectomy) or medically (metyrapone, octreotide, ketoconazole)

Hypercalcemia

This involves production of parathyroid hormone-related protein (PTH-rP) by the tumor.

Cancer types
- NSCLC (15% in squamous cell)
- Head and neck
- Renal
- Bladder
- Other squamous cancers
- Breast
- Small cell
- Ovarian
- Melanoma
- Gynecologic

Presentation
- Nausea, vomiting
- Polyuria
- Dehydration, thirst
- Abdominal pain
- Altered mental status
- Cardiac arrhythmias

Diagnosis
- Elevated serum calcium
- Elevated PTH-rP level
- Hypochloremia
- Hypercalcuria
- High urinary phosphate
- Low or undetectable plasma parathyroid hormone
- Exclude other causes, especially hypercalcemia due to bone metastasis (a more common etiology of hypercalcemia in most cancer).

Management
- IV fluid
- Loop diuretic
- IV bisphosphonate
- Calcitonin

Zolinger-Elison syndrome

This syndrome involves production of gastrin by GI neuroendocrine tumor.

Cancer types
- Gastrinoma located in pancreas or duodenum
- May be associated with MEN-1

Presentation
- Ulcer
- Diarrhea
- Abdominal pain

Diagnosis
- Increased serum gastrin
- Increased acid secretion
- Identification of tumor on imaging (symptoms precede diagnosis)
- Secretin test

Management
- Surgery
- Proton pump inhibitors
- Octreotide

Other neuroendocrine tumors

Additional endocrine syndromes associated with hormone-producing tumors include the following:
- *Hypoglycemia* is due to insulin secreted from insulinoma, most commonly originating from pancreas.
- *Verner-Morrison pancreatic cholera* is due to secretion of vasoactive peptide, leading to watery diarrhea, hypokalemia, and metabolic acidosis, arising from the pancreas.
- *Somatostatin syndrome* is due to somatostatin, with hyperglycemia, gallstones, and weight loss, arising from the pancreas or upper bowel.
- *Glucogonoma syndrome* is due to glucogon secretion, with hyperglycemia and depression, arising from the pancreas.

Neurological paraneoplastic syndromes

- Although rare, these syndromes can affect any aspect of the nervous system.
- Most are due to production of antibodies against tumor antigens that cross-react with nervous system.
  - Some are mediated by antigen-specific T cells.
- Response to treatment varies; many respond poorly to immunosupression (with notable exceptions such as Lambert-Eaton myasthenic syndrome).
- Treatment of underlying malignancy is important in all neurologic PNS.

Paraneoplastic cerebellar degeneration

Cancer types
- Breast (most common PNS)
- Ovary
- SCLC
- HD

Presentation
There is rapid onset and progression of cerebellar dysfunction, including ataxia, dysarthria, visual problems, and late cognitive problems.

Diagnosis
- Radiologic imaging shows cerebellar atrophy.
- CSF has increased lymphocytes.
- Mildly elevated protein with oligoclonal bands
- Anti-Yo antibodies (breast, ovarian)
- Anti-HU, anti-TR (HD)
- Biopsy shows loss of Purkinje cells.

Management
- Response to antitumor treatment
- May be T-cell mediated and respond to T cell-directed therapy

Peripheral neuropathy

Peripheral neuropathy (PN) is caused by antibodies to peripheral nerves. It may be seen alone or as part of a broader PNS.

Cancer types
- SCLC
- Waldenstrom's
- Multiple myeloma
- Thymoma
- HD
- Breast
- GI

Presentation
- Paresthesias
- Pain
- Numbness, weakness

- Cramps
- Sensory ataxia

Diagnosis
- Exclude common causes of neuropathy (drug, B_{12}).
- Electromyography (EMG) or nerve conduction studies
- Nerve biopsy if needed
- Can involve Anti-Hu (most common), Anti-Yo, Anti-Ri, Anti-MAG (Waldenstrom's)

Management
Treat underlying malignancy, and provide immunosuppression.

Encephalomyelopathies

These involve antibody-mediated inflammation or destruction at variable levels of the central nervous system, including the limbic system, brainstem, and spinal cord.

Cancer types
- SCLC
- Testicular
- Breast
- Ovary
- NHL

Presentation
- Altered mental status; depression
- Dementia seizure
- Often slow onset

Diagnosis
- MRI
- CSF pleocytosis
- Elevated protein
- Oligoclonal bands anti-Hu antibody: MRI, anti-MA; ANNA-3, anti-amphiphysin.

Management
Treat underlying malignancy.

Acute necrotizing myopathy

This rapidly progressive proximal weakness can lead to respiratory distress within weeks.

Cancer types
- SCLC
- Breast
- Renal
- Prostate
- GI

Diagnosis
- Marked elevation in creatine phosphokinase (CPK)
- Exclude chemotherapy rabdomyolysis

Management
Treat underlying malignancy.

Paraneoplastic Opsoclonus-Myoclonus syndrome

Cancer types
- Breast
- SCLC
- HD

Presentation
- Occular motor problems
- Myoclonus in head, trunk, and extremities
- Rapid onset and progression of cerebellar dysfunction, including ataxia, dysarthria, visual problems, and late cognitive problems

Diagnosis
- Anti-Ri antibodies

Management
Treat underlying malignancy.

Stiff-man syndrome

Cancer types
- SCLC
- Breast
- Thymoma
- Renal cell
- HD

Presentation
It starts with trunk rigidity, spreading to the extremities and facial muscles, followed by dysphagia, dysphonia, and respiratory distress.

Diagnosis
- Antibodies to GAD or amphiphysin

Management
- Benzodiazepines, baclofen
- Treat underlying malignancy
- Success with plasmapheresis and immunosuppression is reported.

Paraneoplastic (cancer-associated) retinopathy

Cancer types
- SCLC
- Breast
- Gynecological malignancy
- Melanoma

Presentation
- Progressive visual loss, blurred vision
- Photosensitivity
- Changes in color vision
- Peripheral scotomas
- Prolonged dark accommodation

Diagnosis
- Loss of acuity
- Scotomata
- Abnormal electroretinogram
- Antiretinal antibodies
- Antibody to recoverin

Management
- Corticosteroids
- Treat underlying malignancy

Lambert-Eaton myasthenic syndrome

Lambert-Eaton myasthenic syndrome (LEMS) is a disorder of transmission at the neuromuscular junction due to antibodies against the voltage-gated calcium channel.

Cancer types
- SCLC (60–70%)
- Breast
- Ovarian
- Thymus
- GI cancers

Presentation
- Proximal muscle weakness
- Can involve sensory and autonomic neuropathy, diplopia, dry mouth
- Can occur in association with Paraneoplastic cerebellar degeneration

Diagnosis
- EMG with characteristic small-motor unit potentials at rest, increased after exercise
- Antiglial nuclear antibody (AGNA) against SOX1
- Anti-voltage-gated calcium channels

Management
- Treat underlying malignancy
- Corticosteroids
- Plasma exchange (one of the few PNS settings where this has proven efficacy)
- 3,4-Diaminopyridine

Dermatomyositis and polymyositis

These disorders involve inflammatory myopathy, associated with a rash in dermatomyosits. They commonly precede a diagnosis of cancer.

Cancer types
- NSCLC
- SCLC
- Breast
- Ovary
- Prostate
- GI cancers

Presentation
- Proximal weakness
- Decreased tendon reflexes
- Double vision
- Dysphonia
- Respiratory distress
- Dermatomyositis heliotrope rash
- Systemic features include cardiopulmonary conditions, Reynaud's disease, arthralgias, retinopathy, and delayed gastric emptying.

Diagnosis
- Serum: high creatine kinase (CK), LDH, aldolase
- Muscle biopsy: myositis
- EMG: fibrillation, insertion irritability, short polyphasic motor units

Management
- Treat underlying malignancy
- Corticosteroids
- Azathioprine

Hematological paraneoplastic syndromes

Red cell disorders
Erythrocytosis
- Hematocrit (Hct) >50%, due to production of erythropoietin from tumor
- Presents with dizziness, headache, epistaxis, clotting
- Most common in renal cell cancer, hepatoma; rare in other cancers
- Rarely due to testosterone, human placental lactogen
- Treatment is with phlebotomy; treat underlying malignancy.

Hemolytic anemia
- **Autoimmune** form is seen more commonly in hematologic malignancy, rarely with solid tumors. Treat with steroids. It may respond to intravenous immunoglobulin (IVIG), rituximab, spleenectomy, and treatment of underlying malignancy.
- **Microangiopathic** form is characterized by anemia with schistocytes. Most commonly seen in gastric, breast, lung and vascular tumors. Treat underlying malignancy. Consider plasmapheresis.
- **Red cell aplasia** is a classic association with thymoma, also seen in CLL (6%), HD, NHL, and rarely with solid tumors. Treat underlying malignancy, give immunosuppression. There are reports of response to rituximab.

White cell disorders
Sweets syndrome
- Febrile neutrophilic dermatosis
- Most commonly associated with AML
- Also seen with lymphoma, myeloma, rarely with solid tumors

Platelet disorders
POEMS syndrome
POEMS is associated with myeloma:
- Peripheral neuropathy
- Organomegaly
- Endocrinopathy
- Monoclonal plasma cell disorder
- Skin changes
- Edema
- Thrombocytosis

It is treated with radiation, steroids, and chemotherapy.

Thrombocytosis
This is rarely reported with hepatocellular and other solid tumors.

Thrombocytopenia
- A megakaryocytic thrombocytopenia associated with thymoma
- Idiopathic thrombocytopenic purpura (ITP) is associated with solid tumors and hematologic malignancy.

Coagulopathy

Trousseau syndrome

An association between visceral cancer and thrombosis was noted in 1865 by Armand Trousseau. Multiple mechanisms contribute to clotting associated with malignancy:
- Release of procoagulants by tumor cells
- Exposure or release of tissue factor

This syndrome is most commonly associated with mucin-producing carcinomas, although an elevated risk of thrombosis is seen with many malignancies.

Treatment is with anticoagulation.

Dermatologic and skeletal paraneoplastic syndromes

Digital clubbing
- Commonly associated with NSCLC, also with nonmalignant cardiopulmonary disorders
- Loss of angle at nail bed and increased distal soft tissue of phalanges
- Frequently associated with hypertrophic osteoarthropathy

Hypertrophic osteoarthropathy
- Periostial inflammation of the long bones associated with joint pains
- Associated with NSCLC

Pemphigus
Acantholysis with intraepithelial blisters due to autoantibodies

Pemphigus vulgaris
This form is most common, and it often starts with oral lesions.
- Kaposi sarcoma
- HD
- NHL
- CLL
- Thymoma

Paraneoplastic pemphigus
This form is rare and involves mucous membranes. It is painful and widely disseminated.
- NLH
- CLL
- Sarcoma
- Thymoma

Pyoderma gangrenosum
Neutrophilic dermatosis presents as a pustule progressing to ulceration with a necrotic center and raised erythematous margin.
- Frequently on lower extremity, but variable, including visceral
- AML, multiple myeloma, CML, rarely with gastric cancer, solid tumors

Sweets syndrome
Neutrophilic dermatosis presents with
- Fever
- Neutrophilia
- Tender red nodules
- Most commonly associated with AML

This syndrome may be associated with renal, ocular, or pulmonary involvement.

Ichthyosis
This scaling on the trunk and extensor surfaces is associated with HD.

Bazex syndrome
Acral hyperkeratosis presents with psoriaform erythematous lesions, occasionally with pain and itching, strongly in
- Head and neck
- Colon
- Lymphoma
- Bladder
- Prostate
- Gynecological malignancy

Pruritus
Severe itching
- HD
- AML
- NHL
- Insulinoma
- CNS tumors

Acanthosis nigricans
This involves hyperpigmentation, especially in intertriginous areas such as the groin, axillae, and skin folds, with a velvety appearance. It is due to hyperkeratosis.
- Gastric cancer: 90% of paraneoplastic cases are associated with GI malignancy.

Vitiligo
Vitiligo is a sporadic loss of pigmentation, associated with melanoma. It may be a positive prognostic factor.

Sign of Leser-Trelat
This increase in size and number of seborrheic keratoses are associated most commonly with GI malignancy or lymphoma.

Necrolytic migratory erythema
This erythematous rash with blisters and stomatitis typically starts in the groin and lower extremities.
- Glucagonoma
- Rarely seen with other GI malignancy

Erythroderma
Erythroderma is characterized by diffuse redness and inflammation.
- Lymphoma
- AML

Erythema gyratum repens is migratory, with a concentric-ring appearance on the trunk and proximal extremities.
- Lung
- Esophageal
- Breast

Further reading

Altaha R, Abraham J (2003). Paraneoplastic neurologic syndrome associated with occult breast cancer: a case report and review of literature. *Breast J* **9**:417–419.

Kurzrock R, Cohen PR (1995). Cutaneous paraneoplastic syndromes in solid tumors. *Am J Med* **99**:662–671.

Kurzrock R, Cohen PR (1995). Mucocutaneous paraneoplastic manifestations of hematologic malignancies. *Am J Med* **99**:207–216.

Minisini AM, Pauletto G, Bergonzi P, et al. (2007). Paraneoplastic neurological syndromes and breast cancer. Regression of paraneoplastic neurological sensorimotor neuropathy in a patient with metastatic breast cancer treated with capecitabine: a case study and mini-review of the literature. *Breast Cancer Res Treat* **105**:133–138.

Chapter 22

Superior vena cava syndrome and raised intracranial pressure

Christina I. Herold

Superior vena cava syndrome 322
Raised intracranial pressure 326

Superior vena cava syndrome

Etiology

The superior vena cava (SVC) can be obstructed by any combination of the following:
- External compression of the SVC, which accounts for more than 80% of cases of SVC syndrome, e.g., from primary tumor (most commonly in the right paratracheal region) or from metastatic lymphadenoapthy
- Direct invasion of the SVC, from the same causes
- Thrombus within the SVC, e.g., due to central venous catheterization (Hickman or PICC lines etc) or secondary to compression

The most common underlying diagnosis is lung cancer.
- Small cell lung cancer (SCLC) is a particular risk factor for SVC syndrome (up to 20% of patients with SCLC), as these cancers commonly develop within central rather than peripheral airways.
- However, any tumor spreading to the mediastinal lymph nodes can be causative, e.g., lymphoma (typically non-Hodgkin's), thymoma, and mediastinal germ cell tumors.

Benign causes of SVC syndrome are much less common but include sarcoidosis, post-radiotherapy fibrosis, and unusual infections resulting in fibrosing mediastinitis, e.g., aspergillosis, histoplasmosis, and tuberculosis.

Clinical features

Symptoms
- Dyspnea is the most commonly reported symptom. This is due to associated tracheal or bronchial obstruction or compression.
- Swelling of the neck, face, and arms, especially in the morning and often exacerbated by bending forward or lying down
- Cough
- Headache
- Visual disturbance
- Acuteness of presentation depends on the rate at which obstruction of the SVC occurs compared to recruitment of venous collaterals.

Signs
- Fixed engorgement of external and internal jugular veins
- Collateral veins over anterior and lateral chest wall (alternative pathways for the return of venous blood to the right atrium)
- Facial plethora
- Papilledema (late feature)

Differential diagnoses

- Heart failure presents with cardiac signs including jugular vein pulsation, S3 gallop, and dependent edema.
- Cardiac tamponade: Characteristic presentation includes pulsus paradoxus and pericardial friction rub appearances.
- External jugular vein compression is usually caused by supraclavicular lymphadenopathy and present without facial edema or venous collateralization.

Diagnosis

Up to 60% of patients with SVC syndrome due to underlying cancer present without a known diagnosis of malignancy. Unless the patient has severe and life-threatening symptoms (e.g., associated stridor), treatment should not start until a clear diagnosis (including pathology if possible) has been made.

Imaging techniques:
- Chest X-ray typically shows a right paratracheal mass, mediastinal lymphadenopathy, or other indications of lung cancer, e.g., pleural effusion. It is abnormal in >80% of cases.
- CT thorax with contrast, to define the level and degree of venous blockage, assists in identifying the cause of SVC syndrome. It can help with staging of the cancer (especially if the abdomen is also imaged) and hence with appropriate further management. Percutaneous biopsy may confirm the diagnosis.
- MRI is indicated if dye allergy prohibits the use of CT with contrast.
- Upper-extremity ultrasound can help identify venous collateralization and determine the extent of thrombosis.

Venogram is needed if there is no obvious mass causing external compression, or if thrombolysis or stent insertion is planned.

- **Pathologic diagnosis**: The priority is to obtain a tissue diagnosis by the most minimally invasive method possible.
- **Cytology**: Sources include sputum, pleural fluid and fine-needle aspiration from any easily accessible site, e.g., cervical lymphadenopathy.
- Bronchoscopy with biopsy is essential if the clinical picture and imaging suggest lung cancer but no histopathology has been obtained.
- Mediastinal biopsy (via mediastinoscopy, video-assisted thorascopy, thoracotomy, or directed-needle biopsy) provides an alternative method of obtaining pathologic diagnosis if other attempts have failed.
- Bone marrow biopsy may provide both diagnostic and staging information for patients with suspected lymphoma or SCLC.

Management

Most patients present with symptoms of insidious onset and there is time to establish the diagnosis and extent of disease before commencing treatment. Prognosis is dependent on tumor histology and stage of disease at presentation, rather than the presence of SVC syndrome per se.

If a patient is severely compromised, consider the possibility that there is concomitant tracheal compression. In the acute situation:
- Sit the patient up, establish intravenous access, and provide supplemental oxygen if appropriate.
- Consider the use of corticosteroids to reduce peritumoral edema.
- Stenting: An expanding metal stent can be inserted into the SVC at the point of stricture. If an interventional cardiologist or radiologist can provide rapid service, this is the treatment of choice for patients with severe symptoms. Endovascular stenting can also be used for recurrent SVC syndrome in a previously irradiated field.

- Radiotherapy is occasionally used in the absence of a pathologic diagnosis. However, it is important to stress this will *not* provide immediate symptomatic benefit. Anticipated life expectancy must be several weeks to see the full benefit. Radiotherapy may make subsequent pathologic diagnosis difficult to obtain.
- Thrombolysis: In the presence of a clot, thrombolysis can be combined with stent insertion. If thrombus has formed around a central line, removal of the line alone will usually lead to resolution of SVC syndrome.
- Anticoagulation: If thrombolysis is indicated then therapeutic anticoagulation is advised. In the more common scenario where a stent is place without thrombolysis, there is no consensus guideline regarding anticoagulation. Reasonable options include low-dose warfarin or antiplatlet therapy with aspirin and clopiogrel.

In practice it is rare for the clinical situation to be so acute as to prevent an appropriate workup. Therefore, treatment can be tailored according to the underlying diagnosis as in the following examples.

- Small cell lung cancer: These are typically chemosensitive tumors. If the patient has a suitable performance status, systemic chemotherapy is the appropriate first-line management producing palliation of symptoms within 1–2 weeks. Palliative radiotherapy is used in patients of poorer performance status or on relapse after previous chemotherapy.
- Non-small–cell lung cancer: The presence of SVC syndrome is usually associated with locally advanced (and hence incurable) disease. Surgery is unlikely to be appropriate. Occasionally, radical radiotherapy for central, localized cancers may be possible, but generally radiotherapy is palliative in intent.
- Non-Hodgkin's lymphoma: usually chemotherapy
- Mediastinal germ cell tumor: chemotherapy

Raised intracranial pressure

- The rigid bony skull surrounding the brain is resistant to any increase in the volume of its contents, with any such change leading to a rise in intracranial pressure (ICP) and/or displacement of brain structures. The skull contents comprise: Brain and interstitial fluid (80%)
- Intravascular blood (10%)
- Cerebrospinal fluid (CSF) (10%)

An increase in volume of one component may be accommodated by reduction in another to maintain physiological ICP (10–20 cm H_2O).
- When malignancy involves the brain, these physiological regulatory mechanisms are commonly overcome, leading to raised ICP.

Clinical presentation
- Early stages: Typical symptoms include headache, nausea, and vomiting.
- Symptoms are often worse in the morning because cerebral venous congestion is associated with lying supine.
- Coughing or sneezing may aggravate the headache.
- As pressure increases, there may be cognitive impairment and drowsiness, heralding a more rapid neurological deterioration.
- Herniation of cerebral tissue through the tentorium may cause midbrain compression with coma associated with pupillary and oculomotor signs, and altered regulation of respiration and cardiovascular control, with bradycardia and hypertension (Cushing's triad).
- Fundoscopy will reveal papilledema in 50% of cases, and there may be associated neurological deficit.
- Specific signs may suggest the site of pathology, e.g., Parinaud's syndrome, with limitation of upward gaze associated with pineal tumors.
- Raised ICP may cause hyponatremia through SIADH.
- When increase in ICP is more gradual, presentation may be with memory loss, behavioral changes, and altered gait.
- Meningeal malignancy commonly causes cranial nerve palsies in addition to raised ICP.

Pathogenesis
The three most common causes of increased ICP are as follows:
- Space-occupying lesion
- Hydrocephalus (due to obstruction of CSF circulation)
- Benign intracranial hypertension

It should be remembered that patients with malignancy may be at risk of developing nonmalignant raised ICP as a consequence of treatment, e.g., coagulopathy-associated intracranial hemorrhage or CNS infection in an immunocompromised individual.

Of the neoplastic lesions causing raised ICP:
- 50% are due to metastatic disease.
- The remainder are primary brain tumors, of which gliomas are the most common.

Malignant disease in the CNS can produce a rise in ICP through the following:
- Mass effect
- Vasogenic edema: Capillary leakage is associated with the abnormal tumor vasculature.
- Hemorrhage from the tumor (especially melanoma, choriocarcinoma, renal cancer)
- Hydrocephalus
  - Obstruction of CSF flow, e.g., pineal tumor obstructing the aqueduct of Sylvius prevents drainage of CSF from the third to fourth ventricle.
  - Meningeal metastases may reduce the reabsorption of CSF with resulting communicating hydrocephalus.

Diagnosis

Contrast-enhanced CT and MRI scans are the imaging modalities of choice.
- Unenhanced CT may show mass lesion(s) and associated hemorrhage (hyperdense).
- CT with IV contrast demonstrates enhancement in most CNS malignancies.
- MRI has superior sensitivity in the detection of CNS malignancy.
- Where CT shows a solitary tumor, MRI will reveal more than one lesion in at least 20%.
- On MRI, tumor appears iso- or hypodense on T1-weighted images, appears hyperdense on T2, and enhances with contrast.
- MRI gives superior definition of anatomical detail and may demonstrate meningeal spread of malignancy.

Management

Early management is critical.
- Head elevation at 30 degrees above the heart can reduce ICP
- Fluid management and blood pressure control to maintain cerebral perfusion pressure of >60 mmHg
- Steroids are useful when elevated ICP is attributed to brain tumors and CNS infection but are contraindicated in the treatment of intracranial hemorrhage or infarction.
- Consider osmotic diuresis with IV mannitol
- Anticonvulsants are indicated if seizure activity is suspected and may also be considered for prophylaxis
- Fever can elevate ICP and therefore should be treated aggressively

Other considerations to reduce ICP include sedation, the use of propofol and barbituates, mechanical hyperventilation, and therapeutic hypothermia. Additional management will depend on the diagnosis and may include the following:
- Neurosurgical intervention including ventriculostomy for CSF removal and decompressive craniotomy
- Systemic chemotherapy for chemosensitive disease, e.g., CNS lymphoma

- Cranial radiotherapy
- Symptom control alone may be appropriate if there is poor prognosis

Other management considerations:
- In general, CNS tumors presenting with raised ICP require a tissue diagnosis, either by biopsy, which may be stereotactic, or by craniotomy and removal of the tumor.
- Ventricular shunting may be useful in patients with hydrocephalus due to lesions situated in areas difficult to access surgically. However, if at all possible, pathologic confirmation should be sought, because it has major bearing on the therapeutic approach.
- High-grade gliomas may have a substantial cystic component that, in the setting of recurrent disease, may be drained to provide rapid relief of elevated ICP.

Further reading

Edwards P, Arango M, Balica L, et al. (2005). Final results of the MRC CRASH, a randomised placebo-controlled trial of intravenous corticosteroid in adults with head injury-outcomes at 6 months. *Lancet* 365:1957–1959.

Perez-Soler R, McLaughlin P, Velasquez WS, et al. (1984). Clinical features and results of management of superior vena cava syndrome secondary to lymphoma. *J Clin Oncol* 2:260–266.

Rowell NP, Gleeson FV (2002). Steroids, radiotherapy, chemotherapy and stents for superior vena caval obstruction in carcinoma of the bronchus: a systematic review. *Clin Oncol (R Coll Radiol)* 14:338–341.

Wilson LD, Detterbeck FC, Yahalom J (2007). Clinical practice. Superior vena cava syndrome with malignant causes. *N Engl J Med* 356:1862–1869.

Chapter 23

Spinal cord compression

Christina I. Herold

Spinal cord compression *332*

Spinal cord compression

Spinal cord compression is a medical emergency. The symptoms of spinal cord compression vary and often relate to the anatomical site and degree of the compression (see Box 23.1). Treatment must begin within hours, not days. The spinal cord ends at the L1 or L2 level in adults; thecal sac compression with lumbosacral nerve root impingement below this level is known as cauda equina syndrome. The management strategies for true spinal compression and cauda equina syndrome are shared and described below.

Presentation

Spinal cord compression can occur with metastatic spinal involvement from any type of cancer. It is common in these cancers:
- Breast
- Prostate
- Lung
- Myeloma
- Lymphoma

It is less common in these cancers:
- Thyroid
- Kidney
- Bladder
- Bowel
- Melanoma

Other characteristics of spinal cord compression:
- The majority of cases occur in the thoracic cord (60%) with the remainder in the lumbosacral cord and nerve roots (30%) and cervical spine (10%).
- In approximately 20% of cases, spinal cord compression is the patient's initial presentation of malignancy.
- Crush fracture or tumor extension due to bony metastasis in the vertebral spine is the most common mechanism of spinal cord compression and accounts for 85%–90% of cases.

Other less common mechanisms of spinal cord compression include direct extension from retroperitoneal or mediastinal tumors (e.g., lymphoma), extradural compression in the absence of bone involvement, and intramedullary metastases.

Symptoms

- Back pain is often the first neurologic symptom of spinal cord compression. Characteristics of this back pain include radicular pain that is exacerbated by coughing or straining and worsened when lying down.
- Any patient with cancer who develops severe back pain with a nerve root distribution should be considered at risk of spinal cord compression and urgently evaluated.
- Other symptoms may include paraplegia or gait disturbance, weakness of the legs (and arms if the lesion is high in the spine), "saddle" anesthesia (involving the sacral root distributions), urinary symptoms (retention or dribbling from overflow incontinence), bowel symptoms (incontinence or constipation), and impotence.
- Tumors below L1 or L2 may produce cauda equina syndrome with sciatic pain that is often bilateral as well as the symptoms described above.

Box 23.1 Spinal cord compression syndromes

Complete compression
Sensory level just below level of lesion
Loss of all sensory modalities—may be variable at onset
Bilateral upper motor neuron weakness below lesion
Bladder and bowel dysfunction

Anterior compression
Partial loss of pain and temperature below lesion
Bilateral upper motor neuron weakness below lesion
Bladder and bowel dysfunction

Posterior compression
Loss of vibration and position below lesion
Relative sparing of pain, temperature, and touch
Band of dysthesia at level of lesion

Lateral compression (Brown–Séquard syndrome)
Contralateral loss of pain and temperature (touch relatively spared)
Ipsilateral loss of vibration and position
Ipsilateral upper motor neuron weakness

Examination

The spinal lesion may be partial or complete and the nature of the defect may depend on the portion of the cord compressed. The following may be present:
- Visible or palpable gibbus at site of a wedged or collapsed vertebra
- Pain and tenderness on palpation or percussion of the vertebra over the site of compression
- Band of hyperesthesia at the level of the lesion
- Sensory and motor loss (with defects of power and sensation) at and below the level of the lesion
- Loss of anal sphincter tone
- Weakness and wasting of the gluteal muscles

Diagnosis

- Plain X-ray films may demonstrate destruction and/or collapse of a vertebra. Paravertebral masses may sometimes also be shown. In 15%–20% of cases, plain films show no abnormality.
- MRI scanning is the imaging modality of choice. It is particularly useful in cases of cauda equina syndrome.
- If MRI is not available, CT scans may provide useful information. Simultaneous myelography may enhance the diagnostic utility of CT scans.

Management

Speed is critical in the diagnosis and management of spinal cord compression. Optimal management requires urgent consultation and coordination of care between neurosurgery, radiation oncology, and medical oncology. Fewer than 10% of patients with paraplegia from metastatic spinal cord compression walk again. Steroids are critical to reduce peritumoral edema. Dexamethasone (16–20 mg) should be given immediately and continued daily in divided doses.

Indications for surgical decompression of the spine include the following:
- Acute-onset paraplegia
- Fracture dislocation
- Lack of clinical improvement with steroids
- Involvement with a tumor type that is known to display primary resistance to radiation therapy
- Progression or recurrence of spinal cord compression following radiation therapy
- No histological proof of malignancy

Other management considerations:
- If immediate surgery is not indicated, neurological status should be assessed several times daily so that deterioration may be detected early and surgical intervention reconsidered.
- Spinal radiation therapy is useful for patients who are not surgical candidates or as an adjunct to surgical intervention. Radiation-induced edema may exacerbate symptoms, and it is therefore critical to increase the dose of steroids as needed. Chemotherapy may be considered as part of the treatment plan for patients with tumors that are very chemosensitive, including certain lymphomas and germ cell tumors. However, as with all interventions for spinal cord compression, understanding the speed of likely efficacy of the chemotherapy is paramount when planning treatment.

Further reading

Mak KS, Lee LK, Mak RH, et al. (2011). Incidence and treatment patterns in hospitalizations for malignant spinal cord compression in the United States, 1998-2006. *Int J Radiat Oncol Biol Phys* 80:824–831.

Chapter 24

Other obstructive complications

Gary H. Lyman

Bronchial obstruction and stridor *338*
Intestinal obstruction *340*
Obstructive jaundice *344*
Urinary tract obstruction *348*

Bronchial obstruction and stridor

Stridor
Stridor is a high-pitched noise generated by the turbulent flow of air through a partially obstructed airway. Obstruction may be localized above the vocal cords, at the level of the cords, below the cords, or in the trachea.

The timing of stridor may suggest the site of the obstruction.
- Inspiratory stridor, with extrathoracic, supraglottic, or glottic obstruction
- Biphasic stridor, with glottic or subglottic obstruction
- Expiratory stridor, with intrathoracic obstruction of the trachea

Etiology
Malignant
- Primary disease of the upper airway, e.g., laryngeal carcinoma
- Metastatic endobronchial disease affecting the upper airway, e.g., bronchogenic, breast, melanoma, renal cell
- Lymphadenopathy, e.g., from lymphoma or metastatic carcinoma
- Mediastinal neoplasm, e.g., anaplastic thyroid cancer, germ cell cancer

Benign
- Lymphadenopathy, e.g., sarcoidosis, tuberculosis
- Inhaled foreign body, mucus plug, or blood clot
- Tracheal stenosis, e.g. post-tracheostomy, granulation tissue
- Bilateral vocal cord palsy, e.g., post-thyroid surgery
- Infective, e.g. epiglottitis, diptheria

Alternatively, classification may be according to whether obstruction is due to the following:
- Intrinsic upper airway disease, e.g., bulky tumors of the upper airway, larynx, hypopharynx, subglottis, or trachea or local extension of a bronchial tumor invading the carina
- Extrinsic compression, e.g., mediastinal tumors or lymphadenopathy, esophageal carcinoma

Presentation of malignant stridor
Presentation is usually insidious, e.g., with slow compression by mediastinal tumor. Occasionally history is acute, e.g., with rapid deterioration when subcritical obstruction is further compromised by swelling or lower respiratory tract infection.

Symptoms
- Stridor
- Dyspnea
- Dysphagia or drooling
- Cyanosis
- Features of underlying malignancy, e.g., goiter, clubbing, weight loss, disseminated lymphadenopathy

Management and investigation

The priority is to stabilize a distressed patient:
Have the patient sit upright; check ABGs, give 100% O_2, establish intravenous access, involve ENT staff, and consider ICU placement if patient is exhausted or in respiratory failure (P_aO_2 ≤10 kPa, P_aCO_2 ≥6 kPa). Very occasionally, emergency tracheostomy may be required to preserve the airway before appropriate treatment is initiated.

Remember diagnosis and staging of the underlying malignancy may not have been confirmed. *If the patient is stable,* consider the following:
- Chest X-ray may demonstrate mediastinal widening (lymphadenopathy) or primary lung cancer.
- CT scan of the thorax may identify the site of obstruction and indicate the extent of disease (prognostic implications).
- Indirect laryngoscopy shows the mobility of cords.
- Bronchoscopy provides direct visualization, confirming airway obstruction. It differentiates between intrinsic and extrinsic lesions, and may allow histological confirmation of the diagnosis.
- Fiberoptic nasoendoscopy
- Mediastinoscopy

Management of stridor in stable patients
- Supplemental O_2 assess the need to use O_2 with pulse oximetry and ABGs.
- High-dose steroids aim to reduce peritumoral edema and relieve obstruction, e.g., dexamethasone 8 mg bd po/IV.
- Radiotherapy is used for most patients with non-small-cell lung cancer, usually with palliative intent.
  - It is appropriate in some other cancers, e.g., renal cell cancer.
  - It may be initiated in the absence of histology in urgent circumstances. Therapeutic effects are delayed.
  - There is anecdotal concern that radiotherapy may initially worsen peritumoral edema and all such patients should receive steroids.
  - Endobronchial brachytherapy is an option in recurrent obstruction.
- Chemotherapy is the appropriate primary treatment for airway obstruction due to chemosensitive tumors, e.g., small cell carcinoma, lymphoma, germ cell tumors.
- Laser debulking is helpful in treating bulky exophytic laryngeal tumors prior to definitive treatment or if the cancer is radioresistant, e.g., metastatic melanoma. If this is the sole therapy, the effects tend not to be long-lasting.
- Endoluminal stenting may produce useful palliation in cases of recurrent malignancy affecting the trachea or in obstruction due to extrinsic causes.
- Surgical resection has a limited role as salvage therapy for recurrent laryngeal cancer after radiotherapy and, more rarely, primary carcinoid tumor of the trachea or a solitary renal cell metastasis.

Intestinal obstruction

Etiology

- Intestinal obstruction is predominantly associated with pelvic cancers and most commonly found in ovarian (6%–42%), cervical (5%), and colonic cancers (10%–30%).
- The cause is either intraluminal disease (more common in colonic cancer) or extramural compression.
  - In ovarian and cervical cancer there are often multiple levels of obstruction.
  - Obstruction in a patient with previous cancer may also be due to nonmalignant causes such as adhesions or gross constipation.
- Obstruction may be complete, subacute, or functional; it may be intermittent.
- Functional obstruction may be caused by a cancer- or drug-related (vincristine) autonomic neuropathy, by direct involvement of the mesenteric plexus, or ileus (e.g., due to perforation).
- The most frequent cause of intestinal obstruction is the cancer itself, which may invade the lumen of the bowel, extrinsically compress the bowel, or disrupt the neurological supply to the bowel wall muscle.
- The common primary sites causing gastric intestinal problems are colorectal and ovarian cancers.
- Less common but reversible causes include electrolyte disturbances, fecal impaction, postoperative adhesions, or hernia.
- The common electrolyte disturbance is that of hypercalcemia and hypokalemia.

Presentation

Symptoms
- Nausea, vomiting
- Colicky pain
- Constipation

Signs
- Increased bowel sounds
- Distension, dehydration, splash, bowel sounds variable
- Gastric outlet obstruction—large-volume projectile vomiting
- Large-bowel obstruction; feculent vomiting

Investigations

- Erect and supine plain abdominal views may confirm the diagnosis.
- Where the diagnosis is not clear, contrast barium studies may be indicated.
- If surgery is a possibility and there is doubt about the number of levels of obstruction or the site of the lesion, CT or MRI can be helpful.
- Appropriate treatment will be guided by clinical and biochemical assessment of dehydration and electrolyte disturbance.
- Endoscopy of the upper or lower intestinal tract may allow visualization of the area of obstruction.

Management options

- First-line therapy is surgical if active treatment is appropriate.
- Intravenous fluids and nasogastric suction are usually initiated.
- The patient may not wish surgery or surgery may not be appropriate because of the extent of disease.
- Laser therapy may be useful to debulk obstructing esophageal, gastric, and rectal carcinomas.
  - May require repeated treatment.
- Plastic tubes or expandable metal stents can also be considered and are generally of use in esophageal or esophagogastric lesions.

Medical management

Treatment approaches vary depending on whether subacute obstruction or complete obstruction is present. The symptoms to be palliated include nausea, vomiting, pain, and constipation.

Inoperable intestinal obstruction can be managed medically.

- This may permit the patient to be cared for at home.
- The patient can eat and drink small amounts.
- The aim is to remove the debilitating feeling of nausea and to reduce the frequency of vomiting to a level acceptable to the patient.
- Oral medication is poorly absorbed in gastrointestinal obstruction and the subcutaneous (SC) or rectal route should be used.

Pain

- For colic, an antispasmodic (e.g., buscopan 80–120 mg over 24 hours via continuous SC infusion) is usually effective.
- Avoid prokinetic antiemetics (e.g., metoclopramide) if colic is a problem.
- Pain from cancer or metastases usually requires parenteral analgesics, e.g., diamorphine given subcutaneously over 24 hours via a syringe driver, or transdermal fentanyl.

Nausea and vomiting

If partial obstruction without colic is present, metoclopramide 80–120 mg over 24 hours SC may stimulate effective bowel motility.

- This can be combined with high-dose dexamethasone 16 mg/24 hours to reduce peritumor edema and also serve as an antiemetic.
- As vomiting is controlled, introduce oral laxatives as tolerated.

If obstruction is complete or if colic is present, cyclizine 100–150 mg/24 hours SC may be given with buscopan.

- Haloperidol 5–15 mg/24 hours is a suitable alternative.
- Haloperidol, cyclizine, and hyoscine are all miscible with diamorphine in a syringe.

Levomeprazine is a highly specific 5-HT$_2$ antagonist and has inhibitory effects on other emetic pathway receptors. It is a useful alternative to the other antiemetics considered and is also miscible with diamorphine. If vomiting persists then octreotide, a somatostatin analog, 300–600 mg/24 hours via continuous SC infusion can be used.

- This drug is antisecretory and promotes reabsorption of electrolytes and, hence, water from the bowel.

In difficult cases, a nasogastric tube should be considered for short-term use. If all else fails to control the vomiting a venting gastrostomy should be considered, taking into account the patient's prognosis, current condition, and their own wishes. With a gastrostomy the patient can take oral liquids, which can be drawn off via the gastrostomy as needed.

All patients with malignant bowel obstruction who fail to recover bowel function with conservative management should be considered for surgery if the clinical status of the patient permits and the patient wishes further invasive therapy.
- Even in those fit for surgery, 25% will die perioperatively.
- This problem is best managed with a multidisciplinary team, involving surgeons, medical oncologists, and palliative-care physicians, along with discussions with the patient and family.

If the obstruction is due to a very chemosensitive tumor, such as a lymphoma, small cell lung cancer, or testicular cancer, a trial of chemotherapy may be appropriate. This is potentially hazardous, however, and requires close monitoring.

The patient with esophageal obstruction or duodenal obstruction may benefit from local radiotherapy or stent insertion.
- In general, the stent should be inserted first, followed by radiotherapy, because the benefit from the latter may not be seen for 6 weeks.

Surgical treatment

Surgical options include the following:
- Obstruction of the esophagus
  - Esophagectomy in very selected patients
  - Stent insertion
  - Laser treatment
- Duodenum bypass surgery
  - Stent insertion
  - Ileum
  - Resection of obstruction and re-anastomosis
  - Division of adhesions
  - Defunctioning ileostomy
- Colon: resection of obstruction and re-anastomosis
- Defunctioning colostomy: stent

Risks of bowel surgery in patients with advanced cancer
- Multiple levels of bowel obstruction due to intraperitoneal tumor seeding
- Poor anesthetic risk due to generalized debility
- Poor surgical healing due to malnutrition, chemotherapy, or tumor seeding
- High risk of thromboembolic events
- Early mortality and morbidity

Obstructive jaundice

Etiology
There are many causes of jaundice in the patient with malignant disease. They may be divided as follows:
- Increased production of bilirubin, hemolytic anemia
- Decreased uptake of bilirubin
  - Gilbert's syndrome
  - Drugs
  - Portacaval shunts
- Decreased excretion of bilirubin
  - Hepatotoxic drugs
  - Viral hepatitis
  - Malignant infiltration of biliary tree or liver and extrahepatic biliary obstruction

It is important not to focus only on cancer causes in patients with jaundice with a history of cancer. Jaundice is not always due to the recurrence of the cancer or its complications.

Patients must be carefully assessed, ideally by a multidisciplinary team, to ensure that they are adequately investigated so that noncancerous causes of the obstructive jaundice can be dealt with in the appropriate fashion.

History
- Abdominal pain
- Duration of jaundice and whether the jaundice fluctuates
- Fever
- Itching
- Dark stools and pale urine
- It is important to assess whether the patient has signs of sepsis.
- A careful drug history is important because a number of drugs can cause hepatic toxicity: e.g., cisplatin and oxaliplatin can cause cholestasis.
- Likewise, antimetabolites, such as cytarabine, may cause self-limiting abnormalities of liver function, often with a cholestatic pattern.
  - A similar pattern can arise with mercaptopurine and methotrexate.
- Hormonal agents, such as tamoxifen, can occasionally cause abnormal liver function with a fatty liver.
- It is also important to take a detailed history of other drug therapies, such as paracetamol, antibiotics, and antifungal agents, all of which can cause liver abnormalities.
- Total parenteral nutrition can cause fatty infiltration and intrahepatic cholestasis.

Examination

Signs of recurrence of the previous cancer include clinical jaundice, anemia, signs of chronic liver disease, palpable liver, palpable gall bladder, and palpable spleen.

Investigations

Depending on the pointers from the history and the examination, investigations should include the following:

- Routine blood tests, including hemoglobin, white cell count
- Liver function tests, including transaminases, gamma GT, bilirubin, alkaline phosphatase
- Autoantibody screen is important to investigate autoimmune disease.
- Electrophoresis and other investigations for hemolysis in selected patients where indicated
- All patients who are undergoing active management and treatment require coagulation studies, because of deficiency of the vitamin K-dependent coagulation factors.

The most important screening radiological investigation is ultrasound, which can be used to diagnose the following:

- Gallstones
- Intra- or extrahepatic biliary dilatation
- Tumor masses in the region of the pancreas (better seen on CT)
- Liver metastases
- Nodes around the porta hepatis, although the lower end of the common bile duct is not well visualized.

MRI scanning gives a very good view of the biliary tree and is noninvasive. CT scanning is excellent for liver and pancreatic lesions.

In general, endoscopic retrograde cholangiopancreatography (ERCP) is the next step, provided the patient is going to require active management. ERCP is an excellent diagnostic technique.

- ERCP can be used to diagnose pancreatic, intrinsic biliary, extrinsic biliary, and hepatic lesions.
- Brushings for cytology and biopsies can be taken.
- ERCP is an excellent therapeutic modality, which can be used to dilate strictures, place stents, and extract stones from the common bile duct.
- Occasionally, percutaneous transhepatic cholangiography is used in conjunction with ERCP to insert stents for difficult high hilar lesions, either intrinsic, such as cholangiocarcinoma (Klatskin's tumor), or extrinsic (nodes at porta hepatis).

Points of caution

- Intrahepatic duct dilatation does not occur readily in extrinsic biliary obstruction when there are multiple liver metastases compressing the ducts and when there is sclerosing cholangitis or liver cirrhosis.
- Any invasive endeavors around the biliary tree, including ERCP and biliary stenting, must be covered with antibiotics, because there is a high risk of sepsis.
- Serum amylase should be performed pre- and post-ERCP.
- Occasionally, liver biopsy is appropriate. This can be ultrasound guided, laparoscopic, or transjugular in patients with coagulopathies.

Management

Management depends on the cause of the jaundice. It is crucial that patients who are highly complex be managed in a multidisciplinary team setting.

The patient's views should be considered, especially when the jaundice is due to recurrence of a previous carcinoma. Each cause of jaundice should be treated in its own right, depending on the patient's general condition and wishes. For example, a stone in the common bile duct can be removed at ERCP and the patient can undergo laparoscopic cholecystectomy at a later date, should that be appropriate.

Many patients with obstructive jaundice in the setting of cancer require palliation.

If drug causes have been excluded and the patient has an irresectable tumor problem causing the obstruction, often the best mode of palliation is endoscopic stenting. This tends to have a lower early morbidity and mortality than an open surgical bypass. With increasing advances in laparoscopic surgery, laparoscopic biliary bypass is now technically feasible in selected patients, in experienced hands.

The main problem with stents is that they occlude with subsequent recurrence of jaundice and sepsis, although the more modern expandable, metal stents have decreased bacterial colonization and are more resistant to tumor ingrowth.

Hepatorenal syndrome

Classically, this syndrome occurs in obstructive jaundice, and it is essentially acute oliguric renal failure, occurring without intrinsic renal disease. There is intense renal cortical vasoconstriction with increased renal vascular resistance, decreased glomerular filtration rate, peripheral vasodilatation, and sodium and water retention.

This diagnosis should be considered in patients with liver dysfunction, obstructive jaundice, rising serum creatinine in the absence of fluid losses, dehydration, and renal disease, with use of nephrotoxic drugs, and in patients who are not septic.

Investigations should exclude other causes of renal insufficiency, via serum and urinary electrolytes, creatinine clearance, and blood cultures. A urinary tract ultrasound should be obtained to exclude urinary obstruction.

Investigations usually reveal the following:
- High serum creatinine
- Low creatinine clearance
- Low serum sodium
- Low urinary output
- Low urinary sodium

Management is complex and should be done by a multidisciplinary team.
- Nephrotoxic drugs should be withdrawn.
- Sepsis should be corrected.
- Fluid and electrolyte imbalance should be corrected.
- Selected patients may warrant dialysis with correction of the obstructive jaundice.

Prognosis is often poor, however, with only a 10% 3-month survival rate.
- Aggressive therapy in this setting, in the patient with cancer, needs to be very carefully considered.

Urinary tract obstruction

Etiology
The following are the most common causes of urinary obstruction in patients with cancer:
- Carcinoma of the prostate or bladder when the urethra or ureteric orifices become occluded
- Carcinoma of the cervix or other carcinoma involving the pelvis obstructing the lower ureter
- Paraaortic nodes or retroperitoneal tumor compressing the ureters
- Transitional cell carcinoma of one or both ureters
- Fibrosis following surgery, chemotherapy, or radiotherapy

Symptoms
The gradual onset of unilateral ureteric obstruction is often asymptomatic, only diagnosed radiographically as hydronephrosis.

Acute ureteric obstruction may cause painful spasm or dull aching in the flank, and the pain may radiate in the distribution of the L1 nerve root.

Bilateral gradual obstruction becomes symptomatic as the serum urea rises above 25 mmol/L, ultimately leading to anuria and renal failure, with lethargy, drowsiness, confusion, nausea, and twitching.

Investigations
Selective use of abdominal ultrasound, IV urography (contraindicated in the uremic patient), cystoscopy and retrograde ureteric studies, isotope renogram, and CT scan of the abdomen are helpful. CT of the abdomen with IV contrast because a single modality provides the most information by defining any extraureteric pathology, although care must be taken with the use of IV contrast in renal impairment.

Cystoscopy is essential in those patients who are going to require active management.

Management options
Bladder outlet obstruction causes symptoms of acute urinary retention or chronic obstruction, with overflow incontinence relieved by urethral or suprapubic catheterization.

Palliative transurethral resection of a prostate or bladder tumor may be necessary to provide symptomatic relief.

Ureteric decompression can be accomplished by use of the following:
- Percutaneous nephrostomy with or without antegrade stenting
- Cystoscopy and retrograde placement of an internal ureteric stent
- Ureteric stents need to be replaced every 6 months in patients with cancer, although modern stents may last longer.

Percutaneous nephrostomy is a temporary measure, appropriate in the following specific circumstances:
- Undiagnosed malignant disease
- Prostatic or cervical primary tumors, with an available treatment modality with a reasonable chance of response.
- In patients with malignancy in the pelvis, it may be impossible to cannulate the ureters and a nephrostomy may be essential.

Patients with advanced cancer can gain symptomatic benefit from nephrostomy or ureteric stent insertion.
- Because a nephrostomy drain may remain in place for several months, it is prone to dislodgement, infection, and leakage around the site.
- Double pigtail ureteric stents can be inserted in preference to a long-term nephrostomy.
- Complications include transient bacteremia, sepsis, hemorrhage, and obstructive encrustations.
- Care must be taken in these patients to ensure that dehydration, fluid overload, and hyperkalemia are all corrected.
- The latter is a true emergency and will ultimately lead to arrhythmias and cardiac arrest.
- Other problems may include a significant bleeding tendency due to platelet dysfunction.
- Hypertension is occasionally a problem and requires fluid management and/or antihypertensives.
- Any manipulation of the obstructed urinary tract requires antibiotic coverage, because these patients are prone to septicemia.

In selected patients dialysis may be indicated:
- Increasing hyperkalemia
- Fluid overload resistant to diuretics
- Severe renal failure
- Acidosis

Prolonged survival, even with pelvic malignant disease, is still possible.
- In one study series median survival was 26 weeks.
  - Group 1: primary untreated malignancy
  - Group 2: recurrent malignancy with further treatment
  - Group 3: recurrent malignancy with no further treatment
  - Group 4: benign disease as a consequence of previous treatment
- Patients in groups 1 and 2 had similar survival: median survival was 27 and 20 weeks, 5-year survival was 20% and 10%, respectively.
- Patients in group 3 had a poor prognosis, with a median survival of 6 weeks and no patient surviving beyond 1 year.
- Patients in group 4 had the best outlook, with 5-year survival of 64%.
- If the patient has advanced pelvic malignancy for which there is no treatment, quality of life and the patient's own wishes should determine whether or not to intervene.

Chapter 25

Late effects of cancer treatment

Carey K. Anders

Introduction 352
Endocrine and metabolic dysfunction 354
Fertility issues 356
Organ-specific problems 358
Secondary malignancies 359
Neuropsychological consequences 360
Further reading 361

Introduction

In recent decades, significant advances were developed in oncological treatments for many pediatric malignancies and some adult tumors, e.g., germ cell cancer and lymphomas. For the first time, there are long-term survivors who have undergone treatment for advanced malignancy.

The priority for clinicians managing curable cancers is to achieve optimal rates of cure while minimizing long-term toxicity from the treatment. It is important to be aware of the potential long-term consequences of treatment for cancer because many have the potential to significantly detract from future quality of life and some may shorten life expectancy.

Surveillance for complications of therapy needs to be continued for many decades.

Endocrine and metabolic dysfunction

See Table 25.1.

Pituitary dysfunction

This is common after whole-brain radiotherapy. More than 90% of patients become growth hormone (GH) deficient, which can affect bone density, cardiovascular risk, and the sense of well-being.[1]

- Continued surveillance is needed for ≥10 years (initial investigation: serum GH and IGF-1).
- Replacement therapy is an established treatment in children (in the absence of active malignancy) but is more controversial in adults.
- ACTH insufficiency (causing adrenal failure), thyroid dysfunction, and gonadal failure can also occur.

Adrenal failure

Suppression of hypothalamic-pituitary-adrenal function by prolonged administration of synthetic glucocorticoids is the most common cause of adrenal insufficiency. In the absence of ACTH stimulation, the cortisol-producing areas of the adrenal gland atrophy.

- Mineralocorticoid production usually remains near normal. Recovery is usual, but occasionally adrenal failure is permanent.
- Symptoms are typically nonspecific, including chronic malaise and anorexia.
- These patients rarely present with adrenal crisis but may require additional supplementation at times of physiological stress, e.g., sepsis.
- For initial investigation, early-morning cortisol testing is recommended. Values ≤3 µg/dL strongly suggest adrenal insufficiency, while values ≥15 µg/dL predict a normal response to a short ACTH test.

Primary thyroid dysfunction

This is common after total-body or craniospinal irradiation or radiotherapy to the neck; e.g., there was a cumulative incidence of 30% in patients treated for Hodgkins's disease by 20 years postradiotherapy.[2]

- Subclinical syndrome may persist for years before development of overt hypothyroidism.
- Typical symptoms include an insidious-onset, multisystem disorder including fatigue, weight gain, cold intolerance, constipation, and depression.
- Annual screening with thyroid function testing is recommended in high-risk patients.
- Treatment should usually begin once the thyroid-stimulating hormone (TSH) level is elevated, even if T4 levels are normal, to avoid overstimulating the gland.

---

1 Clarson CL, Del Maestro RF (1999). Growth failure after treatment of pediatric brain tumors. *Pediatrics* 103(3):E37.

2 Sklar C, Whitton J, Mertens A, Stovall M, Green D, Marina N, Greffe B, Wolden S, Robison L (2000). Abnormalities of the thyroid in survivors of Hodgkin's disease: data from the Childhood Cancer Survivor Study. *J Clin Endocrinol Metab* 85(9):3227–3232.

Metabolic syndrome

The quartet of insulin resistance, dyslipidemia, hypertension, and abdominal obesity is observed in up to 50% of long-term survivors of childhood bone marrow transplants.

- There is a potential risk of premature cardio- and cerebrovascular events.
- Long-term monitoring should include serum lipids and fasting blood glucose.

Table 25.1 Endocrine and metabolic effects of radiotherapy and chemotherapy

Endocrinopathies	Laboratory Analysis
Pituitary dysfunction	GH, IGF-1, TSH, T4, ACTH, FSH, estrogen (women), testosterone (men)
Adrenal insufficiency	Basal (early morning) cortisol
Hypothyroidism	TSH, free T4
Metabolic syndrome	Serum lipids, fasting glucose

Fertility issues

According to the American Cancer Society[1] and the U.S. Census Bureau, approximately 130,000 cancer patients are diagnosed annually during reproductive years (<45 years of age).

Gonadal dysfunction among both males and females may be due to the following:
- Direct involvement by tumor, e.g., 5% incidence of contralateral carcinoma in situ in testicular tumors
- Surgery, i.e., removal of testicle or ovary
- Radiotherapy affecting pituitary and gonadal function; e.g., total-body irradiation tends to cause infertility in men and women. Lower doses may produce transient oligospermia in men. Radiotherapy is more damaging to ovarian tissue than chemotherapy, which is dose and age dependent.
- Chemotherapy, particularly with alkylating agents (e.g., cyclophosphamide) and cisplatin
- 30% treated for childhood cancers become infertile. Treatment in adulthood can also cause infertility.
- Based on the recently reported American Society of Clinical Oncology recommendations on fertility preservation, *all* cancer patients should be alerted to the risk.[2]

Effects of age

Older age confers a higher risk of premature menopause; e.g., adjuvant cyclophosphamide, methotrexate, 5-fluorouracil (CMF) chemotherapy for breast cancer in a 40-year-old results in an >80% chance of inducing menopause, and in a 25-year-old, <20% chance.

The prepubertal testis seems less susceptible to the effects of chemotherapy than the mature adult testis.

Effects of gender

See Table 25.2 for a summary of options for fertility preservation among cancer survivors.

Post-chemotherapy containing alkylating agents for Hodgkin's disease results in 90% of men being infertile; 50% of women will undergo menopause at an earlier age, but will not necessarily have been infertile.

Fertility versus sexual function

Spermatogenesis is more likely to be disrupted than testosterone production; therefore, men may be infertile without loss of libido or erectile function.

Sperm storage

Sperm storage should be arranged prior to receipt of chemotherapy for *all* men wishing future reproductive potential. Conception rates for stored sperm are approximately 30%. However, certain diagnoses (e.g.,

---

1 www.cancer.org

2 Lee SJ, Schover LR, Partridge AH, et al. (2006). American Society of Clinical Oncology recommendations on fertility preservation in cancer patients. *J Clin Oncol* 20:2917–2931.

Hodgkin's, testicular cancer) may be associated with abnormal pretreatment testicular function.

Strategies for preserving ovarian function include the following:
- Oophoropexy is a surgical procedure to move the ovaries beyond a planned radiotherapy field. Achievement of pregnancy has mixed results. It is probably limited by effects of scatter radiation or surgically induced alterations in the ovarian blood supply.
- Gonadotrophin-releasing hormone (GnRH) analogs to reduce ovarian function reversibly during treatment with chemotherapy have shown mixed results in humans.
- Storage of ovarian tissue and oocytes is increasingly available, after recent reports of successful pregnancies.

Storage of frozen embryos is possible. In general, the woman must have a partner, must delay treatment, and undergo ≥1 cycle of in vitro fertilization (IVF).

Ovarian hyperstimulation after an ER-positive tumor should be avoided if at all possible.

Table 25.2 Standard options for fertility preservation among cancer survivors

Fertility Preservation Options	Males	Females
Sperm banking	X	
Testicular tissue freezing	X	
Embryo freezing		X
Ovarian tissue transposition		X
Radical trachelectomy		X
In vitro fertilization		X
Donor eggs		X
Natural conception	X	X
Adoption	X	X

Organ-specific problems

Heart
Anthracycline exposure (e.g., doxorubicin, epirubicin) is most commonly associated with long-term cardiovascular complications, particularly dilated cardiomyopathy.
- The risk is dose-dependent and effects can be seen many years later.
- Radiotherapy has an additive effect. The maximum lifetime dosing is 550 mg/m^2 for adults; 450 mg/m^2 with prior mediastinal radiation.
- Monitoring via echocardiography or multigated acquisition (MUGA scanning) is appropriate. Abnormal septal movement is usually observed before any decline in ejection fraction. Initial management is usually with an angiotensin-converting enzyme (ACE) inhibitor and referral to a cardiologist.
- Much interest has been focused on the loss of cardiac function after treatment with trastuzumab (Herceptin). Preliminary evidence suggests that this cardiotoxicity is reversible.

Lungs
Bleomycin (e.g., to treat germ cell tumors) can cause pulmonary fibrosis. Presentation with dyspnea, a nonproductive cough, and chest pain may be acute but can also occur many months after treatment.

Kidneys
Several drugs used in oncology have the potential to cause chronic impairment of renal function. These include cisplatin and aminoglycoside antibiotics frequently used during neutropenic sepsis.

Ears
Several treatments can damage hearing permanently, typically causing high-frequency sensorineural loss ± tinnitus, e.g., platinum agents, high-dose radiotherapy, and aminoglycosides.

Nerves
Many chemotherapy drugs can cause cumulative neuropathy, e.g., cisplatin, the taxanes, and vincristine. If treatment is continued, the neuropathy (which is most often sensory) may become chronic.

Eyes
Cataracts can be a consequence of radiotherapy, tamoxifen, or the use of high-dose steroids. Radiotherapy-induced Sjögren's syndrome is a recognized phenomenon.

Bones
Prolonged use of exogenous steroids can cause osteopenia. Induction of premature menopause (i.e., bilateral oophorectomy, GnRH agonist therapy) will also put the patient at risk for this.
- At-risk patients should have bone densitometry and possibly biphosphonate therapy.

Secondary malignancies

Risk factors for development of secondary malignancies include the following:
- Specific treatments previously received, e.g., alkylating agents, topoisomerase II inhibitors, radiotherapy
- Increased inherent genetic risks, e.g., predisposing gene polymorphisms, BRCA1/2 carrier
- Field changes due to carcinogen exposure, e.g., cigarette smoking and risk of lung or urothelial cancers
- Other persisting environmental factors such as smoking

Some 5%–10% of all childhood cancer survivors develop second malignancies. The peak incidence of secondary myeloid malignancies occurs 2–10 years after treatment. Prognosis is extremely poor. Secondary solid malignancies typically occur between 10 and 20 years after treatment for the primary diagnosis.

The risk of a testicular-cancer survivor treated with radiotherapy developing a second solid malignancy is reported to be 2–3 times the rate in the general population.

The incidence of leukemia is also greater in those patients treated with etoposide-containing chemotherapy regimes.

Successful treatment for Hodgkin's disease is associated with an increased incidence of leukemias, non-Hodgkin's lymphomas, and solid tumors, e.g. lung, breast, and thyroid cancers.

The American Cancer Society recommends that women previously treated with radiation therapy to the chest between ages 10 and 30 years (i.e., mantle irradiation for Hodgkin's disease) undergo yearly bilateral breast MRIs as an adjunct to mammography for screening purposes.[1]

---

[1] Saslow D, Boetes C, Burke W, et al. (2007). American Cancer Society for Breast Screening with MRI as adjunct to mammography. *CA Cancer J Clin* 57:75–89.

Neuropsychological consequences

The long-term neuropsychological sequelae of treatment for cancer cannot be underestimated. Some of these are the result of specific treatments.
- Whole-brain radiation therapy in young children is associated with subsequent impairments in short-term memory, attention span, and information processing. Verbal IQ is typically preserved, thus children may give the appearance of coping well.

Other problems are secondary to the process of undergoing intensive, debilitating, and protracted treatments.
- These include social isolation and time away from work or school. Self-esteem can be affected.
- This may be due to problems of integrating back into the peer group and difficulties accepting alterations in appearance or ability.
- Later, there are psychological consequences of adapting to long-term effects on sexual function and employability.

Finally, there are the potential practical considerations of surviving cancer that can have an impact on quality-of-life—for example, difficulty in arranging life insurance or taking out a mortgage.

Further reading

Brown JR, Yeckes H, Friedberg JW, et al. (2005). Increasing incidence of late second malignancies after conditioning with cyclophosphamide and total-body irradiation and autologous bone marrow transplantation for non-Hodgkin's lymphoma. *J Clin Oncol* 23:2208–2214.

Falcone T, Bedaiwy MA (2005). Fertility preservation and pregnancy outcome after malignancy. *Curr Opin Obstet Gynecol* 17:21–26.

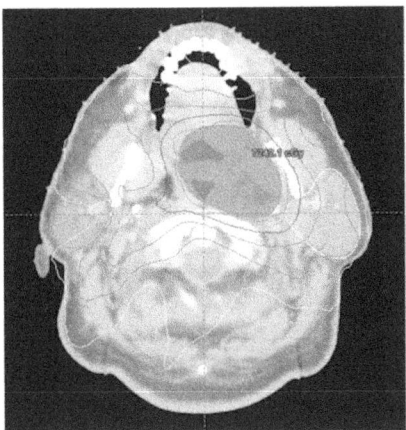

Plate 1 Example of an IMRT plan for a left-sided oropharyngeal head and neck cancer. The primary tumor is covered by the 70 Gy isodose line. Nodal areas at risk receive at least 50 Gy. Note significant sparing of the right parotid, with the 60, 35, and 21 Gy isodose lines curving to avoid the structure. Right parotid is contoured.

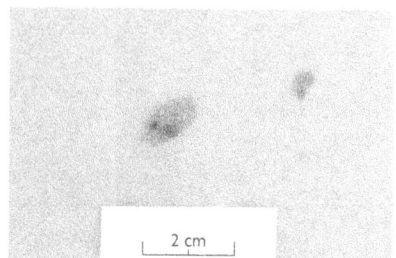

Plate 2 Benign pigmented lesion.

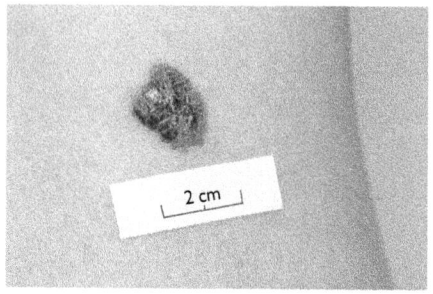

Plate 3 Benign nevus close-up.

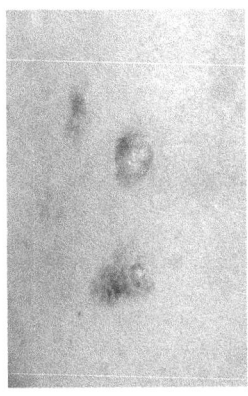

Plate 4 Malignant melanoma close-up.

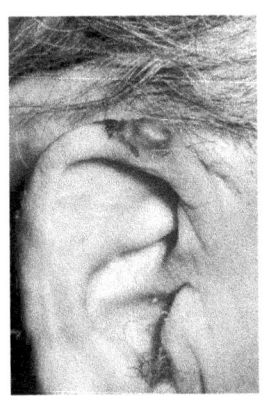

Plate 5 Malignant melanoma close-up.

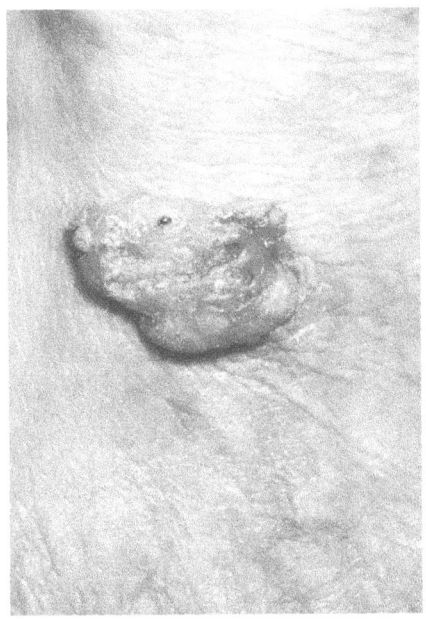

Plate 6 Squamous cell carcinoma.

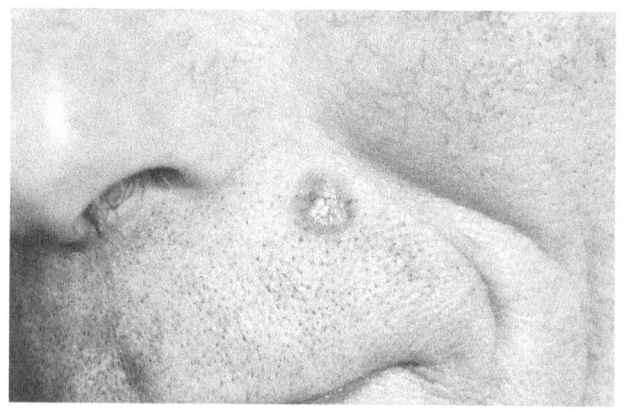

Plate 7 Basal cell carcinoma.

Chapter 26

End-of-life care

Amy P. Abernethy
Thomas W. LeBlanc

Introduction *364*
Management of physical symptoms *366*
  Anorexia and cachexia *366*
  Constipation *367*
  Death rattles *369*
  Delirium *370*
  Dyspnea *371*
  Lymphedema *373*
  Nausea and vomiting *374*
  Nutrition and hydration *379*
Management of psychosocial symptoms *382*
  Communication *382*
  Depression *384*
  Distress (patient) *385*
  Distress (family and caregiver) *386*
  Spiritual suffering *387*
  Terminal agitation *388*
Care in the last days of life *390*
Further reading *392*

Chapter 26 End-of-life care

Introduction

"Palliative care is the active, holistic care of patients with advanced, progressive illness. Management of pain and other symptoms and provision of psychological, social and spiritual support is paramount. The goal of palliative care is achievement of the best quality of life for patients and their families."[1]

Despite major survival advances in cancer overall, the majority of metastatic solid tumors in adults remains incurable. When the advanced-cancer patient enters this setting of life-limiting illness, the appropriate goals of treatment become minimization of the symptom burden on patient and family and caregiver and maximization of quality of life. Importantly, palliative care can coexist with disease-focused treatment, or be the sole focus of care.

Optimal management of patients with terminal cancer requires the involvement of a multidisciplinary care team, including palliative care specialists, to ensure that the patient's physical, psychosocial, and spiritual concerns are well addressed within a coordinated care framework. Ideally, palliative care is integrated into cancer treatment from diagnosis forward, rather than only as the patient nears death.[2]

As disease progresses, the degree of involvement from different members of the care team will shift, but their activities remain integrated around common goals:

- To maximize the patient's physical comfort and mental and emotional well being;
- To optimize the patient's overall quality of life, including psychosocial and spiritual dimensions;
- To minimize distress that may be caused by the transition from "active" care to what is perceived as "terminal care";
- To help the patient live fully and participate in life as meaningfully and actively as possible, regardless of disease stage; and
- To support the patient and family and caregivers during the patient's illness and subsequently to support the family and caregivers in their bereavement.

---

1 World Health Organization (1990). *Cancer Pain Relief and Palliative Care*, World Health Organization technical report series: 804. Geneva: WHO.

2 Smith TJ, Temin S, Alesi ER (2012). American Society of Clinical Oncology Provisional Clinical Opinion: The Integration of Palliative Care into Standard Oncology Care. *J Clin Oncol*. Mar 10;30(8):880–887. doi: 10.1200/JCO.2011.38.5161. Epub 2012 Feb 6

Symptom management in a whole-person care framework

High-quality, end-of-life care in oncology entails a wide range of medical, psychological, spiritual, and social interventions.

Although the focus of the patient and family and caregiver may evolve as disease progresses, the healthcare team must maintain a comprehensive view of the patient's care, monitoring all aspects of his or her status, taking proactive steps to promote comfort and minimize distress wherever possible, and incorporating appropriate care tailored to the individual.

Coordination of care is crucial, to provide a cohesive experience of treatment and of death for the patient and family and caregiver. Attention to key physical symptoms occurs alongside attention to psychosocial and spiritual concerns.

Close communication among members of the healthcare team should ensure that the spectrum of patient and family and caregiver needs is covered, without either duplication or gaps, and that all clinical activities are woven together into a coherent plan of whole-person care.

Management of physical symptoms

Anorexia and cachexia

Anorexia, characterized by reduced or absent appetite for food and consequent weight loss, may be associated with fatigue and wasting away without any other specific cause.

Potentially reversible causes that warrant assessment include the following:
- Inadequate pain control
- Nausea
- Constipation
- Depression
- Metabolic abnormalities, e.g., hypercalcemia, uremia
- Infection, e.g., oral thrush
- Obstruction, ascites

Cachexia, the involuntary increase in basal energy expenditure culminating in loss of both lean muscle and adipose tissue, affects >85% of patients with advanced cancer. It is most commonly seen in patients with advanced solid tumors, particularly those affecting the lungs or GI tract.

The underlying causative mechanisms are unknown; circulating cytokines (e.g., tumor necrosis factor) clearly play a role, causing metabolic abnormalities such as protein breakdown, lipolysis, and increased gluconeogenesis.

Cachexia is often associated with anorexia but differs in that the associated weight loss cannot be reversed by simply increasing caloric intake.

Together, anorexia and cachexia are a major cause of symptoms near the end of life, with multiple associated physical, psychological, and social morbidities. The syndromes distress both the patient and family and caregivers.

Management
The general management approach is to first seek to correct reversible causes. Interventions usually do not influence cachexia.

Nonpharmacological
- **Dietary advice**: Eat small, frequent meals. Eat when hungry. Choose high-calorie, low-volume foods. Drink small amounts of alcohol to stimulate appetite.
- **Education**: Minimize any stress related to food. Encourage family and caregivers not to pressure the patient to eat. Promote enjoyment of food.
- **Activity**: Maximize any potential exercise.

Pharmacological
- **Supplements**: Advise high-protein, high-calorie intake (e.g., Ensure).
- **Corticosteroids** may improve appetite, nausea, and general sense of well-being but do not improve lean muscle (e.g., dexamethasone 0.5–2 mg daily).
- **Progesterones** aid appetite; evidence for useful weight gain is limited. The side effect profile can be troublesome especially for men (e.g., megestrol acetate 160–800 mg daily).

- **Cannabinoids** stimulate appetite and can produce a sense of well being; evidence for useful weight gain is limited. Dronabinol (Marinol) is started at 2.5 mg twice daily (before lunch and dinner)
- **Mirtazapine** (Remeron) can be a useful adjunct in settings where there is concomitant depression or insomnia, as it can improve appetite as well; it should be administered at bedtime. This is an "off label" application.
- *Enteral or parenteral feeding* is occasionally prescribed during active anti-cancer therapy. It is rarely appropriate in the end-of-life setting, and evidence suggests it is not necessary.

Constipation

Constipation in patients at the end of life can be caused by a number of factors. Potential causes in patients with malignancy include the following:
- Drugs, particularly opioid analgesics and some antiemetics (e.g., 5-HT$_3$ antagonists), as well as anticholinergics and tricyclic antidepressants
- Dehydration due to inadequate fluid intake or secondary to vomiting or diuretic therapy
- Anorexia, reduced oral intake, or change in dietary content
- Immobility and/or general weakness
- Hypercalcemia, particularly if accompanied by dehydration, nausea, abdominal pain, and confusion
- Spinal cord compression (usually a late presentation)
- Obstruction, such as malignant, surgical, or post-radiotherapy adhesions, intestinal tumor, or extrinsic compression from pelvic tumor

Presentation
- Difficulty with a bowel movement or bowels not open at all
- Nausea and vomiting
- Abdominal pain, typically colicky
- Overflow diarrhea, history of passing or leaking watery stool
- Urinary retention
- State of acute confusion

Assessment
- **History**: Identify precipitating or potentially reversible causes or difficulties with care at home (e.g., practical issues surrounding toileting).
- **Examination**: Include a digital rectal examination.
- **Abdominal radiography** is only required if the differential is between obstruction and pseudo-obstruction.
- Check serum calcium.

Nonpharmacologic management
- Increase fluid and fiber intake, if possible. Do not add fiber for those whose fluid intake is necessarily reduced, or who have limited gut motility (e.g., the dying patient).
- Mobilize the patient.
- Maximize privacy and dignity.

Pharmacologic management

Prophylaxis

With opioids, always prescribe a laxative from the outset, usually a softener plus stimulant.

- Fentanyl may be less constipating than morphine; consider converting to transdermal fentanyl if pain is stable.

Osmotic agents

Hyperosmolar compounds, which are not absorbed in the GI tract, retain water in the lumen and thus increase stool volume and stimulate peristalsis.

- Side effects include abdominal cramping, thirst, and flatulence (e.g., magnesium salts, nonabsorbable sugars).
- Magnesium and phosphorus salts are contraindicated for patients with renal failure.
- Flavorless polyethylene glycols may be better tolerated than sickly sweet sorbitol and lactulose, which are non-absorbable sugars.
- Polyethylene glycol preparations are now available for daily use (e.g., Miralax, now available over-the-counter).

Stimulant agents

Senna is a commonly prescribed stimulant laxative exerting its effects mainly by altering electrolyte transport within the intestinal mucosa and by increasing motility.

- Dosage begins with one tablet each evening, with a gradual increase to four tablets twice daily, as necessary.
- Senna can cause abdominal cramps and is contraindicated if there is any risk of intestinal obstruction.

Emollients (stool softeners)

These lower the surface tension of the stool, enhancing penetration of water into feces (e.g., docusate).

- Although generally inadequate as a sole agent, they are quite effective when combined with a stimulant such as senna.
- Mineral oil is useful as an enema.

Bulking agents

These are useful in patients who are otherwise well and able to eat and drink relatively normally.

- Require a fluid intake of 2–3 L/day (e.g., ispaghula husk).

Rectal preparations

Use glycerin suppositories to soften and lubricate hard stool palpable within the rectum.

- Use an arachis oil enema to soften stool at night, followed by a high-phosphate enema the next morning to stimulate evacuation.

Opioid receptor antagonists

Methylnaltrexone (Relistor) is a novel agent that selectively blocks the effects of opioids on gut motility.

- Use only for opioid-induced constipation refractory to multiple laxative preparations/enemas listed above.

- Contraindicated in the setting of bowel obstruction; intestinal perforation may ensue.
- Dosing is weight-based; usual dose is 8 or 12 mg as a single subcutaneous injection; result is expected within minutes.

This treatment may be given on an every-other-day schedule if opioid-induced constipation persists despite other therapies.

Death rattles

Noisy ventilation ("death rattles" or "terminal secretions") occur in up to 90% of unconscious dying patients.[1-4] Caused by oscillatory movements of accumulated bronchial mucosa and salivary secretions, death rattles develop when the patient near end of life becomes unable to clear secretions by coughing or swallowing.[1]

Intervention to reduce secretions is often instituted to alleviate the distress of attendant relatives, even when the patient seems settled.[1] Hence, before electing pharmacologic treatment, decide whether the balance of side effects from these medications is reasonable to reduce a symptom that is rarely bothersome to the patient (who is often comatose or nearly so).

A good physical exam is critical to differentiate terminal secretions from other etiologies potentially needing treatment, such as pulmonary edema.

Pharmacologic management

- Anticholinergic agents (i.e., muscarinic receptor blockers), including scopolamine, glycopyrrolate, atropine
- Side effects (varying degrees) include blurred vision, sedation, confusion, delirium, restlessness, hallucinations, palpitations, constipation, and urinary retention.

Nonpharmacologic management

- Perform oropharyngeal suctioning sparingly, as frequent suctioning can unsettle both the patient and visitor. When fluid is inaccessible, brief use of the Trendelenburg position can help.
- Reposition the patient (semiprone, on their side).
- Explain what is happening to the family and caregivers.

---

1 Bennett M, Lucas V, Brennan M, et al. (2002). Using anti-muscarinic drugs in the management of death rattle: evidence-based guidelines for palliative care. *Palliat Med* 16:369–374.

2 Hughes AC, Wilcock A, Corcoran R (1996). Management of "death rattle." *J Pain Symptom Manag* 12:271–272.

3 Bennett MI (1996). Death rattle: an audit of hyoscine (scopolamine) use and review of management. *J Pain Symptom Manag* 12:229–233.

4 Power D, Kearney M (1992). Management of the final 24 hours. *Irish Med J* 85:93–95.

Delirium

Delirium manifests as disturbance of consciousness, cognition, and perception. Observed in 28%–83% of patients nearing end of life, it often distresses patients, families, caregivers, and providers.[1,2] Effects of medications, particularly opioids, are the most common cause of delirium in end-of-life patients.[3]

Two types of delirium occur in this population: agitated/hyperactive delirium and hypoactive delirium. Both are signaled by acute change in the patient's arousal, causing disorientation, visual or auditory hallucination, altered speech pattern, inattention, trouble with memory or language, or sleep–wake cycle disturbance. Symptoms can wax and wane over time.[4]

Assessment using validated tools is highly recommended to help determine specific cognitive dysfunctions.

Assessment instruments
- Delirium Rating Scale
- Confusion Assessment Method (CAM, or CAM-ICU)
- Delirium Symptom Interview
- Memorial Delirium Assessment Scale
- Mini-Mental State Examination (MMSE)—a more general, but widely recognized, tool

General management principles
- Discontinue all medications that are not absolutely necessary.
- Seek to restore the patient to baseline mental state (rather than to suppress agitation or to sedate).
- Provide a calm setting.
- The patient may be helped by the presence of family, friends, caregivers; familiar surroundings; consistent care staff (e.g., nurses); frequent reorientation.

Pharmacologic management
- Haloperidol (intravenous [IV] or oral), starting at 0.5–2 mg twice daily and titrated upward, is the drug of choice.
- Neuroleptic drugs, including IV chlorpromazine, risperidone, and transmucosal olanzapine, can be used.
- Avoid benzodiazepines (lorazepam, midazolam). They may calm the patient but may further sedate, disinhibit, or agitate the patient.
- In cases of severe delirium in actively dying patients, continuous infusion of benzodiazepine (lorazepam) and barbiturate (pentobarbital) may be initiated to alleviate family and caregiver distress.

---

1 Massie M, Holland J, Glass E (1983). Delirium in terminally ill cancer patients. *Am J Psychiatry* 140:1048–1050.

2 Minagawa H, Uchitomi Y, Yamawaki S, Ishitani K (1996). Psychiatric morbidity in terminally ill cancer patients: a prospective study. *Cancer* 78:1131–1137.

3 Bruera E, Miller L, McCallion J, et al. (1992). Cognitive failure in patients with terminal cancer: a prospective study. *J Pain Symptom Manag* 7:192–195.

4 Moryl N, Carver AC, Foley KM (2003). Management of Cancer Pain. In Kufe DW, Pollock RE, Weichselbaum RR, et al. (eds.). *Holland-Frei Cancer Medicine*. 6th ed. Amsterdam: Elsevier, pp. 1113–1123.

Dyspnea

A highly subjective symptom, dyspnea is a sensation of breathlessness that arises from a combination of underlying pathology, signaling of neural pathways, and the patient's perception of physical sensations.[1]

Patients' descriptions of dyspnea vary widely and depend partly on the individual's disease, ethnic or racial background, previous experiences, and emotional state.

Although patients often report dyspnea that seems out of proportion to known underlying lung disease, the clinician must attend to the symptom as reported.

Assessment instruments
- Visual analog scale (VAS)
- Numeric rating scale (NRS)
- Modified Borg scale
- Cancer dyspnea scale
- Medical Research Council dyspnea scale

Causes

Dyspnea in metastatic cancer patients commonly has a multifactorial origin. Full assessment is important to identify potentially reversible causes. Common causes include:

Pulmonary
- Lung tumor
- Pneumonia
- Pleural effusion; if recurrent, consider pleurodesis or tunneled catheter insertion to permit intermittent drainage
- Lymphangitis carcinomatosa
- Obstruction of large airways, with or without distal collapse
- Chronic obstructive pulmonary disease (COPD)
- Post-treatment effects, such as radiation pneumonitis, or drug toxicity

Cardiovascular
- Pericardial effusion
- Congestive cardiac failure
- Pulmonary emboli
- Superior vena cava obstruction
- Anemia
- Arrhythmias
- Pulmonary hypertension

Neuromuscular
- Muscle weakness or fatigue (may be due to or aggravated by anorexia-cachexia syndrome)
- Carcinoma *en cuirasse*, i.e., restrictive malignant infiltration of the chest wall
- Reduced respiratory drive (e.g., due to opiates)

---

1 American Thoracic Society (1999). Dyspnea. Mechanisms, assessment, and management: a consensus statement. *Am J Respir Crit Care Med* 159:321–340.

- Peripheral nerve palsies (e.g., phrenic nerve)
- Malignant infiltration of Xth cranial nerve resulting in hoarse voice ± "bovine" cough should lead to an ENT referral: palliative injection of bulk material into vocal cord may help.

Psychological
- Anxiety
- Fear

General management principles
- Treat reversible causes accordingly.
- Adopt a multidisciplinary approach with nonpharmacological strategies.
- Communicate realistically with patients to help modify expectations.
- Respond according to the patient's place along the end-of-life trajectory and to their preferred goals of care (e.g., managing comfort may be more appropriate than administering blood gas for a patient who is clearly dying).

Pharmacologic management
- Opioids are the mainstay of treatment. Low-dose morphine has been shown to be safe and effective even in elderly patients with COPD.
- In opioid-naïve patients, start with a dose of 15 mg sustained-release morphine once daily (if patient has no contraindications). Increase to twice per day after 5–7 days if the patient tolerates the medication and has residual breathlessness.
- For severe, acute dyspnea give 2–5 mg of morphine IV every 5–10 minutes.
- In patients with contraindication to morphine, use long-acting oxycodone, starting at 10 mg once per day and increasing to twice per day after 5–7 days as tolerated and needed.
- If an opioid-tolerant patient is on a regular dose of morphine or another opioid, sequentially increase opioid by 20% of total daily dose every 3–5 days until breathlessness is relieved or side effects occur.[2]
- Prescribe benzodiazepines for individuals where anxiety causes obvious and substantial aggravation of dyspnea; use alprazolam for short-acting control and clonazepam for longer-acting control. Evidence for benzodiazepines as a primary treatment for dyspnea is lacking.
- There is insufficient evidence to recommend the use of nebulized opioid preparations, although these are used at some centers
- Other drugs that can address specific dyspnea-related symptoms are antitussives (to address coughing), anticholinergics (to minimize secretions), diuretics, bronchodilators, and corticosteroids.

---

[2] Bruera E, MacEachern T, Ripamonti C, Hanson J (1993). Subcutaneous morphine for dyspnea in cancer patients. *Ann Intern Med* 119:906–907.

Oxygen and nonpharmacologic management
- Palliative oxygen may relieve symptoms in patients with refractory dyspnea and PaO_2 >55 mg Hg. Because oxygen is not universally effective, treatment should be based on symptom relief, not on pulse oximetry.[3]
- Patients generally prefer a nasal cannula to a mask; claustrophobic patients may best be served by a face tent. For the dying patient, there is no need to administer >4–6 L/min oxygen via nasal cannula.
- Psychosocial support can alleviate distress and may improve dyspnea when anxiety fuels the patient's experience of it.
- Positioning: Patient leans forward and supports weight with arms and upper body (the so-called "tripod" position).
- Pursed lip breathing: Patient inhales through the nose and exhales slowly (4–6 seconds) through pursed lips
- Air blowing across the face can improve the sensation of dyspnea; try a fan at the bedside.
- Relaxation techniques (e.g., massage, guided imagery)
- Discuss symptom management with the family to alleviate any concerns that treatment, especially opioids, may hasten death.

Lymphedema

Failure of lymph drainage causes an excessive accumulation of interstitial fluid known as lymphedema. Caused by tumor infiltration of lymphatics or by therapy that compromised the lymphatic system (e.g., lymph node dissection, lymph node irradiation), lymphedema most commonly affects limbs, is nonpitting, and may produce disabling symptoms. Lymphedema can be difficult to treat.

The differential diagnosis of limb swelling and edema is usually venous occlusion by thrombus or tumor, impaired lymphatic drainage due to surgery or tumor, fluid overload states, and reduced oncotic pressure from hypoalbuminemia.

It is important to determine the cause, as treatment in each scenario is very different.

Prevention
- This is the best strategy.
- Educate the patient and/or family or caregiver.
- Refer the patient to a specialist lymphedema service, if available.
- Recommend massage and exercise techniques.
- Advise about minimizing risk of infection and trauma (e.g., venepuncture on the other side).
- Treat cutaneous infection aggressively.

Management
- Daily skin care
- Massage or self-massage

---

3 Abernethy AP, McDonald CF, Frith PA, et al. (2010). Effect of palliative oxygen versus room air in relief of breathlessness in patients with refractory dyspnoea: a double-blind, randomised controlled trial. *Lancet* 376:784–793.

- Exercise, to the extent possible
- Fitted gradient compression garments
- Refractory edema may require pressure bandaging before compression garments can be fitted.
- No drugs have been shown to be beneficial.

Nausea and vomiting

- Nausea and/or vomiting (N/V) trouble up to 70% of patients with advanced cancer.
- Appropriate management requires an assessment of the probable underlying mechanisms.

Causes

Iatrogenic

Recent introduction of opioids may suggest opioid-induced N/V (see Figure 26.1).

- Chemotherapy can cause acute or delayed emesis and anticipatory nausea.
- Radiotherapy may also cause N/V, particularly if the CNS or small bowel is within the radiation field.

Metabolic

Hypercalcemia may be accompanied by dehydration, constipation, abdominal pain, and confusion.

- Alternatively, N/V may be the only sign. Uremia also causes nausea often in the absence of other clinical signs.
- Check serum chemistry panel including a corrected calcium and renal function.

Central

Elevated intracranial pressure from metastatic cerebral or meningeal disease can be a cause.

- History may be suggestive (e.g., new headaches). Perform retinal examination to assess for papilledema, and consider brain imaging.

(Sub)-acute obstruction

This occurs particularly if the patient is known to have intra-abdominal malignant disease.

- A history detailing the timing and nature of any vomiting (e.g., shortly after eating, hours after eating, unaltered food, constipation, flatulence, associated pain) will help establish the likely level of obstruction.
- Examine the abdomen and obtain an abdominal X-ray. A CT scan and small bowel series may assist diagnosis of remediable causes.

Dysautonomia and delayed gastric emptying

These have been observed in up to 30% of patients with advanced cancer and may substantially contribute to N/V, especially in patients on opioids.

- A gastric emptying series or other functional bowel study can clinch this diagnosis

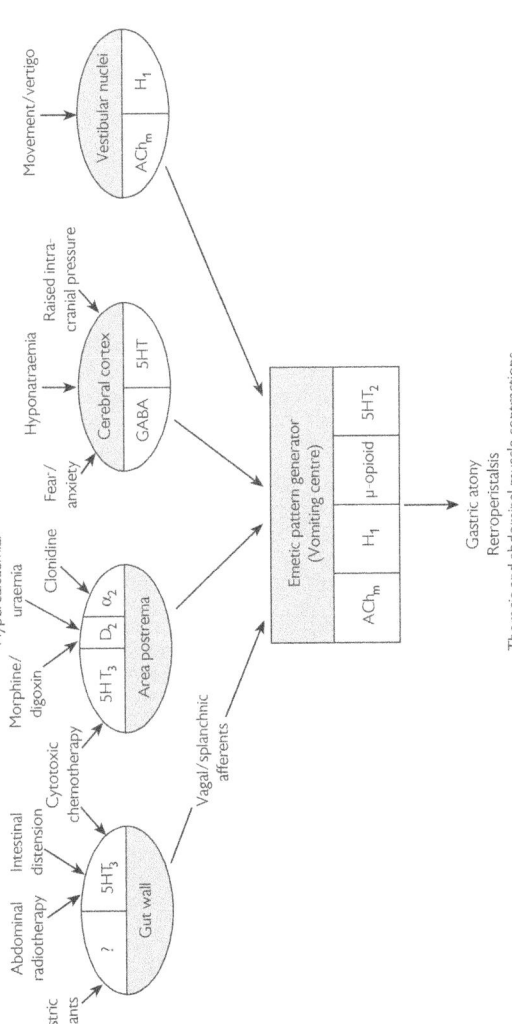

Figure 26.1 Diagram of the neural mechanisms controlling vomiting. (Modified with permission from Twycross R and Wilcock A (2008) Hospice and Palliative Care Formulary 2e. Palliativedrugs.com Ltd. Nottingham, UK. See also www.palliativedrugs.com). Abbreviations refer to receptor types. ACH$_m$, muscarinic cholinergic; A$_2$, alpha-adrenergic type 2; D$_2$, dopamine type 2; GABA, gamma-aminobutyric acid; 5HT, 5HT$_2$, 5HT$_3$, 5-hydroxytryptamine (serotonin) type undefined, type 2, type 3; H$_1$, histamine type 1.

Pseudo-obstruction
- Conduct a rectal examination for assessment purposes.
- A history of very watery stool may suggest potential "overflow" around impacted feces.

Other causes
- **Pain**: Inadequate pain control may present with nausea.
- **Vestibular**: Assess patients for possible vestibular disturbances, which can induce nausea.

Management
Optimal choice of antiemetic requires an understanding of the potential mechanism(s) of N/V and the site(s) of action of the antiemetic selected.

Many neurotransmitter receptors are involved in N/V; most of them lie within different areas of the CNS.

Peripheral pathways are also involved. Table 26.1 summarizes the neural mechanisms controlling N/V.

- Select a first-line antiemetic according to the most likely cause, and administer via a suitable route.
- If vomiting prevents oral administration, other options include sublingual, buccal, rectal, intravenous, intramuscular, and subcutaneous routes.
- Prescribe antiemetics regularly.
- Introduce second-line or combination therapy if symptoms persist after 24 hours.
- Address reversible causes of N/V separately (e.g., correct hypercalcemia, optimize renal function, stop emetogenic drugs if possible, treat delayed gastric emptying, manage bowel obstruction appropriately).
- Metoclopramide is prokinetic and is very useful for many causes of N/V in the advanced-cancer patient. Administer with caution in gastric stasis or subacute obstruction, but discontinue if there is any increase in either vomiting or colicky abdominal pain after administration. Do *not* use in complete obstruction. Watch for extrapyramidal effects.
- Senna products may be beneficial for constipation-related obstruction of the bowel.
- Remember that N/V in patients with cancer is often multifactorial. If the causes are not clear, or first-line therapy fails, then a $5-HT_3$ antagonist (e.g., ondansetron) is an appropriate subsequent choice of antiemetic.
- Anticholinergics (e.g., scopolamine) and antihistamines (e.g., promethazine) may be useful for addressing nausea associated with vestibular disturbances; use with caution, as they may induce delirium or other troublesome side effects
- Metoclopramide, $5-HT_3$ antagonists, and phenothiazines (e.g., prochlorperazine) are useful for opioid-related nausea.

Table 26.1 Selection of antiemetics

Causes of nausea/vomiting	Antiemetic	Class of drug	Example dose schedule	Common side effects
Chemotherapy	*Acute emesis (<24 hours)*			
	Ondansetron	5-HT$_3$ antagonist	16–24 mg po or 8–12 mg IV daily in divided doses	Constipation, headache
	Dexamethasone	Corticosteroid	8–20 mg IV po daily	Agitation/insomnia, gastric irritant
	Delayed emesis (>24 hours)			
	Ondansetron and/or dexamethasone	5-HT$_3$ antagonist Corticosteroid	Ondansetron: 16 mg po, dexamethasone 8 mg, daily in single or divided doses	Constipation, headache Agitation/insomnia, gastric irritant
	Prochlorperazine	Dopamine antagonist	10 mg po or IV every 6 hours	Sedation, extrapyramidal effects
Anticipatory	Lorazepam	Benzodiazepine	1–2 mg slop or SL prn, max 4 mg/24 hours	Sedation
Iatrogenic, e.g., opiates	Metaclopramide	Prokinetic	10 mg po or IV every 8 hours prn	Agitation
	Haloperidol	Dopamine antagonist	1.5–3 mg po every 8 hours prn	Sedation, extrapyramidal effects
Gastric irritation including radiotherapy	Lansoprazole	Proton pump inhibitor	30 mg po daily	Constipation, headache
	Ondansetron	5-HT$_3$ antagonist	4–8 mg po every 8 hours prn	Sedation, extrapyramidal effects
	Prochlorperazine	Dopamine antagonist	10mg po or IV every 6 hours prn	

CHAPTER 26 End-of-life care

Table 26.1 (Cont.)

Causes of nausea/vomiting	Antiemetic	Class of drug	Example dose schedule	Common side effects
Increased intracranial pressure	Dexamethasone	Corticosteroid	Up to 16 mg IV or po daily in single or divided doses	Agitation/insomnia, gastric irritant
Gastric stasis/subacute bowel obstruction	Metoclopramide	Prokinetic	10 mg po or IV every 8 hours prn	Agitation. Discontinue if colicky pain develops.
Obstruction	Cyclizine	Antihistamine & anticholinergic	50 mg three times a day po or IV	Drowsiness, dry mouth, blurred vision, risk of urinary retention
	Haloperidol	Dopamine antagonist	2–5 mg twice daily po or SL	Sedation, extrapyramidal effects
	Dexamethasone	Corticosteroid	Up to 8 mg IV or po daily in single or divided doses	Agitation/insomnia, gastric irritant
	Octreotide	Somatostatin analog	Up to 1000 μg/24 hours SC	Constipation
Metabolic	Correct the cause			

Nutrition and hydration

Nutrition and hydration often become highly charged issues for caregivers and families of a patient nearing the end of life.

Many families request nutrition and hydration support even for terminally ill patients, out of fear that withdrawal of nutrition or hydration will cause hunger, suffering, or a painful death by starvation. Consequently, nutrition and hydration are some of the last therapies to be withdrawn at the end of life.[1,2]

General management principles

- Evidence does not suggest benefit to patients for prevention of aspiration, improved survival, increased activity, or alleviation of cachexia.
- Hunger is not an issue in the vast majority of dying patients.
- Dying patients receiving no hydration or nutrition do not demonstrate an increase in discomfort.
- Nutrition at the end of life is generally not recommended, except in select scenarios such as gastrointestinal complications with limited spread of malignancies, especially involving obstruction.[3]
- Provision of nutrition or hydration near the end of life may cause more discomfort by inducing nausea/vomiting, aspiration, pulmonary edema, ascites, peripheral edema, etc.
- Data on potential benefits versus harm of artificial hydration at the end of life are conflicting.

Management

Discuss the prognosis, goals of care, and possible benefits and harms of hydration and nutritional therapy with patients and caregivers or families.

If patients or caregivers and families insist on therapies that are unlikely to be beneficial, suggest a time-limited trial with explicit, objective criteria for outcomes.

Consider supportive strategies that alleviate anxiety surrounding nutrition and hydration (e.g., use of ice chips or moistened mouth swabs to relieve sensation of thirst).

---

1 Mercadante S, Ferrera P, Girelli D, Casuccio A (2005). Patients' and relatives' perceptions about intravenous and subcutaneous hydration. *J Pain Symptom Manag* 30:354–358.

2 Asch DA, Faber-Langendoen K, Shea JA, Christakis NA (1999). The sequence of withdrawing life-sustaining treatment from patients. *Am J Med* 107:153–156.

3 Duerksen DR, Ting E, Thomson P, et al. (2004). Is there a role for TPN in terminally ill patients with bowel obstruction? *Nutrition* 20:760–763.

Cases where parenteral nutrition may be indicated

For a small subset of advanced-cancer patients, parenteral nutrition may be an appropriate therapy to improve quality of life and/or survival time. Suggested guidelines are to consider parenteral nutrition in the following cases:

- Enteral nutrition (including tube feeding) is not an option or there is a specific benefit expected from parenteral nutrition (e.g., inoperable malignant bowel obstruction, short bowel syndrome, malabsorption). For these patients, the major problem is a nonfunctional GI tract, and not cachexia itself.
- The patient is likely to die from starvation or malnutrition earlier than anticipated from disease progression alone.
- The patient's life expectancy is at least several months, which will allow for a proper trial of parenteral nutrition. These patients have Karnofsky Performance Scale score >50 or Eastern Cooperative Oncology Group (ECOG) performance status ≤2.
- The patient reports good quality of life; prolonging life is consistent with his or her goals of care; and the patient accepts the potential risks of parenteral nutrition.
- Logistics of the home setting will support parenteral nutrition, if the patient is home-based (e.g., a caregiver is able to set up and administer therapy, the patient can be clinically monitored).

When a patient is receiving parenteral nutrition (PN), electrolytes, liver and renal function, and triglycerides require close monitoring. The patient's response to treatment should be carefully assessed, and global clinical course must be monitored to ensure that PN remains an appropriate intervention.

Management of psychosocial symptoms

Communication

A diagnosis of potentially life-limiting cancer transports the patient and family and caregivers into a world of institutional complexity, multiple specialties, numerous professionals, and evolving care plans as disease progresses.

Patients enter this bewildering context at a time when they are grappling with major illness and possibly their own death. Clear and sufficient communication with patients and families and caregivers is essential to alleviate their distress.

Good communication builds trust, reduces uncertainty, and allows appropriate adjustment (practical and emotional) by the patient and family, thus reducing psychological morbidity.

General management principles and practices

- Patients and families consistently mention poor communication and breaking of bad news as sources of stress and dissatisfaction.
- Probably <5% of patients genuinely prefer to have little information and leave everything up to the doctor.
- Patients who are unsatisfied with the amount of information provided are at greater risk for difficulty adjusting to their diagnosis, anxiety, and depression.
- Establish how much information the patient would like at each stage of their illness.
- Tailor information-giving to the individual patient and family and caregivers.
- Make sure that the patient and family and caregivers leave their consultations with a clear understanding of diagnosis and prognosis, and of the likely therapeutic benefits or risks of treatments.
- Ask if the patient or family and caregivers want additional information.

Communication management strategies

Breaking bad news: a 10-step approach

Breaking bad news is not a single, isolated event. The process is ongoing and recurring; it involves conveying the diagnosis, updating the patient and family on changes, and preparing both patient and family and caregivers for death.

The following approach provides a general framework for communication, which can be adapted for specific situations. Remember that a patient has a right, but not a duty, to hear bad news.

1. Preparation: Know the facts. Arrange the meeting and an appropriate location (e.g. private setting). Find out whom the patient wants to be present. Arrange not to be disturbed during the "bad news" conversation (e.g., turn off pager).
2. Establish what the patient already knows. Both doctors and family members generally underestimate the level of the patient's knowledge.
3. Establish whether the patient wants more information.
4. Allow denial. Denial is both a defense and a coping strategy. Allow the patient to control the amount of information he or she receives.

5. At the beginning of the conversation, allow the patient time to consider his or her reactions and whether he or she feels able to take in more information.
6. Explain if requested. Be clear, simple, and compassionate. Avoid stark statements and medical jargon. Check frequently on whether the patient and family or caregivers understand. Be positive, kind, and calm; avoid conveying false optimism.
7. Listen to concerns; empathize.
8. Encourage expression of feelings.
9. Summarize and make a plan, to minimize confusion and uncertainty.
10. Offer availability. Include time for questions. Ideally, provide written information and give details of a contact person (often a nurse specialist) who can be available to answer any queries that arise later. Be clear about the next appointment or investigation—its time, place, and purpose.

Helping the patient and family and caregivers manage uncertainty
Although it is one of the most difficult problems for the human psyche to bear, uncertainty plagues most cancer patients from diagnosis through end of life.

Doctors face the dilemma of how to reassure an anxious patient but also be honest about an enigmatic disease with an uncertain outcome.
- Ask if the patient has had personal experiences of relatives or friends previously diagnosed and treated for advanced malignant disease. This history will, in large part, influence the patient's reaction to uncertainty.
- Discuss potential fears, including discomfort, dependency, resolution of important life themes, and death.
- Reassure the patient that measures will be taken to keep them comfortable.
- Clarify misunderstandings about diagnosis, prognosis, treatment options, and evidence.
- Acknowledge and address valid concerns.

Engaging available palliative care support, e.g., clinical nurse specialist
Palliative care is increasingly recognized as an important component of end-of-life care for cancer patients. Palliative care can be provided by physicians, nurses, or other trained professionals. It is available in many hospitals as a consult service; some institutions have dedicated palliative care beds.

A recent addition to the multidisciplinary care team, the clinical nurse specialist (CNS) occupies a role designed to minimize communication lapses between departments or providers, or due to complicated treatment paths. The CNS ensures continuity between appointments so that patients do not need to repeat their story for multiple providers, understand the purpose of each visit, and know whom to contact should they feel "lost in the system."

Depression

Identifying and differentiating between preparatory grief and depression in a dying patient can be quite difficult, even for seasoned clinicians. In general, depressed patients tend to remain in a consistently sad state, have a poor view of themselves, maintain a sense of hopelessness, show little pleasure in new situations or from memories of prior events, and even actively desire an early death.[1,2]

Patients with normal grief reactions typically experience a progression of feelings, are able to maintain a realistic view of themselves, respond well to social support, are capable of feeling pleasure, and can adjust their goals of care to maintain hope.

Treatment of depression at the end of life is important for 2 reasons:
- First, several studies have shown that untreated depression is associated with increased morbidity and reported sequelae. Depression, hopelessness, loss of meaning in life, and loss of interest in activities are risk factors for desire for hastened death.[3,4] Conversely, patients who have psychosocial needs addressed are less likely to persist in their desire for death.[5]
- Second, depression clearly diminishes quality of life, an agreed goal of treatment at this stage of disease.

Assessment

For the terminally ill patient, diagnosis must rely more heavily on psychological or cognitive symptoms than on somatic symptoms.
- Beck Depression Inventory–Short Form (BDI-SF)
- Hospital Anxiety and Depression Scale (HADS)
- Edmonton Symptom Assessment Scale (ESAS)
- Edinburgh Depression Scale
- Brief Edinburgh Depression Scale (BEDS)

Management

Follow guidelines established for general care of psychiatric illness, with certain adjustments.

Use of pharmacologic therapy must take into account the patient's prognosis. When the patient has limited life expectancy, there may not be time to titrate and achieve effect with SSRIs; psychostimulants may offer a more realistic treatment strategy.

---

1 Periyakoil VS, Hallenbeck J (2002). Identifying and managing preparatory grief and depression at the end of life. *Am Fam Physician* 65:883–890.

2 Noorani NH, Montagnini M (2007). Recognizing depression in palliative care patients. *J Palliat Med* 10:458–464.

3 Breitbart W, Rosenfeld B, Pessin H, et al. (2000). Depression, hopelessness, and desire for hastened death in terminally ill patients with cancer. *JAMA* 284:2907–2911.

4 Schroepfer TA (2007). Critical events in the dying process: the potential for physical and psychosocial suffering. *J Palliat Med* 10:136–147.

5 Ganzini L, Nelson HD, Schmidt TA, et al. (2000). Physicians' experiences with the Oregon Death with Dignity Act. *N Engl J Med* 342:557–563.

Engage psychosocial support from available patient support programs, counselors, therapists, family members and caregivers, and religious community (if applicable).

Distress (patient)

Psychological assessment, and provision of appropriate psychological support, should be an integral part of care for patients with malignant disease. Psychological distress may present as the following:
- Denial or confusion
- Anger
- Anxiety
- Sadness, depression
- Sense of loss
- Alienation
- Poor symptom control

Psychological concerns are frequently overlooked. Set aside time for mental state assessment.
- Heed cues from the patient or family and caregivers.
- Assess the patient; there are many validated, standardized, psychological assessment and quality-of-life instruments available.

Assessment
- Hospital Anxiety and Depression Scale (HADS)
- Functional Assessment of Cancer Therapy (FACT), available in many disease-specific versions (e.g., FACT-Breast Cancer)
- Functional Living Index–Cancer (FLIC)
- European Organization for Research and Treatment Quality-of-Life Questionnaire (EORTC QLQ-C30)

Management

Self-help
Offer patients control over their management. Help them set realistic goals and develop coping strategies.

Informal support
Suggest that sharing of experiences, airing one's feelings in a supportive environment, and exchanging information about the physical, psychological, and social consequences of cancer and treatment can help to reduce the sense of alienation and isolation often associated with cancer (e.g., local cancer support groups).

A religious community can provide spiritual and practical support.

Formal support
Primary care services or hospital-based cancer information centers sometimes provide access, or make referrals, to trained counselors.

Palliative care specialist nurses can assess the need for and provide trained psychological support. They usually have access to psychologists and/or psychiatrists if the patient requires additional help.

Psychological therapies
Cognitive-behavioral therapy and brief psychotherapeutic interventions can be effective for more significant levels of anxiety or depression.

Psychiatric interventions
Recognize when referral to a psychiatrist for drug therapy (e.g., antidepressant, anxiolytic) is required. Psychotropic medication benefits >25% of cancer patients suffering significant anxiety and depression.

Trial of an antidepressant may be worthwhile. A number of selective seritonin reuptake inhibitors (SSRIs) are available generically. Start with a low dose and titrate upwards over time, if tolerated; maximal effects are not expected for 4–6 weeks. Fluoxetine may be a bit more "activating," whereas agents that also block norepinepherine reuptake (SNRIs) can be useful adjuncts for pain relief (venlafexine, duloxetine, etc). Use caution in the setting of thrombocytopenia, as these medications have anti-platelet effects. Always screen for suicidal thinking or behavior and refer to a psychiatrist for cases of severe and/or suicidal/homicidal depression.

Distress (family and caregiver)

Psychosocial problems afflict not only the patient with a terminal illness.
- Up to 50% of caregivers of terminally ill cancer patients experience psychiatric morbidity.[1,2]
- Many families are unprepared for the financial, emotional, and physical commitment of caring for a loved one at the end of life.[3]
- In addition, families often lack the necessary medical knowledge and skills to anticipate care needs.
- Because of the demands of caregiving, many family members are forced to leave their jobs, or to work part-time, thus adding financial strain to an already emotionally intense period.
- Caregivers often neglect their own healthcare and emotional needs because of the burdens of caregiving.[4]
- It is important for physicians to recognize that effective communication, listening, and availability go far toward alleviating suffering of caregivers and patients alike as the patient nears the end of life.

---

1 Pitceathly C, Maguire P (2003). The psychological impact of cancer on patients' partners and other key relatives: a review. *Eur J Cancer* 39:1517–1524.

2 Haley WE, LaMonde LA, Han B, et al. (2001). Family caregiving in hospice: effects on psychological and health functioning among spousal caregivers of hospice patients with lung cancer or dementia. *Hosp J* 15:1–18.

3 Rabow MW, Hauser JM, Adams J (2004). Supporting family caregivers at the end of life: 'they don't know what they don't know'. *JAMA* 291:483–491.

4 Stein MD, Crystal S, Cunningham WE, et al. (2000) Delays in seeking HIV care due to competing caregiver responsibilities. *Am J Public Health* 90:1138–1140.

Management
- Provide effective symptom relief for the patient; when patients are less challenged by symptoms, caregivers are less distressed.
- Seek to alleviate the patient's psychosocial distress. This can also decrease the burden and the psychological effects of terminal illness on caregivers.
- Be present. By being available, discussing difficult topics, and helping manage troublesome symptoms, the physician can provide significant support to caregivers.
- Listen to caregivers' opinions and concerns.
- Provide anticipatory guidance and explanations of what will occur.
- Make appropriate referrals to agencies that can provide assistance, such as hospice.

Spiritual suffering

The spiritual needs of patients and families and caregivers typically become heightened as the patient approaches the end of life.
- Good care of the spirit is thus integral to excellent end-of-life care.
- Spiritual care helps the patient and family and caregivers address nearly unavoidable and sometimes troubling existential issues, such as "What is the meaning of life?," "Why am I here?," "What have I achieved in my life?," "How do I fit into the universe?," and "What will happen to me after my death?"
- Patients' and families' and caregivers' religious and personal beliefs will influence their reactions to these major spiritual questions.

Although physicians are not typically trained to provide spiritual care, patients and families and caregivers often expect that health professionals can adequately introduce and discuss the subject of care of the spirit.

The goal of spiritual care, in the context of end-of-life cancer care, is to support patients in exploring and expressing their spirituality, to the extent that they wish and in the manner that is most meaningful and comfortable for them.

General management principles
- Many people value an expected death as an opportunity to resolve outstanding spiritual issues, and they expect to do so in the context of medical care.
- Patients and families and caregivers may initiate a discussion about spiritual concerns at any time.
- Patients and families and caregivers may react to their circumstances with a variety of emotions: anger, fear, powerlessness, and grief.
- Containing or managing family conflict is crucial to ensure that patients can approach death in a context of full support.

Management
- Do your own inner work. Consider important spiritual and existential questions yourself, to be able to converse meaningfully with patients about their beliefs and concerns.
- Be comfortable with openly exploring and discussing the patient's or family's and caregiver's spiritual issues.
- Raise spiritual themes with the patient as appropriate, but refer certain specific issues to the pastoral care team.
- Do not seek to share your own views, but rather to understand the breadth and complexity of the patient's or family's and caregiver's orientation.
- Use this understanding to identify needs that should be addressed by other professionals (e.g., chaplain, psychotherapist), to guide the delivery of compassionate care, and to incorporate insights into whole-person-focused clinical decisions.

Terminal agitation

To optimize the patient's physical and psychological comfort and to facilitate a dignified and peaceful death, it is sometimes necessary to intervene to preserve mental clarity and calm.

Assessment

Even when death is imminent, it is important to adequately monitor changes in the patient's mental state. Potentially reversible causes of distress and agitation include the following:
- Inadequate pain control
- Urinary retention or the need to have the bowels open
- Nausea
- Breathlessness
- Fear, or existential distress
- Side effects of medication

Symptom assessment at this stage should be achieved with minimal disruption to the patient in terms of examination and investigation.

Management

Discontinue all nonessential medication. In practice, this usually means discontinuing everything except analgesia, anxiolytics, and antiemetics.
- If the patient is unconscious and has entered the terminal phase, it is usually not necessary to continue corticosteroids.

Avoid the oral route. Continuous IV or subcutaneous infusion is often the route of choice and does not necessarily require admission, although it will require significant support from the primary care service, hospice, or community palliative care team.

Make prn doses available so that the nursing team has ready access should any signs of distress develop.
- Ideally, optimal symptom control is achieved by subcutaneous infusion, without the need for additional doses.

Use anxiolytics (e.g., alprozalam or lorazepam), but with frequent review, as many patients will need significantly greater doses.
- Occasionally, agitation persists despite escalating benzodiazepine doses.
- Prn haloperidol, 1–5 mg oral, IV or subcutaneous, is also useful for distress.

Explain to the patient (if conscious) and family or caregivers the goals of care, measures being taken, and steps not being taken.
- Discuss the balance between adequate pain control and likely sedation. Emerging evidence suggests that dexmedetomidine may obviate the need for this trade-off; this medication should be administered under the supervision of a palliative care specialist or anesthesiologist familiar with its dosing and side effect profile.
- Clarify the contents of the subcutaneous infusion. Reassure relatives that the needs of the patient will continue to be reviewed and adjustments made accordingly.
- Time spent at this stage may help the patient's family to understand and subsequently grieve without anger, suspicion, or unanswered questions about the patient's final hours.

Involve specialist palliative care services, either hospital- or community-based.
- Advice on resistant symptoms may be invaluable, as are these professionals' additional skills in managing the needs of relatives before, during, and after the patient's death.
- Remember that the hospice bundle of services includes bereavement support for family members.

Care in the last days of life

Clinicians must be able to recognize the process of dying from cancer, evidenced by continued expected deterioration of a person's overall condition with increasing lethargy, decreasing levels of consciousness, and at times increasing confusion, increasing time asleep, less spontaneous movement, and altered patterns of respiratory effort.

For many people, systemic signs include progressive hypotension, diminishing oxygenation, progressive loss of peripheral perfusion, and autonomic dysregulation (such as wide temperature fluctuations). Alternatively, the terminal phase of cancer may be signaled by a sudden change in condition—an intracerebral bleed, a pulmonary embolus, a perforated viscous, or overwhelming sepsis.

Understanding patients' wishes—often through conversations with their families over both the course of illness and the course of life more broadly—will help determine the best course of action.

General management principles

- The issue of comfort is absolutely paramount. Clearly state this priority to patients and families and caregivers.
- Focus all clinical activities and care management around the goal of comfort.

Management

- **Mouth care**: Ensure that the dying person's mouth is clean and moist.
- **Positioning**: Use an air mattress to shift the person's weight. If an air mattress is not available, reposition the person regularly to relieve musculoskeletal pain from inertia, and to maintain skin integrity to avoid the excruciating (and difficult to control) pain of skin tears and pressure sores.
- **Death rattles**: Gently elevate the head of the bed if noisy upper respiratory tract secretions are a concern.
- **Medications**: Review all medications currently being administered, and continue only those that directly contribute to comfort. Ensure that essential medications are available in a form that can be administered to someone who may not predictably be swallowing (e.g., sublingual, subcutaneous, IV, transdermal, intranasal, or rectal formulation).
- **Hydration/nutrition**: Parenteral hydration and/or nutrition should almost always be stopped, with appropriate advice to the family, to avoid exacerbating respiratory symptoms and inducing vomiting.
- **Agitation**: Ensure that agitation is not due to pain, urinary retention, or constipation. Treatment may include a regular dose of a long-acting benzodiazepine, but use with care because benzodiazepines can precipitate or worsen delirium.

- **Communication**: Clearly, but compassionately, describe the process of dying to the patient and family and caregiver. Reassure patients that, in most cases, the dying person gently slips into a coma and life ebbs away with no dramatic manifestations of death. Family can be educated to expect to see the following:
  - Social withdrawal
  - Decreased need for food and drink
  - Increasing time spent sleeping
  - Disorientation
  - Restlessness
  - Decreased senses (e.g., vision, hearing)
  - Incontinence
  - Physical changes, including perspiration, altered skin color, body temperature changes, irregular breathing, congestion
- Continue to ensure comfort of, and communicate with, a patient who is unconscious.
- Set up a vigil roster and a contact plan if the family wishes to be present at the time of death.

Further reading

American Thoracic Society (1999). Dyspnea. Mechanisms, assessment, and management: a consensus statement. *Am J Respir Crit Care Med* 159:321–340.

Asch DA, Faber-Langendoen K, Shea JA, Christakis NA (1999). The sequence of withdrawing life-sustaining treatment from patients. *Am J Med* 107:153–156.

Back, A, Arnold, R, Tulsky J (2009). *Mastering Communication with Seriously Ill Patients: Balancing Honesty with Empathy and Hope.* New York: Cambridge University Press.

Hughes AC, Wilcock A, Corcoran R (1996). Management of 'death rattle.' *J Pain Symptom Manag* 12:271–272

Kamal AH, Maguire JM, Wheeler JL, et al. (2012). Dyspnea review for the palliative care professional: treatment goals and therapeutic options. *J Palliat Med* 15:106–14.

Kamal AH, Maguire JM, Wheeler JL, et al. (2011). Dyspnea review for the palliative care professional: assessment, burdens, and etiologies. *J Palliat Med* 14:1167–72.

Massie M, Holland J, Glass E (1983). Delirium in terminally ill cancer patients. *Am J Psychiatry* 140:1048–1050.

Periyakoil VS, Hallenbeck J (2002). Identifying and managing preparatory grief and depression at the end of life. *Am Fam Physician* 65:883–890.

Power D, Kearney M (1992). Management of the final 24 hours. *Irish Med J* 85:93–95.

Rabow MW, Hauser JM, Adams J (2004). Supporting family caregivers at the end of life: 'they don't know what they don't know.' *JAMA* 291:483–491.

Schroepfer TA (2007). Critical events in the dying process: the potential for physical and psychosocial suffering. *J Palliat Med* 10:136–147.

Part V
Specific cancers

27	Thoracic cancers	395
28	Breast cancer	429
29	Gastrointestinal cancer I: esophagus, stomach, small intestine, carcinoid	465
30	Gastrointestinal cancer II: pancreas, biliary tract, hepatocellular	483
31	Gastrointestinal cancer III: colorectal, anus	499
32	Endocrine cancers	513
33	Genitourinary cancers I: renal, bladder, ureter, penile carcinomas	535
34	Genitourinary cancers II: prostate cancer	563
35	Genitourinary cancers III: testicular cancer	589
36	Gynecological cancer	605
37	Tumors of the central nervous system	625
38	Head and neck cancers	643
39	Cutaneous malignancies	667
40	Soft tissue and bone sarcomas	687
41	Acute leukemia	717
42	Chronic leukemias and myelodysplastic syndromes	729
43	Multiple myeloma	749
44	Malignant lymphoma	767
45	Cancer of unknown primary	789

Chapter 27

Thoracic cancers

Jeffrey Crawford

Lung cancer *396*
Non-small–cell lung cancer *400*
Surgery for non-small–cell lung cancer *402*
Chemotherapy for non-small–cell lung cancer *406*
Radiation therapy for non-small–cell lung cancer *410*
Small cell lung cancer *413*
Chemotherapy for small cell lung cancer *414*
Radiotherapy for small cell lung cancer *418*
Mesothelioma *420*
Thymic tumors *426*

Lung cancer

Epidemiology

Currently, lung cancer represents the most common cause of cancer mortality in the United States and worldwide (see Table 27.1). Incidence is second only to prostate and breast cancer. It causes more deaths in the United States than colorectal, breast, and prostate cancer combined.
- In 2004, incidence was 67.4 per 100,000 population.
- It is estimated that 214,000 new cases of lung cancer were diagnosed in 2007.
- Approximately 170,000 patients died of lung cancer in 2007.
- Incidence rates have stabilized and are even decreasing among men.
- However, mortality, which has decreased among men, is increasing among women.
- Worldwide, the incidence is continuing to rise, particularly in developing countries, as cigarette smoking becomes more prevalent.

Etiology

Exposure to tobacco smoke accounts for 90% of lung cancers in males and 79% in females. Risk of lung cancer relates to the number of cigarettes smoked, the number of years of smoking, early age starting to smoke, and the type of cigarette (there is greater risk with unfiltered and high-nicotine). Some 2%–10% of lung cancers occur in never-smokers, usually women.

Other exposure risks include the following:
- Asbestos
- Secondhand smoke exposure
- Inhalation of radon
- Previous radiotherapy to the chest
- Rarely, inhalation of polycyclic aromatic hydrocarbons, nickel, chromate, or inorganic arsenicals

Screening and prevention

Lung cancer is a preventable disease; promotion of smoking cessation will likely have the greatest effect on mortality.

Although globally, cigarette consumption is increasing, in the United States cigarette smoking is decreasing. Currently, 23.9% of men and 18.1% of women smoke cigarettes.

Stopping smoking reduces the risk of developing lung cancer. Use of nicotine replacement therapy can improve smoking cessation rates.

There is no mortality benefit for screening with chest X-ray and sputum cytology. Screening at-risk patients with chest CT can detect early and curable lesions, but there has been no demonstrable increase in survival.

Table 27.1 Lung cancer incidence figures

Sex	U.S. incidence and mortality 2000–2004 (age adjusted, per 100,000 population)	
	Incidence	Mortality
All	64.5	54.7
Male	81.2	73.4
Female	52.3	41.1

Pathology

There is evidence that lung cancers may arise in pluripotent stem cells in the bronchial epithelium. This would certainly offer an explanation for the mixed histology that is fairly commonly seen. The WHO pathological classification is as follows:

- Squamous cell carcinoma
- Small cell carcinoma
- Adenocarcinoma
  - Acinar
  - Papillary
  - Bronchioloalveolar carcinoma
  - Solid adenocarcinoma with mucin formation
  - Mixed
- Large cell carcinoma
- Adenosquamous carcinoma
- Carcinomas with pleomorphic, sarcomatoid, or sarcomatous elements
  - Carcinomas with spindle and/or giant cells
  - Pleomorphic carcinoma
  - Spindle cell carcinoma
  - Giant cell carcinoma
  - Carcinosarcoma
  - Pulmonary blastoma
- Carcinoid tumor
- Carcinomas of salivary gland type
  - Mucoepidermoid carcinoma
  - Adenoid cystic carcinoma
- Unclassified carcinomas

Adenocarcinoma, squamous cell carcinoma, large cell carcinoma, and small cell carcinoma account for 85%–90% of all lung cancers.

For the purposes of management, lung cancers are grouped as non-small-cell lung cancer (NSCLC) or small cell lung cancer (SCLC), but within the NSCLC group certain patterns of disease do relate to histological subtype. For example, squamous cancers typically arise in proximal segmental bronchi and grow slowly, disseminating relatively late in their course.

Adenocarcinomas are often peripheral in origin, and even small, resectable lesions carry a risk of occult metastases. Common sites of metastatic spread include the regional lymph nodes, bone, liver, adrenal, lung, central nervous system (CNS), and skin.

For management of patients with advanced NSCLC, it has become useful to categorize patients with squamous NSCLC and non-squamous NSCLC.

The risk of dissemination is greatest in SCLC, where it is estimated that >90% of patients have either overt or occult metastases at presentation. These aggressive tumors, derived from neuroendocrine cells, most frequently arise in large airways but can rarely present as a small peripheral nodule. The latter presentation may be indicative of a different pathology with an inherently better prognosis.

Genetics

Most clinically apparent lung cancers have numerous genetic alterations, acquired in a stepwise fashion, resulting in disruption of cell cycle regulation, chromosomal instability, resistance to apoptosis, anchorage-independent growth, and, finally, invasion and metastasis. Some examples of these genes are listed below.

Inactivation or loss of tumor suppressor genes

- *p53* mutations are present in approximately 90% of SCLCs, 30% of adenocarcinomas, and 50% of squamous cell carcinomas.
- Alterations of the retinoblastoma (*RB*) gene are detected in >90% of SCLCs and only 15%–20% of NSCLCs.
- Allelic loss involving the short arm of chromosome 3 occurs in >90% of SCLCs and approximately 70% of NSCLCs.
- Decreased expression of TGF-β receptor type II gene allows increased proliferation of bronchial epithelial cells.

Overexpression of oncogenes

- The *RAS* oncogene is upregulated in 30% of adenocarcinomas.
- *Myc* oncogene is overexpressed in 75% of SCLCs.
- *EGFR* is overexpressed in 70% of SCLCs and 40% of adenocarcinomas.
- Overexpression of *BCL2* protects against apoptosis in SCLC.
- *TTF-1*, a developmental gene, is unique to the genome of lung adenocarcinomas.

Driver mutations

It has been increasingly recognized that lung adenocarcinomas harbor a genetic mutation that may regulate gene expression and cancer growth. The three most common are K-ras mutation, EGFR mutation, and ALK translocation.

Angiogenesis: tumor progression and metastasis

- VEGF receptor: High levels of VEGF expression are detected in 50% of all lung cancers.
- VEGF may also be induced by hypoxia and COX-2.
- Ang-1 and TIE2 have also been reported in numerous NSCLCs.

Telomerase activation occurs in 100% of SCLCs and 80% of NSCLCs.

Genetic predisposition to development of lung cancer

- Family history of lung cancer in a relative confers a relative risk of 1.8 (1.6–2.0) when age and smoking status are controlled for.
- Rarely, germline mutation of *RB* or *p53*

Presenting symptoms and signs

Typically, presentation is late, with symptoms such as persistent cough and dyspnea being attributed to smoking. Small adenocarcinomas in the periphery of the lung may be asymptomatic.

Symptoms and signs include the following:
- Persistent cough, hemoptysis, dyspnea
- Recurrent chest infections
- Pleural effusion
- Chest pain (constant, progressive)
- Hoarse voice (vocal cord palsy)
- Wheeze, stridor
- Superior vena cava (SVC) obstruction
- Horner's syndrome, arm or hand pain, and neurological deficit (apical cancer)
- Fatigue
- Anorexia, weight loss
- Paraneoplastic syndromes
- Symptoms from metastatic disease

Investigations

After physical examination and chest X-ray, patients with suspected lung cancer require further imaging with a CT scan (chest and upper abdomen). A tissue diagnosis should then be obtained based on imaging findings: it is important that adequate biopsy be obtained to determine histologic subtype with sufficient tissue available for molecular markers. Possible sources include:
- Fine-needle aspiration (FNA) biopsy from palpable disease, most commonly supraclavicular nodes
- Bronchoscopy of endobronchial lesions or ultrasound (EBUS) guided biopsies
- Pleural aspirate cytology with cell block or pleural biopsy
- Transthoracic or transbronchial FNA of lymph nodes or lung lesion
- Mediastinoscopy and lymph node biopsy
- Video-assisted thoracoscopy (VATS) and biopsy
- Rarely, open lung biopsy

Other important assessments include performance status, pulmonary function tests, CBC, and biochemical profile.

Positron emission tomography (PET) scanning with CT is now standard for initial staging of NSCLC. Bone scan plus CT is still satisfactory for SCLC. Brain imaging should also be performed in initial evaluation of both SCLC and NSCLC.

Non-small-cell lung cancer

Staging
Table 27.2 summarizes the TNM staging criteria for non-small cell lung cancer.

The following assessments are required:
- Clinical examination, with particular attention to lymphadenopathy, soft tissue masses, e.g., chest wall
- Bronchoscopy
  - Movement of vocal cords
  - Site of endobronchial tumor in relation to carina and major bronchial divisions
  - Transbronchial needle aspiration of mediastinal lymph nodes
- CT chest and abdomen
  - Size and site of primary tumor
  - Relationship to lung fissures, mediastinum, chest wall
  - Mediastinal or other lymphadenopathy
  - Metastatic disease, in particular lung, pleura, liver, adrenal, bone
  - CT of the brain and an isotope bone scan can be performed if there is clinical suspicion of metastatic disease.

FDG-PET scanning
- Can increase accuracy of preoperative clinical staging and should be routine part of evaluation
- May detect occult malignant metastasis
- Has good negative predictive value, but poor positive predictive value
  - Frequent false-positive results from other inflammatory conditions
- Lesions detected on FDG-PET should be biopsied for accurate staging, where treatment will change based on results.

Treatment modalities

Surgery
- Complete surgical removal of NSCLC offers the best possibility of a cure.
- Appropriate for patients with stage I–II disease and occasionally stage III disease who are fit for surgery (see Surgery for non-small–cell lung cancer, pp. 402–404).

Chemotherapy
- Systemic treatment improves symptoms from advanced disease, and has a modest survival benefit.
- It is appropriate for patients with stage III–IV disease, particularly with good performance status.
- Can be considered before surgery (induction) in certain patients or as adjuvant treatment postoperatively in patients found to have Stage II or III NSCLC a role before surgery and as adjuvant therapy for stage I–II disease.

Radiotherapy
- Effective local treatment, giving prompt symptom relief from advanced disease especially involving large airways
- Can be curative in stage I for patients who are not surgical candidates and can be curative with concurrent chemotherapy in the inoperable patient with Stage III disease.

Table 27.2 TNM staging of lung cancer

Primary tumor characteristics (T)

T1	Tumor 3 cm or less in diameter without invasion more proximal than lobar bronchus
T2	Tumor >3 cm diameter OR tumor of any size with any of the following: • Invades visceral pleura • Atelectasis of less than entire lung • Proximal extent >2 cm from carina
T3	Tumor of any size and any of the following: • Invading chest wall, diaphragm, mediastinal pleura, or pericardium • Tumor in main bronchus <2 cm distal to carina • Atelectasis of the whole lung
T4	Tumor of any size and any of the following: • Invading mediastinum, heart, great vessels, trachea, esophagus, vertebra, or carina • Satellite tumor nodules within the same lobe as primary • Malignant pleural effusion

Nodal involvement (N)

N0	No regional node metastases
N1	Ipsilateral peribronchial or hilar node involvement
N2	Ipsilateral mediastinal or subcarinal nodes
N3	Contralateral mediastinal or hilar nodes OR ipsilateral or contralateral scalene or supraclavicular nodes

Metastasis (M)

M0	Distant metastasis absent
M1	Distant metastasis present (includes tumor in different lobe from primary tumor)

Stage grouping

I	T1–2 N0
II	T1–2 N1; or T3 N0
IIIa	T1–2 N2; or T3 N1–2
IIIb	T4 any N M0; or any N3 M0
IV	Any M1

Surgery for non-small–cell lung cancer

Surgical removal of NSCLC offers the best possibility of cure. Every patient with nonmetastatic NSCLC should be considered for surgical treatment. However, advanced stage, poor pulmonary function, and significant comorbidity will preclude this option in many patients.

Surgery should be supplemented with adjuvant chemotherapy for stage II and IIIA and can be considered for Stage IB with tumors >4 cm.

In the United States, approximately 25% of NSCLC cases are resected.[1] The aim of surgical treatment is cure; in patients in whom this is not possible, suitable nonsurgical treatments should be considered.

Careful preoperative risk assessment and confirmation of diagnosis are crucial before surgery. This should include histological confirmation of diagnosis, along with CT, FDG-PET, sampling lymph nodes, pleural cytology, or pleuroscopy when appropriate

Determination of operable stage of disease involves the following:

- Pathological staging of the mediastinum, usually by mediastinoscopy and lymph node biopsies, is required.
- Lymph nodes that appear normal size (<1 cm diameter) may contain cancer (15%); enlarged lymph nodes can be reactive (45%).
- In the presence of pleural effusion, aspirated fluid for cytology and pleural biopsy should be negative for cancer cells before proceeding with operation.

Stage III disease is defined as locoregionally advanced disease, based on mediastinal lymph node involvement or extension into extrapulmonary structures without distant metastasis. Surgical resection is controversial, but should be considered on the basis of respectability and patient comorbidities.

The following stages should be considered for surgical resection if technically feasible:

- T3N1 disease (Pancoast tumors with hilar nodal involvement should receive chemoradiotherapy followed by surgery)[2]
- T4N0 or T4N1—If there is no malignant effusion
- T1-3 N2 disease with positive mediastinal lymph node status that is converted to negative after induction chemotherapy
- May require preoperative induction therapy to shrink tumors to surgical resectability

Preoperative chemotherapy is recommended for patients with clinical stage IIIa disease. Adjuvant chemotherapy is recommended for patients staged initially as I or II clinically, but then surgically staged as stage III disease.

---

1 Humphrey DW, Smart CR, Winchester DP, et al. (1990). National survey of the pattern of care for carcinoma of the lung. *J Thorac Cardiovasc Surg* 100:837–843.

2 Harpole DH Jr, Healey EA, DeCamp MM Jr, et al. (1996). Chest wall invasive non-small cell lung cancer: patterns of failure and implications for a revised staging system. *Ann Surg Oncol* 3(3):261–269.

Fitness for surgery

Although age alone is not a surgical criteria, performance status, weight loss, and comorbidities that may exclude surgery as a feasible option need to be considered.
- Pulmonary function tests, spirometry, and gas transfer
  - Oxygen saturation <90% is associated with increased mortality.
  - Hypercapnea ($PaCO_2$ >45 mmHg) can contraindicate resection.
  - FEV_1 should be >1.5 L for lobectomy and >2 L for pneumonectomy.
- Cardiac assessment; may require exercise testing

Surgical resection

This may require lobectomy, bi-lobectomy, sleeve resection, or pneumonectomy. The goal is to remove all cancer with clear margins of surrounding normal tissue.

Limited or wedge resection with or without VATS is increasingly used for those patients who cannot tolerate the above procedures. There is increased risk of recurrence, and possibly increased mortality with limited resection compared to that with lobectomy.[1]

The operation should include regional lymph node sampling.

Involvement of chest wall, pericardium, or diaphragm can be dealt with by en bloc dissection along with the primary, but the survival benefit of such extensive surgery is doubtful.

The role of extended lymphadenectomy (mediastinal) is controversial.

Postoperative management

Patients should be managed in an intensive care or high-dependency unit with adequate monitoring of the following:
- ECG
- BP
- Central venous pressure
- Respiratory rate
- Oxygen saturation

Adequate pain control is essential after thoracotomy and can be provided by
- Thoracic epidural anesthesia
- Intravenous opiates administered by patient-controlled analgesia (PCA)
- Intercostal nerve block before wound closure

Oxygen therapy is required in the early postoperative stage, preferably through a nebulizer, and in patients with significant airways obstruction a bronchodilator should be added. Regular chest physiotherapy is essential.

---

1 Ginsburg RJ, Rubenstein LV (1995). Randomized trial of lobectomy versus limited resection for T1 N0 non-small cell lung cancer. Lung Cancer Study Group. *Ann Thorac Surg* 60:615–622.

Postoperative complications

Early (within days)
- Hemorrhage (e.g., after dissection of pleural adhesions) may result in hemothorax.
- Respiratory failure
  - Opiate-induced respiratory depression
  - Pneumothorax with or without surgical emphysema
  - Atelectasis due to retained bronchial secretions
- Prolonged air leak after lobectomy
- Cardiac arrhythmias, particularly atrial fibrillation
- Sepsis
  - Chest infection
  - Wound infection
  - Empyema
- Bronchopleural fistula (particularly on the right after pneumonectomy)
- Pulmonary embolism

Late (within weeks to months)
- Postthoracotomy pain
- Late bronchopleural fistula with empyema
- Tumor recurrence

Results of surgical resection
The postoperative mortality rate should be <3% after lobectomy and <5% after pneumonectomy.

Five-year survival is influenced by a number of factors, the most important of which is pathological staging (see Table 27.3). Overall 5-year survival for patients undergoing resection may be as high as 40%, approaching 70% in cases without nodal involvement (N0). When mediastinal nodes are involved (N2) only 15% of patients will survive 5 years.

Table 27.3 5-year overall survival for NSCLC

Stage at diagnosis	Five-year survival
Localized	49.1%
Direct spread or regional lymph nodes	15.2%
Distant metastasis	3.0%
Unstaged	8.1%

Chemotherapy for non-small–cell lung cancer

Older studies with alkylating agents in advanced NSCLC showed decreased survival with chemotherapy, and until the 1980s no systemic treatments were available, with objective response rates in excess of 20%. Over the last two decades there has been significant progress in this area, with increasing use of chemotherapy in advanced disease, as well as the adjuvant setting.

Local and resectable disease (I, II, IIIa)

Previous trials of patients with stage Ia disease have decreased survival with adjuvant chemotherapy. However, 50% of patients with resected Ib and 70% of patients with resected stage II disease tumors recur, and these patients die despite "curative surgery." Distant metastasis represents a common source of treatment failure.

Adjuvant chemotherapy decreases the risk of distant metastasis. Multiple clinical trials have shown benefit for adjuvant chemotherapy with a cisplatin-based regimen in stage II, and IIIa disease. Stage Ib is more controversial, but patient with tumors greater than 4 cm have improved survival in retrospective analyses. Vinorelbine has been studied the most in combination with cisplatin. Carboplatin and paclitaxel have also shown improved survival in this population.

Neoadjuvant chemotherapy is an alternative to postoperative chemotherapy, but the results of clinical trials are more limited to know if the benefits are comparable. However, the strategy provides an ideal opportunity for evaluating response in relation to survival in clinical trials.

Stage IIIb disease

Approximately 30% of patients with NSCLC present with locally advanced and unresectable disease but no evidence of metastases. This is a heterogeneous group, but it includes patients who may have durable responses to appropriate therapy, including concurrent chemotherapy and radiation treatment.

In general, responses to chemotherapy are more frequent in localized than in metastatic disease, but the benefits of chemotherapy are greater in patients with good performance status.

The same cisplatin or carboplatin chemotherapy doublets are used with the following principles.

- Response to chemotherapy should improve symptoms, reduce locoregional disease before local therapy, and reduce microscopic metastatic disease.
- Platinum-based combination chemotherapy concurrent with radiotherapy gives better survival rates than radiotherapy alone (3-year survival 13%–23% vs. 6%). Sequential chemotherapy followed by radiation is inferior to concurrent treatment, but it can be considered in patients with poorer performance status, where the toxicity of concurrent treatment may be unacceptable.

- Patients unable to receive chemotherapy may be treated with palliative radiotherapy only.
- Selection and coordination of appropriate therapy require close cooperation of medical and radiation oncologists within the multidisciplinary team.

Metastatic disease

Tumor response and survival

Platinum-based chemotherapy produces significant benefits in stage IV disease.
- Symptom relief and improved quality of life in >50%
- Objective response rate of 20%–30% and disease stabilization in 40%–50%.
- Less benefit and increased toxicity in patients with performance status 2 or worse
- Modest impact on survival, which has improved with ____ chemotherapy regimens.
- Initial trials demonstrated 1-year survival is 25% (without chemotherapy, 15%).
- Current regiments demonstrate 1 year survival of 40%–50%.
- Toxicities of treatment include nausea, vomiting, lethargy, myelosuppression, and neuropathy.

During the 1990s, several new drugs demonstrated antitumor activity in NSCLC as single agents and in combination with carboplatin or cisplatin.
- None of the new chemotherapy regimens has proved superior to the others.
- Doublet therapy with the combination of either cisplatin or carboplatin and one of gemcitabine, vinorelbine, paclitaxel, or docetaxel is now accepted as standard therapy for advanced NSCLC.
- Since 2000, the only new cytotoxic agent approved with cisplatin for NSCLC is pemetrexed, which demonstrated a superiority over gemcitabine-cisplatin for nonsquamous NSCLC, but it was inferior in squamous carcinoma. This helped establish the importance of histology-driven treatment in NSCLC.
- Most benefit of chemotherapy occurs in the last 4-6 cycles of treatment.
- Maintenance therapy with a similar nonplatinum agent, such as pemetrexed, may prolong response and survival in some patients.

Single-agent chemotherapy with agents such as gemcitabine or vinorelbine can be of benefit in patients with advanced disease and performance status of 2.

Quality of life

Although cytotoxic regimens produce objective tumor response rates of the order of 20%–50% in advanced NSCLC, symptom improvement can be achieved in a greater proportion of patients, providing important palliative benefit.
- Cough, hemoptysis, and pain are relieved in 70%.
- Anorexia is addressed in 40%.
- Dyspnea is relieved in 30%.

Targeted therapy
Bevacizumab, a monoclonal antibody to vascular endothelial growth factor (VEGF) when combined with carboplatin/paclitaxel, has demonstrated superior survival to chemotherapy alone. However, this agent is contraindicated in patients with squamous cell carcinoma who may develop fatal hemoptysis from the anti-angiogenic drug. Thus, accurately knowing histology of NSCLC is also critical in this setting.

Research in ongoing to identify the development of other agents and tyrosine kinase inhibitors directed at novel agents in NSCLC that have been identified over the last several years.

The best established targets in NSCLC currently include epidermal growth factor receptor (EGFR) mutations and anaplastic lymphoma kinase (ALK) translocations. Both are established drier mutations that have U.S. FDA approved therapies (erlotinib and afitinib for EGFR mutations and crizotinib for ALK translocations). All of these treatments are approved for front line treatment of patients with advanced NSCLC whow tumors demonstrate the appropriate biomarker, truly representing the era of targeted therapy in NSCLC.

As a result, all patients with advanced stage nonsquamous NSCLC should have evaluation of these tumors to see whether they are candidates for these therapies, preferably before chemotherapy. Clinical trial results suggest median survival of 2–3 years with these agents in this population, clearly superior to outcomes with chemotherapy alone.

Toxicities are largely GI and skin related and can be significant, but they can be managed well with preemptive supportive care.

This is a dynamic area in terms of new targets and new agents in NSCLC that can be further improved in the years ahead.

Radiation therapy for non-small-cell lung cancer

External beam radiotherapy is used as the local treatment for thoracic disease in the majority of NSCLC patients, and local tumor control rates correlate with the dose of radiotherapy given.

Radiotherapy with curative intent

Radical radiotherapy is indicated
- For patients with stage I–II NSCLC who are unfit for surgery
- For stage III disease that can be encompassed in a radical volume in patients with good performance status and adequate lung function

Due to the poor functional status of many of these patients, the cost of radical treatment includes
- Frequent hospital attendances
- Acute toxicities, esophagitis, decreased intake, dehydration, and associated comorbidities
- Late toxicities, e.g., lung fibrosis

Patient selection is crucial to minimize the risk of prolonged side effects in patients with poor performance status, while identifying good prognosis patients with Stage III disease who are candidate for aggressive therapy with concurrent chemotherapy and radiation.

Radiotherapy for stage I and II disease

Definitive radiotherapy (RT) is used for patients who refuse resection or who are limited by comorbidities. Overall, 5-year survival ranges from 0% to 42%, based on a review that included 2000 unresectable patients. Poor survival reflects underlying illness and understaging of the disease.
- Stereotactic body radiation therapy (SBRT) uses fixation and is more accurate for treatment planning. SBRT is particularly attractive to treat small node negative lung cancers in a few fractions, while sparing lung tissue and mediastinum.
- Permits high dosage of radiation to more precise area
- The standard dose is 60 Gy in 30 fractions over 6 weeks.
- Attempts to increase tumor dose by giving an increased number of fractions of size <2 Gy given over 6–7 weeks (hyperfractionation without acceleration) have not shown benefit.

Radiotherapy for stage III disease

Definitive RT is used for patients with unresectable disease or those who are not a candidate for comorbidities.
- RT alone results in median 5-year survival of 10 months and a 5-year survival rate of 5%.
- Adjuvant radiation therapy in completely resected patients is controversial, and there is no proven survival benefit, but it decreases local recurrence in patients with previous N2-positive disease.

Treatment volume

No randomized trials have examined the volume that should be irradiated. The standard in most of the world has been the primary tumor and hilar and mediastinal lymph nodes, with a 1–2 cm margin.

Retrospective comparisons have not demonstrated any advantage over volumes encompassing tumor and radiologically involved lymph nodes only.

In dose escalation studies with conformal therapy, adjuvant nodal irradiation constrains the radiation dose delivered to the primary tumor.

Omitting uninvolved nodal groups does not appear to increase local relapse rate. Prospective trials to better evaluate treatment outcome with increased use of PET and CT imaging during ongoing radiation treatment may clarify these issues.

Postoperative radiotherapy

A meta-analysis of randomized trials of postoperative radiotherapy for completely resected NSCLC has shown impaired survival following irradiation in patients with N0 and N1 disease.

There is evidence that radiotherapy affords an improvement in local control for patients with N2 disease. The best results have been reported with 50 Gy in 25 daily fractions.

Palliative radiotherapy

For many patients with advanced NSCLC, radiation therapy is a key component in alleviating symptoms from thoracic disease, in particular:
- Hemoptysis
- Chest pain/bone pain
- Cough
- Large airway obstruction or stridor
- SVC obstruction

Radiotherapy can also produces useful palliation for many metastatic sites including lymph nodes, bone, brain, and soft tissue.
- Survival and symptom control for 1-, 2-, and 10-fraction regimes are equivocal, establishing the shorter courses as the treatment of choice for symptom control in advanced NSCLC, particularly in patients with poor performance status. However, these short schedules are associated with chest pain and flu-like symptoms in up to 40% of patients. A transient reduction in peak expiratory flow rates may occur. Most patients receiving the 2-fraction regimen suffer at least moderate but short-lived esophagitis.
- Higher-dose palliative therapy (39 Gy in 13 daily fractions) offers a modest survival advantage for good-performance status patients with locally advanced NSCLC compared with 2 fractions, but at the cost of greater toxicity, in particular esophagitis.
- The selection of an appropriate radiotherapy regimen requires individual assessment.

Outcomes of radiotherapy treatment

The key prognostic factors are the TNM staging and the patient's performance status. When these are controlled for, treatment-related factors such as chemotherapy and radiotherapy dose can provide modest survival benefits.

Radical radiotherapy
- Stage I–II, 20%–30% 5-year survival.
- Stage III, chemotherapy plus radiotherapy, 25% 2-year survival, 15% 5-year survival

Postoperative radiotherapy

Stage I–II disease

Trials show mixed results, and radiotherapy is not recommended in Stage I–II disease except for positive margins.

Stage III disease

Postoperative radiotherapy may be beneficial to patients with positive margins and N2 disease. It may increase mortality in other patients with stage III disease.

Adjuvant chemotherapy is recommended postoperatively, and sequential radiation can be considered in selected patients.

Small cell lung cancer

Introduction

Small cell lung cancer (SCLC) accounted for 13%–14% of all lung cancers in the United States. It occurs almost exclusively in smokers.

Staging and management are quite distinct from NSCLC because
- Almost all SCLC demonstrate rapid growth and early dissemination.
- >90% have systemic disease at presentation.
- Surgery is inappropriate in the vast majority; <10% are operable.
- However, for clinical Stage I and II SCLC, surgical staging and surgery if no mediastinal node involvement, is appropriate and can be associated with substantial 5-year survival.
- Adjuvant chemotherapy and prophylactic cranial radiation should be considered for these patients as well.
- Chemotherapy is the key primary treatment and has an important impact on survival.

Staging and prognostic factors

A much-simplified staging system is used for SCLC, as the vast majority of patients are initially treated with chemotherapy irrespective of disease extent. A two-stage system was drawn up by the Veterans Administration Lung Group, decades ago and remains in standard use today.

Limited-stage disease

Tumor is confined to one hemithorax and regional lymph nodes, and can be covered by tolerable radiotherapy fields.

Note: the presence of a malignant pleural effusion is considered extensive stage disease.

Extensive-stage disease

Disease is beyond these bounds. Within these broad categories, subgroups may be defined according to one or more of the following prognostic factors:
- Performance status
- Sex (females have better prognosis)
- Lactate dehydrogenase (LDH)
- Alkaline phosphatase
- Serum Na (hyponatraemia carries a poor prognosis)

Chemotherapy for small cell lung cancer

Before the introduction of systemic treatment with chemotherapy in the 1970s, the outlook for patients diagnosed with this disease was dreadful, with a median survival of 6 weeks for patients with extensive disease and 3 months for those with limited disease.

Combination chemotherapy leads to objective response in the majority, with improved survival times, and is now the standard primary treatment for both stages of disease.

Principles of treatment

- Etoposide plus cisplatin or carboplatin (EP or EC) has been established as the best first-line treatment. Platinum plus irinotecan can be comparable, but it is associated with increased toxicity in Western populations.
- These regimens have demonstrated superior response rates and tolerability compared with older anthracycline regimens, e.g., cyclophosphamide, doxorubicin, vincristine (CAV).
- Etoposide platinum chemotherapy is compatible with concomitant thoracic irradiation.
- Standard chemotherapy treatment comprises 4 cycles of EP or EC.
- No benefit from maintenance treatment or increased dose intensification or high-dose chemotherapy has been demonstrated in randomized trials.

Benefits of treatment

Limited disease
- 80%–90% response rates with chemotherapy and radiotherapy
- 50%–60% complete response
- Thoracic radiotherapy improves local control from 10% up to 50% and is associated with improved survival.
- 2-year survival is 20%–40%.
- 5-year survival is 10%–13%.

Extensive disease
- 60%–80% response with chemotherapy alone (radiotherapy not indicated)
- 15%–20% complete response
- 2-year survival is <5%.

Other features
- Response lasts 6–8 months.
- Median survival is 4 months after disease recurrence.
- There is a high risk of CNS relapse after chemotherapy, and this can be reduced by prophylactic cranial irradiation in both limited and extensive stage patients.

Risks of treatment
- Febrile neutropenia is common and increased with increased tumor burden, comorbidities and poor performance status. Myeloid growth facts such as G-CSF are well documented to decrease this risk and should be considered as primary prophylaxis in patients at increased risk.
- DVT and thromboembolic disease
- Nausea, vomiting, diarrhea, renal failure, neuropathy
- Esophagitis and pneumonitis from radiotherapy

Specific problems of small cell lung cancer

Poor performance status
Unlike NSCLC, SCLC patients with performance status of 2–3 may benefit from chemotherapy, if they were previously fit and deterioration is due to rapid tumor progression, but initial dose reduction and supportive care are vital in being able to get these patients through chemotherapy successfully.

Superior vena cava obstruction
- Relatively common with locally advanced right-sided central tumors, mediastinal lymphadenopathy
- Initial treatment with chemotherapy is appropriate for most patients and leads to prompt resolution of superior vena cava obstruction (SVCO) in the majority.

Elderly patients
- The majority of patients with SCLC are >70 years of age.
- There is good evidence to support the use of primary chemotherapy in these patients if there are no other contraindications to treatment, again with appropriate supportive care.

Central nervous system disease at presentation
Chemotherapy may be given as initial treatment in fit patients with asymptomatic disease, followed by RT postchemotherapy. For patients with symptoms, initial cranial radiotherapy is preferable.

Surgery
In general, resection is reserved for mediastinal node negative SCLC, less than 5% of patients.
- Rarely, patients present after resection of a small peripheral tumor, without evidence of regional lymphadenopathy or metastasis.
- If SCLC is treated by primary surgery, the systemic relapse rate is high, and adjuvant chemotherapy with four cycles of EP or EC is recommended, as well as prophylactic cranial radiation.

Second-line chemotherapy

This cancer can remain chemosensitive at relapse after primary chemotherapy ± radiotherapy.

Treatment options with response rates of approximately 20% include
- CAV
- Topotecan
- Taxanes
- For patients with prolonged front line responses (>6–12 months) retreatment with this initial platinum/etoposide regimen has a high likelihood of achieving a second response.

Despite the chemosensitivity of this disease, only limited progress has been made in long-term survival (see Table 27.4).

Currently, clinical trials are evaluating the potential benefits of, for example,
- Drugs that interfere with autocrine growth-factor loops and signal transduction pathways
- Angiogenesis inhibitors
- Tumor vaccines

Table 27.4 Outcome of chemotherapy for SCLC

Stage of disease	Median survival (months)	1-year survival	3-year survival
Limited	18–24	50%–70%	10%–20%
Extensive	8–10	20%	
Relapsed*	6		

* Limited to patients who remain fit to receive chemotherapy for relapsed diseases.

Radiotherapy for small cell lung cancer

Background
The primary treatment for most patients with SCLC is combination chemotherapy. More than 90% of patients have systemic disease (either overt or microscopic) at presentation.

Although SCLC is a highly chemosensitive disease, many patients with SCLC benefit from radiotherapy.
- Concurrent chemotherapy with radiation of the thorax (TI) improves the survival of patients with localized disease.
- Palliative radiotherapy is effective treatment in patients relapsing after, resistant to, unable to receive chemotherapy.

Thoracic irradiation
- 60% of relapses after chemotherapy are in the thorax.
- Therefore, consideration can be given to sequential radiation to the chest in patients with extensive stage SCLC who have good control of metastatic disease after chemotherapy.
- The optimum dose is approximately 60 Gy delivered once daily in fractions of 1.8–2.0

Prophylactic cranial irradiation (PCI)
- SCLC has a high propensity for brain metastases.
  - 20% have brain involvement at diagnosis.
  - 50% will develop CNS involvement with 2 years
- The blood-brain barrier limits access of chemotherapy to the CNS. Although chemotherapy may suppress CNS progression during therapy, consolidative radiation is needed for patients with known CNS involvement either before or after chemotherapy.
- For patients without CNS involvement, prophylactic cranial radiotherapy (PBI) can substantially reduce the risk of CNS disease and improve survival in both limited and advanced stage SCLC. Prophylactic cranial irradiation (PCI) should be reserved for patients who have not responded to front line chemotherapy. Patients at increased risk of CNS toxicity from PCI and risk/benefit must be carefully considered.
- PCI is recommended in patients for whom thoracic irradiation (TI) is appropriate, but it is given at the end of chemotherapy in an effort to minimize CNS toxicity.
- The optimum treatment regimen is uncertain.
- Examples include 25–30 Gy/10 fractions, 36 Gy/18 fractions.

Palliative radiotherapy
A short course of irradiation to either the primary tumor or metastases can provide useful symptom control even in frail patients.

Mesothelioma

Malignant pleural mesothelioma (MPM) is an aggressive tumor arising from the serosal lining of the chest and characterized by poor survival rates.

Epidemiology
- Rare, approximately 2200 cases each year in the United States
- Incidence has increased by 50% in the past decade.
- Peak age is 60–70 years.
- Male-to-female ratio 5:1.

Etiology
- Caused by asbestos exposure in the vast majority of cases
- 90% of patients have an occupational history of exposure; there is high risk in, e.g., builders, shipyard workers.
- Nonoccupational exposure leads to increased risk in the partners of these at-risk workers, e.g., by washing their clothing.
- All types of asbestos fibers are implicated.
- There is a prolonged latent period after exposure, so that clinical presentation is often 20–40 years later.
- Rarely caused by other agents
  - Erionite fibers (Turkey)
  - Thorium dioxide

Prevention
Recognition of the hazards of asbestos and improved protection of workers at risk should result in a falling incidence of mesothelioma after 2020.

Pathology
Mesothelioma arises from the parietal or visceral pleura and grows diffusely within the pleural space, commonly associated with pleural effusion, and often leads to encasement of the lung by solid tumor.

Tumor invades directly into the lung and mediastinum, and it may cross the diaphragm to involve the peritoneum. There is metastatic spread to other organs, e.g., liver in advanced disease.

Malignant mesothelioma has three distinct histological subtypes:
- Epithelial (approximately 50%)
- Sarcomatoid
- Biphasic

Malignant tumors may be localized or diffuse and are more commonly associated with asbestos exposure and symptoms such as chest pain and dyspnea.

Differentiation from other intrathoracic malignancies such as adenocarcinoma requires the assistance of an experienced pathologist.

Primary mesothelioma of the peritoneum is rare, associated with heavy exposure and ingestion of asbestos.

Clinical presentation

Late presentation is common, with only insidious development of the classic symptoms:
- Nonpleuritic chest pain
- Dyspnea
- Systemic symptoms of fatigue, weight loss, sweating, and fever

Physical examination frequently demonstrates signs of pleural effusion or solid pleural tumor.
 Signs of advanced disease may include the following:
- Palpable chest wall mass
- Hoarse voice, vocal cord palsy
- Ascites due to extension of tumor into peritoneum

Occasionally early disease, which is asymptomatic, is picked up on chest X-ray for another cause, as unexplained pleural effusion.

Investigations

Laboratory results in mesothelioma are usually unremarkable. No serological tumor marker is reproducibly identified.
 Radiological appearances are often nonspecific:
- Pleural effusion or thickening on chest X-ray
- 20% of cases have associated pulmonary fibrosis (asbestosis).
- CT scan demonstrates the extent of pleural mass and effusion, and encasement of the lung and with concurrent techniques, is sensitive to detection of chest wall or transdiaphragmatic extension.

Histological diagnosis should be obtained in
- Aspiration cytology can be considered, but it is notoriously difficulty to differentiate mesothelioma from reactive mesothelial cells on cytology.
- CT-guided biopsy
- Thoracoscopy and biopsy (80% positive)

Each of these carries a risk of implantation of tumor in the chest wall which must be addressed subsequently if surgery is entertained.

Staging

The TNM classification (Table 27.5) was adopted by the American Joint Committee on Cancer in 2002. Staging is vital if patients are to be considered for surgery.
 The Brigham staging system (see Table 27.6) provides an alternative straight forward method, based on key disease characteristics, that stratifies survival.
 Accurate preoperative pathological staging is best achieved by thoracoscopy for pleural evaluation, mediastinoscopy for mediastinal nodal involvement, and laparoscopy to rule out peritoneal seeding or diaphragmatic involvement when indicated.

Table 27.5 TNM staging system for malignant pleural mesothelioma

Stage	Description
TX	Primary tumor cannot be assessed
T0	No evidence of primary tumor
T1	Ipsilateral pleura
T1a	Limited to ipsilateral parietal, mediastinal, or diaphragmatic pleura
T1b	Involvement of ipsilateral parietal, mediastinal, diaphragmatic pleura + visceral pleura
T2	Ipsilateral lung, diaphragm, confluent involvement of visceral pleura
T3	Endothoracic fascia, mediastinal fat, focal chest wall, non-transmural pericardium
T4	Contralateral pleura, peritoneum, rib, extensive chest wall or mediastinal invasion, myocardium, brachial plexus, spine, malignant pericardial effusion
NX	Cannot assess regional lymph nodes
N0	No regional lymph node involvement
N1	Ipsilateral bronchopulmonary or hilar nodes
N2	Subcarinal, ipsilateral mediastinal nodes
N3	Contralateral mediastinal or internal mammary nodes or any supraclavicular nodes
M0	No metastasis
M1	Distant metastasis

Stage grouping			
Stage I			
IA	T1a	N0	M0
IB	T1b	N0	M0
Stage II	T2	N0	M0
Stage III	T3	Any N	M0
	Any T	N1	M0
	Any T	N2	M0
Stage IV	T4	Any N	M0
	Any T	N3	M0
	Any T	Any N	M1

Table 27.6 Brigham staging system for malignant pleural mesothelioma

Stage	Description
I	Disease completely resected within the capsule of the parietal pleura without adenopathy; ipsilateral pleura, lung, pericardium, diaphragm, or chest wall disease limited to previous biopsy sites
II	All of stage I with positive resection margins and/or intrapleural adenopathy
III	Local extension of disease into the chest wall or mediastinum, heart, or through diaphragm into peritoneum; or with extrapleural lymph node involvement
IV	Distant metastatic disease

Management

Without treatment, the average patient with MPM survives less than 1 year from the time of diagnosis.

Patient selection is crucial for the appropriate use of treatment such as surgery and chemotherapy, and all patients should be discussed at a multidisciplinary meeting.

Surgery

For the vast majority of patients, the extent and spread of disease at presentation precludes complete surgical removal of the disease.

Perhaps 5% of patients present with localized disease for which radical surgery with extrapleural pneumonectomy (EPP) may be followed by prolonged survival. In the rare patient in whom this is possible, 46% 5-year survival is reported, if margins are negative for tumor, and mediastinal nodes are negative.

The mortality of EPP has fallen from 31% in 1970 to 3.8% in specialized centers in 2000.

Pleurectomy and decortication control effusions in 80% of cases if the patient is fit.

Pleurodesis

Talc pleurodesis is effective in many patients in delaying the reaccumulation of the pleural effusion.

Radiotherapy

Early irradiation of chest drain, biopsy, or thoracoscopy wounds prevents the development of chest wall tumors (e.g., 21 Gy/3 fractions).

Short-course palliative radiotherapy is used for painful chest disease and masses.

Chemotherapy

Objective responses occur in 20%–30% of patients with advanced disease. When treated with platinum and pemetrexed. Second line agents to consider include gemcitabine and navelbine.

In patients who are candidates for EPP, platinum/pemetrexed can be considered either as neoadjuvant or adjuvant therapy. Because local recurrence remains high, some centers also include radiation delivered by IMRT (intensity undetected) after surgery.

Palliative care

Symptom control is often difficult, in particular, pain and dyspnea, and early involvement of specialist palliative care services may be beneficial.

Treatment outcome

Overall median survival is poor, at 8–14 months. There is a better prognosis with epithelioid pathology.

Single-center results from a carefully selected group of patients undergoing radical surgery followed by chemotherapy and radiotherapy are better, particularly in patients in whom early disease is excised with clear pathological margins:
- Perioperative mortality rate 3.8%
- Median survival 26 months
- 2-year survival 38%
- 5-year survival 15%

Thymic tumors

Tumors derived from the thymus (thymomas) comprise approximately 20% of all mediastinal tumors and are the most common tumor in the anterior mediastinum (less common pathologies include lymphoma and teatime).

Epidemiology

Thymomas occur at any age but are rare before the age of 20 and peak between 40 and 60 years, with similar frequency in both sexes.

The incidence varies somewhat in different countries, being more frequent in the Far East. The average incidence in the United States is approximately 0.15 new cases per year per 100,000. There is a slight male predominance.

Etiology

The cause is unknown.

Pathology

Most thymomas are slow-growing, "low-grade," malignant tumors. It is believed that they derive from epithelial elements, but the tumors retain the capacity for production of T cells. The T cells are generally of normal phenotype.

According to the relative abundance of epithelial and lymphocytic cells, histological subgroups have been described:
- Epithelial
- Lymphocytic
- Mixed

These cellular characteristics have no clear influence on prognosis. In contrast, the gross appearance of the resected tumor is related to clinical prognosis.

The presence or absence of an intact capsule is of prognostic importance and local invasion remains the most consistent factor in predicting outcome.

The following classification is of practical benefit.
- Encapsulated thymoma has benign cytology and biological behavior (50%).
- Invasive thymoma has benign cytology but is capable of local invasion and, rarely, distant metastasis (40%).
- Thymic carcinoma (10%) demonstrates cytological and biological features of cancer.

However, recurrent disease can occur after complete excision of a histologically bland thymoma. Metastatic spread can involve pleura, lung, lymph nodes, and other viscera.

Clinical presentation

- 30% are diagnosed with an asymptomatic mediastinal mass.
- 40% have local symptoms, e.g., chest pain, cough, dyspnea, or SVC obstruction.

- 30% have paraneoplastic syndromes, most being associated with an immunological phenomenon.
- Myasthenia gravis is the most common paraneoplastic effect; it occurs in 15%–25% of patients with thymoma.
  - Antibodies target the acetylcholine receptor.
  - 10%–25% of patients with myasthenia have a thymoma.
- Red-cell aplasia occurs in 5% of thymomas.
  - In 30%, low platelets or low white-cell count
  - 30%–50% of patients with red-cell aplasia have a thymoma.
- Hypogammaglobulinemia occurs in 5%–10% of thymomas.

Investigations

- Imaging by CT or MRI is essential to stage and plan therapy.
- There are no specific tumor markers.
- CT-guided core biopsy is preferred to FNA cytology.

Management and staging

Ninety percent of patients present with localized disease for which surgery is the preferred treatment. Thymectomy is performed through a median sternotomy, although bilateral anterolateral thoracotomy, with transverse sternotomy (clam shell approach), is better for advanced tumors.

Modern surgical techniques allow complete resection of invasive thymomas, e.g., lung resection, SVC removal and reconstruction, but debulking alone is of little benefit. Video-assisted thoracoscopic approaches are possible but unproven.

Complete resection gives an 82% 7-year survival. Subtotal resection gives a 71% 7-year survival. Without surgical treatment, survival is 26% at 7 years. Operative mortality was 2% in the year 2005.

Staging of disease is based on the surgical findings and radiology:
- Stage I: tumor confined within intact capsule
- Stage II: pericapsular growth into the mediastinal fat tissue
- Stage III: invasive growth into the surrounding organs
- Stage IV: disseminated disease

In stage I disease, adjuvant treatment is not recommended.

Postoperative radiotherapy is recommended for stage II and III disease, particularly where excision has been incomplete, and for local recurrence of thymoma.
- 50–60 Gy in 20–30 fractions

Chemotherapy

Malignant thymoma is chemosensitive, with objective response rates in advanced disease of 60%. Most regimens include cisplatin, e.g., CAP (cisplatin, doxorubicin, and cyclophosphamide).

Indications for chemotherapy include the following:
- Metastatic disease
- Bulky recurrent disease
- Recurrence postradiotherapy
- Preoperative treatment of locally advanced disease

Treatment outcomes

Overall survival rates are good (see Table 27.7). Patients with autoimmune disorders such as myasthenia are diagnosed with relatively small tumors. However, thymectomy leads to remission in paraneoplastic syndromes in only 30%–50%.

Patients with persistent symptoms, e.g., myasthenia, require ongoing medical treatment with anticholinesterases and/or immunosuppressants.

Table 27.7 Treatment outcomes for thymoma

Stage of disease	Recurrence rate	10-year survival
I	4%	88%
II	14%	70%
III	26%	57%
IV	46%	38%

Chapter 28

Breast cancer

Christina I. Herold

Introduction 430
Epidemiology 432
Genetics of breast cancer 434
Pathology 436
Prognostic factors 438
Breast cancer screening 440
Presentation and staging 442
Management of noninvasive breast cancer 446
Management of early breast cancer 448
Management of locally advanced breast cancer 456
Follow-up of early-stage breast cancer patients 458
Management of metastatic breast cancer 459

Introduction

Among women, breast cancer is the most common solid tumor and is second only to lung cancer in terms of cancer-related mortality.

Breast cancer research efforts have yielded significant advances in our knowledge regarding many relevant aspects of oncology:
- Epidemiology
- Medical genetics
- Screening of average- and high-risk women
- Management of early breast cancer, including breast conservation
- Neoadjuvant and adjuvant therapy
- Management of advanced breast cancer

Large clinical trials have enabled meta-analyses and evidence-based clinical guidelines. Our enhanced knowledge of breast oncology has translated directly into improved clinical care, as evidenced by a significant fall in breast cancer deaths over the past 30 years.

Epidemiology

Key facts about breast cancer
- The risk of breast cancer correlates with socioeconomic status.
- The lifetime risk in the United States for developing invasive breast cancer is approximately one in eight women and is among the highest in the world.
- Breast cancer is the most common female cancer in the United States, with a projected incidence of 232,340 cases in 2013 representing 29% of all malignancies
- After decades of steady increases, the incidence of breast cancer stabilized from 2001 to 2003. This stabilization has been attributed to saturation of screening mammography as well as decreased use of hormone replacement therapy (HRT).
- In the United States, breast cancer is second only to lung cancer as a leading cause of cancer-related deaths among women. There are 39,620 deaths projected from breast cancer in 2013 representing 14% of all cancer-related deaths.
- Breast cancer is the leading cause of cancer mortality among women aged 20–59 years.
- Breast cancer mortality rates have declined since 1975 in response to improved screening with earlier diagnosis and improved adjuvant treatment.
- Male breast cancer is rare, with approximately 2,240 new cases and 410 deaths projected in the United States in 2013.

Etiology
Several risk factors have been identified by epidemiological studies.

Age
- Breast cancer is very rare before the age of 20 and rare below 30 years.
- Incidence of breast cancer doubles every 10 years until menopause.
- After 50 years, the rate of increase slows and in some countries plateaus.

Geography
- There is a 7-fold variation in incidence between high- and low-risk countries, with the highest rates in Northern America and Western Europe and the lowest rates in Asia and Africa.
- Migrants from low-incidence countries assume the risk in the host country within two generations.

Age at menarche and menopause
- Early menarche and late menopause increase the risk.
- Ovarian ablation before 35 years reduces the risk of breast cancer by 60%.
- Menopause after the age of 55 years doubles the risk.

Age at first pregnancy
- Nulliparity and late age at first pregnancy increase the risk.

- A woman whose first pregnancy is at age 30 years has double the risk of breast cancer compared with a woman whose first pregnancy is at <20 years.

Family history
Inheritance of genetic mutations, such as *BRCA1*, *BRCA2*, *p53*, *ATM*, *CHEK2*, and *PTEN*, accounts for approximately 5%–10% of breast cancers.

Exogenous estrogens
- Use of oral contraceptives for >4 years before the first pregnancy increases the risk of premenopausal breast cancer.
- Combined HRT preparations increase the risk of breast cancer.
- The use of unopposed estrogens in HRT has a less clear effect.

Diet
Associations have been shown with high dietary fat intake, obesity, and alcohol consumption.

Benign breast disease
Previous breast surgery for severe, atypical epithelial hyperplasia is associated with a 4-fold increase in risk.

Radiation
- Exposure to ionizing radiation at an early age, e.g., treatment of Hodgkin's disease.
- Mammographic screening is associated with a decrease in breast cancer deaths but the effects of screening younger women (<50 years) are uncertain.

Male breast cancer
- Peak incidence is 10 years later than in women.
- It may occur in association with Klinefelter's syndrome.

Genetics of breast cancer

- 5%–10% of female breast cancer is due to inheritance of a mutated copy of either *BRCA1* or *BRCA2*.
- Women who inherit a mutated copy of either gene have an elevated lifetime risk of breast cancer—up to 70% by the age of 70 years.
- Particular risk of premenopausal breast cancer, often before the age of 40 years.
- Associated risk of ovarian cancer (greater with *BRCA1*).
- Male carriers are at risk for breast cancer and, for *BRCA2* carriers, melanoma, prostate and pancreatic cancers.
- Some ethnic groups are at particular risk for carriage of these mutations (an estimated 2% of U.S. Ashkenazi Jews).

Other genes contribute less often to familial breast cancer.
- Risk is associated with mutation in *PTEN* (Cowden disease), *p53* (Li–Fraumeni syndrome), *CHEK2* (particularly *1000delC), *STK11* (Peutz–Jegers syndrome), *CDH1* (hereditary diffuse gastric cancer syndrome), and *PALB2*.
- Whole genome association studies are increasingly identifying genes of low and moderate penetrance.

The management of hereditary breast cancer is essentially that of non-hereditary disease.
- Controversial issues include management of the contralateral breast of index cases and care of asymptomatic female family members.
- Published guidelines define groups of women at higher risk for breast cancer (see Box 28.1) and recommend referral to medical genetic clinics for counseling, consideration of genetic testing, and further management.

Currently, the following options are available for women at higher risk for breast cancer.

Prophylactic surgery
Bilateral subcutaneous mastectomy (usually with immediate reconstruction) reduces the incidence of breast cancer in these women, but has no established impact on survival. It may be offered in conjunction with prophylactic oophorectomy.

Screening
In addition to annual screening mammography, recent guidelines recommend annual screening with breast magnetic resonance imaging (MRI) for women who carry, or are untested but have a first-degree relative who carries, a genetic mutation as listed above.

Breast cancer prevention trials
Clinical trials utilizing the selective estrogen receptor modulators (SERMs) tamoxifen and raloxifene as well as the aromatase inhibitor exemestane have demonstrated that these drugs reduce the incidence of breast cancer by approximately 50% in higher-risk populations of women. There is no evidence that any of these breast cancer prevention drugs reduce breast cancer mortality.

Box 28.1 Summary of NCCN Guidelines for Breast and/or Ovarian Cancer Genetic Assessment

An affected individual with one or more of the following:
- A known mutation in a breast cancer susceptibility gene within the family
- Breast cancer diagnosis ≤ age 50
- Triple-negative (i.e., ER/PR/HER2-negative) breast cancer
- Two breast cancer primaries
- Ovarian cancer
- Male breast cancer
- Breast cancer at any age and a concerning family history (examples include ≥1 relative with breast cancer ≤ age 50 or epithelial ovarian cancer at any age)

An unaffected individual with a family history of one or more of the following:
- A known mutation in a breast cancer susceptibility gene within the family
- ≥2 breast primaries in a single individual
- ≥2 individuals with breast primaries on the same side of the family
- Ovarian cancer
- Male breast cancer
- Other concerning family history patterns (examples include first- or second-degree relative with breast cancer ≤ age 45; and ≥1 family members with a combination of cancers)

Citation

National Comprehensive Cancer Network. *NCCN Practice Guidelines, Genetic/Familial High-Risk Assessment: Breast and Ovarian Cancer.* Available at: August 27 2014, www.nccn.org.

Pathology

Approximately 50% of breast cancer cases arise in the upper outer quadrant. The most common pathology is ductal carcinoma (see Table 28.1).

Ductal carcinoma in situ

Ninety percent of breast carcinomas arise in the ducts of the breast. It begins as atypical proliferation of ductal epithelium that eventually fills and plugs the ducts with neoplastic cells. As long as the tumor remains within the confines of the ductal basement membrane, it is classified as ductal carcinoma in situ (DCIS).

Localized DCIS is not palpable but is often visible on mammography as an area of microcalcification.

Not all DCIS will inevitably progress, but the probability of development of invasive cancer is estimated at 30%–50%.

Lobular carcinoma in situ

These preinvasive lesions carry a risk not only of ipsilateral invasive lobular carcinoma but also of contralateral breast cancer. Typically, they are neither palpable nor contain microcalcification.

Invasive ductal carcinoma

This accounts for 75% of breast cancers. Tumor invades through breast tissue into the lymphatics and vascular spaces, to gain access to the regional nodes (axillary and, less often, internal mammary) and the systemic circulation. Systemic spread can involve almost any organ, but most commonly bone, other lymph nodes, lung or pleura, liver, skin, and CNS.

The histological grade (I–III) of the tumor predicts tumor behavior and is assessed from three features:
- Tubule formation
- Nuclear pleomorphism
- Mitotic frequency

Estrogen and progesterone receptor status is commonly assessed by immunohistochemistry. Hormone receptor positivity confers a more favorable prognosis and allows for treatment with endocrine therapies such as tamoxifen and aromatase inhibitors.

HER2 amplification or overexpression occurs in approximately 18%–20% of breast cancer and is associated with a more aggressive phenotype. This subtype of breast cancer can be treated with anti-HER2 agents such as trastuzumab, lapatinib, pertuzumab, and trastuzumab emtansine (T-DM1).

Basal-like or triple-negative breast cancer has no hormone receptor or HER2 expression, is more common in patients with African ancestry, and has a poor prognosis.

Special types of ductal carcinoma

A number of pathological variants are identified with relatively good prognosis, namely medullary carcinoma, tubular carcinoma, and mucinous carcinoma.

Paget's disease of the breast presents clinically with scaly, often erythematous, involvement of the nipple and is defined pathologically by the presence of intraepithelial malignant adenocarcinoma cells within the nipple-areolar complex. The vast majority (estimated at 97%) of patients who present with Paget's disease are diagnosed with underlying invasive or in situ breast cancer.

Invasive lobular carcinoma

Lobular carcinomas account for 5%–10% of breast cancers. About 20% of patients develop contralateral breast cancer.

Unusual patterns of spread are recognized, including propensity for spread to the peritoneum, gastrointestinal tract, orbit, meninges, ovaries, and uterus.

Table 28.1 Histological types of breast malignancy

Invasive ductal carcinoma
No special type
Combined with other type
Medullary carcinoma
Mucinous carcinoma
Paget's disease
Invasive lobular carcinoma
Mixed lobular and ductal carcinoma
Sarcoma (various)
Lymphoma
Metastases (e.g., breast cancer, small cell lung cancer)

Prognostic factors

Survival after a diagnosis of breast cancer depends on the following:
- Eradication of the primary tumor
- Eradication of any locoregional disease, particularly involved axillary, internal mammary, or supraclavicular lymph nodes
- Successful treatment of any systemic micrometastases
- Currently, macroscopic metastatic disease is incurable but is often compatible with several years of good-quality life, especially if the disease is confined to bone.

The three most important independent prognostic factors are commonly combined in the Nottingham Prognostic Index (NPI; see Box 28.2):
- Tumor size
- Tumor grade
- Number of histologically positive axillary lymph nodes

Other prognostic factors include the following:
- Hormone receptor status: estrogen receptor (ER) and progesterone receptor (PR)
- HER2 status
- Histological subtype
- Lymphovascular invasion
- Proliferative index

For women with N0 or N1 ER-positive and HER2-negative breast cancer, the recurrence score (RS), generated using genomic techniques through a 21-gene assay (16 cancer and 5 reference genes), can be used to differentiate women at low, intermediate, and high risk of recurrence. Beyond the prognostic yield, the RS also predicts the benefit associated with adjuvant chemotherapy.

Rather than viewing breast cancer as one disease with uniform prognosis, enhanced knowledge of biologic and molecular characteristics is increasingly being used to define subtypes of disease. Subtype classification is quickly supplanting traditional staging as a means of estimating prognosis.

> **Box 28.2 Nottingham Prognostic Index (NPI) calculation**
>
> $$\text{NPI} = (0.2 \times \text{pathological tumor size (cm)} + \text{grade (1–3)} + \text{axillary node score})$$
>
> | Axillary node status | Score |
> | --- | --- |
> | No lymph nodes positive | 1 |
> | 1–3 lymph nodes positive | 2 |
> | >3 lymph nodes positive | 3 |
>
> | NPI | Prognosis |
> | --- | --- |
> | <3.41 | Good |
> | 3.41–5.4 | Intermediate |
> | >5.4 | Poor |

Breast cancer screening

There have been at least seven randomized controlled trials of mammographic screening over the last 30 years. Meta-analysis of all the published trials confirms a significant mortality benefit for screening women over 50 and weaker evidence to support screening women aged 40–49.

Current consensus guidelines support annual screening mammography for women over 50: the U.S. Preventive Services Task Force (USPSTF) found insufficient evidence to define a screening interval for women aged 40–49.

Imaging modality

The aim of screening for breast cancer is to identify preinvasive disease or invasive disease before dissemination (through the lymphatics or blood).

There is no evidence that breast self-examination is an effective means of screening for breast cancer.

Mammography
- Is a sensitive technique for detecting breast cancer and is also the most specific
- Is most sensitive once involution of the breast tissue has occurred (i.e., postmenopausal women)
- Is less sensitive in women with dense breasts; that is, those with predominantly glandular tissue or residual stromal tissue

Breast ultrasound
This is useful for assessment of focal abnormalities. It is also useful for detecting lesions that are not palpable.

Breast magnetic resonance imaging
Magnetic resonance imaging (MRI) is a very sensitive technique, but widespread application of it has been limited by a high false-positive rate (often leading to unnecessary biopsies), cost, and variable standards of use.

Recommended use of screening MRI is currently limited to high-risk women, defined as having a lifetime risk of breast cancer of at least 20%.

Mammographic technique
- The breast is compressed to flatten the breast tissue to reduce movement, overlapping shadows, and radiation dose.
- The uniform thickness of tissue improves image quality and contrast.
- Low-energy radiation is passed through the breast, resulting in a high-contrast image.
- Standard mammography is recorded on X-ray film, whereas digital mammography is recorded and displayed on a high-resolution computer screen.
- Two views of each breast are performed: one in the mediolateral oblique (MLO) position diagonally across the chest, the other in the craniocaudal (CC) position.

Radiation dose
- Low radiation dose (2 mGy per examination)
- The radiation risk is 1–2 excess cancers per million women screened after a latent period of 10 years in the postmenopausal age group but is higher in women under 30.
- Radiation dose to the breast is 5 times that of a chest X-ray.

Interval cancers
These are cancers that occur in the interval between two screening episodes. They fall into five categories.
- **True interval cancer** appears in the screening interval and was not present on the previous mammogram.
- **False negative**: the lesion was present on the previous screening mammogram.
- **Technical**: cancer was not on the film because of its position.
- **Mammographically occult** cancer is not visualized on either the screening mammogram or at the time of diagnosis.
- **Unclassifiable**: no mammogram was taken at the time of diagnosis.

Screening for high-risk groups
In addition to mammography, annual screening MRI is recommended for the following high-risk women:
- Known *BRCA* mutation
- Untested, but with a first-degree relative carrying a *BRCA* mutation
- Lifetime risk for developing breast cancer of at least 20% as defined by a model weighted to include family history (such as BRCAPRO)
- History of chest radiation between ages 10 and 30 years
- Personal history or first-degree relative with specific genetic breast cancer familial syndromes (such as Li-Fraumeni and Cowden syndromes).

Features of screen-detected breast cancer
The reduction in breast cancer deaths resulting from mammographic screening is attributed to the following:
- Diagnosis and effective treatment of asymptomatic preinvasive disease (DCIS)
- Diagnosis and effective treatment of early invasive breast cancer, which would otherwise not present until systemic spread had occurred.

A number of studies have found good evidence to support this, including the following observations:
- 10%–20% of screen-detected lesions are noninvasive.
- >30% screen-detected invasive cancers are <10 mm.
- <20% are grade 3.
- 70%–80% are node negative.

Presentation and staging

The most common presentations include the following (see Box 28.3):
- Abnormal screening mammogram
  - Now accounts for approximately 25% of cases
  - Microcalcification, mass lesion, distortion
- Breast lump or thickening
- Axillary mass
- Breast skin changes: dimpling, puckering, erythema
- Nipple changes: inversion, discharge, rash (Paget's disease)
- Persistent breast tenderness or pain
- Infrequently, symptoms from metastatic disease, e.g., bone pain, spinal cord compression

Diagnosis

The diagnosis of breast cancer is often made through a combination of physical examination and imaging leading to diagnostic biopsy.
- Full clinical examination
  - Calliper measurement of any lump in either breast, and clinical assessment of tumor, including whether the mass is fixed to adjacent skin or pectoral muscle
  - Lymphadenopathy, in particular axillary and supraclavicular
- Bilateral mammography usually combined with ultrasound
- Core biopsy under stereotactic or ultrasound; image guidance is the preferred diagnostic approach.
  - Core biopsy differentiates between carcinoma in situ and invasive cancer in most patients.
  - Fine-needle aspiration (FNA) may be still appropriate for some clinical situations.

This combined approach to assessment has >90% sensitivity and specificity.
- In cases where there is still uncertainty, excision biopsy of the breast lesion may be required.
- The axilla is staged surgically in patients with invasive disease.
- Serum tumor markers, such as CEA, CA 15-3, and CA 27.29, exhibit low sensitivity and specificity and are not useful in the diagnosis of breast cancer.
- Assessment of circulating tumor cells is also not indicated.
- In the absence of locally advanced disease (see Management of locally advanced breast cancer, pp. 448–449) or symptoms or signs of metastatic disease, routine radiological staging such as chest X-ray, bone scan, or CT scan have not been found to be beneficial.

Box 28.3 Indications for referral to breast clinic

- Screen-detected breast cancer
- Breast lump
  - Any new discrete lump
  - New lump in preexisting nodularity
  - Asymmetrical nodularity persisting after menstruation
  - Abscess or inflammation that does not settle after one course of antibiotics
  - Persistent or recurrent cyst
- Pain
  - Associated with a lump
  - Intractable pain that interferes with the patient's life and fails to respond to simple measures (well supporting bra, simple analgesics, abstention from caffeine, evening primrose oil)
  - Unilateral persistent pain in postmenopausal women
- Nipple discharge
  - In any women age >50 years
  - In younger women if blood-stained, persistent single duct or bilateral, sufficient to stain clothes
- Nipple retraction, distortion, or eczema
- Change in breast skin contour

TNM staging system

Recent changes have been made in the staging system to take account of improvements in the pathological assessment of this disease.

Pathological assessment of the extent of disease may differ considerably from clinical staging (see Box 28.4).

Box 28.4 TNM staging system for breast cancer

T stage
Tis — In situ disease only
T1 — ≤2 cm
  T1mic — ≤0.1 cm
  T1a — >0.1–0.5 cm
  T1b — >0.5–1 cm
  T1c — >1–2 cm
T2 — >2–5 cm
T3 — >5 cm
T4 — Any size of tumor with involvement of chest wall or skin
  T4a — Direct extension into chest wall
  T4b — Direct extension into skin, with edema, ulceration, or nodules
  T4c — Both chest wall and skin involvement
  T4d — Inflammatory breast cancer

N stage
NX — Lymph node status has not been assessed
N1 — Mobile axillary lymphadenopathy
  pN1mi — Micrometastasis, >0.2 mm ≤2 mm
  pN1a — 1–3 positive axillary nodes
  pN1b — Internal mammary nodes with micrometastasis
  pN1c — 1–3 positive axillary nodes and internal mammary micrometastasis
N2a — Fixed axillary lymph nodes
  pN2a — 4–9 positive axillary nodes
N2b — Internal mammary nodes clinically apparent
  pN2b — Internal mammary nodes positive, clinically apparent, negative axillary nodes
N3a — Infraclavicular lymphadenopathy
  pN3a — ≥10 positive axillary nodes or positive infraclavicular node
N3b — Internal mammary and axillary lymphadenopathy
  pN3b — Positive axillary and internal mammary nodes
N3c — Supraclavicular lymphadenopathy
  pN3c — Supraclavicular node positive

M stage
M1 — Positive evidence of distant metastasis

Management of noninvasive breast cancer

DCIS and lobular carcinoma in situ (LCIS) are rarely symptomatic, although extensive preinvasive disease may present with a mass or thickening of breast tissue.

Management options

Simple mastectomy

In situ breast cancer was rarely diagnosed before the advent of mammographic screening. Standard treatment until the 1980s was mastectomy. After mastectomy, relapse rates are very low (2%–3%).

Locoregional recurrence and metastatic disease are attributed to undiagnosed microinvasive cancer.

Surgical assessment of the axillary lymph nodes for staging is not indicated because of the low risk of positive nodes.

Mastectomy remains standard treatment for large in situ cancers and for multifocal disease (with breast reconstruction, if desired).

Wide excision alone

With the increased diagnosis of small, localized, noninvasive cancers by mammographic screening, breast-conserving surgery has been adopted for the majority of cases. With breast-conserving therapy alone, 20%–30% develop local recurrence within 5 years.

The highest risk of recurrence is associated with high-grade DCIS and involved or close surgical margins (<1 mm clear)—an excision margin of 1 cm is preferable. Half of the recurrences are noninvasive, and the rest have invasive cancer.

Wide excision and postoperative radiotherapy

Three large, randomized studies have now confirmed the benefit of radiotherapy in this setting.
- Whole breast is irradiated 50 Gy/25 fractions
- Risk of recurrence <10% at 5 years

Adjuvant hormone therapy

Tamoxifen for 5 years reduces the frequency of recurrence of DCIS by approximately 30%. Subset analysis suggests that this benefit is only for patients with ER-positive DCIS.

Clinical trials with aromatase inhibitors are underway.

The management of LCIS is controversial. Many are managed by wide local excision and postoperative radiotherapy. Problems include the following:
- LCIS is commonly missed on mammograms.
- Risk of multifocal ipsilateral disease
- Risk of contralateral disease

Many breast specialists now view LCIS as a risk marker and local excision alone as adequate.

For all patients with early breast cancer, the key to selection of the optimum treatment is multidisciplinary discussion including staff from radiology, pathology, and surgical, radiation and medical oncology. Appropriate treatment options can then be presented to the patient to help determine an individualized treatment plan.

Management of early breast cancer

- Early breast cancer is defined as disease that can be completely removed by surgery. The management of this disease includes the following: Surgical treatment of the breast and axilla
- Pathological assessment and staging to direct adjuvant therapy
- Adjuvant therapy
  - Chemotherapy
  - Radiotherapy
  - Endocrine therapy

Multidisciplinary discussion and planning of treatment is essential to optimize treatment outcomes.

Consensus guidelines do not recommend extensive radiographic staging, although this is commonly performed in practice for patients with high-risk disease.

Recent studies support the use of breast MRI for enhanced locoregional staging in selected cases of early-stage breast cancer.

Breast surgery

All patients require complete removal of the primary tumor by either wide local excision (lumpectomy) or mastectomy.

Halsted mastectomy, also known as radical mastectomy, in which the breast, axillary contents, and pectoralis major and minor muscles are removed, was extensively applied during the first half of the 20th century, but it has gradually been replaced by a variety of less disfiguring operations.

Total mastectomy and axillary dissection preserves the pectoralis major muscle and its neurovascular bundle.

Quadrantectomy, introduced at the beginning of the 1970s, is a breast-conserving operation in which the primary cancer with a margin of 2.0 cm of normal breast tissue is removed. It is infrequently performed now because of the poor cosmetic result.

Wide local excision or lumpectomy provides for removal of the tumor mass with a limited margin of normal tissue (0.5–1 cm). This is now the most commonly performed procedure for early breast cancers.

Breast-conserving surgery alone was followed by local recurrence of breast cancer in up to 30% of patients. However, several large randomized trials comparing breast-conserving surgery followed by breast radiotherapy with mastectomy alone have demonstrated similar local control rates and survival.

Wide local excision followed by breast irradiation is the preferred treatment for the majority of T1–2 breast cancers.

Breast conservation therapy is not always medically appropriate; common examples include cases in which there is

- Multifocal disease
- Large tumor in a small breast
- Contraindication to breast irradiation

Some patients simply prefer mastectomy, not least because of the possible avoidance of radiotherapy. Regardless of the choice of local treatment, it should result in a local recurrence rate of <10% after 10 years follow-up.

Breast reconstruction can be offered after mastectomy, either at the time of primary surgery or at a later date. A variety of reconstruction techniques are available these broad categories: pedicled musculocutaneous flaps (i.e., transverse rectus abdominus myocutaneous [TRAM] flap, latissimus dorsi flap), "free" perforator flaps (i.e., deep inferior epigastric perforator (DIEP) flap, gluteal artery (GAP) flap) and implants (either saline or silicone).

Axillary surgery

- Clinical assessment of axillary nodes is inaccurate.
- At least 30% of positive nodes are impalpable.

Aims of axillary surgery

- Provide pathological staging of axillary lymph nodes
- May clear the axilla of disease so that radiotherapy is not required to treat positive nodes

Side effects include lymphedema, arm pain, sensory deficits, and limited range of motion.

Sentinel node biopsy

- Dye and radiolabeled colloid is injected around the tumor and nipple and any blue-stained node(s) with radioactivity count >10 times the background is excised (there may be more than one sentinel node).
- Identification and removal of the first draining lymph node
- Aim is to identify patients with negative sentinel lymph nodes and to spare them axillary lymph node dissection (ALND).
- Patients with positive sentinel lymp nodes are then often treated with ALND with the intent of clearing any residual lymph node involvement. However, there is interest in identifying women with limited sentinel lymph node involvement who may safely be spared ALND. In the phase III Z11 study, women with 1–2 involved sentinel lymph who were treated with breast conserving therapy (lumpectomy and adjuvant radiation therapy) and appropriate systemic therapy but without completion ALND had equivalent overall survival and locoregional recurrence to women who underwent completion ALND.

Axillary lymph node dissection

- Complete clearance and staging of the axilla
- Higher morbidity and lymphedema rates than sentinel lymph node biopsy

Locoregional radiotherapy

Breast irradiation reduces the risk of local recurrence after breast-conserving surgery from approximately 30% to <10% at 10 years. Breast irradiation is recommended for all patients after wide local excision for invasive breast cancer. The whole breast is treated with tangential fields to a dose of 50 Gy in 25 fractions (or an equivalent dose-fractionation regimen).

- Care is taken to minimize the volume of lung and heart irradiated.
- A boost of 10–15 Gy is commonly delivered to the tumor bed, using electrons or ^{192}Ir implant.

Partial breast irradiation techniques are currently investigational.

Postmastectomy radiotherapy to the chest wall reduces the risk of locoregional recurrence. It is recommended for discussion with patients with positive axillary nodes and for patients with T3 node-negative disease in whom there is a modest survival benefit when given in conjunction with systemic therapy.

Axillary radiotherapy is certainly indicated after a lymph node sampling is positive. In general, it should be avoided after axillary clearance because of the high risk of lymphedema and brachial plexopathy. Supraclavicular fossa may be irradiated after axillary clearance if nodes are positive.

In general, radiotherapy should begin as soon as possible after surgery. Enhanced normal tissue damage can result when radiotherapy and adjuvant chemotherapy are given together, and radiotherapy is often postponed until completion of chemotherapy.

Adjuvant systemic therapy

Despite effective local therapy with surgery and radiotherapy, many women with early breast cancer harbor occult micrometastases. If left untreated, these may give rise to overt metastatic disease, which may lead to the eventual death of the patient.

There is now a large body of evidence that effective, systemic treatment directed against micrometastatic disease at the time of diagnosis of breast cancer conveys a significant survival benefit in most women.

The risk of micrometastatic disease correlates well with the recognized prognostic factors, simply summarized by the Nottingham prognostic index (NPI). Likewise, the potential gains from systemic therapy in terms of improved survival are greatest in patients with a poor prognosis.

There have been many trials among women with operable breast cancer that have examined the effects of systemic treatment, either endocrine therapy, chemotherapy, or both, on the survival of these patients. The basis of all these therapies is the reduction or eradication of microscopic systemic, metastatic disease in women in whom all of a macroscopic local tumor has been effectively removed.

In 1992, the Early Breast Cancer Trialists' Collaborative Group (EBCTCG) published an overview of 133 randomized trials involving 75,000 women with early breast cancer. Updated at regular intervals, these meta-analyses continue to have major impact insetting the standards of care for adjuvant therapy for breast cancer.

Adjuvant chemotherapy

In 2012, the EBCTCG published an overview of long-term outcomes from 123 randomized trials involving 100,000 women treated with adjuvant chemotherapy. This analysis showed that, compared with no chemotherapy, the CMF and anthracycline-based regimens are associated with approximately 30%–35% relative improvements in distant recurrence and 20%–25% improvements in breast cancer mortality. In aggregate analysis, the addition of four cycles of a taxane to anthracycline-based chemotherapy resulted in 13% relative improvements in both breast cancer recurrence and mortality compared with anthracycline-based chemotherapy alone.

Until recently, the standard adjuvant regimens were 6 months of CMF or 12 weeks (4 cycles) of AC (see Table 28.2). Given improved efficacy as described above, other regimens that are now more commonly used in the adjuvant setting include 4 cycles of AC followed by 4 cycles of a taxane (paclitaxel or docetaxel), 6 cycles of TAC, 6 cycles of FEC, 3 cycles of FEC followed by 3 cycles of Taxotere, and 4 cycles of TC.

Regarding the optimal use and scheduling of taxanes after AC, E1199, a four-arm trial, compared paclitaxel and docetaxel given either weekly or every 3 weeks. Compared to every 3 week paclitaxel, weekly paclitaxel was associated with approximately 30% relative improvements in both disease-free survival (DFS) and overall survival (OS).

Significant controversy exists regarding the role of taxanes in ER-positive disease, due to limited evidence of additional therapeutic benefit and the risk of significant additional toxicity. Concern for cardiotoxicity has prompted the development of non-anthracycline-containing regimens such as 4 cycles of TC, which has compared favorably to 4 cycles of AC in a single multicenter trial, US Oncology 9735.

The Intergroup 9741 trial studied "dose-dense" scheduling, in which chemotherapy is given every 2 weeks rather than every 3 weeks. Compared with AC x4 followed by paclitaxel x4 with the standard 3-week intervals between treatments, dose-dense scheduling of the same regimen was associated with a 25% relative improvement in DFS and a 30% improvement in OS. Use of granulocyte colony-stimulating factor (G-CSF, filgrastim or pegfilgrastim) is recommended to reduce the risk of febrile neutropenia.

For HER2-positive disease, results from several large cooperative trials indicate significant survival benefits when 1 year of trastuzumab, a monocolonal antibody that targets the HER2 receptor, is added to adjuvant chemotherapy. Combined analyses of the N9831 and B-31 studies show that trastuzumab-based systemic therapy is associated with a 50% relative improvement in DFS and 40% relative improvement in OS compared with adjuvant chemotherapy alone. Recently, the HERA trial showed no benefit of continuing trastuzumab for 2 years compared to 1 year.

Results from BCIRG 006, a three-arm study in which AC x 4 cycles followed by docetaxel x 4 cycles was compared to the same regimen with trastuzumab and to TCH x 6 cycles, show equivalence in outcomes between the two trastuzumab-containing arms and reduced cardiotoxicity in the TCH arm compared with the combined anthracycline and trastuzumab regimen.

Chemotherapy should be considered in all premenopausal women with breast cancer and in postmenopausal women with breast cancer who have intermediate or poor prognoses.

Estimates of benefit from adjuvant chemotherapy may be calculated for individual patients, via www.adjuvantonline.com. Of note, this model does not include HER2 status and therefore cannot be used to predict the benefit of trastuzumab-based systemic therapy for women with HER2-positive breast cancer.

Table 28.2 Examples of adjuvant chemotherapy regimens

CMF, 6 cycles over 24 weeks			
Cyclophosphamide plus	100 mg/m² oral	d1–14	q 4/52
	or	d1, 8	q 4/52
	600 mg/m² IV		
Methotrexate	40 mg/m² IV	d1, 8	q 4/52
5-fluorouracil	600 mg/m² IV	d1, 8	q 4/52
AC, 4 cycles over 12 weeks			
Doxorubicin	60 mg/m²	d1	q 3/52
Cyclophosphamide	600 mg/m²	d1	q 3/52
AC, 4 cycles, followed by taxane for 4 cycles over 24 weeks			
AC as above followed by			
Paclitaxel (weekly)	80 mg/m²	d1, 8, 15	q 3/52
Paclitaxel (every 3 weeks)	175 mg/m²	d1	q 3/52
Docetaxel (weekly)	35 mg/m²	d1, 8, 15	q 3/52
Docetaxel (every 3 weeks)	100 mg/m²	d1	q 3/52
TAC, 6 cycles over 18 weeks			
Docetaxel	75 mg/m²	d1	q 3/52
Doxorubicin	50 mg/m²	d1	q 3/52
Cyclophosphamide	500 mg/m²	d1	q 3/52
FEC, 6 cycles over 18 weeks			
5-flourouracil	500 mg/m²	d1	q 3/52
Epirubicin	100 mg/m²	d1	q 3/52
Cyclophosphamide	500 mg/m²	d1	q 3/52
FEC, 3 cycles, followed by docetaxel for 3 cycles over 18 weeks			
FEC as above followed by			
Docetaxel	100 mg/m²	d1	q 3/52
TC, 4 cycles over 12 weeks			
Docetaxel	75 mg/m²	d1	q 3/52
Cyclophosphamide	600 mg/m²	d1	q 3/52
For HER2-positive disease			
AC, 4 cycles, followed by paclitaxel for 4 cycles. Trastuzumab is started with paclitaxel and given for 1 year			
AC as above followed by			
Paclitaxel	175 mg/m²	d1	q 3/52
Trastuzumab	Loading 4 mg/kg	d1	q 1/52
	Followed by 2 mg/kg	d1	q 1/52

Table 28.2 (Cont.)

TCH, 6 cycles. Trastuzumab is started during chemotherapy and given for 1 year			
Docetaxel	75 mg/m^2	d1	q 3/52
Carboplatin	AUC 6	d1	q 3/52
Trastuzumab (weekly during chemotherapy then every 3 weeks)	Loading dose 4 mg/kg	d1	q 1/52
	Followed by 2 mg/kg	d1	q 1/52
	Then 6 mg/kg	d1	q 3/52
"HERA style": Trastuzumab is given for 1 year following chemotherapy			
Trastuzumab	Loading dose 8 mg/kg	d1	q 3/52
	Followed by 6 mg/kg		

For women with N0 or N1 ER-positive and HER2-negative breast cancer, the recurrence score (RS) can be used to predict the benefit associated with adjuvant chemotherapy. In brief, women with low-risk RS are predicted to have no benefit from adjuvant chemotherapy whereas those with high-risk RS are projected to benefit. For women with intermediate-risk RS, the benefit of chemotherapy is unknown and is being investigated in two ongoing multicenter trials for node-negative and node-positive patients, the TAILORx and RxPONDER trials, respectively.

Active areas of current breast cancer research include the development and optimization of adjuvant regimens that include targeted therapies for specific subtypes of disease, such HER2-positive, and triple-negative disease.

Adjuvant endocrine therapy

- 75% of breast cancers are hormone receptor (HR)-positive (estrogen [ER] and/or progesterone [PR] receptor). Options for adjuvant endocrine therapy include tamoxifen and the aromatase inhibitors.
- Tamoxifen is a selective estrogen receptor modulator (SERM) that blocks estrogen from binding to estrogen receptors on breast cancer cells. Tamoxifen is effective for all women regardless of menopausal status.
- The aromatase inhibitors (AIs) such as letrozole, anastrozole and exemestane, act by blocking conversion of adrenal androgens to estrogen. AI therapy is only effective in women who are postmenopausal. Menopause can be natural, surgical, or chemically induced via suppression of the GnRH/LH axis.
- AIs are not effective in premenopausal women because these drugs reduce circulating estrogen that releases negative inhibition of the pituitary gland resulting in increased FSH/LH secretion and ovarian stimulation counteracting the initial reduction in circulating estrogen.
- For hormone receptor (HR)-positive patients, adjuvant endocrine therapy confers significant benefits including both reduced recurrence rates and improved OS. The benefit of tamoxifen is significant even for weakly HR-positive disease.

- For HR-negative patients, there is no benefit associated with adjuvant endocrine therapy.
- Tamoxifen given simultaneously with chemotherapy reduces its benefit. Adjuvant endocrine therapy should only be commenced after completion of chemotherapy.
- Both tamoxifen and the AIs are associated with menopausal side effects such as vasomotor symptoms and vaginal dryness.
- Tamoxifen is also assocated with the rare but serious toxicities of venous thromboembolism and uterine cancer (both <5%).
- The AIs are associated with bone thinning and risk of osteoporosis and related complications such as fractures. Tamoxifen is relatively protective of bone density.
- Results from the EBCTCG analysis demonstrate that 5 years of tamoxifen is associated with 10-year reduced risk of breast cancer recurrence (by approximately 50%) and 15-year improved breast cancer related mortality (by approximately 30%).
- Regarding duration of tamoxifen therapy, results from prior trials, including NSABP B-14, had demonstrated that continuation of tamoxifen past 5 years was associated with inferior DFS and increased risk of uterine cancer. However, more recent results from two large phase 3 randomized clinical trials (ATLAS and aTTom) have shown that 10 years of adjuvant tamoxifen is superior to 5 years of tamoxifen with regard to both breast cancer recurrence and breast cancer mortality.
- In postmenopausal women, the benefit of AIs as compared tamoxifen has been evaluated in multiple large prospective randomized clinical trials. Latest guidelines by the American Society of Clinical Oncology (ASCO) recommend that an AI be incorporated into the adjuvant hormone therapy of postmenopausal women with HR-positive cancers.
- One of the pivotal trials that established the superiority of aromatase inhibitor therapy over tamoxifen therapy for postmenopausal women was the Breast International Group (BIG) 1-98 study. In this trial, approximately 8,000 women were enrolled and randomized to one of the four following treatment arms: tamoxifen monotherapy for 5 years, letrozole monotherapy for 5 years, letrozole for 2 years followed by tamoxifen for 3 years, or tamoxifen for 2 years followed by letrozole for 3 years. With median follow-up of over 8 years, the letrozole monotherapy arm was superior to the tamoxifen monotherapy arm with significantly superior DFS (by approximately 20%) and OS (also by approximately 20%). Further comparisons between the arms show no difference in these outcomes between the letrozole monotherapy arm and either of the two arms that involved sequential switching strategies.
- Regarding the optimal duration of adjuvant endocrine therapy, the NCIC CTG (National Cancer Institute of Canada Clinical Trials Group) MA.17 trial randomized over 5,000 postmenopausal women who had completed 5 years of tamoxifen therapy to receive either letrozole or placebo for 5 more years. At initial publication, and with a median follow-up of 2.4 years, there was a statistically significant improvement in estimated 4-year DFS associated with the use of letrozole compared with placebo (93% vs 87%; hazard ratio 0.57, $P \leq .001$).

- Women who present with higher-risk disease (larger tumors, involved lymph nodes) at diagnosis are at higher risk for breast cancer recurrence. The proportional benefit of extending adjuvant endocrine therapy past 5 years of treatment is greater among these higher-risk patients.
- The long-terms benefits extending adjuvant endocrine therapy must be balanced with the associated risks, such as the rare but serious complications of venous thromboembolic disease and uterine cancer with tamoxifem and cumulative bone loss potentiating osteoporosis with the AIs. In light of these considerations, the optimal sequencing and duration of adjuvant endocrine therapy for premenopausal and postmenopausal women remains an active area of research.

Neoadjuvant therapy

Neoadjuvant therapy (also known as primary or preoperative therapy) with chemotherapy or endocrine therapy for operable breast cancer provides early systemic treatment and allows assessment of the response to treatment. By definition, this is impossible with adjuvant therapy (see Table 28.3). The disadvantages of neoadjuvant therapy are the delay in definitive local surgery and risk of overtreatment with chemotherapy in the absence of pathological staging (e.g., postmenopausal, ER-positive, node-negative tumor).

Multiple large, randomized trials (including NSABP B-18 and B-27) have shown no difference in survival when pre- and postoperative chemotherapy were compared.

Preoperative treatment does downstage the primary tumor and, in some women, facilitates breast-conserving surgery where mastectomy would otherwise be required.

Table 28.3 Comparison of adjuvant and neoadjuvant therapy

	Adjuvant therapy	Neoadjuvant therapy
Advantages	Pathological staging available for patient selection Immediate surgical removal of all macroscopic disease	Tumor response is visible to both clinicians and patient Reduction in tumor volume can facilitate breast conservation Lack of response gives opportunity to change chemotherapy
Disadvantages	No visible benefit in individual patients No means of assessing efficacy of treatment regimen in individual patients Mastectomy required for many tumors >3 cm diameter	Risk of overtreatment, particularly for low-risk postmenopausal women Disease progression may occur before surgery (clinical trials have shown this is a rare event)

Management of locally advanced breast cancer

Locally advanced disease is defined by the presence of infiltration of the skin or the chest wall or fixed axillary nodes. It is represented in the TNM system by disease stages IIIA–C (see Table 28.4).

Inflammatory breast cancer (IBC) is a subtype of locally advanced breast cancer, designated T4d and carries a poor prognosis. Histologically, the classic finding of IBC is dermal lymphatic invasion by tumor cells. However, the diagnosis of IBC is clinical and includes the following characteristic findings:
- Rapidly enlarging, warm, tender breast
- Skin changes are the classic "peau d'orange" appearance with redness and thickening of the skin

With locally advanced breast cancer, the probability of metastatic disease is high and exceeds 70%. However, long-term survival is possible and the median survival of these patients exceeds 2 years. Staging investigations should include comprehensive radiographic staging of the chest, abdomen, pelvis and bones with either PET/CT or a combination of CT torso with radionucleotide bone scan.

Local control of the tumor and prevention of tumor fungation are of major importance to the quality of life of these women, irrespective of the presence of metastases. A combination of primary systemic treatment and radiotherapy is commonly used.

For elderly patients with indolent ER-positive locally advanced breast cancer, it is reasonable to begin treatment with the endocrine therapy. First-line therapy in this group should be with one of the aromatase inhibitors (anastrozole, letrozole, or exemestane), which have been shown to be superior to tamoxifen in advanced breast cancer.

The standard of care for younger patients and patients with ER-negative locally advanced disease is treatment with primary chemotherapy, usually with an anthracycline- and taxane-containing regimen. For patients with HER2-positive disease, incorporation of trastuzumab facilitates tumor control. In patients with a good response to systemic treatment, surgery may be feasible, followed by locoregional radiotherapy.

Similar to the adjuvant treatment approach for earlier-stage breast cancers, for locally advanced ER-positive tumors, adjuvant endocrine therapy is started after completion of chemotherapy.

Table 28.4 Treatment outcomes: breast cancer survival rates

Stage	10-year survival*
0	>95%
I	75–95%
IIA	45–85%
IIB	40–80%
IIIA	10–60%
IIIB	0–35%
IIIC	0–30%
IV	<5%

*There is a wide range of survival rates, and individual prognosis is determined by TNM stage, grade, ER status, and treatment, e.g., chemotherapy.

Follow-up of early-stage breast cancer patients

Given declining mortality rates in breast cancer, there is an ever-increasing population of breast cancer survivors. The approach to following this group of patients is an important issue in primary care.
- There are ~2.5 million breast cancer survivors in the United States.
- Long-term effects of breast cancer treatment include hormonal deprivation and menopausal side effects (i.e., hot flashes, risk for accelerated or premature bone loss), loss of fertility, cardiac toxicity, peripheral neuropathy, risk of secondary leukemia, and bone marrow dysfunction.
- Ongoing concerns about recurrence can be disabling.

Follow-up should focus on a careful history and physical examination. Consensus guidelines recommend the following:
- Clinic visits every 3–6 months for the first 3 years; every 6–12 months in years 4 and 5; annual follow-up after year 5.
- Annual breast imaging with mammography; no routine blood work or tumor markers for surveillance.
- Randomized studies have demonstrated no improvement in DFS or OS for intensive imaging surveillance (i.e., CT scans, PET/CT, bone scans). These studies should be done only for diagnostic evaluation of symptoms.

Recurrence patterns differ significantly by breast cancer subtype:
- Triple-negative and HER2-positive breast cancers have higher likelihoods of recurring in the years close to diagnosis, with recurrences stabilizing after 5 years.
- ER-positive breast cancer has a much longer risk-of-recurrence time period, with more than half of recurrences occurring after 5 years.

Management of metastatic breast cancer

Approximately 10% of patients present with metastatic breast cancer (MBC), and currently approximately 30% of patients with operable breast cancer will ultimately relapse with metastatic disease.

Despite advances in the systemic treatment of breast cancer, MBC is incurable with current therapies; the median survival is approximately 2 years.

Principles of the management of MBC include the following:
- The major aims of treatment are prolongation of life and palliation of symptoms.
- ER-positive disease often metastasizes to bone and commonly demonstrates relatively indolent growth with prolonged survival compared with the other subtypes of MBC.
- Common sites of MBC include lung and pleura, liver, bone, brain, skin.
- Rarer sites include the peritoneum (lobular carcinoma), choroid, and pituitary
- For ER-positive MBC first-line therapy with either an endocrine agent or chemotherapy may be options. Relevant considerations include the aggressiveness, including symptoms and degree of visceral involvement at presentation in that tumor response to chemotherapy may be quicker to chemotherapy than to endocrine therapy. Endocrine therapies are generally better tolerated than chemotherapy and responses can be durable. Although most ER-positive tumors will initially respond to endocrine therapy, and may in fact to multiple lines of endocrine therapy as outlined below, the natural progression of this disease is the eventual development of endocrine resistance eventually necessitating a transition to chemotherapy. The mainstay of HER-2 positive MBC is targeting the HER2 receptor with HER2-directed targeted therapies, often in combination with either chemotherapy or endocrine therapy (if ER-positive)
- Triple-negative MBC often presents with aggressive visceral involvement and is treated with sequential use of chemotherapy, either in combinations or as sequential monotherapies.

Endocrine therapy

Treatment for ER-positive MBC with first-line endocrine therapy is generally preferred over chemotherapy in older patients, and for those with more indolent clinical courses including those with metastatic involvement that is predominantly nonvisceral. Disease response to first-line endocrine therapy is approximately 50%–60%. Disease that responds to first-line endocrine therapy and then progresses has a 25% response rate with second-line treatment; the response to a third agent is 10%–15%.

Endocrine therapy options for MBC include the following:
- Aromatase inhibitors (for postmenopausal women or in combination with ovarian ablation or suppression for premenopausal women)
- Estrogen receptors antagonists (tamoxifen)
- Estrogen receptor downregulator (fulvestrant)
- Ovarian ablation or suppression (for premenopausal women)
- Progestins (megestrol acetate)
- Estrogens (estradiol)
- Exemestane plus everolimus

For postmenopausal women the AIs are superior to tamoxifen for first-line treatment for ER-positive MBC. A meta-analysis demonstrated that AI therapy was associated with an 11% relative risk reduction for death compared with tamoxifen (95% confidence interval [CI], 1%–19%; $P = .03$). Thus, the AIs are the mainstay of early-line therapy for postmenopausal women with MBC. Clinical trials have sought to define whether front-line combination therapy with an AI and fulvestrant is superior to AI monotherapy with conflicting results.

Active areas of breast cancer research include potentiating cancer cell responsiveness and overcoming resistance to ER-directed therapies. A recent example of this effort is illustrated by the phase 3 BOLERO-2 trial in which postmenopausal women who had recurrence or progression while receiving a nonsteroidal AI (letrozole, anastrozole) were randomized to the steroidal AI exemestane with or without the oral mammalian target of rapamycin (mTOR) inhibitor everolimus. The combination therapy group had improved progression-free survival (PFS) of 10.6 months compared to 4.1 months with exemestane alone (hazard ratio 0.36, 95% CI, 0.27–0.47; $P <.001$).

Intravenous bisphosphonates

Zolendronic acid and pamidronate have important roles in patients with bone metastases from breast cancer:
- Treatment and prevention of malignant hypercalcemia
- Healing of osteolytic metastases
- Reducing bone pain
- Delaying progression of bone disease with reduced requirement for

Radiotherapy and reduced fractures

Major side effects include osteonecrosis of the jaw (ONJ) and renal insufficiency. Risk factors for development of ONJ include older age, recent dental extractions, and prolonged use of intravenous bisphosphonates.

The optimal scheduling and duration of bisphosphonate therapy for MBC to bone is currently being defined by ongoing clinical trials. Recent trials are also exploring the adjuvant use of the bisphosphonates in women with early breast cancer with the aims of preventing both the developments of metastatic disease and bone thinning leading to osteoporosis.

Radiotherapy

Low-dose directed radiotherapy provides effective
Palliation for:
- Painful bone metastases
- Soft tissue disease such as symptomatic chest wall involvement
- Spread to brain or choroid

Stereotactic radiosurgery techniques are finding application, particularly in the treatment of brain metastases.

Chemotherapy

Advanced breast cancer is among the most sensitive solid tumors to chemotherapy. The response rate to first-line chemotherapy is approximately 60%. However, response rates to later-line therapy progressively diminish; for example approximately 30% and 15% response rates to second-line and third-line therapies, respectively. Although combination chemotherapy can be considered when a patient presents with rapidly progressive metastatic involvement, for example in visceral crisis with respiratory distress or liver impairment, in general chemotherapy for MBC involves sequential use of single agents.

Active agents include the following:
- Anthracyclines (doxorubicin, pegylated liposomal doxorubicin, epirubicin)
- Taxanes (paclitaxel, nab-paclitaxel, docetaxel)
- Alkylating agents (cyclophosphamide)
- Antimetabolites (5-fluorouracil, capecitabine, methotrexate, gemcitabine, pemetrexed)
- Platinum agents (carboplatin, cisplatin)
- Vinca alkaloids (vinorelbine)
- Nontaxane microtubule inhibitors including the epothilones (ixabepilone) and halichondrin B analogs (eribulin)
- Topoisomerase I inhibitor (topotecan)
- Topoisomerase II inhibitor (etoposide)

There is no prescribed algorithm for selecting the sequence of chemotherapy agents. In general, the anthracyclines and taxanes are among the most active agents and should be considered. Multiple considerations can guide rational drug selection:
- Prior adjuvant chemotherapy regimen and time to relapse. For example, a patient who relapses during or within 6 months of taxane exposure is unlikely to respond to further taxane therapy in the metastatic setting.
- Understanding of likely toxicity profiles with reference to coexisting illnesses and impairments such as neuropathy or kidney dysfunction.
- Ease of administration including impact on the patient's quality of life

Targeted therapies

A classic example of the success of targeted therapies in oncology is HER2-directed therapies against HER2-positive breast cancer. Approximately 20% of breast cancers are HER2-positive. Trastuzumab, the original HER2-directed therapy, is a monoclonal antibody directed against the HER2 receptor. In a seminal proof-of-concept study involving first-line therapy of MBC, patients with HER2-amplified disease experienced a significantly longer time to progression with trastuzumab monotherapy compared with those with HER2-non-amplified disease, 4.9 months versus 1.7 months (P <.0001).

Trastuzumab is commonly administered in tandem with a chemotherapy backbone with multiple safe and effective options including the taxanes, vinorelbine, and capecitabine. Combined use of trastuzumab with an anthracycline is generally avoided due to risk of cardiotoxicity.

In recent years, the treatment of HER2-positive MBC has been revolutionized with the development of other HER2-directed targeted therapies including:
- Lapatinib (an oral tyrosine kinase inhibitor against EGFR and HER2)
- Pertuzumab (a monoclonal antibody that inhibits HER2 dimerization)
- Ado-trastuzumab emtansine or T-DM1 (an antibody drug conjugate of trastuzumab with the microtubule inhibitor DM1, a maytansine derivative)
- These targeted agents can be paired with trastuzumab, with chemotherapy or endocrine therapies (if co-positive for ER/PR expression) or given as monotherapies.
- Index studies demonstrating the potency of these approaches include the phase 3 randomized CLEOPATRA and EMILIA studies.
- In the CLEOPATRA study, women were randomized to receive first-line therapy with trastuzumab and docetaxel or to the same doublet with the addition of pertuzumab. The median PFS was significantly longer in the group that received pertuzumab, 18.5 months versus 12.4 months.
- The EMILIA study randomized women who had previously received trastuzumab and a taxane for HER2-positive MBC to second-line therapy with either capecitabine with lapatinib or T-DM1. The group that received T-DM1 had significantly improved median PFS: 9.6 months versus 6.4 months. Median OS was also significantly better: 30.9 months versus 25.1 months.

Further reading

Siegel R, Naishadham D, Jemal A (2013). Cancer Statistics, 2013. *CA Cancer J Clin* 63:11–30.

Voegl VG, Costantino JP, Wickerham DL, et al. (2010). Update of the National Surgical Adjuvant Breast and Bowel Project study of tamoxifen and raloxifene (STAR) P-2 trial: preventing breast cancer. *Cancer Prev Res* 3:696–706.

Goss PE, Ingle JN, Alés-Martínez JE, et al. (2011). Exemestane for breast-cancer prevention in postmenopausal women. *N Engl J Med* 364:2381–2391.

Paik S, Shak S, Tang G, et al. (2004). A multigene assay to predict recurrence of tamoxifen-treated, node-negative breast cancer. *N Engl J Med* 351:2817–2826.

Paik S, Tang G, Shak S, et al. (2006). Gene expression and benefit of chemotherapy in women with node-negative, estrogen receptor-positive breast cancer. *J Clin Oncol* 24:3726–3734.

Giuliano AE, Hunt KK, Ballman KV, et al. (2011). Axillary dissection vs no axillary dissection in women with invasive breast cancer and sentinel node metastasis. *JAMA* 305:569–575.

Early Breast Cancer Trialists' Collaborative Group (EBCTCG) (2012). Comparisons between different polychemotherapy regimens for early breast cancer: meta-analyses of long-term outcome among 100,000 women in 123 randomised trials. *Lancet* 379:432–444.

Mamounas EP, Bryant J, Lembersky B, et al. (2005). Paclitaxel after doxorubicin plus cyclophosphamide as adjuvant chemotherapy for node-positive breast cancer: results from NSABP B-28. *J Clin Oncol* 23:3686–3696.

Sparano JA, Wang M, Martino S, et al. (2008). Weekly paclitaxel in the adjuvant treatment of breast cancer. *N Engl J Med* 358:1663–1671.

Berry DA, Cirrincione C, Henderson IC, et al. (2006). Estrogen-receptor status and outcomes of modern chemotherapy for patients with node-positive breast cancer. *JAMA* 295:1658–1667.

Jones S, Holmes FA, O'Shaughnessy J, et al. (2009). Docetaxel with cyclophosphamide is associated with an overall survival benefit compared with doxorubicin and cyclophosphamide: 7-year follow-up of US Oncology Research Trial 9735. *J Clin Oncol* 27:1177–1183.

Citron ML, Berry DA, Cirrincione C, et al. (2003). Randomized trial of dose-dense versus conventionally scheduled and sequential versus concurrent combination chemotherapy as postoperative adjuvant treatment of node-positive primary breast cancer: first report of Intergroup Trial C9741/Cancer and Leukemia Group B Trial 9741. *J Clin Oncol* 21:1431–1439.

Edith A, Perez EA, Edward H, et al. (2011). Four-year follow-up of trastuzumab plus adjuvant chemotherapy for operable human epidermal growth factor receptor 2-positive breast cancer: joint analysis of data From NCCTG N9831 and NSABP B-31. *J Clin Oncol* 29:3366–3373.

Goldhirsch A, Gelber RD, Piccart-Gebhart MJ, et al. (2013). 2 years versus 1 year of adjuvant trastuzumab for HER2-positive breast cancer (HERA): an open-label, randomised controlled trial. *Lancet* 382:1021–1028.

Slamon D, Eiermann W, Robert N, et al. (2011). Adjuvant trastuzumab in HER2-positive breast cancer. *N Engl J Med* 365:1273–1283.

Early Breast Cancer Trialists' Collaborative Group (EBCTCG) (2011). Relevance of breast cancer hormone receptors and other factors to the efficacy of adjuvant tamoxifen: patient-level meta-analysis of randomised trials. *Lancet* 378:771–784.

Fisher B, Dignam J, Bryant J, et al. (2001). Five versus more than five years of tamoxifen for lymph node-negative breast cancer: updated findings from the National Surgical Adjuvant Breast and Bowel Project B-14 randomized trial. *J Natl Cancer Inst* 93:684–690.

Davies C, Pan H, Godwin J, et al. (2013). Long-term effects of continuing adjuvant tamoxifen to 10 years versus stopping at 5 years after diagnosis of oestrogen receptor-positive breast cancer: ATLAS, a randomised trial. *Lancet* 381:805–816.

Gray RG, Rea D, Handley K, et al. (2013). aTTom: long-term effects of continuing adjuvant tamoxifen to 10 years versus stopping at 5 years in 6953 women with early breast cancer. *J Clin Oncol* 31(Suppl) abstr 5.

Burstein HJ, Prestrud AA, Seidenfeld J, et al. (2010). American Society of Clinical Oncology clinical practice guideline: update on adjuvant endocrine therapy for women with hormone receptor-positive breast cancer. *J Clin Oncol* 23:3784.

Regan MM, Neven P, Giobbie-Hurder A, et al. (2011). Assessment of letrozole and tamoxifen alone and in sequence for postmenopausal women with steroid hormone receptor-positive breast cancer: the BIG 1-98 randomised clinical trial at 8.1 years median follow-up. *Lancet Oncol* 12:1101–1108.

Goss PE, Ingle JN, Martino S, et al. (2003). A randomized trial of letrozole in postmenopausal women after five years of tamoxifen therapy for early-stage breast cancer. *N Engl J Med* 349:1793.

Rastogi P, Anderson SJ, Bear HD, et al. (2008). Preoperative chemotherapy: updates of National Surgical Adjuvant Breast and Bowel Project protocols B-18 and B-27. *J Clin Oncol* 26:778–785.

Mauri D, Pavlidis N, Polyzos NP, et al. (2006). Survival with aromatase inhibitors and inactivators versus standard hormonal therapy in advanced breast cancer: meta-analysis. *J Natl Cancer Inst* 98:1285–1291.

Jonas Bergh J, Jönsson PE, Lidbrink EK, et al. (2012). FACT: an open-label randomized phase III study of fulvestrant and anastrozole in combination compared with anastrozole alone as first-line therapy for patients with receptor-positive postmenopausal breast cancer. *J Clin Oncol* 30:1919–1925.

Mehta RS, Barlow WE, Albain KS, et al. (2012). Combination anastrozole and fulvestrant in metastatic breast cancer. *N Engl J Med* 367:435–444.

Baselga J, Campone M, Piccart M, et al. (2012). Everolimus in postmenopausal hormone-receptor–positive advanced breast cancer. *N Engl J Med* 366:520–529.

Vogel CL, Cobleigh MA, Tripathy D, et al. (2002). Efficacy and safety of trastuzumab as a single agent in first-line treatment of HER2-overexpressing metastatic breast cancer. *J Clin Oncol* 20:719–726.

Baselga J, Cortés J, Kim SB, et al. (2012). Pertuzumab plus trastuzumab plus docetaxel for metastatic breast cancer. *N Engl J Med* 367:109–119.

Verma S, Miles D, Gianni L, et al. (2012). Trastuzumab emtansine for HER2-positive advanced breast cancer. *N Engl J Med* 367:1783–1791.

Chapter 29

Gastrointestinal cancer I: esophagus, stomach, small intestine, carcinoid

Esophageal cancer 466
  Epidemiology and etiology 466
  Staging and Her2Neu testing 466
  Surgical considerations 468
  Treatment 468
Gastric cancer 472
  Epidemiology and etiology 472
  Staging and Her2Neu testing 472
  Surgical considerations 472
  Treatment 474
Small intestine and carcinoid tumors 478
  Introduction 478
  Pathology 478
  Management 480
  Future directions 481

Esophageal cancer

Ivy Altomare

Esophageal cancer is a highly aggressive malignancy, usually advanced at diagnosis. Approximately 90% of patients will ultimately die of their disease.

Treatment should be multidisciplinary, and early involvement of thoracic surgery, radiation oncology, nutritionists, and social workers is necessary for optimal outcomes.

Epidemiology and etiology

Esophageal cancer is the eighth most common malignancy worldwide. Although not in the top 10 in the United States for incidence (1% of all cancers), it is the seventh leading cause of cancer deaths in men in the United States.

Squamous histology is most common worldwide, and is endemic in Asia and Southeast Africa. However, esophageal adenocarcinoma has the fastest rising incidence of any malignancy in the United States and Europe.

Risk factors include male gender, age, and Caucasian heritage.

- **Squamous**: Smoking, alcohol
- **Adenocarcinoma**: Smoking, obesity, gastroesophageal reflux disease (GERD), Barrett's esophagus
- If high-grade dysplasia is diagnosed, approximately 50% of patients will already have invasive cancer and the treatment of choice is resection (versus close surveillance every 3 months with esophagogastroduodenoscopy [EGD])
- Higher response rates are seen with squamous cell carcinoma after treatment, but long-term outcome is not statistically different among histologies.

Staging and Her2Neu testing

- Pretreatment workup: history and physical examination (H&P), complete blood count (CBC), basic metabolic profile (BMP), prothrombin and partial prothrombin time (PT/PTT), EGD or double-contrast barium study, PET ± CT of the chest and/or abdomen
- Endoscopic ultrasound (EUS) (if there is no distant metastasis) is a valuable tool to assess the depth of invasion, pathological stage (FNA of celiac, mediastinal or perigastric nodes) and plan treatment (resection versus neoadjuvant).
    - Consider bronchoscopy if tumor is located above carina
    - Consider laparoscopic staging of peritoneum if there is gastroesophageal junction (GEJ) tumor
- Staging is TNM as per *AJCC Staging Manual*, 7th edition (2010) (see Table 29.1).

Table 29.1 TNM staging of esophageal cancer

Stage	T	N	M	Primary tumor (T)	Lymph nodes (N)	Distant metastases (M)
0	Tis	N0	M0	TX: cannot be assessed	Nx: cannot be assessed	Mx: cannot be assessed
I	T1	N0	M0	T0: no evidence of primary tumor	N0: no regional lymph node metastasis	M0: no distant metastases
IIA	T2	N0	M0	Tis - carcinoma in situ	N1: regional lymph node metastasis	M1: distant metastases
	T3	N0	M0	T1: invades lamina propria or submucosa		Lower thoracic esophagus:
IIB	T1	N1	M0	T2: invades muscularis propria		M1a: celiac lymph node metastasis
	T2	N1	M0	T3: invades adventitia		M1b: other distant met
III	T3	N1	M0	T4: invades adjacent structures		Mid-thoracic esophagus:
	T4	Any N	M0			M1a: n/a
						M1b: nonregional lymph nodes or
IV	Any T	Any N	M1			Other distant metastases
IVA	Any T	Any N	M1a			Upper thoracic esophagus:
IVB	Any T	Any N	M1b			M1a: cervical lymph node met
						M1b: other distant met

- Her2Neu testing should be performed on locally advanced, recurrent or metastatic adenocarcinomas of the esophagus and EGJ
- Her2Neu overexpression occurs in approximately 20%–25% of adenocarcinomas of esophagus or EGJ
  - Testing is done by IHC and/or FISH
  - consider testing many biopsy specimens for more accurate results

Surgical considerations

Choice of technique is a subject of great debate (transthoracic, transhiatal esophajectomy); R0 resection is the goal (negative margins). At minimum, 15 lymph nodes must be resected. Newer, minimally invasive techniques include endoscopic mucosal resection (EMR), endoscopic cryoablation, RFA, and photodynamic therapy.
- May be appropriate for early stage (T1a with no venous or lymphatic invasion) or Barrett's/high grade dysplasia
- Used widely in Japan
- May offer lower mortality, especially in more experienced centers but has high recurrence rates and close surveillance (q3 month EGD x1 year) is required. EMR/endoscopic ablation has not been compared with standard techniques in randomized trials.

Treatment

Treatment for localized (resectable) disease

Acceptable strategies include resection ± adjuvant treatment, neoadjuvant treatment followed by resection, resection with perioperative chemotherapy, and definitive chemoradiotherapy. All are supported by the literature in certain clinical situations, and treatment plans must be multidisciplinary.

For T1/T2 disease consider upfront resection-preferred for:
- Thoracic tumors >5 cm from cricopharyngeus, intraabdominal esophagus, and EGJ cancers.

Adjuvant treatment is indicated for positive margins (R1 resection) or macroscopic residual disease (R2 resection), "high-risk T2" (poorly differentiated, lymphovascular or neurovascular invasion, younger patient), or T3 disease.
- Adjuvant combined-modality chemoradiotherapy is preferred. Data are extrapolated from INT 0116 (Macdonald trial) where 20% of patients had tumors of the GEJ. Patients who were randomized to 5 treatments of postoperative 5-fluorouracil-leucovorin (5-FU/LV) with concurrent radiotherapy had a 10% improvement in 5-year overall survival versus surgery alone.
- There is no survival advantage for adjuvant radiotherapy alone (based on results of RTOG 85-01, showing 0% survival at 3 years). However, intensity-modulated radiotherapy (IMRT) and brachytherapy techniques are under investigation.

Neoadjuvant chemotherapy alone is not recommended, as there is an unclear survival benefit and little improvement in curative resection rate.
- In a randomized trial by Stahl et al, there was a trend toward inferior outcomes with neoadjuvant chemo alone with cis/5FU versus chemo/XRT but this did not reach significance due to poor trial accrual.
- Trials with newer agents and combinations are ongoing.

Perioperative chemotherapy is appropriate for adenocarcinomas given results of the MAGIC trial, in which 26% of patients had GEJ or lower esophageal tumors.
- Patients randomized to epirubicin, cisplatin, 5-FU (ECF) followed by surgery followed by ECF had a 4-month improvement in median overall survival (mOS) and a 5-year overall survival of 36% (versus 23% for surgery alone).

Combined-modality treatment is the current NCCN standard for:
- surgical candidates with >T2 disease to increase curative resection rates
- as definitive treatment without surgical resection, especially for cervical cancer with squamous cell histology.
- Use is supported by RTOG 85-01 and two meta-analyses showing improvement in 3-year mortality with 5-FU, cisplatin, and radiotherapy versus surgery alone.
- Neoadjuvant chemoradiotherapy is a new standard of care based on the CROSS trial, which randomized resectable patients to surgery alone versus weekly carbo/taxol/XRT (41.4Gy in 23 fractions): R0 resections 69% versus 92%; mOS 24mos versus 49.4mos, HR 0.657
- Combined treatment was prospectively studied in CALGB 9781: patients randomized to neoadjuvant 5-FU, cisplatin, and radiotherapy versus surgery alone had significantly better median survival (4.5 years versus 1.8 years) and 5-year overall survival (39% versus 16%).
- Pathologic complete response (pCR) is a strong predictor of survival in nearly all trials (5-year survival is as high as 50%–60%).
- Combined 5-FU-cisplatin and radiotherapy is the regimen supported by the literature, historically, but Phase II data support other combinations such as docetaxel/cis, carbo/paclitaxel, FOLFOX and docetaxel/oxaliplatin/capecitabine (for adenoca). Randomized phase III trials are ongoing.
- Induction of chemotherapy prior to combined-modality treatment does not seem to improve outcome.

Patients must be informed to expect toxicities of enteritis, mucositis, and nausea. Consider prophylactic J-tube placement for nutritional support.

Esophagectomy after combined definitive treatment:
- Two European randomized trials suggest improvement in local control but no impact on overall survival.
- Most strongly indicated for nonresponders to neoadjuvant treatment.
- PET can be used to identify patients with early treatment failure who would most benefit from resection.

Treatment for recurrent and metastatic disease
Salvage esophagectomy is recommended, if possible. Chemotherapy is not known to improve survival but can be palliative and should be offered to patients with ECOG PS of 2 or less.
- No single standard regimen; 5-FU and cisplatin most historically supported; reserve three drug regimens for fit patients.
- Various combinations have been tested in the phase II setting with response rates of mostly 40%–50% (docetaxel-cisplatin-5FU (DCF), cisplatin-CPT 11, carboplatin-paclitaxel; gemcitabine–cisplatin; fluorouracil-leucovorin-oxaliplatin [FOLFOX]; 5-FU–CPT-11; docetaxel–CPT-11+/- cisiplatin).

REAL-2, a recently published large, randomized phase III trial, supports the use of capecitabine and oxaliplatin in advanced gastric and esophageal cancer. In this noninferiority trial with 2 x 2 design, ECF, epirubicin-oxaliplatin-fluorouracil (EOF), epirubicin–cisplatin–capecitabine (ECX), and epirubicin-oxaliplatin-capecitabine (EOX) regimens were found to have similar RR (40%) and mOS (~10 months), with EOX having a statistically superior overall survival versus ECF.

The TOGA trial confirmed trastuzumab plus cisplatin-5FU (or capecitabine) offers a 3 month survival benefit versus chemo alone in patients with locally advanced or metastatic esophagogastric adenocarcinomas that overexpress Her2Neu by IHC or FISH. Treatment with trastuzumab is now standard of care in this subset of patients.

Other palliative techniques to treat symptoms of obstruction, dysphagia, bleeding, and fistulas and to preserve eating function should be integrated into treatment:
- Balloon dilatation, thermocoagulation, laser therapy, ethanol injection, stent, photodynamic therapy, and radiation therapy

Further reading

Al-Sarraf M, Martz K, Herskovic A, et al. (1997). Progress report of combined chemoradiotherapy versus radiotherapy alone in patients with esophageal cancer: an intergroup study. *J Clin Oncol* 15:866.

Cunningham D, Allum, WE, Stenning SP, et al. (2006). Perioperative chemotherapy versus surgery alone for resectable gastroesophageal cancer. *N Engl J Med* 355:11–20.

Cunningham D, Starling N, Rao S, et al. (2008). Capecitabine and oxaliplatin for advanced esophagogastric cancer. *N Engl J Med* 358:36–46.

Enzinger PC, Mayer RJ (2003). Esophageal cancer. *N Engl J Med* 349:2241–2252.

Macdonald JS, Smalley SR, Benedetti J, et al. (2001). Chemoradiotherapy after surgery compared with surgery alone for adenocarcinoma of the stomach or GEJ. *N Engl J Med* 345:725–730.

Tepper JE, Krasna M, Niedzwiecki D, et al. (2006). Superiority of trimodality therapy to surgery alone in esophageal cancer: Results of CALGB 9781. ASCO meeting abstracts. 24(18 Suppl):4012.

Bang YJ, Van Custem E, Feyereislova A, et al. (2010). Trastuzumab in combination with chemotherapy vs. chemotherapy alone for treatment of HER2-positive advanced gastric or gastro-oesophageal junction cancer (ToGA): a phase 3, open label, randomized controlled trial. *Lancet* 376:1302.

Van Hagen P, Hulshof MC, van Lanschot JJ, et al. (2012). Preoperative chemoradiotherapy for esophageal or junctional cancer. *N Engl J Med* 366:2074–2084.

Gastric cancer

Ivy Altomare

Gastric cancer is the third most common cancer killer worldwide, with 50% of patients having locally advanced disease at diagnosis. Even after curative resection, 80% of patients will experience recurrence. Thus referral to experienced centers is indicated for optimal treatment.

Epidemiology and etiology
- More common in Asian countries; screening is routinely done in Japan and Korea
- In Western countries, location shifts proximally to GEJ, cardia, and lesser curvature
- Risk factors include *Helicobacter pylori*, smoking, and high-salt diet.
- *Hereditary diffuse gastric cancer*: Autosomal dominant mutation in E-cadherin (*CDH1*) with varying penetrance- accounts for 25% of familial gastric cancer. Consider prophylactic gastrectomy.

Staging and Her2Neu testing
Pretreatment workup
- H&P, CBC, SMA 12, chest X-ray, EGD, CT of abdomen, PET ± CT (if there is no evidence of metastatic disease)
  - EUS if potentially resectable, to assess depth of invasion and/or to FNA perigastric lymph nodes
  - Consider laparoscopic staging of peritoneum (even if patient is unfit for surgery) as it aids in making the decision for or against combined modality treatment, especially for T3 or N1 disease.
- Staging is TNM as per *AJCC Staging Manual*, 7th edition (2010) (see Table 29.2).
- Her2Neu testing should be performed on unresectable locally advanced, recurrent or metastatic gastric tumors
- Her2Neu overexpression is variable and occurs in approx 20% of gastric tumors
- Testing is done by IHC and/or FISH

Surgical considerations
Subtotal versus total gastrectomy is a subject of great debate, as is D2 (celiac axis) versus D1 (perigastric) lymph node dissection.
- Japanese literature supports D2 (more extensive) resection, but large, randomized trials, including the Dutch Study, found higher postoperative morbidity and mortality and no survival benefit with D2.
- Experienced centers may still prefer D2 dissection. High-volume centers have low morbidity/mortality rates with modified D2 lymphadenectomy without pancreatectomy and splenectomy.
- D0 resection (incomplete removal of N1 nodes) is unacceptable.
- At minimum, 15 lymph nodes must be resected.
- 4 cm margins are preferred.

Table 29.2 TNM staging of gastric cancer

Stage	T	N	M	Primary tumor (T)	Lymph nodes (N)	Distant metastases (M)
0	Tis	N0	M0	TX: cannot be assessed	Nx: cannot be assessed	Mx: cannot be assessed
IA	T1	N0	M0	T0: no evidence of primary tumor	N0: no regional lymph node metastasis	M0: no distant metastasis
IB	T1	N1	M0	Tis- carcinoma in situ	N1: 1 to 6 regional lymph node metastases	M1: distant metastases
	T2a/b	N0	M0	T1: invades lamina propria or submucosa		
II	T1	N2	M0	T2a: invades muscularis propria	N2: 7–15 regional lymph node metastases	
	T2a/b	N1	M0	T2b: invades subserosa	N3: >15 regional lymph node metastases	
	T3	N0	M0	T3: penetrates serosa (visceral peritoneum) without invasion of adjacent structures		
IIIA	T2a/b	N2	M0	T4: invades adjacent structures		
	T3	N0	M0			
	T4	N1	M0			
IIIB	T3	N2	M0			
IV	T4	N1–3	M0			
	T1–3	N3	M0			
	Any T	Any N	M1			

Newer, minimally invasive techniques include endoscopic mucosal resection (EMR), endoscopic submusocal dissection (ESD) and laparoscopic wedge resection.
- May be appropriate for early stage (T1N0, well-differentiated, <30 mm, without ulceration, venous or lymphatic invasion)
- These techniques may offer lower mortality, especially in more experienced centers, but they have not been compared with standard techniques in randomized trials and must be considered investigational.

Treatment

Treatment for localized resectable disease

T1 disease or bleeding
Consider upfront resection.

T2+ disease
- **Adjuvant chemotherapy alone**: Meta-analyses suggest a small survival benefit, but this approach is not standard. Trials with newer agents are ongoing.
- **Neoadjuvant combined chemoradiotherapy**: Attractive in the phase II setting, and phase III trials are ongoing.
- **Perioperative chemotherapy**: Preferred approach, per NCCN guidelines and a current standard of care based on results of the MAGIC trial.
  - Patients randomized to ECF followed by surgery followed by ECF had a 4-month improvement in mOS and a 5-year overall survival of 36% (versus 23% for surgery alone).
- **Adjuvant combined chemoradiotherapy**: Also a standard of care. It is indicated after resection for positive margins (R1 resection) or macroscopic residual disease (R2 resection), "high-risk T2" (poorly differentiated, lymphovascular or neural invasion, younger patient), or T3 disease.
  - Use is supported by INT 0116 (Macdonald trial), where patients randomized to 5 treatments of postoperative 5-FU/LV with concurrent radiation therapy during cycles 2 and 3 had a 10% improvement in 5-year overall survival versus surgery alone.
  - Institutional preferences may exist for active regimens supported by phase II data (taxane, CPT-11, capecitabine-based), and trials are ongoing for the use of targeted agents in the adjuvant setting.

Treatment for localized unresectable disease

An aggressive approach may benefit medically fit patients. Combined chemoradiotherapy is preferred, based on small trials showing modest survival benefit with 5-FU and radiotherapy versus radiation alone.
- Platinum-, taxane-, and CPT-11-based regimens were most often used, based on phase II data with higher response rates.
- In patients with a strong clinical response, consider salvage gastrectomy.

Treatment for recurrent and metastatic disease
Randomized trials confirm that palliative chemotherapy offers a survival benefit in both the first and second line settings (3 months in older studies) and improves quality of life.
- There is no one standard firstline regimen; ECF is most historically supported (found superior to FamTX in a phase III trial).
- Combination chemotherapy is indicated even in the palliative setting (higher response rates).
- Trastuzumab-containing regimens are standard of care in patients with Her2Neu-overexpressing tumors
- The TOGA trial confirmed trastuzumab plus cisplatin-5FU(or capecitabine) offers a 3 month survival benefit versus chemo alone in patients with locally advanced or metastatic esophagogastric adenocarcinomas that overexpress Her2Neu by IHC or FISH.
- The COUGAR-2 trial supports use of single agent docetaxel as second-line therapy with a survival benefit of 5.2 versus 3.6 months and improved symptom control when randomized against best supportive care.

Other key trials in treating metastatic esophagogastric cancer include the following:
- In the V325 study, doxetaxel-cisplatin-5-FU (DCF) was compared with cisplatin-5-FU (CF) and showed a significant improvement in mOS (9.2 versus 8.6 months) and TTP (5.6 versus 3.7 months), with higher toxicity, leading to approval of docetaxel for gastric cancer in combination with 5-FU and cisplatin.
- A multicenter phase II study of cisplatin, CPT-11, and bevacizumab in patients with advanced gastric or GEJ cancers cited a RR of 65% and mOS 12.3 months.
- REAL-2, a recently published large, randomized phase III trial supports the use of capecitabine and oxaliplatin in treating advanced gastric and esophageal cancer.
  - In this noninferiority trial with a 2 x 2 design, ECF, EOF, ECX, and EOX regimens were found to have similar RR (40%) and mOS (~10 months), with EOX having a statistically superior overall survival to that of ECF.
- Capecitabine was also found to be noninferior to 5-FU in the ML17032 trial.
  - The capecitabine-cisplatin arm had a higher response rate and equal mOS to the 5-FU-cisplatin arm (~10 months).

Other palliative techniques to treat symptoms of bleeding, obstruction, pain, and fistulas and to improve nutritional status should be integrated into treatment.
- Palliative surgery, gastrojejunostomy, endoscopic tumor ablation, ethanol injection, stent, photodynamic therapy, radiation
- Intraperitoneal chemotherapy for peritoneal metastases: there are no randomized trials, and this is offered in only a few highly specialized centers worldwide.

Further reading

Bonenkamp JJ, Hermans J, Sasako M, et al. (1999). Extended lymph-node dissection for gastric cancer. Dutch Gastric Cancer Group. *N Engl J Med* 420:908–914.

Cunningham D, Allum WE, Stenning SP, et al. (2006). Perioperative chemotherapy versus surgery alone for resectable gastroesophageal cancer. *N Engl J Med* 355:11–20.

Cunningham D, Starling N, Rao S, et al. (2008). Capecitabine and oxaliplatin for advanced esophagogastric cancer. *N Engl J Med* 358:36–46.

Jansen EP, Boot H, Verheij M, et al. (2005). Optimal locoregional treatment in gastric cancer. *J Clin Oncol* 23:4509–4517.

Macdonald JS, Smalley SR, Benedetti J, et al. (2001). Chemoradiotherapy after surgery compared with surgery alone for adenocarcinoma of the stomach or GEJ. *N Engl J Med* 345:725–730.

Shah MA, Ramanathan RK, Ilson DH, et al. (2006). Multicenter phase II study of irinotecan, cisplatin and bevacizumab in patients with metastatic gastric or gastroesophageal junction adenocarcinoma. *J Clin Oncol* 24:5201–5206.

Van Cutsem E, Moiseyenko VM, Tjulandin S, et al. (2006). Phase III study of docetaxel and cisplatin plus fluorouracil compared with cisplatin and fluorouracil as first-line therapy for advanced gastric cancer: a report of the V325 study group. *J Clin Oncol* 24:4991–4997.

Bang YJ, Van Custem E, Feyereislova A et al. (2010). Trastuzumab in combination with chemotherapy vs. chemotherapy alone for treatment of HER2-positive advanced gastric or gastro-oesophageal junction cancer (ToGA): a phase 3, open label, randomized controlled trial. *Lancet* 376:1302.

Small intestine and carcinoid tumors

Karen E. Bullock
Johanna C. Bendell

Introduction

These tumors constitute ~2% of gastrointestinal neoplasms. Approximately 65% of all small bowel tumors are malignant. Their incidence is 1–15 per 100,000, with slight male predominance. Peak incidence is at age 50–70 years.

Diagnosis is often late due to varying nonspecific signs and symptoms: crampy intermittent abdominal pain, anorexia, weight loss, obstruction, and occult bleeding.

Risk factors include dietary factors, smoking and alcohol use, immunodeficiency (including AIDS), Crohn's disease, celiac disease (lymphoma), and heritable diseases, such as the following:
- Peutz-Jeghers syndrome (benign hamartomas in jejunum/ileum; rare malignant transformation)
- Familial adenomatous polyposis (FAP)
- Gardner's syndrome (adenomas)
- Von Recklinghausen's neurofibromatosis
- MEN-1 (carcinoid)

Up to 25% of patients with small bowel cancers have synchronous malignancies in the colon, breast, endometrium, prostate, and other sites.

Imaging may include small bowel barium series, CT/MRI, endoscopy (standard and/or capsule if no obstruction), and enteroclysis.

Some 50% of these tumors are not accurately diagnosed until exploratory laparoscopy or laparotomy.

Pathology

Adenocarcinoma (45%)
- Usually found in proximal small bowel (80%); 65% are periampullary
- Thought to develop from adenomas similar to colorectal cancer. Villous adenomas should be treated similarly to those found in the colon.
- Staging is the same as that for colorectal cancer (see Colon TNM, AJCC).
  - T3 includes subserosal and/or retroperitoneal (<2 cm) invasion.
  - T4 includes perforation of visceral peritoneum or local structures.
- More distal tumors have a worse prognosis.
  - Duodenal (resectable): 5-year survival is 65%, like colon cancer.
  - Jejunal/ileal: 5-year survival is 20%–30%; there is more nodal involvement.

Carcinoid tumors (29%)
- Rare neuroendocrine tumor found in bowel, stomach, lung
- 90% are in the ileum or appendix: over 50% have metastasized to the liver at diagnosis.

- Usually found within 60 cm of ileocecal valve
- Most frequently found incidentally during appendectomy
- 30%–40% of patients have multiple nodules at diagnosis, so the entire bowel and colon should be examined before or during surgery.
- Cause intense desmoplastic reaction in surrounding tissue, which can result in obstruction
- Carcinoid syndrome: Watery diarrhea, sweating, flushing, wheezing, dyspnea, abdominal pain, right heart failure symptoms
- 10% of patients present with carcinoid syndrome due to serotonin and vasoactive peptides in the following settings:
  - Hepatic metastases
  - Retroperitoneal disease
  - Extraintestinal primary tumors
- Can cause tricuspid or pulmonic valve disease due to fibrosis; 10%–20% of patients with carcinoid syndrome have this at presentation.
- Measurement of the level of 24-hour urinary 5-HIAA is the initial diagnostic test; sensitivity decreases from 75% if disease is asymptomatic or nonmetastatic. Usually >100 mg/day accompanies metastatic disease.
- Serum or plasma chromogranin A has excellent sensitivity (though poor specificity), andalthough usually not used for diagnosis, it is often followed during treatment if there is metastatic disease.
- Octreoscan (somatostatin analogue scintigraphy) can be used in diagnosis and staging along with CT/MRI. Sensitivity is >90%.
- Risk for metastasis increases sharply if tumors are over 2 cm.
- 5-year survival for localized disease is 75%–95%; regional node disease, 40%–60%; and metastatic disease, 20%–30%.

Lymphoma (16%)
- More prevalent distally, along with sarcomas
- The GI tract is the most common extranodal site of lymphoma and lymphoma here may occur alone or with systemic disease.
- May be low or high grade, B- or T-cell predominant.
- Extranodal marginal zone B-cell lymphoma of MALT type and mantle cell are most common.
- Stomach is the most common site of GI lymphoma in the United States (75%), followed by small bowel (9%). Small bowel lymphoma is more common in the Middle East.
- Incidence is increasing in United States along with the increased number of immunocompromised patients (HIV/AIDS, transplants).
- Perforation is more common, in up to 25% of patients.
- 5-year survival is 20%–33%, and relapse at up to 5–10 years is common.
- See section on lymphomas for staging (p. 752).

Sarcoma (10%)
- Very rare, 75% leiomyosarcoma
- TNM staging is used.

- Watch for hematogenous metastasis.
- Survival rates vary depending on grade and stage.
- See discussion of gastrointestinal stromal tumors (GIST) in Chapter 40 (p. 692–3).

Metastases (rare) from lung, breast, gastric, colon, renal cell cancers
The small intestine is the #1 site of GI metastasis for melanoma.

Management

Surgery is the primary therapy for all small bowel tumors.

All benign tumors are cured by adequate resection with negative margins if endoscopic polypectomy will not suffice (e.g., large villous adenomas). Malignant disease requires adequate lymph node dissection for staging.

Advanced metastatic lesions may benefit from palliative surgery if bleeding or obstruction is of concern.

Adenocarcinoma

Surgery
- Duodenal: frequent pancreaticoduodenectomy (Whipple)
- Distal ileum: right colectomy

Chemotherapy
Chemotherapy, both adjuvant and for metastatic disease, is extrapolated from trials in colorectal cancer, as there are few studies addressing this disease. Retrospective reports from three large trials show no survival advantage for small bowel adenocarcinoma with adjuvant therapy.
- 5-FU, capecitabine, oxaliplatin, irinotecan, and, if metastatic, bevacizumab or the EGFR inhibitors may be used. See Chapter 31 for regimens.
- Cisplatin and gemcitabine are also active, unlike in colon cancer.

Adjuvant radiation
Radiation (usually in combination with chemotherapy) may also be used for local control of positive retroperitoneal margins in small bowel adenocarcinomas, particularly of duodenal and ampullary origins.

Carcinoid tumors

Surgery
- **Small bowel**: Wide en bloc resection is needed, as tumors are more likely to metastasize even when under 1 cm.
  - Often excised even when metastatic:
  1. to improve disease-free survival
  2. decrease carcinoid syndrome
  3. avoid extensive fibrosing mesenteritis
  4. there is no known survival benefit
- **Appendix**: Size matters:
  - <1.5 cm can have appendectomy alone, unless it involves mesoappendix, vessels, or suspicious nodes.
  - >1.5 cm or these characteristics, right hemicolectomy

Chemotherapy
- Has poor activity, although regimens of cisplatin and etoposide or streptozocin/5-FU or doxorubicin are used for palliation in metastatic disease

Radiation
Radiation therapies may be used focally for hepatic metastasis via:
- Radiolabeled indium111-octreotide
- MIBG
- Yttrium-90 labeled microspheres (SirSpheres or Theraspheres) delivered by interventional radiology/nuclear medicine.

Somatostatin analogues
These are used for treatment of carcinoid syndrome but may also stabilize disease in 50% of patients.
- Available in monthly depot injection
- Should be given preoperatively in metastatic patients undergoing resection to avoid carcinoid crisis (massive release of vasoactive peptides)

Interferon
IFN (subcutaneous) is decreasing in use for carcinoid syndrome palliation because of its own significant side effects.

Lymphoma
- **Surgery**: Requires frozen section evaluation and en bloc resection of mesentery with nodes due to high frequency of involvement
- **Chemotherapy**: Even stage I disease is usually treated if it is high grade or if regional nodes are involved.
  - CHOP (cyclophosphamide, doxorubicin, vincristine, prednisone) along with rituximab is the most common regimen.

Sarcoma
- **Surgery**: Lymphadenectomy is not required; there is no survival benefit.
- **Chemotherapy**: Adjuvant therapy is not recommended; doxorubicin-containing regimens are most common for metastatic disease.

Future directions

Adenocarcinoma
There is a need for trials in both the adjuvant and metastatic setting at centers of excellence to establish chemotherapy guidelines for all of these rare tumors.

Currently, randomized phase II trials using bevacizumab, multitargeted tyrosine kinase inhibitors (sunitinib, sorafenib), and inhibitors of the mTOR system are ongoing.

Carcinoid
PET-CT using serotonin or levodopa as metabolic enhancers instead of glucose may aid in the diagnosis of carcinoid tumors. Efforts are being made to enhance the histological grading system for prognostic significance with genomics.

Radiolabeled therapies targeting the somatostatin receptor are underway. As with small bowel adenocarcinomas, preliminary data suggest that VEGF inhibitors and mTOR inhibitors may have efficacy in this disease.

Further reading

Dabaja BS, Suki D, Pro B, et al. (2004). Adenocarcinoma of the small bowel: presentation, prognostic factors, and outcome of 217 patients. *Cancer* 101:518.

Frost DB, Mercado PD, Tyrell JS. (1994). Small bowel cancer: a 30-year review. *Ann Surg Oncol* 1:290.

Lepage C, Bouvier AM, Manfredi S, et al. (2006). Incidence and management of primary malignant small bowel cancers: a well-defined French population study. *Am J Gastroenterol* 101:2826.

Modlin IM, Oberg K, Chung DC, et al. (2008). Gastroenteropancreatic neuroendocrine tumours. *Lancet Oncol* 9:61–72.

Chapter 30

Gastrointestinal cancer II: pancreas, biliary tract, hepatocellular

Pancreatic cancer *484*
   Introduction *484*
   Evaluation and staging *485*
   Pathology *486*
   Management *486*
Cancers of the biliary tract *490*
   Cholangiocarcinoma *490*
   Gallbladder cancer *491*
Hepatocellular carcinoma *494*
   Epidemiology *494*
   Symptoms *494*
   Diagnosis and prognosis *494*
   Pathology and staging *495*
   Management *495*

Pancreatic cancer

Karen E. Bullock
Johanna C. Bendell

Introduction

Anatomy

The pancreas is divided into the head (including uncinate process), neck, body, and tail. Its retroperitoneal location provides contact with many organs and structures that can be involved with direct tumor extension.

Tumors of the pancreas may be exocrine (>95%) or endocrine (<5%). Approximately 66% of cancers are found in the pancreatic head, 15% in the body, and 10% in the tail. Generalized peritoneal spread is more common with body and tail tumor locations.

Epidemiology

- #5 cancer killer of Americans (2007), although not in top 10 for incidence
- 2007 U.S. incidence was 37,170, with 33,370 deaths.
- From 2000 to 2004, mean age at diagnosis was 72, with male predominance.
  - Risk dramatically increases after age 45.
  - Black men have the highest risk and death rate.

Risk factors include the following:
- Smoking (30% risk)
- Obesity and low exercise state
- Occupational exposure to benzidine and betanapthylamine
- Familial cancer syndromes are associated with 5%–10% of incidence (see Table 30.1).

Familial pancreatitis confers 40–70 times increased risk. Saturated fat, alcohol use, and caffeine intake, as well as chronic pancreatitis and diabetes, remain controversial factors.

- Molecular abnormalities in $p16$, $p53$, $DPC4$, and $BRCA2$ account for 50%–95% of tumors.
- K-ras activation is 90%.

Presentation depends on location

- Pain, weight loss, painless jaundice, steatorrhea, anorexia
- New-onset atypical diabetes, acute pancreatitis, or thromboses may herald the diagnosis.
  - Trousseau's syndrome = migratory thrombophlebitis

An abdominal mass, supraclavicular node, and ascites are late findings.

- Courvoisier's sign = painless, palpable gall bladder
- Virchow's node = enlarged left supraclavicular node (also seen in gastric cancer)
- Sister Mary Joseph's node = periumbilical lymph node or tumor nodule.

Table 30.1 Familial cancer syndromes

Syndrome	Associated gene
Peutz-Jeghers	STK11
Li-Fraumeni	p53
HNPCC II, or Lynch II	MSH and MLH
Familial adenomatous polyposis (FAP)	APC
BRCA-1 and -2	BRCA1, BRCA2
Ataxia-telangectasia	ATM
Familial atypical multiple mole melanoma	CDKN2A
Familial pancreatitis	PRSS1, SPINK1

Evaluation and staging

Computed tomography scan with contrast
Using this modality, 90% of patients are appropriately determined to undergo surgery or not.
- May be used for fine needle aspiration for diagnosis.
- MRI and PET are not presently considered superior for imaging the pancreas, and PET has been shown lacking in detecting nodal disease.

Endoscopic ultrasound
- Accurate staging with operator expertise
- FNA for diagnosis, without potential seeding of peritoneum

Staging laparoscopy
Although out of favor, it can be used to assess resectability by direct examination of the liver and peritoneal surfaces, biopsy if indicated, and peritoneal washings. If any are positive, surgery may be aborted and the patient directed to appropriate systemic therapy.

Cancer antigen 19–9
This has diagnostic sensitivity (80%) and specificity (90%) in larger tumors.
- Not recommended as a screening test.
- Higher baseline levels have been linked with poorer prognosis.
- It helps in following disease response, although imaging is decisive.

Tumor-node-metastasis staging
Practically, patients are staged according to whether they have resectable tumors or not.

Survival by stage at diagnosis
Localized disease survival may be closer to a 30% 5-year survival, according to current 3-year data. (see Table 30.2)

Table 30.2 Survival by stage at diagnosis, adapted from SEER database

	Localized	Locally advanced	Metastatic	Unknown
Stage	7%	26%	52%	15%
5-year survival	20.3%	8%	1.7%	4.1%
Median survival	13–20 months	9–13 months	3–6 months	—

Pathology

- Adenocarcinoma (ductal): 90%
- Others: 10% (islet cell tumors, cystadenoma or cystadenocarcinoma)
  - Slower growth and history
- Periampullary tumors may be of diverse origin and can have different patterns of progression and prognosis.

Management

Surgery

Whipple procedure, or pancreaticoduodenectomy

This procedure can be performed with or without pylorus-sparing. Patients may be taken directly to surgery if the tumor is resectable. Unresectability differs by center but distant metastases and SMA, celiac, IVC, and aorta encasement are universal definitions.

- Lymph node involvement may be resectable. Involvement of the SMV or its confluence is not always a marker of unresectability.
- Offers only means of cure, but only 5%–25% are resectable at presentation
- Should be performed in centers with high volume and extensive experience
- Age is not a strict contraindication.
- Radical pancreatectomy with extensive node dissection has not been found superior for long-term survival.
- Palliative surgeries are used when indicated, such as biliary diversion or gastrojejunostomy.
- The best predictors of survival after surgery are stage, grade, and margin status.

Recurrence tends to be in the local pancreatic bed, peritoneal cavity, or liver. Local recurrence tends to be retroperitoneal because of the difficulty achieving a clear resection plane near the great vessels.

Concurrent chemoradiation therapy

Concurrent chemoradiation therapy (CRT) is used for locally advanced disease and adjuvant therapy. The usual dose is 45–50.4 Gy in 1.8 Gy fractions to tumor or tumor bed.

Radiosensitizing chemotherapy agents include the following:
- Infusional 5-FU (maximum tolerated dose 250 mg/m^2 per day) OR
- Oral capecitabine (1600 mg/m^2 per day) as available
- Newer trials include gemcitabine, oxaliplatin, and/or paclitaxel with EBRT and have shown tolerability and similar survival to that of 5-FU.

Locally advanced disease (unresectable, nonmetastatic)
Chemoradiation offers the possibility of improved local control.
- Trial results have been mixed as to whether chemoradiation therapy or chemotherapy alone is the optimal treatment in this setting.
- 50%–80% of patients have a decrease in cancer-related pain.

Some centers have adopted neoadjuvant CRT for several reasons:
- It ensures that CRT is given in conjunction with surgery, as 25% of patients do not receive intended adjuvant therapy post-Whipple.
- It includes radiotherapy for local control and chemotherapy for potential systemic disease, with better-oxygenated tumor tissue and less bowel in radiation fields (decreased toxicity).
- It allows time for metastatic disease to become evident before potentially unnecessary surgery. An estimated 25% of patients who undergo resection have occult metastatic disease.
- It offers potential down-staging for more curative resections, although this is rare.

Adjuvant CRT is controversial; however, it remains a viable option.
- Radiation dose in this setting is 45–54 Gy.
- It is supported by one randomized clinical trial and retrospective results from several institutions, including the Johns Hopkins Medical Institute (1990s), yielding improved median survival compared with that with surgery alone (20 vs. 14 months).

Chemotherapy alone

Adjuvant
Gemcitabine has been shown to significantly improve 3-year disease-free survival (14.2 vs. 7.5 months). Overall survival is unchanged.
- Gemcitabine dosing: 1000 mg/m^2 weekly for 3 weeks every 28 days for 6 cycles is commonly used.

Metastatic disease
Gemcitabine is the first-line standard of care therapy.
- 1- year survival is 18% vs. 2% for 5-FU.
- Clinical benefit response (palliative measures) was also significant (23.8 vs. 4.8%) for gemcitabine.

A randomized phase III trial of gemcitabine plus erlotinib (either 100 or 150 mg po daily) showed statistically significant improvement in overall survival, although by approximately only 2 weeks.
   Second-line therapy has no established agent.
- Capecitabine monotherapy is often used.
- Other agents used in further lines of therapy include irinotecan and docetaxel.

Clinical trial enrollment is especially recommended, given the poor prognosis and limited treatment options for this disease.

Radiotherapy
Improved precision, multifield techniques have yielded more tolerable, higher-dose therapy by limiting the dose to off-target abdominal organs.
- Rarely given without concurrent chemotherapy
- Intraoperative radiotherapy (IORT) has shown promise in small studies of selective patients with locally advanced disease.

Targeted biological therapy
Epidermal growth factor receptor inhibition
Erlotinib is currently the only targeted therapy of known benefit, although only improving overall survival by 2 weeks when added to gemcitabine.

Cetuximab failed to improve disease-free and overall survival in final results from the phase III Southwestern Oncology Group (SWOG) S0205 study.

Vascular endothelial growth factor inhibition
Bevacizumab has been shown in the phase III CALGB 80303 trial to be of no additional benefit in the advanced setting.

Symptomatic therapies
- **Diarrhea**: Enzyme supplementation for exocrine insufficiency
  - Usually 2–4 capsules of current formulations per meal
- **Pain**: Aggressive opioid therapy
  - Gabapentin or pregabalin are often added for neuropathic pain.
  - Celiac plexus neurolysis (block) may be an excellent adjunct and can now be done via endoscopic ultrasound.
- *Jaundice, pain, cholangitis*: ERCP with stenting, percutaneous biliary drains
- *Bowel obstruction*: Enteral stenting, palliative gastrojejunostomy
- *Nausea/vomiting* from delayed gastric emptying: Metoclopromide
- *Depression*: SSRI or SNRI (especially duloxetine or venlafaxine for concurrent pain therapy) and psychotherapy. Palliative medicine consults are encouraged.

Future directions
Conformal therapy and IMRT are being explored for more precise radiotherapy. New combinations of radiosensitizers in the locally advanced setting are underway. Additional targeted agents to be tested include src and mTOR inhibitors, and TRAIL death receptor agonists.

Biomarker analysis will be vital as in all areas of oncologic drug development.

Further reading

Burris HA 3rd, Moore MJ, Andersen J, et al. (1997). Improvements in survival and clinical benefit with gemcitabine as first-line therapy for patients with advanced pancreas cancer: a randomized trial. *J Clin Oncol* 15:2403–2413.

Ghaneh P, Costello E, Neoptolemos JP (2007). Biology and management of pancreatic cancer. *Gut* 56:1134–1152.

House MG, Choti MA (2005). Palliative therapy for pancreatic/biliary cancer. *Surg Clin North Am* 5:359–371.

Moore MJ, Goldstein D, Hamm J, et al. (2007). Erlotinib plus gemcitabine compared with gemcitabine alone in patients with advanced pancreatic cancer: a phase III trial of the National Cancer Institute of Canada Clinical Trials Group. *J Clin Oncol* 25:1960–1966.

The NCCN Pancreatic Adenocarcinoma Clinical Practice Guidelines in Oncology (Version 1.2008). 2006 National Comprehensive Cancer Network, Inc. Available at: http://www.nccn.org. Accessed 15 January 2008.

Willett CG, Czito BG, Bendell JC, Ryan DP (2005). Locally advanced pancreatic cancer. *J Clin Oncol* 23:4538–4544.

Yeo C, Yeo T, Hruben R, et al. (2007). Cancer of the pancreas. In DeVita V, Hellman S, Rosenberg S (eds.), *Cancer: Principles and Practice of Oncology*, 7th ed. Philadelphia, PA: Lippincott Williams & Wilkins.

Cancers of the biliary tract

Michael Morse
Phuong L. Doan

Cholangiocarcinoma

Annual incidence is approximately 0.7–1.5 per 100,000 in the Western world; it is rare below age 40. Classified as intra- or extrahepatic, 60%–70% of cases arise at the bifurcation of the hepatic ducts (Klatskin tumors), 20%–30% in the distal common bile duct, and 5%–10% within the intrahepatic ducts of the liver peripherally.

The most important predisposing risk is sclerosing cholangitis. Other risk factors include intrahepatic stones, choledochal cysts, carcinogens, and liver fluke infections.

Cholangiocarcinomas infiltrate along the walls of the ducts and the perineural tissue before obstructing the lumen. Metastases to the lymph nodes are seen in 13%–30% of patients undergoing surgery. Direct duodenal invasion and peritoneal carcinomatosis occur late.

More than 90% of cholangiocarcinomas are adenocarcinomas.

Symptoms
- Painless jaundice (occasionally intermittent)
- Palpable gall bladder (Courvoisier's sign)
- Weight loss
- Fatigue
- Pruritus

Diagnosis
Simple blood tests can indicate obstructive jaundice:
- Elevated bilirubin and alkaline phosphatase
- Elevated transaminases with cholangitis
- Elevated CA19–9 and, in some cases, CEA
- Prolonged prothrombin time if vitamin K deficient or liver failure

Imaging modalities include ultrasound, computed tomography (CT), MRI cholangiography, and percutaneous transhepatic cholangiopancreatography (PTC).

Endoscopic retrograde cholangiopancreatography (ERCP) with brushings of the biliary ducts offers both diagnostic information and a mechanism for therapeutic biliary decompression.

An angiogram may be needed to assess vessel involvement.

Management
These should be resected if there are no distant metastases and no involvement of the hepatic artery and portal vein. Resection of extrahepatic cholangiocarcinomas requires complex surgery:
- For tumors in the proximal third of the duct l lymphadenectomy with or without en bloc liver resection
- For tumors in the distal third of the duct l pancreaticoduodenectomy with lymphadenectomy

Five-year survival for resected intrahepatic cholangiocarcinoma is 20%–40%, for hilar, it is 11%–25%, and for distal, it is 28%.

A few centers will perform liver transplantation in very select patients with small cholangiocarcinomas.

Adjuvant chemoradiotherapy is recommended on the basis of retrospective data for extrahepatic cholangiocarcinomas, particularly if there are positive margins or there is lymph node involvement. Observation or chemoradiotherapy is considered if lymph nodes are not involved and the margins are negative.

For unresectable cholangiocarcinomas, patients should be offered best supportive care, chemotherapy with 5-fluorouracil with or without radiation, or gemcitabine-based combinations of therapy. All patients should undergo palliative biliary drainage if obstruction is observed.

Gallbladder cancer

Epidemiology
- Most common biliary tract cancer
- Majority of cases present over age 70
- Women are affected 3:1 more often than men
- The most important risk factor for gallbladder cancer is gallstones and associated chronic cholecystitis.
- Other risk factors include calcified gallbladder, gallbladder polyps, typhoid carriers, and exposure to carcinogens.

Symptoms and clinical presentation
- Obstructive jaundice
- Abdominal pain
- Right upper quadrant mass

Diagnosis and prognosis
The diagnosis of gallbladder cancer is often made in advanced stages, usually at cholecystectomy.
- Liver function tests, CEA, and CA19–9 may be increased.
- Ultrasound may reveal a suspicious mass.
- CT or MRI can define the following:
  - Invasion of ducts
  - Lymphadenopathy
  - Secondary liver lesions
- For tumors detected in early stages, the 5-year survival rate is 90%.
- For tumors detected in advanced stages and that are resectable, the 5-year survival rate is 20%–40%.

Pathology and staging
Histologic subtypes
- Adenocarcinoma is the most common subtype (glandular, medullary, scirrhous, papillary, colloid). Papillary form carries a better prognosis.
- Epidermoid, 6.5%; adenoacanthomas, 4%
- Others: Small cell, carcinoid, anaplastic

Staging is based on the degree of muscle and vessel invasion and lymph node involvement.

Management

Surgery is the only treatment that offers cure. Prophylactic surgery should be considered in patients with a porcelain gall bladder and patients with polyps over 1 cm in size (risk of malignancy is significant).

Patients with incidentally identified gallbladder cancer after a cholecystectomy should be considered for hepatic resection (gallbladder bed) and lymphadenectomy.

Adjuvant 5-fluorouracil and radiation (and/or gemcitabine) is recommended for almost all patients with resectable disease. One phase III clinical trial showed that adjuvant therapy doubles 5-year survival.

For unresectable tumors, treatment options are as follows:
- Enrollment in clinical trial
- Best supportive care
- 5-fluorouracil and radiation
- Gemcitabine-based chemotherapy
- Palliative biliary decompression

Current trials are investigating the role of capecitabine, oxaliplatin, and bevacizumab in gallbladder cancer.

Further reading

Rajagopalan V, Daines WP, Grossbard ML, et al. (2004). Gallbladder and biliary tract carcinoma: a comprehensive update. Part I. *Oncology* 18:889–896.

Reid KM, Ramos-De la Medina A, Donohue JH (2007). Diagnosis and surgical management of gallbladder cancer: a review. *J Gastrointest Surg* 11:671–681.

Yonemoto N, Furuse J, Okusaka T, et al. (2007). A multicenter retrospective analysis of survival benefits of chemotherapy for unresectable biliary tract cancer. *Jpn J Clin Oncol* 37:843–851.

Hepatocellular carcinoma

Michael Morse
Phuong L. Doan

Epidemiology
- Hepatocellular carcinoma (HCC) is the seventh most common cancer and third-ranked cause of cancer death globally.
- Estimated 1 million deaths annually, 5-year survival rate is 5%
- Incidence is 2.4 cases per 100,000 people in Western countries and 120 per 100,000 in Asia and Africa.
- The majority of cases present under age 50.
- Men are affected more frequently than women; African Americans more often than Caucasians.
- Chronic hepatitis B accounts for a proportion of cases, but hepatitis C infection is increasingly becoming a cause.
  - The latency period between hepatitis B or C exposure and HCC is 30 years.
- Patients with cirrhosis have 1%–2% annual risk of developing HCC.
- Other risk factors include hereditary hemochromatosis, aflatoxin exposure, a_1-antitrypsin deficiency, NASH, and alcoholic cirrhosis.

Symptoms
Symptoms present in advanced disease and are due to mechanical effects of tumor growth and paraneoplastic syndrome (see Table 30.3).

Diagnosis and prognosis
The diagnosis of HCC is made on the basis of history, laboratory, and radiological findings of a mass lesion within the liver. Immunohistochemistry can distinguish between HCC and other primary and metastatic liver cancers.

Initial lab studies include complete blood count, hepatitis serologies, liver chemistries, prothrombin, albumin, creatinine, and lactate dehydrogenase. α-Fetoprotein is elevated in 60%–90% of patients with advanced HCC.

CT or MRI can be used to define the following:
- Number and size of lesions
- Vascular anatomy and tumor involvement
- Extrahepatic disease

Positron emission tomography (PET) has a lower sensitivity than that of CT for detecting HCC. Tumor size and vascular invasion are the most important prognostic factors.

Biopsy of liver mass should be deferred if there is potential for surgical resection, because of the risk of tumor seeding.

Table 30.3 Symptoms of hepatocellular carcinoma

Mechanical effects of tumor growth	Paraneoplastic syndrome
Right upper-quadrant pain is the most common symptom	Hypoglycemia
Weight loss and anorexia	Erythrocytosis
Abdominal distension	Hypercalcemia
Intraperitoneal hemorrhage and ascites	Hypercholesterolemia

Pathology and staging

Disease may appear as a large, solitary tumor or as a central mass with satellite lesions. Histologic subtypes include trabecular, pseudoglandular or acinar, compact, scirrhous, clear cell, and fibrolamellar. Of these subtypes, the fibrolamellar variant carries the best prognosis and is often resectable.

Many staging systems exist, based on clinical and radiographic features:
- Cancer of the Liver Italian Program (CLIP) is the most commonly used staging system for unresectable HCC.
- Okuda staging assesses adverse predictors: larger tumor size, ascites, hypoalbuminemia, and hyperbilirubinemia
- Barcelona Clinic Liver Cancer staging system accounts for performance status, liver function, extent of tumor, and treatment.

Management

Surgery

Surgical resection and transplantation are the only treatments that offer cure. In transplanted patients, 5-year survival is 75%.

Resection is not possible in many patients because of low performance status, comorbidity, or extent of liver disease.

Laparoscopic surgery is gaining acceptance, with less postoperative morbidity and low mortality.

In cirrhotic patients with hepatitis C with HCC lesions <3 cm, liver transplantation is preferred to resection because of a high likelihood of developing new tumor lesions with resection alone.

Nonsurgical management

Enrollment in clinical trial is recommended.

Liver-directed approaches
- Radiofrequency ablation
- Transarterial embolization with or without chemotherapy deprives tumor of vascular supply and induces tumor necrosis.
- Transarterial, intrahepatic radiolabeled spheres
- Percutaneous absolute alcohol injection directly into the tumor

Sorafenib
This is an inhibitor of cell proliferation and vascular endothelial growth factor receptor (VEGFR)
- Offers improved median overall survival when compared with placebo
- Should be considered first-line therapy in patients with unresectable HCC
- Major adverse reactions are diarrhea, anorexia, fatigue, and bleeding.

Systemic chemotherapy
- Monotherapy with doxorubicin or in combination with cisplatin and 5-FU
- No survival advantage in single-drug or combination chemotherapy
- Capecitabine offers modest antitumor benefit.

Best supportive care
Other investigative therapies
- Erlotinib is an epidermal growth factor receptor (EGFR) inhibitor. Most HCCs overexpress EGFR.
- EGFR inhibition with erlotinib can delay disease progression, with acceptable toxicities of skin rash and diarrhea.
- Bevacizumab and sunitinb are VEGF inhibitors that have improved time to disease progression in nonrandomized clinical trials compared with historical data.

Further reading

Carr B (2005). *Hepatocellular Cancer: Diagnosis and Treatment*. Totowa, NJ: Humana Press.

Khan MA, Combs CS, Brunt EM, et al. (2000). Positron emission tomography scanning in the evaluation of hepatocellular carcinoma. *J Hepatol* 32:791–797.

Llovet J, Ricci S, Mazzaferro V, et al. (2007). Sorafenib improves survival in advanced hepatocellular carcinoma (HCC): results of a phase III randomized placebo-controlled trial (SHARP trial). *J Clin Oncol* 2007 ASCO Annual Meeting Proceedings Part I. 25 (June 20 Suppl):LBA1.

Thomas M, Chadha R, Glover K, et al. (2007). Phase II study of erlotinib in patients with unresectable hepatocellular carcinoma. *Cancer* 110:1059–1067.

Villa E, Colantoni A, Cammà C, et al. (2003). Estrogen receptor classification for hepatocellular carcinoma: comparison with clinical staging systems. *J Clin Oncol* 21:441–446.

Chapter 31

Gastrointestinal cancer III: colorectal, anus

S. Yousuf Zafar
Gerard Blobe

Colorectal cancer 500
  Introduction 500
  Staging 500
  Surgery for colorectal cancer 500
  Adjuvant chemotherapy for colorectal cancer 502
  Radiotherapy for rectal cancer 503
  Palliative therapy for metastatic colorectal cancer 504
Anal cancer 508
  Introduction 508
  Staging 509
  Workup 510
  Initial treatment 510
  Palliative treatment 510
  Rarer tumors 511
  Practical points 511

Colorectal cancer

Introduction

Epidemiology
- Colorectal cancer is the third most common cancer in the United States (over 140,000 cases/year), and it is the second most common cause of cancer death.
- It affects men and women equally.
- Mean age at diagnosis is 71 years.
- Primarily adenocarcinoma

Risk factors
- Average-risk patients have a lifetime incidence of 5%.
- 90% of cases occur after age 50.
- 1/3 of cases are associated with familial clustering.
- One affected first-degree relative increases risk to 1.7x that of the general population.
- Patients with familial adenomatous polyposis (FAP) have a 90% risk of colorectal cancer by age 50.
- Patients with hereditary nonpolyposis colorectal cancer (HNPCC) have an 80% lifetime risk of developing colorectal cancer.
- Diets high in fat and low in fruits and vegetables, decreased physical inactivity, and obesity have been associated with an increased risk.

Survival
- 5-year overall survival rate is approximately 60%.
- 5-year survival rate for localized disease is 90%.
- 5-year survival rate for metastatic disease is 10%.

Staging
See Table 31.1
- Stage I: T1-2, N0
- Stage IIA: T3, N0
- Stage IIB: T4, N0
- Stage IIIA: T1-T2, N1
- Stage IIIB: T3-T4, N1
- Stage IIIC: Any T, N2
- Stage IV: Any T, any N, M1

Surgery for colorectal cancer

Surgery is the mainstay of curative therapy for colorectal cancer. Curative resection requires the excision of the primary tumor and its lymphatic drainage with a margin of normal tissue.

Preoperative workup
- Precise site and local extent of the tumor should be known before laparotomy.
- Full colonoscopy (in the absence of obstruction or perforation) should be performed prior to laparotomy.
- CT of the chest, abdomen, and pelvis should be obtained to assess for distant disease.

Table 31.1 Colorectal cancer TNM staging system

T—primary tumor	
Tis	Carcinoma in situ
T1	Tumor invades submucosa
T2	Tumor invades muscularis propria
T3	Tumor invades through muscularis into subserosa, or into nonperitonealized pericolic or perirectal tissue
T4	Tumor invading adjacent organ(s) and/or perforates visceral peritoneum
N—Regional lymph nodes	
N0	No regional lymph node metastasis
N1	Metastasis in 1–3 regional nodes
N2	Metastasis in ≥4 regional nodes
M—Distant metastasis	
M1	Distant metastasis

- Preoperative CBC, chemistry profiles, and carcinoembryonic antigen (CEA) level should be obtained.
- For rectal cancer, endorectal ultrasound (EUS) or pelvic MRI should be obtained to assess stage and the depth of invasion.
- An enterostomal therapist should be consulted as needed for site marking and patient education.

Primary surgical resection

Colectomy with en bloc removal of regional lymph nodes is the procedure of choice for resectable colon cancer. At least 12 lymph nodes should be examined for accurate staging.

Minimally invasive colon cancer surgery is becoming more common but should only be performed by experienced surgeons in selected cases.

Rectal cancer

Transanal resections should only be performed for small (<3 cm), T1–T2, well to moderately differentiated, mobile tumors located within 8 cm from the anal verge, and in the absence of lymphadenopathy.

Transabdominal resection via abdominoperineal or low anterior resection should be performed using total mesorectal excision (TME). TME reduces the incidence of positive surgical margins and resects draining lymphatics.

Resection of metastatic or recurrent disease

Resection of liver or lung metastases should generally not be considered in the setting of additional, unresectable extrahepatic or extrapulmonary disease. Solitary liver metastases have a better postresection prognosis than that of multiple liver lesions.

No definitive criteria exist (e.g., number or size of tumors) to determine eligibility for liver resection. Eligibility should instead be determined by likelihood of achieving negative margins while preserving liver function.

Five-year survival rates in selected patients following resection of liver metastases are approximately 30%–50%.

Adjuvant chemotherapy for colorectal cancer

Rationale

Approximately half of patients undergoing apparently curative resection of colorectal cancer are destined to relapse and eventually die with either locally recurrent or distant metastatic disease due to the presence of residual micrometastases at the time of surgery. The aim of adjuvant chemotherapy is to eradicate these micrometastases and thereby decrease the risk of relapse.

Indications

Adjuvant chemotherapy is an exercise in risk reduction. Multidisciplinary team discussion is essential. Questions to be considered after a potentially curative operation are the following:
- What is the probability of micrometastases?
- Will adjuvant therapy prevent or delay relapse?
- What are the side effects of chemotherapy?

After surgery, the risk of micrometastases is estimated by examining the pathological features of the primary cancer.

Stage III cancers, which have spread to the nearby lymph nodes, carry a much higher risk (~50%). There is substantial evidence that this risk is reduced by adjuvant chemotherapy, which is the standard of care in the absence of a strong contraindication.

Stage II cancers, which have breached the muscle layers but not spread to lymph nodes, carry an intermediate risk of ~30%. There is limited evidence to support the use of adjuvant chemotherapy in these patients. However, the use of adjuvant chemotherapy should be discussed in high-risk stage II patients (T4 tumor stage, bowel perforation, or clinical obstruction).

Rectal cancer presents some special considerations. A relative lack of a barrier to lateral spread and increased technical difficulty of surgery in the pelvis combine to increase the risk of local recurrence. Radiotherapy, targeted to the pelvis either before or after surgery, reduces local recurrence rates. Adjuvant therapy for rectal cancer may therefore include both radiotherapy and chemotherapy, determined by the preoperative regimen used.

Chemotherapy used in the adjuvant setting

5-fluorouracil (5-FU) given in combination with folinic acid, by bolus intravenous (IV) injection, was standard of care until 2004.

In 2004, the addition of oxaliplatin (platinum analog) to infusional 5-FU and leucovorin (FOLFOX) was shown to result in longer disease-free survival (and longer overall survival among stage III patients) at the cost of some (mainly short-lived) extra toxicity. Six months of FOLFOX therapy is now the standard adjuvant therapy.

Single-agent capecitabine is equivalent to 5-FU-leucovorin for adjuvant treatment of resected stage III patients, but it should be reserved for those unable to tolerate FOLFOX.

Studies investigating the addition of agents that target EGF or VEGF receptors in the adjuvant setting have not provided support for use of these agents outside the context of a clinical trial.

Toxicity

The clinical activity of 5-FU and its side effects are both dependent on the dose and schedules used, which vary considerably from patient to patient. The side-effect profile should, for most patients, be quite tolerable and consistent with continuing normal activity, including work. Treatment is feasible and effective even in the elderly.

Common side effects
- Nausea and vomiting
- Oral mucositis
- Diarrhea
- Red, painful palms, and soles (with capecitabine, the oral formulation of 5-FU, or continuous infusion of 5-FU)
- Peripheral neuropathy (due to oxaliplatin)
- Cytopenias (due to oxaliplatin)

Radiotherapy for rectal cancer

For colon cancer, radiotherapy is limited to the palliative setting. However, the rectum is immobile and fixed within the pelvis, providing a more suitable target for radiotherapy. Radiotherapy has been used in both the preoperative and postoperative setting in rectal cancer.

5-FU is also a radiosensitizer. For patients with rectal cancer, pelvic radiotherapy is often given concurrently with a fluoropyrimidine to harness this effect. Chemoradiotherapy may be followed by a more prolonged course of adjuvant chemotherapy aimed at distant micrometastases. The treatment course for rectal cancer is dependent on stage:
- T1–2, N0: Resection followed by observation
- T3, N0 or T any, N1–2: Preoperative chemoradiotherapy (approximately 5 weeks) with continuous infusion 5-FU, followed by surgery, followed by adjuvant chemotherapy (FOLFOX) for 4 months
- T4, or initially unresectable: Preoperative chemoradiotherapy, followed by resection, if possible, followed by FOLFOX for 4 months
- Patients who do not receive preoperative chemoradiotherapy may receive it postoperatively, followed by additional adjuvant chemotherapy.

Palliative therapy for metastatic colorectal cancer

In the absence of further therapy, metastatic colorectal cancer has a poor prognosis with a median survival time of 6 months. The goals of therapy are palliation and prolongation of survival. With current therapy, median survival is increased to approximately 2 years.

In most cases chemotherapy is the primary modality used, but this does not preclude the use of combined modalities such as surgery, localized radiotherapy, or ablative techniques for liver metastases.

A small proportion of patients have oligometastatic disease, disease that is potentially resectable or could be made so by volume reduction using chemotherapy (down-staging). These highly selected patients should be identified and treated within a multidisciplinary team setting with a view toward surgical resection and potential cure.

First-line chemotherapy
See Table 31.2

Infusional 5-fluorouracil or oral capecitabine forms the backbone of therapy.
- 5-FU/leucovorin alone or capecitabine alone is usually reserved for patients unable to tolerate combination therapy.
- Combination therapy includes a fluoropyrimidine with either oxaliplatin or irinotecan.
- Chemotherapy can be combined with targeted therapy against VEGF (bevacizumab) or EGFR (cetuximab or panitumumab). Note that EGFR targeted therapy should not be used for KRAS mutant tumors.

Oxaliplatin synergy with fluoropyrimidines has been demonstrated in clinical trials.
- Combination studies with 5-FU-based regimens versus the same regimen without oxaliplatin have confirmed a higher response rate, with some studies also demonstrating a survival benefit.
- A striking feature of these studies is the number of patients who are "down-staged" by the combination therapy and then go on to have salvage surgery, with some achieving long-term remission.
- Potential toxicities are neurotoxicity and neutropenia.
- Dose reduction of oxaliplatin should be initiated with the onset of neuropathy, with discontinuation considered with ≥grade 3 neuropathy.

Irinotecan is a topoisomerase inhibitor. In combination with 5-FU, first-line trials confirmed a higher response rate and overall survival.
- Potential toxicities are diarrhea and neutropenia.
- Either oxaliplatin or irinotecan are acceptable in combination with 5-FU for first-line therapy. Selection of either agent should be based on prior therapy and toxicity profile.

Capecitabine, an orally administered prodrug of 5-FU, is an effective part of combination therapy in the metastatic setting.
- In advanced colorectal cancer, capecitabine has shown equivalent survival to that with a 5-FU regimen.
- The convenience to the patient of replacing infusional regimens of 5-FU with oral medication is an important factor.

Table 31.2 Chemotherapy regimens

Regimen	Agents	Interval
mFOLFOX6-bevacizumab	Oxaliplatin 85 mg/m^2, day 1; leucovorin 400 mg/m^2, day 1; 5-FU 400 mg/m^2 bolus, day 1, then 2400 mg/m^2 continuous infusion over 46 hours; bevacizumab 5 mg/kg, day 1	Every 2 weeks
FOLFIRI-bevacizumab	Irinotecan 180 mg/m^2, day 1; leucovorin 400 mg/m^2, day 1; 5-FU 400 mg/m^2 bolus, day 1, then 2400 mg/m^2 continuous infusion over 46 hours; bevacizumab 5 mg/kg, day 1	Every 2 weeks
CapeOX-bevacizumab	Oxaliplatin 85–130 mg/m^2, day 1; capecitabine 850–1000 mg/m^2, twice daily for 14 days; bevacizumab 7.5 mg/kg, day 1.	Every 3 weeks
5-FU/LV ± bevacizumab	Leucovorin 400 mg/m^2, day 1; 5-FU 400 mg/m^2 bolus, day 1, then 2400 mg/m^2 continuous infusion over 46 hours; bevacizumab 5 mg/kg, day 1	Every 2 weeks

- Studies combining capecitabine with irinotecan or oxaliplatin have shown favorable response rates, although greater toxicity is seen with the combination of capecitabine with irinotecan than with oxaliplatin.
- Higher doses are tolerated by Europeans than by Americans.

Bevacizumab, an antivascular endothelial growth factor (VEGF) monoclonal antibody, has been shown to improve survival in the metastatic setting.
- The most common toxicities are hypertension, proteinuria, and delayed wound healing.
- Less common—though severe—toxicities are hemorrhage, gastrointestinal perforation, stroke, myocardial infarction, and arterial thromboembolism.

Cetuximab, a chimeric antiepidermal growth factor receptor (EGFR) monoclonal antibody, and panitumumab, a human anti-EGFR monoclonal antibody, have both been shown to improve outcomes in the first line metastatic setting in combination with chemotherapy for patients with *KRAS* wild-type tumors.

KRAS mutation status of tumor tissue should be assessed before treatment with an EGFR inhibitor, because *KRAS* mutation has been associated with lack of response to EGR inhibitors in advanced colorectal cancer.
- The most common toxicities are rash, skin fissures, paronychia and hypomagnesemia.
- For cetuximab, infusion reactions, which can be quite severe, are also a significant concern.

Combinations of the agents listed above have been tested in a large number of clinical trials.
- Consensus exists that combination therapy offers higher response rates at the cost of some increase in subjective toxicity.
- Extended, planned treatment breaks (not related to toxicity) should not be a part of standard therapy.
- Dosing should be adjusted for toxicity.

Second-line chemotherapy

Patients who progressed on first-line therapy with oxaliplatin and bevacizumab should be treated with irinotecan with or without 5-FU, and with or without bevacizumab, cetuximab or panitumumab (if *KRAS* wild-type). In *KRAS* wild-type tumors, cetuximab and panitumumab have both shown efficacy as single agents and in combination with irinotecan. Cetuximab or panitumumab and bevacizumab should not be used in combination outside of a clinical trial.

Patients who progressed on first-line therapy with irinotecan and bevacizumab should be treated with oxaliplatin and 5-FU (FOLFOX or XELOX), with or without cetuximab or panitumumab (if *KRAS* wild-type).

A recent study has provided support for aflibercept, a VEGF receptor trap, in the second line in combination with FOLFIRI. It is unclear whether aflibercept provides any benefit in this setting relative to bevacizumab.

Potential second-line regimens (assuming first-line treatment with oxaliplatin) include FOLFIRI-bevacizumab, FOLFIRI-cetuximab or panitumumab, FOLFIRI-aflibercept, irinotecan-cetuximab or panitumumab, single-agent irinotecan, or single-agent cetuximab or panitumumab.

Subsequent chemotherapy

With increasing survival, colorectal cancer patients are exposed to multiple lines of therapy. Clinical-trial participation should be encouraged for patients with good performance status.

Single-agent therapy with cetuximab or panitumumab (fully humanized monoclonal antibody to the EGFR) is acceptable if the patient has not yet been treated with these agents and does not have a *KRAS* mutation.

Head-to-head comparisons of cetuximab versus panitumumab are not yet available, although they might be considered equivalent. Current data do not support treating patients who have progressed on cetuximab with panitumumab (or vice versa).

Recent data provide support for the use of regorafenib, a multityrosine kinase inhibitor (VEGR, PDGFR, RET, c-Kit), in refractory metastatic colon cancer patients. However, in the clinical trial, the benefit was modest, and toxicity was a concern.

Toxicities of regorafenib include hand-foot syndrome, fatigue, hypertension, diarrhea, and rash.

Anal cancer

Introduction

Epidemiology
- This is a rare cancer, with 6000 cases in the United States in 2011.
- Anal tumors comprise 1.7% of all digestive system malignancies.
- The anal canal extends from the perianal skin (anal verge) to rectal mucosa, approximately 3–4 cm.
- Most anal tumors arise from the epidermal elements of the anal canal lining (squamous cell—85% of anal tumors), although some arise from the glandular mucosa of the uppermost part of the anal canal or from the anal ducts and glands (adenocarcinomas—10% of anal tumors).
  - Adenocarcinomas should be treated as rectal cancers.
- The anal margin includes the perianal skin. Anal margin tumors are staged and treated slightly differently than anal canal tumors.

Etiology
- Anal cancer is strongly associated with human papillomavirus (HPV).
- Sexually transmitted disease
- Risk factors include: receptive anal intercourse; >10 sexual partners; prior cervical, vulvar, or vaginal cancer; immunosuppression after solid organ transplant; HIV infection; and cigarette smoking.

Pathology and natural history
Included within the category of epidermal derived anal canal cancers are squamous cell carcinomas, basaloid carcinomas, transitional (or cloacogenic) carcinomas, and mucoepidermoid cancers. The anal sphincter and the rectovaginal septum, perineal body, and the vagina are common sites of direct invasion.

Anal cancers above the dentate line are likely to drain to internal iliac lymph nodes. More proximal tumors drain to inferior mesenteric or perirectal nodes. Tumors below the dentate line drain to the superficial inguinal nodes.

- 60%–70% present with early-stage disease (stages I–II).
- 10%–40% of patients will present with inguinal lymph node involvement.
- 5-year survival for tumors <5 cm is 80%, but drops to 50% for tumors >5 cm.

Clinical presentation
Common symptoms include the following:
- Pain, mass sensation (30%)
- Bleeding (45%), often attributed to hemorrhoids
- No symptoms (20%)

Staging
See Table 31.3.

Anal cancer
- Stage I: T1, N0
- Stage II: T2–3, N0
- Stage IIIA: T1–3, N1 or T4, N0
- Stage IIIB: T4, N1 or any T, N2–3
- Stage IV: Any T, any N, M1

Anal margin cancer
- Stage I: T1, N0
- Stage II: T2–3, N0
- Stage III: T4, N0 or any T, N1
- Stage IV: Any T, any N, M1

Table 31.3 TNM staging system

Cancer of the anal canal	
T—primary tumor	
Tis	Carcinoma in situ
T1	Tumor 2 cm or less in greatest dimension
T2	Tumor >2 cm but not >5 cm in greatest dimension
T3	Tumor >5 cm in greatest dimension
T4	Tumor invading adjacent organ(s) (vagina, prostate, pelvic wall)
N—Regional lymph nodes	
N0	No regional lymph node metastasis
N1	Regional lymph node metastasis
N2	Metastasis in unilateral internal iliac and/or inguinal lymph node(s)
N3	Metastasis in perirectal and inguinal lymph nodes and/or bilateral internal iliac and/or inguinal lymph nodes
Cancer of the anal margin	
T—primary tumor	
Tis, T1, -2, -3	Identical to cancer of the anal canal
T4	Tumor invades deep extradermal structures (cartilage, skeletal muscle, or bone)
N—regional lymph nodes	
N0	No regional lymph node metastasis
N1	Regional lymph node metastasis

Workup
- Digital rectal exam
- Careful examination under anesthetic with biopsy of lesion, documentation of length, site, and extent of primary tumors
- Inguinal lymph node evaluation, biopsy/FNA cytology of enlarged inguinal lymph nodes
- CT or MRI scan: chest, abdomen, and pelvis
- Consider HIV testing
- Gynecological exam and cervical cancer screening for women

Initial treatment
Over the last 20 years, treatment of this cancer has moved from surgery (abdominoperineal resection) to organ-conserving therapy. Chemoradiation is now a standard treatment for most patients (T1–4, and all node-positive patients).

- Chemotherapy consists of the combination of 5-FU (1000 mg/m^2 per day on days 1–4 and 28–31 of radiation) and mitomycin (10 mg/m^2 on days 1 and 28, with a maximum of 20 mg/cycle)
- Radiation is given to 45 Gy in 1.8 Gy fractions over 5 weeks.
- 5-FU alone has been shown to result in worse colostomy-free and disease-free survival than the 5-FU-mitomycin combination.
- The use of cisplatin in place of mitomycin results in worse overall survival, worse disease-free survival, higher rates of colostomy, and more days spent receiving chemotherapy. As a result, cisplatin is not used.
- Limited data suggests that adjuvant chemotherapy after definitive chemoradiation does not improve rates of complete response.
- For anal margin cancer (as opposed to anal canal cancer), initial treatment is as follows:
  - T1, N0: local excision
  - T2–T4, N0 or any T, N+: 5-FU and mitomycin with concurrent radiotherapy

Palliative treatment
Surveillance
- Response should be evaluated in 8–12 weeks posttreatment by physical exam (including inguinal node palpation), digital rectal exam, ± biopsy.
- Patients should be observed every 3–6 months for 5 years, with annual chest/abdomen/pelvis imaging.

Recurrence
- Local failure occurs in approximately 40% of patients.
- Patients with tumors >5 cm are at highest risk for local recurrence (40%–64%)
- Preferred treatment for recurrent disease after chemoradiotherapy is abdominoperineal resection.
- Postoperative complications are greater in those who have received chemoradiotherapy.
- Salvage chemoradiotherapy with 5-FU, cisplatin, and radiotherapy had unexceptional results but remains the standard treatment for recurrent disease.

Metastatic disease
- 10%–17% of patients treated with chemoradiotherapy develop metastases.
- The most common sites of metastases are the liver, lung, and lymph nodes outside the pelvis.
- Published data to treat metastatic disease are limited, but the standard treatment is 5-FU-cisplatin.
- Clinical trial participation should be encouraged.

Rarer tumors

Adenocarcinoma

Adenocarcinoma in the anal canal is usually a very low rectal cancer that has spread downward to involve the canal and is thus treated as a rectal cancer. True adenocarcinoma of the anal canal can occur, probably arising from the anal glands that are found around the dentate line and pass radially outward into the sphincter muscles. This is a very rare tumor; although it is radiosensitive, it is still usually treated by radical surgery.

Malignant melanoma

This tumor is exceedingly rare, accounting for just 1% of anal canal malignant tumors. The lesion may mimic a thrombosed external hemorrhoid because of its color, although amelanotic tumors also occur. It has a worse prognosis than melanoma at other sites. Because the chances of cure are minimal, radical surgery as primary treatment is infrequently attempted.

Practical points

- Rectal bleeding and anal pain are common: a high degree of suspicion is required to diagnose anal cancer correctly.
- Multifocal anal and genital disease may coexist: be sure to examine the anal and genital areas.
- Examination under anesthetic is essential for adequate staging and permits a generous biopsy.
- Biopsy or needle aspiration of enlarged inguinal lymph nodes is essential before treatment.
- Local excision may be appropriate for small anal-margin cancers.
- Chemoradiotherapy is the treatment of choice for most anal squamous carcinomas.

Chapter 32

Endocrine cancers

Gary H. Lyman

Thyroid cancer 514
Surgery for thyroid cancer 520
Radioiodine treatment for thyroid cancer 522
External beam radiotherapy for thyroid cancer 524
Chemotherapy for thyroid cancer 525
Surveillance, follow-up, and prognosis for thyroid cancer 526
Adrenal cancer 528
Neuroblastoma 532

Thyroid cancer

Epidemiology and etiology
- Thyroid cancer accounts for approximately 1% of all malignancies and 0.5% of all cancer deaths.
- Annual cases (deaths) in the United States:
  - 28,410 (910) in women
  - 8930 (680) in men
- Female preponderance is 3:1.
- Preponderance is in the fourth and fifth decades.
- Relatives of patients with thyroid cancer have a 10-fold increased risk.

Papillary including mixed papillary-follicular carcinomas
- 75%–80% of thyroid cancers
- Peak age 30–50 years
- The only well-established risk factor is previous head and neck irradiation, particularly in early childhood.
- ≥1 affected first-degree relative in approximately 5%
- Occurs in a few rare inherited syndromes, e.g., familial adenomatous polyposis, Gardner's syndrome
- Lymph node involvement in >50%
- Cure rate is close to 100% for small tumors in patients.

Follicular and/or Hurthle cell carcinomas
- 15%–20% of thyroid cancers
- Peak age is 40–60 years.
- Less common with radiation exposure
- Lymph node involvement in approximately 10%
- Cure rate is 95% for small tumors in younger patients.

Anaplastic (undifferentiated) carcinomas
- 1%–2% of all thyroid cancers
- Typically in older population than that with differentiated tumors; mean age at presentation is 65 years. They occur in females more than in males.
- More than 1 in 5 patients will have a previous history or coexisting diagnosis of differentiated carcinoma.
- Up to 50% have a history of multinodular goiter.
- There is increased risk for these carcinomas after radiation exposure.
- More than 90% have lymph node involvement at diagnosis.
- Very poor prognosis: 3-year survival 10%

Medullary carcinoma
- 5% of all thyroid cancers
- Typically in fifth to sixth decade of life
- Slight female preponderance
- Not associated with radiation exposure
- 80% of cases are sporadic.

- 20% of cases are familial, tending to occur in younger age groups, i.e., the third decade. If there is more than one case within the family, always consider the possibility of familial disease, e.g.:
  - Multiple endocrine neoplasia (MEN) types 2a (Sipple syndrome) and 2b
  - Isolated familial medullary thyroid cancer
- Lymph node involvement occurs early in the disease course.
- Prognosis is poor with MEN-2b, particularly in men >50 years and with distant metastases.

Pathology and genetics

Papillary including papillary-follicular carcinomas

These carcinomas arise from follicular cells of the thyroid and typically respond to TSH by taking up iodine and producing thyroglobulin. Typically they are unencapsulated with or without cystic components.

Papillae consist of a few layers of tumor cells surrounding fibrovascular core. Follicles and colloid are usually absent. 50% contain calcified psammoma bodies (scarred remnants of tumor papillae).

More than 50% of sporadic cases have somatic gene rearrangements, e.g., of the *RET* oncogenes, producing chimeric proteins with tyrosine kinase activity that contribute to the development of malignancy. No germline mutations have been identified so far.

There are several histological subtypes, most of which are rare. Examples include the following:
- Follicular variant
  - Most common subtype (15%)
  - Microscopically small to medium-sized follicles with near-total absence of papillae
  - Prone to hematogenous spread but less likely to show lymphatic invasion
- Tall-cell variant
  - ~1% of papillary cancers
  - More aggressive than common-type papillary tumors. There is a higher incidence of local invasion and distant metastases at presentation.

Follicular carcinomas

Like papillary carcinomas, neoplastic elements arise from follicular cells of the thyroid and typically respond to TSH by taking up iodine and producing thyroglobulin.
- Typically round, encapsulated neoplasms
- Fibrosis, hemorrhage, and cystic changes are commonly found.
- Differentiated from benign follicular adenomas by tumor capsule invasion and/or vascular invasion (distinction can be difficult with fine needle biopsy and frozen-section evaluation).
- Nearly always immunohistochemistry (IHC) positive for thyroglobulin and cytokeratin

Anaplastic (undifferentiated) carcinomas

These are undifferentiated tumors of the thyroid follicular epithelium.

Medullary

This unencapsulated neuroendocrine tumor arises from the parafollicular C cells (the cell of origin of calcitonin). They have variable histological appearance within a single tumor, with 80% showing amyloid deposition; 98% are calcitonin positive.

MEN type 2 autosomal, dominantly inherited syndromes arise from different mutations in the *RET* proto-oncogene.
- *MEN type 2a*: 100% of patients get medullary thyroid cancer, 50% develop pheochromocytomas, and 30% get hyperplasia of the parathyroid glands.
- *MEN type 2b*: Medullary carcinoma of the thyroid, which is often bilateral, more aggressive, and occurs at an earlier age. There is also Marfanoid appearance and pheochromocytomas, but normal PTH.
- *Familial medullary thyroid cancer* is a variant of MEN type 2a with a similar high risk of medullary carcinoma without the other associated diseases.

Half of sporadic cases have somatic *RET* gene mutations as well.

Other thyroid tumors
- Lymphoma
- Metastases, e.g., from breast or colon cancer

Screening and prevention

Medullary carcinoma

Prophylactic thyroidectomy at an early age is often appropriate if the patient is a known carrier of predisposing gene mutation, e.g., in MEN 2.
Screening with serum calcitonin:
- Supranormal serum calcitonin response to intravenous calcium suggests C-cell hyperplasia or overt medullary carcinoma, but can also be a false positive result, e.g., in autoimmune thyroid disease.

Screening is now usually by molecular analysis for germline *RET* gene mutations. Approximately 7% of apparently sporadic cases are also positive for germline mutations in the *RET* proto-oncogene with significant implications for family members.

Presentation

Papillary and follicular carcinomas
- Incidental microcarcinomas (<1 cm) are a common finding at autopsy.
- The most common clinical presentation is with a painless lump in the neck, i.e., solitary thyroid nodule.
- Clinical regional lymph node involvement at diagnosis is more common in children than in adults.
  - Occult nodal involvement in 40%–90% of adults
- 2%–10% have disseminated disease at presentation, most commonly pulmonary or bony metastases.
- Most patients are clinically and biochemically euthyroid.
  - Graves' disease or toxic nodular goiter may coexist.
  - Carcinomas synthesizing functioning T3/T4 are rare.

Anaplastic (undifferentiated) carcinoma
- Rapidly enlarging neck mass that may be painful
- Confluent bilateral lymphadenopathy
- 90% have regional or distant spread at diagnosis.
- The most common sites of metastases are the lungs and bones.
- They may be accompanied by superior vena cava obstruction and/or Horner's syndrome.

Medullary
- Painless lump in the neck, i.e., solitary thyroid nodule (>75%)
- Usually unilateral
- 20% have locally advanced disease at presentation, e.g., symptoms of upper aerodigestive tract compression.
- 50% have clinically detectable cervical lymph node involvement at diagnosis and 15% have distant metastases.
- Large tumors may have an associated paraneoplastic syndrome, e.g., Cushing's syndrome due to corticotrophin secretion.

Investigations

The investigation of patients with suspected thyroid cancer and their subsequent management should be coordinated by a specialist multidisciplinary team with expertise and interest in the management of thyroid cancer.

The team will usually comprise a surgeon, endocrinologist, oncologist, pathologist, radiologist, medical physicist, and nurse specialist.

Depending on the clinical situation, the following investigations may be considered.
- Full blood count and liver function tests
- Renal function, especially if considering iodine-131 therapy
- Thyroid function tests
- Calcitonin is produced by C cells. Its role in the initial diagnostic evaluation of patients remains controversial because of the frequency of falsely high serum levels. Once a diagnosis of medullary carcinoma is confirmed, a baseline level will establish whether the tumor is capable of hypersecreting calcitonin, to assist with postoperative monitoring.
- High-resolution thyroid ultrasonography and fine needle aspiration have false negative rates varying from 0 to 5%; the false positive rate is usually <5%.

If there is a high risk of local disease extension (e.g., presentation with hoarseness, stridor, dysphagia, or hemoptysis) consider the following:
- CT scan of neck or mediastinum—assess for laryngeal involvement, invasion of the great vessels, etc.
- MRI scan of neck—evaluate any soft tissue invasion.
- CT of the chest or liver
- Skeletal scintigraphy for any suspicion of bony disease. The typical appearances are lytic lesions.

Staging

Papillary or follicular (differentiated) carcinomas
The staging system for differentiated carcinoma of the thyroid is based on the TNM system:
- T, primary tumor. This generally reflects the size of the tumor, any invasion beyond the thyroid capsule (T4).
- N, involvement of regional lymph nodes
- M, absence (0) or presence (1) of distant metastases or inability to assess for their presence (X)

Anaplastic (undifferentiated) carcinoma
These tumors have a very poor prognosis and all are effectively stage IV.

Medullary
The staging system is based on the following:
- Tumor size
- Local invasion
- Nodal disease
- Metastases

Unlike in differentiated thyroid cancer, age is not a factor in the staging of medullary thyroid cancer (see Table 32.1).

Table 32.1 Staging system for medullary carcinoma of the thyroid

Stage I	Primary tumor <1 cm with no evidence of disease outside the thyroid gland
Stage II	Primary tumor >1 cm or the presence of extrathyroidal invasion without nodal or distant metastases
Stage III	Local or regional nodal metastases
Stage IV	Distant metastases

Surgery for thyroid cancer

Papillary and follicular (differentiated) carcinomas

For the primary tumor (papillary, follicular)
Surgery is the primary mode of treatment. The aim must be to perform definitive surgery at the outset.
- The prognosis following incomplete surgery and subsequent further surgery may be poorer than if a total thyroidectomy had been performed at the start.
- Minimally, a total lobectomy must be performed on the side of the tumor.

Surgical options include the following
Unilateral total lobectomy may be appropriate for selected low-risk patients, e.g., pT1 (<1 cm) N0 women <45 years old.

Total thyroidectomy is the procedure of choice in most cases. Advantages include the following.
- Many papillary tumors are multicentric.
- Up to 1 in 5 will recur after partial thyroidectomy.
- Local recurrence is associated with a poor prognosis with up to 40% risk of death from metastatic disease. Others argue that this can be treated with radioactive iodine.
- There is a small risk of progression to anaplastic carcinoma.
- Subsequent monitoring for recurrence is more straightforward (it allows diagnostic and therapeutic radioactive iodine scans).
- Up to 50% of completion thyroidectomies are tumor positive.

More extensive resection is involved in pT4 tumors, with the following options:
- Extensive resection of all involved structures, e.g., larynx, esophagus, with potential loss of organ function, *or*
- Conservative surgery with preservation of local structures but residual foci of disease followed by external beam radiotherapy.

Rates of local control and disease-free survival are similar, but quality of life appears better following the more conservative surgery. Long-term data (30 years) from the Mayo Clinic show a 2% 30-year mortality irrespective of extent of surgery.

Those arguing for total lobectomy quote the increased risk of recurrent laryngeal nerve damage and hypocalcemia after total thyroidectomy.

Potential complications of thyroid surgery
- Hypoparathyroidism
- Recurrent laryngeal nerve injury with hoarse voice and "bovine" cough
  - This should be <1% in experienced hands.
- Superior laryngeal nerve injury with inability to reach higher registers with the voice

Selective neck dissection
The extent of neck dissection should depend on the following:
- Size of primary tumor, e.g., up to 80% of pT4 tumors will have regional nodal involvement at presentation

- Clinical examination, e.g., presence of palpable nodes
- Intraoperative findings, e.g., suspicious nodes at surgery with or without histological examination of frozen section
- Gross cervical metastatic disease should be treated with a modified radical neck dissection.

Recurrent or metastatic disease

If there is metastatic disease at presentation, radical thyroidectomy and ablation are usually still required.
- Optimal management is based on the ability of most differentiated cancers to concentrate radioiodine.
- Re-excision can be considered for locally recurrent disease.

Occasionally, resection may also be appropriate for a solitary metastatic deposit. Further surgery is usually followed by ^{131}I therapy with or without external beam radiotherapy (EBRT).

Anaplastic (undifferentiated) carcinomas

- These are usually inoperable at presentation.
- 50% have lung metastases at presentation.
  - If localized, surgery offers the best chance of a prolonged period of symptom-free survival.
- Total thyroidectomy may not result in any survival advantage over ipsilateral lobectomy with wide margins of adjacent soft tissue.

Medullary

Preoperative screening for pheochromocytoma (MEN type 2) and hyperparathyroidism is with iCa^{2+} (MEN type 2a).

All patients should be treated by *total* thyroidectomy.
- Surgery is the only potentially curative intervention.
- 20% have intraglandular lymphatic spread.
- 20% are *RET* oncogene positive, even if the case is "sporadic."
- Hereditary background may not be known.
- Radioactive iodine is not effective.

The quality of lymph node dissection is paramount and appears to be the sole surgical factor that can improve prognosis. The size of the primary tumor correlates with the chances of metastatic lymphatic spread:
- <1 cm: 11%–50%
- >2 cm: 60%
- Palpable tumor: 85%

Usually surgery involves total thyroidectomy and central and ipsilateral neck node dissection. Surgery with palliative intent can also produce long-term survivors, e.g., reoperation for local recurrence or even resection of solitary metastases.
- Screening for disseminated disease prior to further surgery should include laparoscopy to assess for liver metastases.
- Up to 20% of patients with no hepatic disease identified on conventional imaging will have liver metastases seen at laparoscopy.

All familial cases (frequently bilateral) must have total thyroidectomy.

Radioiodine treatment for thyroid cancer

^{131}I is used in the diagnosis and treatment of differentiated thyroid carcinoma for the following:
- Ablation of residual thyroid tissue
- Assessment of possible disease recurrence
- Treatment of residual or recurrent disease

Postthyroidectomy there is typically up to 2 g of functioning thyroid tissue.

^{131}I is administered at doses sufficient to ablate residual thyroid tissue, including microscopic foci of malignancy.
- ^{131}I treatment reduces the risk of local recurrence by approximately 60% compared with thyroid suppression alone.
- It prolongs overall and disease-free survival.
- It is effective against microscopic disease only. It is not a treatment for macroscopic residual cancer.
- It increases the sensitivity and specificity of the subsequent screening program to identify persistent or recurrent disease. Screening may be by:
  - Monitoring changes in serum thyroglobulin (TG) levels. TG is secreted by normal and >90% of cancerous thyroid cells, so ablation of all active thyroid tissue should mean that TG is undetectable.
  - Diagnostic ^{131}I scans

Preparation for treatment with ^{131}I includes the following:
- Total thyroidectomy approximately 1 month previously
- No thyroid hormone replacement, a low-iodine diet, and no iodine-containing medication to maximize the chance of avid uptake of the iodine (be aware of the iodine load of CT contrast agents)
- Confirm hypothyroid status before administration (the patient is likely to be feeling unwell by this stage).
- Explain to the patient that they will be confined to a single room during their admission; interaction with nurses will be minimal, and visitors will be limited.

Postablation diagnostic ^{131}I scans are performed to confirm the absence of residual active thyroid tissue. The serum TG level should become undetectable.

Potential acute toxicity of therapeutic ^{131}I treatment includes nausea, sialadenitis, radiation cystitis, or gastritis. Very rarely it may precipitate hemorrhage into metastases.

Late effects include a persistent dry mouth, accelerated dental caries, and a very small risk of late second malignancies, particularly if repeated cycles of treatment have been necessary, e.g., leukemias, salivary gland tumors. Men should be offered sperm storage, particularly if repeated administrations are likely.

Replacement thyroid hormone therapy should be commenced following ablation of active glandular tissue. The aim is for lifelong suppression of TSH, i.e., the dose of exogenous hormone aims to maintain biochemical hyperthyroidism to avoid theoretical overstimulation of occult residual tissue.

Diagnostic ^{131}I scans can be repeated as part of posttreatment surveillance; >60% of differentiated thyroid cancers take up enough iodide to be detected by radioiodine imaging.

Treatment doses of ^{131}I can be repeated if:
- Serum TG begins to rise
- Further activity is observed on a diagnostic ^{131}I whole-body scan indicating inoperable or metastatic disease, e.g., pulmonary metastases

There is no role for ^{131}I treatment in medullary or anaplastic carcinoma, because these tumors are not iodine avid.

External beam radiotherapy for thyroid cancer

Differentiated (papillary and follicular) carcinoma

After complete resection

Adjuvant external beam radiotherapy (EBRT) should be offered to selected patients whose tumors do not concentrate radioiodine.

It should also be considered after surgery and ^{131}I therapy if:
- The primary tumor is large (pT4).
- There is extracapsular spread or lymph node involvement.
- There are other poor prognostic features.

A typical treatment regime would involve 60 Gy administered in 30 fractions.
- Treatment is usually in two phases, with lead shielding in the second phase to avoid exceeding spinal cord tolerance.
- Conformal techniques and CT planning allow reduction in the dosage to normal tissue.
- Potential side effects include cutaneous erythema, mucositis, and dysphagia.

Palliation

There is a role for external beam radiotherapy
- After incomplete resection, to improve local control of residual tumor
- For symptomatic metastatic disease, e.g., painful skeletal metastases

Undifferentiated (anaplastic) carcinoma

Consider postoperative radiotherapy for the small number of patients whose tumors are completely resected. This is more frequently used with palliative intent for local control of inoperable tumors or for symptomatic metastatic disease. Up to 80% will have a partial response for a short period of time.

Stridor and superior vena cava obstruction (SVCO) are urgent indications for radiotherapy.

Medullary carcinoma

Postoperative EBRT is used for macroscopic remnants to maximize local control. Alternatively, preoperative radiotherapy may cause an inoperable tumor to become operable.

Occasional avidity of uptake to meta-iodo-benzyl-guanidine (MIBG) makes radioiodinated MIBG therapy a possibly useful therapeutic modality.

Chemotherapy for thyroid cancer

- This has a very limited role.
- It is used only if surgery, ^{131}I, or external beam radiotherapy is no longer appropriate and the patient remains fit.
- Response rates are poor (<30%), incomplete, and of short duration.
- There is no evidence for improvement in overall survival.
- The standard first-line agent is doxorubicin.
- Other options are largely trial based.

Surveillance, follow-up, and prognosis for thyroid cancer

Surveillance and follow-up

Differentiated (papillary and follicular) carcinomas
- Most recurrences occur within 5 years.
- Regular physical examination particularly of the neck
- Serum T4, TSH, and TG at each visit. ↑TG in the presence of a suppressed serum TSH requires investigation.
- Approximately 5% of recurrent disease is not associated with ↑TG.
- Chest X-ray, ultrasound scan of the neck, and diagnostic radioiodine imaging can be used, depending on risk factors.

Medullary
- Clinical examination
- Serial serum calcitonin levels
- Screen for familial disease
  - New cases of medullary carcinoma should be offered genetic testing.

Prognosis

Differentiated
- Most patients with follicular and papillary carcinomas do not die of their disease.
- >90% 10-year survival
- Prognosis for the follicular subtype is worse than for common-type papillary carcinoma, e.g., 92% versus 98% 10-year survival.
- Stage IV disease still has a 5-year survival of approximately 25%.

Poor prognostic features include the following:
- >45 years old
- Larger primary tumor, e.g., >7 cm
- Bilateral or mediastinal lymph node involvement or distant metastases
- Lymphocytic infiltration
- Male sex
- Soft tissue or regional organ invasion, e.g., trachea, esophagus

The most common site of initial relapse is local neck lymph nodes. Treatment is further surgical resection followed by ^{131}I therapy.

Undifferentiated (anaplastic) carcinoma
- Aggressive cancer with very poor prognosis
- Median time from first symptom to death is 3–7 months
- 1-year survival is 20%–35% and 5-year survival is only 5%–14%.

Medullary
There is no effective treatment for advanced disease. However, patients may live for years despite a high metastatic load, e.g., median survival for stage III/IV disease is 3–5 years.

Patients with MEN type 2b are more likely to have invasive disease at diagnosis and fall into a worse prognostic group. Stage-for-stage there is no difference in prognosis between sporadic and hereditary disease.

Adrenal cancer

The adrenal gland is composed of the following:
- Outer cortex, which is mainly controlled by the renin-angiotensin system that regulates the release of aldosterone
- Inner cortex, which is mainly controlled by the corticotrophin-releasing hormone-corticotrophin (ACTH) system that regulates the release of cortisol and adrenal androgens
- Medulla, which is part of the sympathetic nervous system.

Tumors arising in the cortex and the medulla are etiologically and functionally different, reflecting their cells of origin.

Epidemiology and etiology

Adrenocortical tumors
- Rare: incidence is approximately 1.0 per 10^6 population
- Etiology generally unknown: rare familial cases
- Carcinomas are even less common: bimodal age distribution
  - Peak incidence is before 5 years of age and in the fourth to fifth decades.

Medullary tumors
- Even rarer: incidence is approximately 0.6 per 10^6 population
- 10% are currently identified as familial, although this is likely to increase with improvements in genetic analysis.
- Associated with MEN type 2 (germline mutation in *RET* proto-oncogene; see Medullary carcinoma of the thyroid, p. 500) and occasionally von Hippel-Lindau disease

Pathology

Adrenocortical tumors
- Adenomas or adenocarcinomas of the adrenal cortex
- If malignant, spread is via
  - Local invasion of lymph nodes and liver
  - Distant dissemination
- 60% of all adrenocortical tumors are nonfunctioning.
- 40% are functioning, secreting steroids that may include estrogens, testosterone, and/or aldosterone.

Medullary tumors
- The most common adrenomedullary tumor is a pheochromocytoma, which has a golden or tan-colored appearance macroscopically.
- The majority are benign. Approximately 10% are malignant.
- 10% of pheochromocytomas are extra-adrenal, i.e., arise elsewhere in the sympathetic chain; 10% are multiple.
- Hereditary pheochromocytomas
  - Often occur in younger age groups
  - Are more likely to be bilateral and benign
- Tumoral hypersecretion of epinephrine, norepinephrine, and/or dopamine

Table 32.2 Endocrine syndromes associated with adrenocortical tumors

Syndrome	Steroid
Cushing's syndrome (ACTH-independent)	Cortisol
Conn's syndrome/primary hyperaldosteronism	Aldosterone
Virilization syndrome	Androgen
Feminization syndrome	Estrogen
Precocious puberty syndrome/adrenogenital syndrome	Sex hormones
Nonfunctioning	None

Presentation

Adrenocortical tumors

See Table 32.2.
- Often an incidental finding
- Pressure symptoms, e.g., pain in the abdomen or symptoms from metastatic disease

In functioning tumors, symptoms and signs will vary according to the predominant steroid hormone produced:
- Virilization: most common presentation in children
- Cushing's syndrome: most common presentation in adults
- Feminization: very rarely
- Hypertension

Medullary tumors
- Often an incidental finding during screening for associated familial syndromes
- Intermittent, severe hypertension or essential hypertension
- Classical presentation: episodic symptoms of
  - Headache
  - Sweating
  - Tachycardia and palpitations
  - Pallor or tremor

Investigations

- Careful family history
- Hemoglobin, electrolytes, urea, liver function tests
- Plasma catecholamines
- Plasma aldosterone-to-renin activity ratio
- Urinary VMA and urinary catecholamines
- Chromogranin assays
- Serum and urinary cortisols
- Blood estrogen and testosterone
- Chest X-ray, ultrasound, CT, MRI abdomen to assess for potential metastatic disease
- Ultrasound of the thyroid gland (MEN)
- ^{123}I-MIBG, octreoscan for medullary tumor
- Selenocholesterol imaging for cortical tumor

Surgery

Surgery is the only treatment likely to achieve cure in benign disease or in the small group of patients with localized malignant disease without occult micrometastases.

It may still be appropriate to resect the primary tumor in the presence of metastases if it is slow-growing or where there are a small number of metastases, to achieve local control. Radical resection with adjacent nephrectomy, if necessary, is essential for cure.

Special preoperative considerations include the following:
- Correction of electrolyte abnormalities;
- Appropriate blood pressure control.

Surgery may be
- **Open**: preferable for larger adenomas and carcinomas. There are early, encouraging results for laparoscopic adrenalectomy with small cancers.
- **Laparoscopic**: longer operating time, less postoperative pain, shorter hospital stay postoperatively. There is a long learning curve.

Nonsurgical options

Adrenocortical tumors

Mitotane is an orally administered adrenocorticolytic drug with some efficacy in patients with adrenal carcinoma. It is first-line treatment in patients with unresectable or metastatic tumors.
- Common side effects include nausea and anorexia.
- It may also cause cortisol and aldosterone deficiency, necessitating replacement therapy.
- Control of disease is usually transient, with symptomatic or biochemical progression typically occurring after only 6–12 months.

Metyrapone, aminoglutethamide, and ketoconazole are potential second-line medical therapies that can also reduce excessive cortisol secretion.

Chemotherapy has limited benefit. There are no randomized clinical trials. The most active drugs appear to be cisplatin and etoposide.

Radiotherapy has no established role in the management of adrenal carcinoma, as it is rarely effective. Occasionally, it is used for the treatment of symptomatic metastases, usually in bone.

Medullary tumors

Antihypertensive medication may be required for pheochromocytomas with residual or unresectable disease to control the blood pressure.

If the tumor takes up the radionuclide MIBG, a therapeutic dose of ^{131}I-MIBG may be administered. Symptomatic, hormonal, and radiological improvements can be seen, although these are transient. Treatment can be repeated.

Radiotherapy is appropriate for painful skeletal metastases.

Chemotherapy may be considered for tumors that will not take up MIBG. A combination of dacarbazine, vincristine, and cyclophosphamide shows activity.

Prognosis

Adrenocortical tumors
Almost all patients with benign disease are cured by surgery (usually laparoscopic).

Prognosis is poor for patients with malignant disease. Untreated, the median survival is 3–9 months. Even if the carcinoma is small volume and apparently confined to the adrenal gland, survival after surgery may be as little as 14–36 months. It may be better in children.

Medullary tumors
Surgical resection is not always curative even in benign disease. Long-term monitoring is therefore required. Subsequent recurrence may have malignant characteristics.

5-year survival for malignant pheochromocytoma is <50%, although some patients live for many years without significant symptoms.

Neuroblastoma

This is the most common extracranial solid tumor in childhood, with incidence peaking at age 1–3 years.
Tumors arise in sympathetic nervous tissue:
- 60% are adrenal or elsewhere within the abdomen, producing pain, abdominal distension, and general malaise.
- 15% are intrathoracic, causing cough, pain, and Horner's syndrome, and are an incidental finding on chest X-ray.
- Bone or bone marrow metastases may result in nonspecific limb, joint, or back pain often misdiagnosed as arthritis or an irritable hip. It may also become pancytopenic from marrow involvement.

Investigations include abdominal ultrasound, CT/MRI of the chest and abdomen, MRI of the spine, urinary catecholamines, blood tests including serum LDH (elevation is a poor prognostic sign), serum neuron-specific enolase (NSE), and techetium or I^{123} MIBG scan.

Pathology ranges from an undifferentiated, small, round-cell tumor (that may be difficult to distinguish from rhabdomyosarcoma, primitive neuroectodermal tumor [PNET], or non-Hodgkin's lymphoma [NHL]) to a highly differentiated ganglioneuroblastoma.

Biopsy can be done percutaneously, thorascopically, or with the laparoscope.

Management

Management depends on tumor stage and the presence of certain genetic features that may indicate a less good prognosis, e.g., amplification of the n-myc oncogene.

A watch-and-wait policy is an option for tumors of early stage with favorable biology. Spontaneous regression can be seen.

Surgical clearance
This should be done, if possible. Most thoracic, pelvic, and cervical primaries, and those abdominal tumors that do *not* cross the midline, are resectable. Even subtotal resection in infants is beneficial.

Neoadjuvant chemotherapy
This treatment may be used with the aim of making localized but inoperable tumors resectable. Chemotherapy is also used in disseminated, high-risk disease. Occasionally, high-dose chemotherapy followed by autologous hemopoietic stem cell rescue may be considered.

Radiotherapy
Radiotherapy is used following incomplete resection or for tumors that remain unresectable after induction chemotherapy.

Prognosis

Prognosis depends on the stage of tumor (see Table 32.3), tumor genetics, and age at diagnosis. Children <1 year old have a good prognosis even in the presence of widely disseminated disease, e.g., 85% overall survival for stage 4S. This compares with an overall survival of <40% in children >5 years old with neuroblastoma of any stage.

Table 32.3 International staging system for neuroblastoma

Stage	
Stage 1	Localized tumor with complete gross excision, with or without microscopic residual disease. Representative ipsilateral and contralateral lymph nodes are negative for tumor microscopically (nodes attached to and removed with the primary tumor may be positive).
Stage 2a	Localized tumor with incomplete gross excision. Representative ipsilateral and nonadherent lymph nodes are negative for tumor microscopically.
Stage 2b	Localized tumor with complete or incomplete gross excision, with ipsilateral nonadherent lymph nodes positive for tumor. Enlarged contralateral lymph nodes must be negative microscopically.
Stage 3	Unresectable unilateral tumor infiltrating across the midine, with or without regional lymph node involvement; or localized unilateral tumor with contralateral regional lymph node involvement; or midline tumor with bilateral extension by infiltration or by lymph node involvement
Stage 4	Any primary tumor with dissemination to distant lymph nodes, bone, bone, marrow, liver skin, and/or other organs (except as defined in stage 4S)
Stage 4S	Localized primary tumor as defined for stage 1, 2a, or 2b with dissemination limited to skin, liver, and/or bone marrow (limited to infants <1 year old only).

Chapter 33

Genitourinary cancers I: renal, bladder, ureter, penile carcinomas

Prateek Mendiratta
Andrew J. Armstrong
Phillip Febbo
Daniel George

Renal cancer *536*
Cancer of the bladder and ureter *548*
Penile cancer *558*
Further reading *562*

Renal cancer

Epidemiology and etiology
- 51,000 new cases of renal cancer were expected in 2007, nearly 13,000 U.S. deaths annually. Renal cancer accounts for approximately 2% of all malignancies.
- Median age at diagnosis is 65 years.
- It is 1.6 times more common in men.
- Incidence increased from 2.3% to 4.9 % annually from 1975 to 1995.
- It is associated with smoking (relative risk [RR] 2x, 20%–30% attributable risk [AR]).
- Other major associations include obesity (30%–40% AR), family history (2%–5% AR), hypertension, long-term dialysis (8–10 years), phenacetin use, and increasing age.
- There are relatively weak associations with urban geographic location, occupational exposure (e.g., asbestos, benzenes, cadmium, nitrosamines, petrols).
- No strong associations with alcohol consumption, dietary factors, oral contraceptive use, or modern analgesic use have been found.

Genetics
The vast majority of adult renal cancers are sporadic, but an inherited predisposition causes 2%–5%, and these may be multifocal or bilateral.

Von Hippel-Lindau (VHL) syndrome
VHL occurs in 1 per 36,000 births.
- The *VHL* gene on chromosome 3 is a tumor suppressor gene.
- Germline loss or mutation of this gene leads to a multiorgan syndrome including cerebral and retinal hemangioblastomas, endolymphatic sac tumors, and risk of renal cell carcinoma.
- In sporadic renal cell cancer, both parental alleles are inactivated by acquired mutations or epigenetic silencing, unlike VHL syndrome, in which the first mutation is inherited.
- Loss of *VHL* function is seen in over 60% of sporadic clear cell carcinomas. Loss of function leads to activation of hypoxia-inducible genes, including vascular endothelial growth factor (VEGF), platelet-derived growth factor receptor (PDGFR), erythropoietin, and others genes implicated in tumorigenesis.

Hereditary clear cell carcinoma
This carcinoma is caused by germline mutation in chromosome 3 and is without other features of VHL.

Hereditary papillary renal carcinoma syndrome (type 1 papillary)
Hereditary papillary renal carcinoma syndrome (HPRCC) has increased predisposition to multiple, small bilateral tumors.
- Usually found later in life and is less likely to have metastatic spread.
- Found to involve mutations in the *c-met* oncogene located on chromosome 7 and linked to several other malignancies (GI, melanoma).

Hereditary leiomyoma and papillary renal cell carcinoma (type 2 papillary renal cell carcinoma)
- Increased predisposition to unilateral large aggressive renal tumors, skin and uterine leiomyomas, and linked to chromosome 1q42 (fumarate hydratase gene in Krebs cycle)

Birt-Hogg-Dube syndrome
- Patients have increased risk for lung cysts leading to pneumothorax, a predisposition to kidney neoplasms (chromophobe and oncocytoma subtype), and prominent skin findings (fibrofolliculomas).
- The defect is due to loss of function of the *BHD* (folliculin) gene found on the short arm of chromosome 17.

Other diseases
- Increased risk is also found in autosomal dominant polycystic kidney disease and tuberous sclerosis.
- Pediatric renal cell carcinoma (RCC): translocation of 1:X chromosomes; very rare

Pathology

Adenocarcinomas make up 85% of renal cancers and arise from the renal tubular epithelium. The next most common type is transitional cell carcinomas of the renal pelvis (78%). These renal cell carcinomas demonstrate several histological types:

- **Clear cell** (75%): Usually found to have mutations of *VHL* (in both sporadic and inherited cases)
  - PAS-positive cells, +RCC antigen, often CD10 positive, + cytokeratins
  - Likely derived from proximal tubule cell or progenitor
- **Type 1 papillary** (5%): Usually found to have mutations in *c-Met*, with basophilia and small nuclei. Usually favorable prognosis
- **Type 2 papillary** (10%): Usually found to have mutations in the fumarate hydratase gene in familial cases, linked to *c-myc* activation in sporadic cases
  - Eosinophilic with large nuclei and nucleoli, pseudostratified epithelium
  - Aggressive tumor with unfavorable prognosis
  - Unclear derivation of PRCC, but likely proximal tubule or progenitor
- **Chromophobe** (5%): Usually found to have loss of function of the *BHD* gene in familial cases, widespread chromosomal instability in sporadic cases (loss of chromosomes 1, 6, 10, 11, 17, hypodiploidy), and positive Hale's iron stains, + c-kit expression, PAS negative, and likely derived from intercalated cells
- **Oncoctyoma** (5%): Usually found to have loss of function of the *BHD* gene, packed with mitochondria on electron microscopy
- **Collecting duct (Bellini tumor)** (<1%): Very rare transitional cell carcinoma; very aggressive and usually presents with metastatic disease
- **Spindle cell or sarcomatoid**: Highest grade variant of clear cell or other pathologic subtypes, poor prognostic feature
- Overlapping and coexisting histologies are common.
- **Medullary carcinoma**: Rare aggressive tumor arising in African Americans with sickle cell trait, likely ductal origin
- **Mucinous or multilocular cystic carcinomas**: Rare, typically benign

RCC typically arises as a solitary mass in one pole of the kidney, with <4% being bilateral renal masses. As it progresses, it may invade directly through the renal capsule, along the renal vein toward the IVC or even right atrium, and via lymphatics to regional nodes (para-aortic).

Systemic metastases are common; locally advanced and macroscopic spread is present in 25% of cases at presentation, typically to lung or bone, but also liver, adrenal, and brain.

Transitional cell carcinomas (TCCs) can arise within the urothelium of the renal pelvis and represent the majority of the remaining tumors. They vary from low-grade superficial papillary tumors to high-grade invasive TCC with a propensity for direct invasion into perinephric tissues and lymphovascular spread.

Investigations

Many RCC tumors are identified on ultrasonography, but CT is the preferred imaging modality. Increasing incidence is likely linked to increasing use of CT imaging and incidental discovery.

Contrast-enhanced CT scan of the abdomen characteristically shows an enhancing mass, at least partly solid. CT should also be used to image the following:

- Chest, for lung and mediastinal lymph node metastases
- Extrarenal direct tumor extension, e.g., into psoas muscle
- Regional para-aortic lymph nodes
- Spread to other organs, e.g., liver, adrenals

MRI of the abdomen may be preferred to look for involvement of the collecting system and inferior vena cava or renal vein invasion.

Biopsy is usually omitted prior to surgical treatment (nephrectomy or partial nephrectomy) of renal cancer because of the risk of hemorrhage and tumor seeding along the biopsy tract. Biopsy may be appropriate if no nephrectomy is to be performed for advanced or metastatic disease.

Other recommended investigations include the following:

- CBC (searching for anemia or erythrocytosis), liver and kidney function tests
- LDH and serum calcium levels as prognostic factors
- Bone scan in patients with poor-risk disease or in patients with bone pain or elevated alkaline phosphatase or calcium
- CT/MRI of the brain if poor risk or clinical evidence of CNS spread
- Isotope renogram to assess function of contralateral kidney if renal function is impaired
- PET scanning does not have a currently defined role.

Staging

The American Joint Commission of Cancer (AJCC) staging is commonly used (Table 33.1).

Table 33.1 TNM staging of renal cancer

Primary tumor	
Tx	Primary tumor cannot be assessed
T0	No evidence of primary tumor
T1	Tumor <7 cm in greatest dimension, limited to kidney
T2	Tumor >7 cm in greatest dimension, limited to kidney
T3	Tumor extends into major veins or invades the adrenal gland or perinephric tissues, but not beyond Gerota's fascia
T3a	Tumor invades the adrenal gland or perinephric tissues but not beyond Georta's facsia
T3b	Tumor grossly extends into the renal vein(s) or vena cava below the diaphragm
T3c	Tumor grossly extends into the renal vein(s) or vena cava above the diaphragm
T4	Tumor invades beyond the Gerota's fascia
Regional lymph nodes	
Nx	Regional lymph nodes cannot be assessed
N0	No regional lymph node metastases
N1	Metastases in a single regional lymph node
N2	Metastases in more than one regional lymph node
Distant metastases	
Mx	Distant metastases not assessed
M0	No distant metastases
M1	Distant metastases
Stage group	
Stage I	T1N0M0
Stage II	T2N0M0
Stage III	T1N1M0 T2N1M0 T3AN0M0
	T3AN1M0 T3BN0M0 T3BN1M0
	T3CN0M0 T3CN0M1
Stage IV	T4N0M0 T4N1M0
	Any T N2M0 or any M1

Presenting symptoms and signs
Up to 30% are asymptomatic and are discovered coincidentally during abdominal imaging for other reasons. Symptoms may relate directly to the primary tumor, but paraneoplastic effects are not uncommon:
- Hematuria (50%)
- Groin pain (50%)
- Palpable mass (30%)
- Anemia (40%)
- Weight loss (35%)
- Pyrexia (20%)
- Hypertension (37%)
- Hypercalcemia (6%)
- Polycythemia (<5%) due to elevated erythropoietin
- Elevated liver function tests in absence of metastasis (Stauffer syndrome)

Renal tumors may invade directly into adjacent psoas muscle or lumbar spine causing pain, or may present de novo with symptoms from metastatic disease in the lungs, lymph nodes, bone, or brain.

Surgery
Resection of the entire tumor is the only potentially curative treatment and should be offered to patients with operable disease without metastases who are fit for surgery for stage I–III disease.

Anatomic extent of disease is the most consistent factor determining prognosis in newly diagnosed patients with metastatic renal cell cancer.

Patients with metastatic disease but good performance status and resectable primary tumor may benefit from nephrectomy as a palliative procedure, with two randomized trials demonstrating a survival benefit (3–7 months) with nephrectomy.

These trials were performed in the era of interferon (IFN) systemic therapy, and it is unclear why nephrectomy was done prior to the use of current targeted VEGF- or mTOR-based therapy. Most patients in clinical trials of these agents had undergone prior nephrectomy.

The reasons to consider nephrectomy in the face of metastatic disease include the following:
- To provide control of local symptoms (pain, hematuria)
- Although there are documented cases of regression of metastases following nephrectomy, this is extremely rare. Nephrectomy cannot be justified on this basis in patients who are frail or have extensive metastatic disease.
- Improvement in response to immunologic therapy (high-dose IL-2)

Partial nephrectomy is occasionally performed for small, localized tumors or in patients without a second kidney, or in the rare case of bilateral renal cancer.

Radical nephrectomy includes removal of Gerota's fascia and its contents, including the kidney and the adrenal gland, and removal of regional lymph nodes.

Some surgeons believe that adrenal-gland and lymph-node dissection can remain optional, although for upper pole lesions the unilateral adrenal gland is typically removed. Lymph node status can serve as prognostic information; however, most patients with nodal involvement experience recurrence with distant metastasis.

Laparoscopic nephrectomy is becoming increasingly established to decrease the morbidity of the open procedure—morbidity is less, and early survival seems to equate to the open procedure. Unless patients are frail or very elderly, even small tumors should be resected.

Surgery for metastases (e.g., lung, brain) is indicated for isolated metastases or oligometastatic disease that occurs after a long disease-free interval, and can result in prolonged survival in up to 30% of patients.

Although surgery is the cornerstone of management of localized disease, some patients are unfit for nephrectomy or their tumor is unresectable. Cryotherapy and/or radiofrequency ablation may provide some tumor control for patients with small tumors. In some elderly asymptomatic patients, conservative management is appropriate, and tumor growth may be slow.

Neoadjuvant systemic therapy remains unproven but may be used in select cases that are currently unresectable. Appropriate holding of anti-VEGF/mTOR-based therapy prior to nephrectomy should be considered to prevent wound healing complications.

Adjuvant therapy

Adjuvant therapy of any type has not been proven to offer a survival benefit or decreased time to relapse when combined with nephrectomy.

Cytotoxic chemotherapies, endocrine therapy, radiotherapy, and immunotherapy have been tested. Randomized clinical trials of targeted therapy approved in the metastatic setting and immunotherapy alone or in conjunction are ongoing.

The current standard of care is observation after complete nephrectomy or a clinical trial for intermediate- to high-risk disease (T3, node positive, high grade).

Radiotherapy

In general, renal cancer is relatively radioresistant. Palliative radiotherapy is appropriate for
- Painful or bleeding primary tumor
- Nonresectable metastatic disease, e.g., bone, brain, soft tissue, isolated nephrectomy bed recurrences (with or without surgery)

Higher palliative doses than those used in other malignancies may be appropriate to give durable control of disease, particularly for isolated nonresectable metastases after nephrectomy in patients with good performance status.

Supportive care

Bisphosphonate (zoledronic acid) therapy should be used for patients with bone metastatic disease to prevent skeletal-related events (hypercalcemia of malignancy, fracture, bone pain, need for radiation), according to evidence from randomized controlled trials.
- The studied schedule for this agent is 4 mg (renally dose adjusted) every 3 weeks, but alternative, less-frequent schedules may also be effective.
- Side effects include osteonecrosis of the jaw (ONJ), renal insufficiency, and bone and joint pains.

Anemia may be treated with transfusional support, iron supplementation if deficient, and/or erythropoiesis-stimulating agents (ESA). However, renal cell carcinoma expresses erythropoietin and has functional erythropoietin receptors on the cell surface.

Numerous clinical trials for other tumor types have demonstrated evidence of increased tumor progression and lower survival when these agents were used in the absence of chemotherapy-induced anemia. Given these concerns, future studies in RCC are warranted for the safe use of these agents.

General supportive care for pain control, nausea, diarrhea, fatigue, depression, weight loss, and psychosocial stress is recommended. The reader is referred to National Comprehensive Cancer Center (NCCN) guidelines for standard management of these symptoms.

Prognostic features determining recurrence

Multiple prognostic models have been created to categorize patients with clinically relevant differences in prognosis.

For predicting recurrence in patients with localized cancer, the most common model is the UCLA integrated system, which focuses on three factors: TNM staging, Fuhrman's histological grade, and ECOG performance status. Another model has been created by the Cleveland clinic, which also uses the number of metastatic sites as an additional validated poor prognostic factor.

A validated European nomogram has been developed for the prediction of long-term outcome in RCC. For more information on these nomograms, please refer to the references under the future readings.

For patients with metastatic disease and who have had a previous nephrectomy, the prognostic model most commonly used in clinical trials and that has shown the ability to predict a shorter survival is the Memorial Sloan Kettering Cancer Center model (Motzer criteria). This model identifies patients as poor-, intermediate-, or good-prognosis patients, with difference in overall survival by 6 months or more. Those defined as poor prognosis included patients with ≥3 of the following poor prognostic features: high LDH, low performance status, elevated corrected calcium, anemia, and absence of prior nephrectomy or <1 year from nephrectomy to recurrence.

Poor-risk patients have a median survival of 4 months in the pretargeted therapy era. Intermediate-risk patients have 1–2 risk factors and have a median survival of 10 months in the pretargeted therapy era.

Good-risk patients (zero risk factors) have a median survival of 20 months. These estimates are likely to be increased upward in the current era of VEGF- and mTOR-based systemic therapy.

Other risk factors that may be important include the number of metastatic sites of disease, pathologic subtypes (chromophobes favorable), and prior radiation therapy.

Chemotherapy

Cytotoxic drugs are of little value in treating clear cell renal carcinoma. The chemoresistance may be in part due to the high expression of a multidrug resistance phenotype in both normal and malignant renal tissue.

Response rates for single agents are generally under 10%. Chemotherapy may be indicated for transitional cell carcinomas (collecting duct tumors), using traditional cisplatin-based regimens.

Biological therapy

The goal of management of patients with advanced and/or metastatic renal cancer is palliative. However, there is good evidence that a small subset of patients (7%–10%) who have complete responses to biological therapy may enjoy long-term, disease-free survival with intensive immunologic therapy.

In general, these patients tend to fall into the good-risk Motzer subgroup. Most studies have shown that only patients with clear-cell pathology respond to biological therapy, leaving limited treatment options for patients with nonclear-cell pathology.

Biological therapy has been extensively tested in renal cancer, partly because of this cancer's chemoresistance, but mainly because of the presumption that immunological mechanisms underlie
- Occasional spontaneous regression of metastases
- Very late relapses in some patients
- Increased incidence of renal cancers in immunosuppressed patients

Interleukin-2

Interleukin-2 (IL-2) is the most widely tested biological agent in the treatment of advanced renal cancer. It induces complete responses in 10%–25% of patients with advanced metastatic disease.

Patients with a complete radiological response have a significant survival benefit, with sustained remissions of several years in up to 70%.

Studies have shown that high doses of intravenous IL-2 given in an inpatient ICU setting, compared with subcutaneous dosing, showed no difference in overall survival, but decreased response rate with the subcutaneous dose. These regimens are associated with serious mortality (up to 4%) and morbidity, in particular capillary leak syndrome, including hypotension and pulmonary edema, renal failure, and hemorrhage.

Other toxicities include flu-like symptoms and effects on bone marrow, hepatic and renal function, and the CNS (delirium, psychosis), and thyroid dysfunction.

There is some evidence in the melanoma literature that the induction of autoimmunity with IL-2 is associated with a survival benefit.

Interferon-α
- As a single agent, subcutaneous interferon (IFN) provides a response rate of ~15%–20% but without prolonged remissions.
- In clinical trials comparing IFN to progesterones, IFN was demonstrated to have a 2- to 4-month survival benefit.
- Dosing of this agent is initially 9 mU subcutaneously three times weekly, escalating as tolerated to 18 mU.
- Toxicities of this drug are significant but not life threatening, in particular flu-like symptoms, lethargy, anorexia, and nausea.
- Other side effects include deranged LFTs, and effects on bone marrow and renal function, hypothyroidism, neuropathy, and CNS symtoms (depression and psychosis).

Combined biological and chemotherapy

Although phase II studies have reported higher objective response rates with combinations of IL-2 and IFN, with or without chemotherapy, so far, phase III studies have failed to demonstrate a significant benefit with any combination regimen.

Management of transitional cell carcinoma

These tumors arise in the renal collecting system and may be associated with transitional cell carcinoma (TCC) in the ureter and bladder. Their biology, management, and prognosis are similar to that of TCC of the ureter.

Medullary tumors are typically chemorefractory, with some case reports indicating prolonged responses to proteasome inhibition (bortezomib) or anthracycline therapy.

Treatment outcomes

Most of the data used to determine treatment outcomes was determined in the pretyrosine kinase inhibitors era (which will be discussed in detail later). Using the previously defined Motzer criteria, one could estimate the median time to death in the favorable risk (zero risk factors: 20 months), intermediate risk (one or two risk factors: 10 months), and poor risk (three or more risk factors: 4 months). Data are limited in the posttyrosine kinase inhibitor era in each of these groups; yet, one could state that these figures can likely be adjusted upwards 2–6 months in the current era.

Molecular targeted treatments for renal cancer

Recent advances in the understanding of the pathogenesis of renal cell cancer have led to recent U.S. FDA approval of three targeted therapies for patients with advanced renal cell cancer.

By focusing on patients with loss of function of the *VHL* gene (which is actually seen in approximately 60%–80% of patients with sporadic clear cell pathology), it has been discovered that renal cell cancer progression is dependent on angiogenesis and its downstream and upstream effectors.

Table 33.2 shows agents that target specific members of this pathway, their approved indication, and their major side effects.

Given that these agents are not likely to be curative, enrollment in clinical trials remains a priority in first- and second-line settings and beyond.

Combination therapy or novel approaches to targeted therapy may provide additional benefit compared with the agents listed below.

Table 33.2 Targeted therapies for renal cancer

Target	Agent	Indication	Side effects
VEGF (vascular endothelial growth factor)	Bevacizumab	Not currently U.S. FDA approved	Bleeding, impaired wound healing, proteinuria, hypertension, venous thromboembolism, GI perforation
mTOR	Temsirolimus (Torisel)	Approved for patients with advanced RCC	Fatigue, hyperlipidemia, rash, stomatitis, anemia, hyperglycemia
VEGF/PDGF (platelet-derived growth factor)	Sunitinib (Sutent)	Approved for patients with advanced RCC	Fatigue, hypertension, hand-foot syndrome, diarrhea, rash, skin discoloration
	Sorafenib (Nexavar)	Approved for patients with advanced RCC	Hypertension, rash, fatigue, hand-foot syndrome, diarrhea

Sunitinib (Sutent), U.S. Food and Drug Adminstration-approved dose 50 mg for 4 weeks daily and then 2 weeks off by mouth

Sunitinib was recently approved after a phase III trial compared this agent with IFN in newly diagnosed patients with renal cell cancer (clear-cell pathology).

- Progression-free survival (PFS) was 11 months (sunitinib arm) vs. 5.1 months (IFN arm) and overall response rate (ORR) was 31% (sunitinib arm) vs. 6% (IFN arm).
- Significant ORR and significant increased time to progression were shown in the sunitinib arm.
- A trend toward improved overall survival (not statistically significant) was shown in those treated with sunitinib. Crossover was permitted.
- This agent was studied and showed similar activity in previously treated (cytokine-refractory) patients and was approved for this indication as well.
- A 2008 update at the American Cancer Society Oncology Annual meeting in 2008 showed a clear advantage in overal survival in the sunitinib arm (28 months) vs the IFN arm (14 months) in those patients who did not receive and poststudy treatment. The calculated P value was .0033.

Sorafenib (Nexavar), U.S. Food and Drug Adminstration-approved dose 400 mg twice a day by mouth

This was studied in a large placebo-controlled trial in patients who failed previous cytokine-based therapies.

- Median PFS was 5.5 months (sorafenib arm) vs. 2.8 months (placebo), P value <.01.
- Sorafenib reduced the risk of death compared with a placebo (hazard ratio = 0.72, P value <.02), but this did not meet the prespecified

cutoff for significance. Patients crossed over from IFN to sorafenib in this study.
- In newly diagnosed patients, the conclusions are less clear.
- A phase II trial comparing this agent with IFN showed improved tumor shrinkage, 68% (sorafenib arm) vs. 39% (IFN arm); no statistical benefit was seen in time to progression, 5.7 months (sorafenib arm) vs. 5.6 months (IFN arm).
- Randomized phase II studies have not supported a routine role for sorafenib in the first line setting for metastatic RCC.

Temsirolimus (Torisel), U.S. Food and Drug Adminstration-approved dose 25 mg IV weekly

This intravenous agent was studied in a large phase III trial of previously untreated patients. Temsirolimus was compared with IFN or the combination of temsirolimus and IFN. The study was focused on poor-risk patients categorized by Motzer criteria or multiple metastatic sites (modified criteria).

The study showed an increase in overall survival (OS), 10.9 months (in the temsirolimus arm) vs. 7.3 months (in the INF arm), $P = .008$. The study also showed an increased PFS, 5.5 months (in the temsirolimus arm) vs. 3.1 months (INF arm). The objective response rate was also increased in the temsirolimus vs. INF arm (8.6% vs. 4.8%).

The drug was also studied in the previously treated setting in a phase II trial and showed a rather long time to progression and overall survival in heavily pretreated individuals.

Bevacizumab (Avastin)

A phase II trial of previously treated patients or cytokine-refractory patients showed that this agent was able to increase time to progression compared with placebo; however, no benefit in overall survival was seen.
- High doses (10 mg/kg every 2 weeks) seemed to confer a greater progression-free survival advantage.
- A recent phase III trial in previously untreated patients compared IFN-α + bevacizumab with IFN-α alone:
- The ORR was 31% (IFN-α with bevacizumab arm) vs. 13% (IFN-α-alone arm), $P < .0001$.
- PFS was 10.2 months (IFN-α with bevacizumab arm) vs. 5.4 months (IFN-α-alone arm), $P < .0001$.
- A trend toward improved OS was observed with the addition of bevacizumab to IFN-α2a ($P = .0670$).
- This drug is currently not U.S. FDA approved for the treatment of patients with advanced renal cell cancer.
- Two randomized phase III studies have shown improved PFS with Avastin/IFN vs. IFN (CALGB 90206 and the AVOREN study) and that this agent is approved in the European Union for RCC therapy.

Future directions

Further investigations are looking at different dosages of these molecular agents (including continuous dosage) and combinations of these agents along with other molecular agents to improve response. Investigators are also looking at the potential of using allogenic stem cell transplant and vaccine therapy to improve survival in these patients. An oral mTOR inhibitor RAD001 (everolimus) has recently shown promise in heavily treated patients (including tyrosine kinase inhibitors) in the second/third line setting with data showing improved PFS but that this agent is not currently approved. Future combination therapy with these agents and novel agents are being actively explored.

At this time, allogeneic bone marrow transplantation remains an unproven therapy in renal cell carcinoma, with recent findings indicating a lack of sufficient graft-versus-tumor effect in this disease.

Ongoing clinical trials are also being pursed to determine the best therapy for patients with nonclear-cell pathology, as most clinical trials have focused on clear-cell pathology.

Novel agents focused on upstream events that control VEGF production (HIF, VHL) are also being evaluated.

Cancer of the bladder and ureter

Epidemiology
An estimated 67,000 new cases are diagnosed each year, and 14,000 patients are expected to die from this disease. It remains the fourth most common male cancer diagnosed.
- Male-to-female ratio is 73:1.
- 80% occur in patients aged >60 years.

Etiology
- Cigarette smoking increases the relative risk by 6–10.
- Pelvic radiation
- Occupational exposure to a number of carcinogens including aromatic amines is associated with increased risk and latency of 20–30 years.
- Other agents with increased risk include aluminum, paint, petroleum, diesel exhaust, older hair dyes, artificial sweeteners, analgesic abuse (phenacetin), and possibly the amount of arsenic in drinking water.
- Water consumption >1.5 L/day may be protective.
- Family history may rarely contribute, because hereditary nonpolyposis colorectal cancer (HNPCC) is associated with upper-tract TCC.

Occupations putting individuals at risk include the following:
- Aniline dye and the rubber industries
- Gas works
- Rodent care and other laboratory work
- Sewage treatment
- Textile printing
- Firelighter manufacturers

Chronic irritation of the bladder usually leads to nontransitional cell carcinomas such as squamous cell carcinoma. Such irritation can be due to the following:
- Infection
- Stones
- Long-term catheter
- Schistosomiasis
- Chronic inflammation
- Cyclophosphamide therapy
- Previous pelvic radiotherapy
- Spinal cord injury

Persistent urachus (allantois) or bladder extrophy may predispose to adenocarcinoma in the dome of the bladder (rare).

Pathology
Most (>90%) urothelial tumors presenting in the United States are transitional cell carcinomas. Less common pathologies include the following:
- Squamous carcinomas associated with chronic irritation
- Adenocarcinomas arising from urachal remnants in the bladder dome
- Metaplasia in a TCC may give rise to carcinomasarcoma or neuroendocrine carcinoma (small or large cell), both of which are associated with poor outcome.

The majority (>90%) of urothelial tumors originate in the urinary bladder, with the rest arising from the renal pelvis, ureter, and urethra.

Typically, the disease presents with superficial tumor involving only the bladder epithelium, but in 25% there is tumor invasion into the detrusor muscle of the bladder, and 5% present with metastatic disease to the regional lymph nodes, lung, liver, or bone. Pathological grading (I–III) correlates well with the natural history of the disease.

Multifocal disease is not uncommon, and a history of TCC of bladder carries an increased risk of TCC arising anywhere in the urothelium.

Genetics and molecular biology

Studies focusing on familial aggregates of patients with bladder cancer have shown that hereditary predisposition may exist.

Transitional carcinomas have a number of characteristic chromosomal abnormalities including, in particular, deletion of 17p, 18q, 13q, and chromosome 9.

Other common abnormalities include mutation of the *p53* gene and overexpression of EGFR (epidermal growth factor receptor), both of which are found more often in advanced cancers and have been associated with an increased risk of treatment failure.

Ras pathway activation is also commonly found along with retinoblastoma (*Rb*) tumor suppressor loss, leading to increased proliferation and survival. The number of pathway alterations (p53, Rb, Ras) may be prognostic.

Further work is being done to examine other molecular and epigenetic alterations that would lead to possible biomarkers and/or targets for therapy in this disease.

Staging

The management and prognosis of transitional cell carcinoma of the bladder are largely determined by the stage of disease and its pathological grading. There is a strong association between well-differentiated tumors and early stage.

Seventy percent of new patients present with superficial disease, of which at least half have papillary (Ta) noninvasive tumors. Although approximately 50% of these develop recurrent superficial bladder cancers, few progress to advanced disease.

Carcinoma in situ has a worse outlook, with up to 60% of cases progressing to invasive disease if recurrent disease is not eradicated. There is a significant risk of metastatic disease with high-grade T1 disease, and this rises with increasing stage of muscle-invasive disease.

A full urological evaluation of the urinary tracts includes cystourethroscopy, urine cytology, examination under anesthesia, and evaluation of the upper tracts, because the disease could present with multifocal involvement.

Evaluation of the upper tract can be accomplished by CT scan of the abdomen or pelvis (CT urogram) or intravenous pyelography (IVP) plus renal ultrasound or MR urography. Staging per the American Joint Committee on Cancer (AJCC) is provided in Table 33.3.

Table 33.3 Staging of TCC of the bladder

Stage	Description
Tx	Primary tumor cannot be assessed
T0	No evidence of primary tumor
Ta	Noninvasive papillary carcinoma
Tis	Carcinoma in situ, dysplasia confined to epithelium
T1	Invades subepithelial connective tissue
T2a	Invades superficial muscle (inner half)
T2b	Invades deep muscle (outer half)
T3a	Invades perivesical tissue microscopically
T3b	Invades perivesical tissue with a palpable mass
T4a	Invades prostate, uterus, or vagina. Invades pelvic
T4b	wall or abdominal wall
Nx	Regional lymph nodes cannot be assessed
N0	No regional lymph node metastasis
N1	Metastasis in one lymph node up to 2 cm
N2	Metastasis in one or more lymph nodes, none >5 cm
N3	Metastasis in one or more lymph nodes >5 cm
M0	No distant metastasis
M1	Distant metastasis present
Stage group	
Stage 0a	TAN0M0
Stage 0IS	TISN0M0
Stage I	T1N0M0
Stage II	T2AN0M0
	T2BN0M0
Stage III	T3AN0M0
	T3BN0M0
	T3BN1M0
	T4AN0M0
Stage IV	T4BN0M0
	Any T any N M0
	Any T any N M1

Investigation
- CBC, liver and renal function tests, calcium and alkaline phosphatase. A bone scan should be performed if there are bony symptoms or elevated alkaline phosphatase or calcium levels.
- Upper tract evaluation (CT urogram, MRI urogram, IVP or ultrasound)

Cystoscopy with examination under anesthesia and adequate transurethral resection of bladder tumor (TURBT)
- Provide pathological diagnosis and stage
- Should include resection through underlying detrusor muscle to confirm or refute muscle invasion

Biopsy other areas of abnormal-looking epithelium (in situ carcinoma often appears as a red patch). After cystoscopic resection, pelvic examination under anesthesia should confirm the presence or absence of a residual pelvic mass (presence indicates at least T3 disease) or fixation to pelvic structures.

For low-grade superficial tumors no further imaging is required. High-grade superficial tumors do carry a significant risk of synchronous disease in the upper urinary tract and should have IVP after diagnosis.

Urine cytology should be performed for noninvasive disease.

For G3 pT1 and muscle-invasive disease, staging with chest X-ray and either CT or MRI scan of the abdomen and pelvis is required, looking particularly at the following:
- Tumor extent in the bladder and extravesical extension of tumor into adjacent fat or organs
- Pelvic and para-aortic lymphadenopathy
- Ureteric obstruction
- Liver and lung metastases

Presentation
- 80%–90% have frank or microscopic hematuria, usually painless.
- Irritative symptoms, e.g., frequency and dysuria, may be associated with muscle-invasive disease or carcinoma in situ.
- Asymptomatic disease may be picked up at routine cystoscopy in a patient with previous bladder cancer or upper tract TCC.

Management options
Superficial tumors (70%–5% newly diagnosed cases)
Treatment options for superficial bladder cancer involves TURBT, intravesical chemotherapy, immunotherapy, and, in selected patients with multiple recurrences, cystectomy.

Most of these patients have recurrence of disease; however, most of this can be treated locally. Prediction of muscle invasive disease is based on pathological stage and grade.

Grading of the tumor (G1, well differentiated, to G4, undifferentiated) plays a more important role in patients with noninvasive tumors than in those with muscle-invasive tumors.

Tables derived from large series of patients (EORTC) are available for the individual prediction of recurrence risk and risk of progression to muscle-invasive disease.

Ta and low-grade (G1–2) T1 tumors are resected cystoscopically. A single postresection infusion of intravesical chemotherapy reduces the risk of recurrence.

Because of the risk of recurrent disease, regular cytologic and cystoscopic follow-up is required (usually every 3 months). Recurrent disease is managed by intravesical therapy with bacillus Calmette-Guérin (BCG) and chemotherapy such as IFN, or through participation in clinical trials. Although maintenance BCG therapy after initial induction therapy may delay the time to recurrence or progression it remains controversial.

Tis commonly responds to intravesical BCG but recurrences are common and may be multifocal. Refractory Tis is best managed by cystectomy given the risk of progression.

Refractory Ta and low-grade (G1–2) T1 tumors are best managed by cystectomy.

G3T1 tumor management is controversial.
- >50% risk of recurrence, up to half of which may be invasive TCC
- Significant risk of regional and metastatic disease
- Initial treatment of solitary tumor often comprises TURBT followed by intravesical therapy.
- Multifocal or recurrent disease requires staging and management as for muscle-invasive disease.
- Radiotherapy is not of benefit in preventing recurrence.
- Multimodality therapy (chemotherapy, chemoradiation, and possible surgery) may be useful in select patients who wish to keep their bladder, but it has not been studied in controlled trials.
- Options would involve intravesical therapy with BCG or chemotherapy or cystectomy.

Muscle-invasive bladder cancer

Given the high rate of recurrence after TURBT, all patients with invasive disease should be considered for further treatment. Options should be discussed by the multidisciplinary team and with the patient:
- Radical cystectomy
- Chemoradiotherapy and bladder conservation
- Neoadjuvant or adjuvant chemotherapy with focus on bladder-sparing options

Radical surgery

The usual procedure is cystoprostatectomy in male patients or anterior bladder exenteration in female patients (with removal of the fallopian tubes, uterus, and anterior vaginal wall), with dissection of local lymph nodes.

The number of lymph nodes removed is prognostic, with a higher number of resected nodes conferring a more favorable prognosis. Generally, at least 10–15 lymph nodes should be removed at the time of surgery for adequate staging.

Bladder resection is associated with urinary diversion, most commonly a nonrefluxing ileal conduit and urinary bag. Another option would be creation of a continent reservoir by making a neobladder from detubularized loops of intestine, which would eliminate the need for an external stoma. However, the patient may need to perfom intermittent catheterizations.

Complications from urinary diversion include and are not limited to electrolyte disturbances, pyelonephritis, infection, and increased formation of urinary calculi.

Complications from the surgery include loss of erectile function in the male and shortening of the vagina in the female. It is important for patients to recieve advice from a stoma therapist before surgery.

Increasingly, excellent results can be achieved in selected patients treated by radical cystectomy with continent diversion based on urinary tract reconstruction by ileocystoplasty. This can produce urinary continence and, in experienced centers, the surgical complication rates are less than 10% and operative mortality less than 2%.

The large proportion of patients with muscle-invasive disease will have local or metastatic recurrence, depending on prognostic factors (node status, grade, stage, and presence of lymphovascular invasion).

Meta-analyses of studies of cisplatin-based chemotherapy regimens used in the metastatic setting have shown an increase in overall survival and an acceptable morbidity for patients with muscle-invasive disease when the chemotherapy was given either before or after surgery. This coordinated approach with medical oncologists and urologists is being more commonly used for patients with newly diagnosed muscle-invasive disease.

Radiation therapy alone

Traditionally, many patients outside the United States with invasive TCC of bladder have been treated with radiotherapy. Most studies have shown that use of radiation therapy alone is inferior to results seen with combined chemoradiation and surgery.

In the United States, radiation has not been standard care and is used only in the subset of patients who cannot tolerate chemotherapy or a cystectomy due to medical comorbidities.

Neoadjuvant and adjuvant radiation therapy alone also has not been shown to add any significant benefit. Further discussion regarding combined chemoradiation is discussed under Bladder conservation.

- Radiotherapy is planned using a CT scan to define the target volume.
- The entire bladder and prostatic urethra are treated using a 3- or 4-field plan.
- Common treatment regimens include 64 Gy/32 fractions or 52.4 Gy/20 fractions.
- Side effects include cystitis and diarrhea, and late reduction in bladder capacity.
- Frail patients unfit for radical surgery or radiotherapy may benefit from palliative radiotherapy to the bladder, ideally CT planned, e.g., 21 Gy/3 fractions/5 days.

Chemotherapy in neoadjuvant and adjuvant settings
Chemotherapy has been extensively studied in the neoadjuvant setting (see Table 33.4).

Multiple trials using cisplatin-based regimens have shown benefits and large recent meta-analyses of neoadjuvant and adjuvant trials have shown an overall survival benefit. There are no single definitive trials in these settings; however, meta-analysis has consistently shown a clear benefit to systemic therapy either before or after surgery.

In general, cisplatin-based neoadjuvant chemotherapy (MVAC, gemcitabine–cisplatin, others) has shown a 15% relative improvement in survival, translating into a 5% absolute 5-year survival advantage. This benefit is also seen in the adjuvant setting (20%–25% relative risk reduction).

In general, 4 cycles of cisplatin-based chemotherapy is typically given, with the most common U.S. regimen being gemcitabine and cisplatin on a 3- to 4-week cycle schedule.

Bladder conservation
Multiple efforts have focused on bladder conservation, which would allow patients to keep their bladder and prevent the complications of cystectomy.

The combining of multimodality therapy with chemotherapy and radiotherapy has been extensively studied. Results with chemotherapy and radiation alone have not proved to be as successful as combined modality therapy.

The most commonly used regimen is complete TURBT followed by cisplatin-based chemotherapy and chemoradiation with a cisplatin-based regimen. Studies have shown that patients respond fairly well to this regimen; yet many patients do have relapses, requiring additional therapy, and approximately 1/3 of patients will ultimately require cystectomy. Further studies are investigating responses with other radiation sensitizers.

Randomized trials are in progress to evaluate the role of this bladder-sparing approach. The patient most likely to respond to this approach has T2 pathology without hydronephrosis or carcinoma in situ and has a complete response to induction chemoradiation therapy. These patients usually have a 5-year overall survival of 50%, and 70% are able to maintain their bladder function.

Interval cystoscopy during radiotherapy to assess for primary refractory disease is recommended in this setting. Cystectomy is reserved for those patients not in a complete remission.

Table 33.4 Examples of chemotherapy regimens for bladder cancer

MVAC		
Methotrexate	30 mg/m² d1, 8, 15	
Vinblastine	3 mg/m² d2, 8, 15	q4/52
Doxorubicin	30 mg/m² d2	
Cisplatin	70 mg/m² d2	
CMV		
Methotrexate	30 mg/m² d1, 8	
Vinblastine	4 mg/m² d1, 8	q3/52
Cisplatin	100 mg/m² d2	
Gemcitabine-cisplatin		
Gemcitabine	1000 mg/m² d1, 8,	q4/52
Cisplatin	15 70 mg/m² d2	
	or	
	1000 mg/m² d1, 8	q3/52
	70 mg/m² d1	

Chemotherapy in the metastatic setting

Combination chemotherapy has an established role in the palliation of patients with advanced bladder cancer. Therapy is usually indicated for metastatic (stage 4) disease.

Cisplatin-based regimens such as MVAC were developed in the 1980s and found to have high objective response rates (750%), although few patients survive beyond 2 years. These regimens can be toxic, especially for patients with poor performance status and impaired renal function. Life-threatening toxicity (up to 5%), e.g., neutropenic sepsis, is not uncommon.

The combination of gemcitabine and cisplatin has been shown to be as effective as MVAC, with reduced toxicity, and has largely superseded the older regimen.

Prognostic factors in the metastatic setting include presence of node-only disease, presence of visceral metastases, and performance status. The median survival for node-only metastatic TCC is 18–20 months with a 20% long-term survival, indicating that node-positive TCC may still be a curable disease.

However, the median survival for patients with visceral metastatic disease is 10–12 months, with a 5%–10% 5-year survival. Thus, gemcitabine with cisplatin is the preferred regimen for metastatic disease, based on similar palliation and long-term survival and improved cost-effectiveness and safety compared with that of MVAC.

There appears to be no major survival benefit to a three-drug regimen of gemcitabine-cisplatin with paclitaxel. Other drugs being studied include taxanes, ifosfamide, and targeted (EGFR) therapy with trastuzumab (Herceptin) or cetuximab.

Even with high response rates, most patients with metastatic disease have a poor prognosis, with an average survival of 12 months even with chemotherapy.

Limited data exist for determining the optimal therapy for patients with nontransitional cell pathology.

Future treatments
- Other cytotoxics, including the taxanes, are active in this disease.
- Molecular-targeted therapies are being investigated.
- Molecular markers are being sought that may optimize selection of treatment for individual patients.

Treatment outcomes

The prognosis for superficial disease is good, with 5-year survival rates in excess of 80%.

The outlook for invasive disease is less good, with the following estimated 5-year survival rates after cystectomy:
- T2, 50%–70%
- T3, 30%–40%
- T4, 20%

Many patients treated with radiotherapy would not be candidates for radical surgery, but may still achieve successful bladder conservation.

The best results with radical radiotherapy appear to follow TURBT for a solitary T2 tumor. Poor results are obtained with T4 disease, and squamous carcinomas.

For metastatic disease, treatment with chemotherapy is associated with a median survival time of ~1 year, but <10% survive 2 years. These data depend on prognostic factors, with node-only disease having a 20% 5-year survival rate.

Renal pelvis and ureteric TCC
These uncommon tumors range from superficial low-grade disease to aggressive muscle-invasive cancer with a high propensity for distant spread.

Presentation may be with ureter obstruction, hematuria, or symptoms related to advanced disease. The tumor is commonly visible on IVP, and may be biopsied via a flexible ureteroscope.

Staging requires a CT or MRI scan of the abdomen and pelvis, as well as cystoscopy to look for synchronous bladder TCC.

Localized disease is usually treated by nephroureterectomy with removal of a cuff of bladder.

Adjuvant therapy has no proven benefit, but advanced disease may be treated with chemotherapy and palliative radiotherapy as for TCC of bladder.

Meta-analyses of adjuvant chemotherapy regimens did not show any difference in benefit according to the primary tumor site (bladder vs. upper tract). Thus cisplatin-based regimens are recommended for T2 or higher upper-tract tumors.

Penile cancer

Epidemiology
- This is an uncommon cancer, with approximately 1200 cases per year in the United States and an estimated 290 deaths from the disease.
- The incidence is close to 0.2 cases per 100,000 males and accounts for only 0.4% of all malignancies.
- Up to 23% of patients with penile cancer die of their disease.
- Most cases occur in the over-60 age group, although up to 20% occur under the age of 40.
- The disease is relatively more common in Africa, India, and South America, where the disease accounts for 10%–20% of all malignancies.

Etiology
- Age
- Human papilloma virus (HPV 16 and 18) infection
  - Prevention of disease with HPV vaccination or sexual abstinence may be possible.
- Associated with poor hygiene and phimosis
- Premalignant lesion—carcinoma in situ:
  - On the glans: erythroplasia of Queyrat
  - On the shaft: Bowen's disease
  - Progresses to invasive carcinoma in 710%
- There is increased risk with cigarette smoking and immunosuppression, including HIV infection.
- Neonatal circumcision gives lifelong protection (in uncircumcised men, the lifetime risk of penile cancer is as high as 1 in 600).

Pathology
The vast majority of cases are squamous carcinomas, which may be exophytic or locally invasive and destructive, and can spread initially via lymphatics to inguinal and then pelvic lymph nodes.

Locally advanced disease can spread to other organs, including the liver, lungs, bone, and skin.

Other types of cancers seen include basal cell carcinoma, melanoma, sarcoma, Kaposi's sarcoma, and rare metastatic lesions.

Staging
The TNM system is commonly used (see Table 33.5). Some of the older literature uses the Jackson staging system. See Table 33.5 for full staging parameters.

Table 33.5 TNM staging for penile cancer

Tx	Primary tumor cannot be assessed
T0	No evidence of primary tumor
Tis	Carcinoma in situ
Ta	Noninvasive verrucous carcinoma
T1	Tumor invades subepithelial connective tissue
T2	Tumor invades corpus spongiosum or cavernosum
T3	Tumor invades urethra or prostate
T4	Tumor invades other adjacent structures
Nx	Regional lymph nodes cannot be assessed
N0	No regional lymph node metastases
N1	Single superficial inguinal lymph node metastases
N2	Multiple or bilateral superficial inguinal lymph node metastases
N3	Deep inguinal or pelvic lymph node metastases
Mx	Distant metastasis cannot be assessed
M0	No distant metastasis
M1	Distant metastasis
Jackson staging system	
Stage I	Tumor confined to the glans or prepuce
Stage II	Tumor invasion into shaft or corpora; no nodal or distant metastasis
Stage III	Tumor confined to the penis; inguinal nodal metastasis not operable
Stage IV	Tumor involves adjacent structures (extending off the shaft); inoperable regional nodes and or/distant metastases
Stage group	
Stage I	T1N0M0
Stage II	T1N1M0
	T2N0M0 T2N1M0
Stage III	T1N2M0 T2N2M0 T3N0M0
	T3N1M0 T3N2M0
Stage IV	T4 any N M0 any T N3 M0
	Any T any N M1

Investigations

Careful examination of the penis includes cytological assessment or biopsy (punch, incisional, or excisional) of any lesion.

General examination includes palpation of inguinal lymph nodes.

- >50% have inguinal lymphadenopathy, but less than half of these have metastatic disease within the nodes: reactive lymphadenopathy is more common.
- FNA shows suspicious lymph nodes or review lymph nodes after treatment of the primary carcinoma.

Further staging, e.g., cross-sectional imaging of the abdomen and pelvis, is only required if inguinal nodes are involved or there is clinical suspicion of metastatic disease.

Newer approaches in evaluation of lymph nodes are currently underway (including sentinel lymph node sampling).

Presentation

At least 50% of cases arise on the glans, appearing as an area of erythema, warty tumor, or ulceration; 20% involve the foreskin only. In advanced disease there may be considerable destruction of the penis.

Patients not uncommonly conceal the diagnosis until there is advanced locoregional disease with considerable secondary infection.

Patients may present with metastatic disease, e.g., inguinal and pelvic lymphadenopathy.

Management

Primary tumor

Early-stage disease may be successfully managed with organ conservation.

- **Tis**: Topical 5-FU, laser therapy, Mohs microsurgery, cryotherapy, and local excision are all reasonable options with excellent local control rates and good cosmetic results.
- **T1**: Excision or radiotherapy

More advanced disease or local recurrence often requires at least partial amputation of the penis. Patients with inoperable disease may be treated with chemotherapy and radiotherapy.

New advancements include development of penile-sparing procedures such as Mohs microsurgery or surgical laser treatment.

Radiation has been extensively studied but not in a randomized fashion.

High doses of radiation are needed, but with increased side effects (meatal stenosis, fistula, skin necrosis), because most squamous cell carcinomas are radioresistant.

Penectomy-sparing radiation or brachytherapy has been used with success in many cases where the tumor is <4 cm with minimal corporal invasion.

Definitive inguinal radiation in the adjuvant setting adds to morbidity (lymphoceles, edema) but may improve local control.

Regional lymph nodes

Penile cancer is one of the few cancers in which regional lymhadenectomy is curative; however, the indications and timing for this procedure remain controversial.

Inguinal lymph nodes may be managed by surveillance if impalpable after completion of local treatment to the primary. However, with high-grade T2 and more advanced cancers, the incidence of positive regional lymph nodes is 60% or higher, and prophylactic bilateral inguinal lymphadenectomy may be considered.

Patients with persistent lymphadenopathy, after clearance of the primary tumor and any infection, should be considered for bilateral inguinal lymphadenectomy.

The extent of lymph node involvement has very important prognostic information. The majority of patients (>90%) found to have microscopic involved inguinal nodes have an excellent chance for a long-term cure through the use of preemptive lymphadenoctomy.

New techniques being studied to minimize the morbidity of lymph node dissection include modified inguinal lymphadenctomy, sentinel lymph node dissection, and selective lymphadenectomy.

Patients who are unfit for surgery or have inoperable disease may benefit from chemotherapy and radiotherapy. Adjuvant chemotherapy with platinum-based regimens is reasonable but understudied and no randomized trials are available.

Regimens studied in the metastatic disease setting are preferred, and combined modality regimens with radiotherapy are encouraged for patients with high-risk node-positive disease.

There are limited large-number trials for patients with metastatic disease receiving systemic chemotherapy. Treatment in the metastatic setting is mostly palliative and very rarely curative.

The disease is moderately chemosensitive, and active regimens include methotrexate, bleomycin, and cisplatin (MBP). The response rate in the metastatic setting has been as high as 35%, yet there was significant toxicity to this regimen. In the adjuvant setting, no clear randomized trials have shown benefit; however, some studies have shown that therapy has prevented relapse in 21 of 25 patients.

Other regimens are platinum-based regimens consisting of carboplatin and paclitaxel, cisplatin and paclitaxel, 5-FU and cisplatin, and the three-drug regimen of 5-FU, cisplatin, and paclitaxel.

Further studies are examining the role of chemotherapy in the neoadjuvant setting to enable treatment of resectable disease.

Outcomes

Overall, 50% of patients survive disease-free beyond 5-years, with better results for patients with node-negative (60%) than with node-positive (30%) disease.

Most relapses occur in the first 2 years, and close follow-up is recommended during this time.

Further reading

References

DeVita VT, Hellman S, Rosenberg SA (2005). *Cancer: Principles & Practice of Oncology* (7th ed.). Philadelphia: Lippincott Williams & Wilkins.

Dreicer R (2007). Chemotherapy for muscle-invasive bladder cancer in the perioperative setting: current standards. *Urol Oncol* 25:72–75.

Escudier B, Eisen T, Stadler WM, et al. (2007). Sorafenib in advanced clear-cell renal-cell carcinoma. *N Engl J Med* 356:125–134.

Govindan R (2008). *The Washington Manual of Oncology* (2nd ed.). Philadelphia: Lippincott Williams & Wilkins.

Greene FL, American Joint Committee on Cancer, American Cancer Society (2002). *AJCC Cancer Staging Manual* (6th ed.). New York: Springer-Verlag.

Grossman HB, Natale RB, Tangen CM, et al. (2003). Neoadjuvant chemotherapy plus cystectomy compared with cystectomy alone for locally advanced bladder cancer. *N Engl J Med* 349:859–866.

Hudes G, Carducci M, Tomczak P, et al. (2007). Temsirolimus, interferon-α, or both for advanced renal-cell carcinoma. *N Engl J Med* 356:2271–2281.

Jemal A, Siegel R, Ward E, et al. (2007). Cancer statistics. *CA Cancer J Clin* 57:43–66.

Karakiewicz PI, Briganti A, Chun FK, et al. (2007). Multi-institutional validation of a new renal cancer-specific survival nomogram. *J Clin Oncol* 25:1316–1322.

Lotan Y, Gupta A, Shariat SF, et al. (2005). Lymphovascular invasion is independently associated with overall survival, cause-specific survival, and local and distant recurrence in patients with negative lymph nodes at radical cystectomy. *J Clin Oncol* 23:6533–6539.

Motzer RJ, Hutson TE, Tomczak P, et al. (2007). Sunitinib versus interferon-A in metastatic renal-cell carcinoma. *N Engl J Med* 356:115–124.

Motzer RJ, Mazumdar M, Bacik J, et al. (1999). Survival and prognostic stratification of 670 patients with advanced renal cell carcinoma. *J Clin Oncol* 17:2530–2540.

Advanced Bladder Cancer Meta-analysis Collaboration (2003). Neoadjuvant chemotherapy in invasive bladder cancer: a systematic review and meta-analysis. *Lancet* 361:1927–1934.

Parekh DJ, Bochner BH, Dalbagni G (2006). Superficial and muscle-invasive bladder cancer: principles of management for outcomes assessments. *J Clin Oncol* 24:5519–5527.

Pizzocaro G, Piva L, Bandieramonte G, Tana S (1997). Up-to-date management of carcinoma of the penis. *Eur Urol* 32:5–15.

Rintala E, Hannisdahl E, Fossa SD, et al. (1993). Neoadjuvant chemotherapy in bladder cancer: a randomized study. Nordic Cystectomy Trial I. *Scand J Urol Nephrol* 27:355–362.

Shammas FV, Ous S, Fossa SD (1992). Cisplatin and 5-fluorouracil in advanced cancer of the penis. *J Urol* 147:630–632.

von der Maase H, Hansen SW, Roberts JT, et al. (2000). Gemcitabine and cisplatin versus methotrexate, vinblastine, doxorubicin, and cisplatin in advanced or metastatic bladder cancer: results of a large, randomized, multinational, multicenter, phase III study. *J Clin Oncol* 18:3068–3077.

Yang JC, Haworth L, Sherry RM, et al. (2003). A randomized trial of bevacizumab, an anti-vascular endothelial growth factor antibody, for metastatic renal cancer. *N Engl J Med* 349:427–434.

Zisman A, Pantuck AJ, Dorey F, et al. (2001). Improved prognostication of renal cell carcinoma using an integrated staging system. *J Clin Oncol* 19:1649–1657.

NCCN Guidelines

NCCN Clinical Practice Guidelines in Oncology: Bladder Cancer. V.2.2008. National Comprehensive Cancer Network, 2008.

NCCN Clinical Practice Guidelines in Oncology: Kidney Cancer. V.1.2008. National Comprehensive Cancer Network, 2008.

Chapter 34

Genitourinary cancers II: prostate cancer

Rhonda L. Bitting
Andrew J. Armstrong

Prostate cancer *564*
Management of prostate cancer *574*
Treatment outcomes *580*
Future directions *586*
Further reading *587*

Prostate cancer

Cancer of the prostate gland is one of the most controversial malignancies. The clinical states of prostate cancer include clinically localized disease, recurrent disease with rising prostate-specific antigen (PSA) (when salvage therapy is typically given), clinical metastases in a noncastrate state, castration-resistant progression, and progression after chemotherapy. Death from prostate cancer is usually confined to only the latter two states.

Much work is being done to further understand each of these progression points and the development of therapies to prevent progression along this continuum.

Despite its high incidence—now the most common noncutaneous male cancer in the United States—for many men with this diagnosis, the optimum management is uncertain, with a spectrum of treatment options ranging from observation to complex surgery, radiation therapy, hormonal manipulation, and chemotherapy for metastatic disease.

Epidemiology

Prostate cancer is the most common male cancer in the United States and the second leading cause of cancer-related deaths.
- >230,000 new cases per annum with incidence continuing to rise
- Lifetime risk is 15%–20% and risk of death from prostate cancer is 3.6%.
- It is rarely diagnosed in men <50 years, although autopsy studies show clinically latent prostate cancer in 30%–50% of men under 50.
- 85% of men are diagnosed at age 65 or older.
- Autopsy studies have estimated that 70% of men >80 years have histological evidence of cancer in the prostate.
- 27,000 deaths per year are caused by prostate cancer in the United States, making it the second leading cause of cancer death among U.S. men; however, many men with this diagnosis die of other causes, and only 1 in 8 men with prostate cancer will die of their disease.

Etiology

Its pathogenesis is likely androgen dependent, and men who are castrated or develop hypogonadism before 40 years rarely develop prostate cancer.
- Age is the most important risk factor, and recent data indicate that young men with prostate cancer are more likely to have androgen-driven genomic breakpoints, suggesting differences in pathogenesis based on age.
- Genetic factors also play a factor, because studies have shown that having an affected first-degree relative increases the risk 2-fold and monozygotic concordance of 25%.
- 5%–10% of cases seem to be linked to inheritance of a susceptibility gene, particularly cases arising at a young age. Linkages to the insulin growth factor (IGF), inflammatory response axis, and the androgen receptor are notable.
- There is no particular association with alcohol or tobacco, although smoking may be a risk factor for aggressive prostate cancer.

Recent analysis of genome-wide association studies showed that a region on chromosome 8q24 leads to an increased risk of prostate cancer in patients of European and African-American ancestry; however, the exact gene or genes have not been discovered.

Further work is being done to investigate genes responsible for oxidative stress and inflammation that may lead to increased susceptibility to the development of prostate cancer.

- At present, linked genes include *BRCA1* and *BRCA2*, but these do not account for the majority of cases with a family history.
- Linkage analysis suggests that there is a hereditary prostate cancer locus on chromosome 1q 24–25 (RNASEL) that may be associated with retroviral infection and a higher risk of prostate cancer.

Race is a factor, because there is a 60% increased incidence among African Americans, often with poor prognosis and an earlier age of onset than that of Caucasian Americans. Prostate cancer is uncommon in Asian men.

Dietary factors (high animal fat, low cruciferous vegetables) may also lead to increased development of aggressive prostate cancer.

- Obesity is linked to advanced prostate cancer, PSA recurrence, and lower PSA levels (hemodilution), thus underdiagnosis, but is not associated with prostate cancer incidence.
- Tomato sauce consumption, low-calcium intake, exercise, low body mass index, nonsmoking status, and high intake of cruciferous vegetables with low consumption of red meats are potential modifiable risk factors for aggressive prostate cancer.

Height is also linked to increased risk. Statin use is linked to a decreased risk of high-grade prostate cancer

Pathology

The vast majority (95%) are adenocarcinomas; rare pathologies include neuroendocrine and transitional cell carcinomas, ductal carcinomas, foamy carcinomas, mucinous carcinomas, and small cell tumors. Seventy percent arise in the peripheral zone of the gland and many are multifocal.

The natural history of the disease correlates well with its histological grade assessed by Gleason score. Low-grade cancers (Gleason 6 or less) are typically small and slow growing and confined to the prostate gland.

High-grade cancers (Gleason >7) have a higher proliferative index and frequently invade through the prostate capsule. They can directly infiltrate adjacent organs (seminal vesicles, bladder, rectum) and may disseminate to regional lymph nodes and by vascular invasion, typically to bone, but also occasionally to the lung and liver.

The Gleason score combined with other factors such as performance status (PS), clinical stage, PSA velocity, the presence of Gleason 5 components (poorly differentiated), and the percentage of gland involvement have proven to have significant predictive prognostic impact in patients diagnosed with prostate cancer.

Screening for prostate cancer

The rationale for screening is to detect the disease at an early stage in asymptomatic men, which then will lead to decreased morbidity and mortality. Ten-year prostate cancer survival is clearly improved in patients with localized disease (close to 75%) compared with survival for those with metastatic disease (close to 15%).

Since the development of assays to measure serum PSA to diagnose prostatic disease, the condition has been increasingly diagnosed at an earlier stage. This stage migration has led to approximately 75% of cancers being diagnosed as local disease when therapies are most effective.

Over the last 10 years, the mortality rate from prostate cancer in the United States has fallen, and advocates of PSA screening have claimed this as evidence of success of screening.

The issue of screening in prostate cancer is still very controversial. Those who advocate for regular screening believe that finding prostate cancer early offers men with more treatment options. Those who recommend against regular screening argue that most prostate cancers grow very slowly, and the side effects of treatment would likely outweigh any benefit from detecting the cancer at an early stage. Most groups recommend that physicians have individual discussions with patients regarding risks and benefits of screening and individualize decisions on the basis of the patient's life expectancy, underlying prostate cancer risk, and other medical comorbidities.

Many worldwide studies have investigated the benefits of screenings, and no randomized trials have clearly shown a decrease in overall mortality with screening, although prostate cancer specific mortality was reduced by 20%–30% in the large European screening trial. The harms of screening include overdiagnosis of disease (diagnosing clinically insignificant disease), biopsy complications, and the potential side effects of therapy.

Recent studies in large U.S. and European populations have suggested that the benefit of screening occurs 10 or more years after screening, given the long natural history of prostate cancer. These studies indicate that 500-1,000 men will need to be screened to save one life from prostate cancer. As such, in 2012, the U.S. Preventative Task Force recommended against the use of PSA screening for healthy men of all ages, stating that the harms of screening outweigh the benefits. In contrast, however, physician-led groups such as the American Society of Clinical Oncology and the American Urological Association maintain that PSA screening should be considered in the context of a man's life expectancy and other medical conditions and based on individual risk/benefit assessments. Most experts agree that there is no role for PSA screening for men expected to live less than 10 years. If screening is chosen, then the recommendations are for a yearly digital rectal exam (DRE) and PSA beginning at age 50 until life expectancy <10 years. Screening should begin earlier (age 40) for patients with increased risk (first-degree relative and black men). The NCCN recommends a baseline PSA at age 40 to establish risk over time and inform upon the appropriate intervals for screening. However, this practice has not been prospectively validated.

We will discuss the potential modalities used in screening currently in the Unites States.

Prostate-specific antigen, % free prostate-specific antigen, velocity, age-specific prostate-specific antigen

Measurement of serum PSA has limitations as a screening test for prostate cancer. Conventionally, PSA >4 ng/mL is viewed as an indication for prostatic biopsy. However
- PSA may be elevated in the absence of prostate cancer, e.g., in benign prostatic hyperplasia, prostatitis.
- One in 4 men with a PSA >4 ng/mL will be found to have cancer on biopsy of the prostate, but approximately one third of prostate cancers will have a PSA <4 ng/mL.
- Sensitivity is generally low, on the order of 40%–60% depending on the populations studied. Specificity may range from 50% to 90% depending on the population studied.
- Higher levels of PSA (>10 ng/mL) correlate with tumor stage and grade but also with prostate volume.
- Free PSA has also been recently approved as an adjunct to help improve total PSA in diagnosing men with prostate cancer. Using a cutoff at <25%, free PSA has been shown to help increase the sensitivity for the diagnosis of prostate cancer in patients with a PSA of 4–10 ng/mL.
- PSA velocity (rate of change of PSA over time) has also been shown to help determine patients more likely to have prostate cancer. Different studies have shown that different values are most predictive, with the range being 0.5 ng/mL per year to 0.75 ng/mL per year. A recent study also showed that patients with a PSA velocity of 2.0 ng/mL per year, during the year of prostate cancer diagnosis, have decreased overall survival.
- To reduce the risk of false-positive and false-negative biopsies, studies have shown that use of age-specific PSA cutoff criteria may improve biopsy results.

Potential new biomarkers

Analysis of genomic, proteomic, and epigenetic changes in the progression from normal prostate epithelium to prostate cancer has led to the discovery of new biomarkers that may be approved in the future to help diagnose men with prostate cancer

Potential biomarkers being used and tested in serum and urine include the following:
- ETS family transcription factors (ERG and ETV1) and the TMPRSS2-ERG gene fusion (urine fusion detection), urine RNA profiles or exosomes
- AMACR
- Autoantibodies

Further work is required to validate these markers for use in combination with PSA to help prevent the large number of false-positive biopsies in prostate cancer.

Investigations

Patients with lower urinary tract symptoms should have DRE and PSA testing offered. All patients having PSA tested should be counseled that
- The test may detect cancer in 15%–75% of men aged 50–65.
- The test will fail to detect up to 25% of cancers.
- Biopsy and further treatment of cancer, if found, carry the risk of some morbidity, with no guarantee of improved life expectancy.

Asymptomatic patients with elevated PSA should also be assessed by digital rectal examination (40% of palpable nodules are malignant).

Transrectal ultrasound scan and prostatic biopsy are required for patients with PSA >4 µg/L and in patients with normal PSA but a palpable abnormality in the gland. In younger men, this threshold could reasonably be lowered to 2.5 ng/mL, given the lack of confounding by BPH. However, lowering this threshold would raise the risk of over-detection and false-positive biopsies.

Current guidelines recommend at least a 12-core biopsy along the prostate gland with antibiotic coverage. The prostate volume is measured by ultrasound, and urinary flow rate may also be measured.

In patients with biopsy-proven cancer, further investigation depends on the stage, grade, and PSA, and the planned treatment. Staging evaluation includes bone scan and CT scan of the chest, abdomen, or pelvis for intermediate- to high-risk men with prostate cancer.
- MRI scan of the prostate and pelvis provides the most accurate estimate of locoregional tumor extent.

CNS imaging is not recommended in the absence of symptoms. Risk-based staging (CT or bone scan) evaluations are based on the following risk groups:
- Low risk: T1c–T2a OR Gleason <7 OR PSA <10: no staging scans needed
- Intermediate risk: Gleason 7 OR PSA 10–20 OR T2b: consider staging scans particularly for Gleason 7 and PSA >10 or based on nomogram calculated probabilities of lymph node involvement >5%–10%
- High risk: T2c–T3 disease OR PSA>20 OR Gleason >7: staging recommended

However, these risk groups do not take into account the PSA velocity, percentage of gland involvement with tumor on biopsy, or presence of tertiary Gleason 5. Individual risk staging and treatments may be guided by these factors in addition to current risk models and nomograms.

It is not recommended that cross-sectional imaging or bone scan be performed in patients with clinically T1–2, Gleason grade 6 or less, and PSA <10 ng/mL, because of the low probability of disease spread beyond the prostate gland. Locally advanced disease (T2c to T4), high-grade cancer, and high PSA level (>10 ng/mL) at presentation are all indications for more complete staging, initially with bone scan, and if the bone scan is clear, either MRI or CT to examine pelvic and para-aortic nodes.

Presenting symptoms and signs
- >50% are asymptomatic with elevated PSA (T1c).
- Urinary symptoms, e.g., frequency, nocturia, poor stream, retention, hematuria
  - These are commonly due to coincident benign prostatic hyperplasia (BPH).
  - Symptoms may be scored, e.g., using the International Prostate Symptoms Score (IPSS).

Locally advanced disease may cause the following:
- Impotence due to neurovascular bundle infiltration
- Hemospermia
- Ureteric obstruction and renal failure
- Rectal symptoms, e.g., tenesmus, bleeding
- Lymph node spread with lymphedema in legs and genitals
- Bone metastases with pain, fracture, nerve root or spinal cord compression, or malignant hypercalcemia
- Rarely liver, pleura, or lung metastases

Staging and prognostic factors

The TNM staging system is used and recent AJCC 2010 staging of prostate cancer additionally incorporates Gleason sum and PSA (Table 34.1). Independently, the PSA value, Gleason's score, and clinical staging are all prognostic; however, when they are combined they are able to prognosticate more accurately. Thus each are incorporated into modern staging assessments.

Multiple nomograms and tables (i.e., Partin tables, Memorial Sloan Kettering Cancer Center [MSKCC] nomograms) have used these parameters to accurately predict pathological stage from preoperative clinical stage (helping the urologist plan the extent of surgery and probability of organ-confined disease) and prostate cancer recurrence after radical prostatectomy and radiation therapy.

In stratifying patients once they are initially diagnosed, the standard usually involves stratification along three groups, with low, intermediate, and high risk of recurrence (Table 34.2).
- The low-risk group consists of patients with any of the following: T1–T2a disease, Gleason score 2–6, and PSA <10 ng/mL; 83% 10-year disease-free survival (free of PSA recurrence)
- The intermediate-risk group consists of patients with any of the following: T2b–T2c disease, Gleason score 7, or PSA 10–20 ng/mL; 40%–50% 10-year disease-free survival
- The high-risk group consists of patients with any of the following: T3b–T4 disease, Gleason score 8–10, and PSA >20 ng/mL; 30% 10-year disease-free survival.

The 5-year biochemical recurrence-free survival for these patients is 94.5%, 76.6%, and 54.6% for the low-, intermediate-, and high-risk groups, respectively, based on commonly used nomograms.

Table 34.1 TNM clinical staging of prostate cancer

Primary tumor	
TX	Primary tumor cannot be assessed
T0	No evidence of tumor
T1a	Tumor, incidental histologic finding at resection (<5%)
T1b	Tumor, incidental histologic finding at resection (>5%)
T1c	Nonpalpable tumor identified by needle biopsy and elevated PSA
T2a	Tumor involves less than half of one lobe
T2b	Tumor involves more than half of a lobe but not both lobes
T2c	Tumor involves both lobes
T3a	Unilateral or bilateral extracapsular extension
T3b	Tumor involves seminal vesicles
T4	Tumor invades bladder neck, rectum, pelvic side-wall
Clinical lymph nodes	
Nx	Regional lymph nodes were not assessed
N0	No regional lymph nodes metastasis
N1	Metastasis in regional lymph nodes
Pathologic	
pNx	Regional nodes sampled
pN0	No positive regional nodes
pN1	Metastasis in regional nodes
Distant metastases	
Mx	Distant metastasis cannot be assessed
M0	No distant metastasis
M1a	Nonregional lymph nodes
M1b	Metastasis to the bone
M1c	Metastasis to other site(s) with or without bone metastasis

Table 34.2 Estimate of risk of prostate cancer-specific survival after biochemical recurrence following radical prostatectomy

PSA doubling time, months	Recurrence >3 years after surgery		Recurrence <3 years after surgery	
	Gleason Score <8	Gleason Score >8	Gleason Score <8	Gleason Score >8
5-year estimate				
>15	100	99	99	98
9–14.9	99	98	97	94
3–8.9	97	94	91	81
<3	92	83	74	51
10-year estimate				
>15	98	96	93	86
9–14.9	95	90	85	69
3–8.9	84	68	55	26
<3	59	30	15	1

Adapted from Freedland SJ, Humphreys EB, Mangold LA, et al. (2005). Risk of prostate cancer-specific mortality following biochemical recurrence after radical prostatectomy. *JAMA* 294:433–439. Reprinted with permission of the American Medical Association.

The most common preoperative and postoperative nomograms are briefly discussed below.
- In the Kattan preoperative nomogram, 60-month recurrence-free probability is based on points assigned for the following risk factors: pretreatment PSA, biopsy Gleason sum, and clinical stage.
- In the Kattan postoperative nomogram, 84-month recurrence-free probability is based on points assigned for the following risk factors: preoperative PSA, Gleason sum, prostatic capsule invasion, surgical margins, seminal vesicle invasion, and lymph nodes.

Clinicians are able to determine the best management for patients depending on where they fall in the above risk groups.
- It is essential to identify high-risk patients to target more aggressive multimodality strategies useing surgery and/or radiation therapy, or clinical trials involving systemic therapy before or after local therapy.
- The goal of therapy is to prevent development of metastatic disease.

In patients with relapse after radical prostatectomy, one of the strongest surrogates determining increased mortality is PSA doubling time. Studies have shown that patients with a PSA doubling time of <6 months have the highest prostate cancer mortality, and that men with PSA doubling times >15 months are equally likely to die of other nonprostate cancer causes.

When combining PSA doubling time, pathological Gleason score, and time from surgery to biochemical recurrence, clinicians are able to more accurately predict patients who are more likely to develop metastasis and prostate cancer mortality.

The men in these studies typically had hormonal therapy withheld until symptomatic or metastatic progression, which provides a good natural history estimate for 5-, 10-, and 15-year outcomes, but may not be generalizable to men treated with androgen deprivation earlier in the disease course based on PSA level.

In the metastatic setting and hormone refractory/castration-resistant setting, prognostic factors leading to decreased overall survival include rapid PSA doubling time, poor performance status, presence of visceral metastases, elevated LDH, circulating tumor cells ≥5, low albumin, the type of progression (bone scan, PSA only, measurable disease), presence of significant pain requiring narcotics, elevated baseline PSA, presence of anemia, and elevated LDH.

PSA nadir following initiation of androgen deprivation therapy (ADT) is also highly prognostic.

Several nomograms have been developed (MSKCC, Halabi, and Armstrong) that allow for risk stratification even in this uniformly fatal disease state.

Management of prostate cancer

Organ-confined prostate cancer

For patients diagnosed with early-stage prostate cancer, several treatment options may be considered (Table 34.3).

Selection of the most appropriate option depends on consideration of the following:
- Life expectancy of the patient, taking into account age and comorbidities
- Predicted natural history of the prostate cancer, determined by stage, PSA, Gleason score, and other risk factors
- Patient preferences, often with consideration of toxicities of treatment

Prostate disease is commonly categorized as follows:
- *Low risk*: T1–2a and PSA <10 µg/L and Gleason score 6 or less
- *Intermediate risk*: T2b–c, or PSA 10–20 µg/L, or Gleason score 7
- *High risk*: T3–4, or PSA > 20 µg/L, or Gleason score >7

Active surveillance

However, active surveillance (AS) is also a very reasonable option in men with low risk disease. The recent PIVOT trial randomized men with localized PC to immediate RP vs. initial observation and did not demonstrate an improvement in PC specific or overall survival despite 10 years of follow up. In low-risk men in particular, there was evidence of harm rather than benefit, suggesting that immediate RP should be reserved for men with higher risk disease in which the probability of PC specific mortality with active surveillance is high (i.e., intermediate to high-risk men, low comorbidity, >10 year life expectancy). The ideal candidate for AS is currently not known, given a lack of long-term followup in most series. However, currently, men with low-risk PC and low volume disease (PSA density <0.15, <4 cores involved, <50% of a single core involved) are reasonable candidates for initial active surveillance, which usually entails a period of serial PSA and DRE measures every 3–6 months and repeat biopsies every 12 months and then based on changes over time. A worsening of Gleason sum or tumor volume or a rapid rise in the PSA are often triggers for treatment of localized disease but a consensus definition for when to stop AS and move to definitive therapy is not yet known. Approximately 10%–15% of men per year on AS will progress or move to radical therapy, indicating that progression does occur over time; however, a large minority of men may remain on AS long term (5–10 years) without progression and free of the side effects of radical interventions.

Radical prostatectomy

For patients <70 years, without significant comorbidities, and with low- or intermediate-risk disease, radical surgery gives excellent disease-free survival rates.
- The approach may be retropubic or perineal, the former allowing pelvic lymph node sampling. Robotic or laparoscopic or standard open procedures are all reasonable options.

- Lymph node sampling may be performed laparoscopically, avoiding major surgery in patients who have positive lymph nodes.
- Postoperative problems have been reduced with improvements in surgical technique but may include:
  - Urinary incontinence, rarely (75%) persists beyond 6 months
  - Impotence, previously inevitable after prostatectomy, with nerve-sparing procedures may be prevented in 50%.

After prostatectomy the PSA should fall promptly within 4–6 weeks to <0.1. Patients with positive resection margins with slowly rising PSA levels may benefit from postoperative adjuvant or salvage radiotherapy to the prostate bed.

Increasingly, radical prostatectomy is being undertaken laparoscopically with early excellent results (in some centers aided by robotic surgery).

The benefits of robotic surgery include less intraoperative blood loss and quicker recovery time; however, no randomized trials have been done comparing the two approaches. Current recommendations are that the most critical factor in the success of a robotic approach lies in the skill and volume of robotic cases done by the urologist.

Patients with positive lymph nodes on surgery can be treated with androgen deprivation therapy or watchful waiting, but it is unclear whether surgical removal of the prostate is necessary for local control in this situation. Long-term survival has been seen in some node-positive patients who underwent surgery and prolonged ADT.

There have been no neoadjuvant or adjuvant trials showing successful use of ADT and surgery in high-risk, node-negative patients.

Further neoadjuvant trials are currently being done with combination hormonal therapy, chemotherapy, and targeted therapy to decrease time to recurrence and overall survival in patients diagnosed with intermediate- and high-risk local prostate cancer.

Radiotherapy

For patients with low-, intermediate-, or high-risk disease in which metastatic disease has been excluded by isotope bone scan and MRI or CT scan of the pelvic and retroperitoneal lymph nodes, radical radiotherapy offers an alternative curative treatment option.

Although there are no randomized trials comparing surgery and radiotherapy for early prostate cancer, stage-for-stage rates of disease-free survival after radiotherapy compare favorably with surgery. In addition, many patients treated by radiotherapy are unfit or have disease too extensive for surgery.

New advances in the delivery of radiation, such as intensity-modulated radiation therapy (IMRT), have allowed delivery of higher doses of targeted radiation with less damage to normal tissues.

Table 34.3 Treatment options summarized

Risk	Option	Comments
Low	Active surveillance, brachytherapy, external beam radiation therapy, or radical prostatectomy	Consider baseline urinary, sexual, and bowel function. Two randomized trials have shown that higher doses of radiation decreases risk of prostate cancer recurrence and one randomized trial showed that surgery may lead to increased survival and decreased cancer-related death over that with watchful waiting.
Intermediate	Active surveillance, brachytherapy, external beam radiation therapy, or radical prostatectomy	One randomized trial showed that use of neoadjuvant and concurrent hormonal therapy for 6 months may prolong survival for patients who receive radiotherapy. One randomized trial showed that radical prostatectomy may lead to increased survival and lower risk of cancer recurrence and cancer-related death than active surveillance. Two randomized trials showed that higher doses of radiation may decrease risk of prostate cancer recurrence.
High	Active surveillance not recommended. Brachytherapy combined with external beam radiation therapy, or radical prostatectomy. Prostate cancer recurrence rates are high with all these options.	One randomized trial has shown that radical prostatectomy may be associated with improved survival and lower cancer recurrence risk and cancer-related death than that with active surveillance, and one trial showed use of adjuvant and concurrent hormonal therapy leads to increased prolonged survival in patients receiving radiation.

Adapted from Walsh PC, DeWeese TL, Eisenberger MA (2007). *N Eng J Med* 357: 2696–2705. Copyright © 2007 Massachusetts Medical Society. Reprinted with permission.

External beam radiotherapy
High doses of ionizing radiation are needed to eradicate prostate cancer.
- Using CT-planned, conformal radiotherapy, doses of 78–79 Gy can be safely delivered to the prostate, with acceptable normal tissue reactions and a high rate of disease-free survival.
- Prior treatment with 3–6 months of anti-androgen therapy reduces the prostatic volume and is commonly used in intermediate- and high-risk disease to decrease the risk of prostate cancer mortality and local/PSA recurrences.

In high-risk disease there is now good evidence to support the continuation of adjuvant anti-androgen therapy (usually an LHRH agonist) for 2–3 years after radiotherapy, with improvement in survival at least in locally advanced disease.
- Radiotherapy fields can encompass tumor that is invading through the prostate capsule. It remains unclear if whole pelvic radiotherapy is beneficial in the modern era of IMRT and long-term ADT.
- Common toxicities of radiotherapy to the prostate include the following:
  - Acute-radiation cystitis or urethritis with urinary frequency, poor stream, and dysuria
  - Acute-radiation proctitis with tenesmus, pain, and passage of mucus and blood
  - Late effects include impotence in 75% (and all patients receiving anti-androgen therapy) and rectal bleeding from telangiectasia.

Proton beam radiotherapy may improve the delivery of focused radiation to the prostate and avoid normal structures, but the safety and efficacy of this modality is unproven over IMRT alone.

There is evidence that irradiation of the pelvic lymph nodes as well as the prostate gland reduces the risk of relapse in men with intermediate- or high-risk disease.

Many centers are currently using IMRT techniques to facilitate irradiation of lymph nodes and prostate with reduced normal tissue damage, in particular bowel and rectum.

Brachytherapy
Permanent implantation of radioactive iodine seeds (^{125}I or ^{103}Pd) under transrectal ultrasound control may be used to deliver a dose of 7140 Gy to the prostate, again with excellent results in organ-confined prostate cancer. This treatment is contraindicated in those with large volume disease, very small or large prostate volumes, or previous TURP.

It avoids the inconvenience of 7–8 weeks of external beam radiotherapy, and it has similar toxicities:
- Radiation urethritis, may require a urinary catheter for some days
- Radiation proctitis
- Impotence, probably less frequent than with external beam radiotherapy

Neoadjuvant and adjuvant hormone therapy may be used with brachytherapy as with external beam radiotherapy. Randomized controlled trials comparing brachytherapy to other modalities are lacking but single-arm series suggest excellent long-term control with combination external beam and brachytherapy.

Cryotherapy

There is ongoing research into the use of this modality for the primary treatment of patients diagnosed with local prostate cancer. Currently, its indications are for patients unable to tolerate radical prostatectomy or radiation therapy with low-risk disease and poor sexual dysfunction.

Salvage cryotherapy for local failure after radiation or surgery may also be considered. Trials are ongoing to evaluate this modality in both the primary and recurrent setting.

Hormone therapy alone

Androgen deprivation has been used for many years to treat patients with localized prostate cancer if they are unfit for radical surgery or radiotherapy. However, such treatment has only temporary impact in terms of delay of tumor progression, and, although normal PSA levels may be maintained for a number of years, hormone-refractory disease eventually develops. In men who are candidates for radiotherapy, ADT alone is not recommended.

There is some controversy surrounding the timing of hormone therapy for nonmetastatic prostate cancer, particularly when this is asymptomatic. Treatment is typically guided by the absolute level of PSA and the rate of PSA rise over time.

Cardiovascular risk and comorbidities should be considered, given the known risks of ADT. For patients with high-risk disease for which radical treatment is not appropriate or feasible, immediate treatment with androgen deprivation may be preferred to watchful waiting.

Watchful waiting

Particularly for patients >70 years with low-risk, low-volume cancers, a policy of expectant management is appropriate. This approach is distinct from active surveillance in that local therapy is not applied in a deferred fashion typically, and therapy is usually used only if disease spreads or becomes symptomatic. Therapy such as ADT or radiation is typically applied palliatively.

The Scandinavian Prostate Cancer Group has published 10-year results of their randomized study of watchful waiting versus radical prostatectomy.

- This study clearly demonstrates benefits of radical treatment for prostate cancer, in terms of reduction in the risk of local recurrence, metastatic disease, need for hormone therapy, and death from prostate cancer.
- However, these benefits appear to be in patients <65 years, often with intermediate-risk disease. Thus, initial AS or WW in elderly men with localized low or intermediate risk PC is reasonable.

Patients who develop progressive disease (based on PSA or biopsy) on watchful waiting should be considered for radical treatment or androgen deprivation therapy.

PSA failure

A rising PSA level after a radical prostatectomy (detected on two or more visits) or radical radiotherapy (a rise >2 ng/mL or more above the nadir PSA) may herald the development of local recurrence or metastatic disease. Predictors of the latter are the following:
- A short interval from treatment to PSA rise (<2–3 years)
- PSA doubling time <6–12 months
- Involved pelvic lymph nodes or seminal vesicles at surgery
- Baseline Gleason score >8
- Positive margins

Patients with features suggesting local recurrence (positive seminal vesicles, extracapsular disease, and positive margins) after surgery may be candidates for adjuvant radiotherapy. It remains unclear if adjuvant radiation surgery is equivalent to waiting until PSA recurrence and then giving salvage radiotherapy. Treating all men with these high-risk features may be overtreatment, thus exposing a large population to unnecessary side effects including impotence and urinary complications.

Rising PSA after radiotherapy may be managed expectantly, with androgen deprivation, or with salvage local therapy, e.g., prostate cryotherapy. There is controversy surrounding the benefits and timing of these interventions. For men with node + disease at surgery, immediate ADT has shown a survival benefit compared with deferred ADT based on metastatic progression. However, many men do well with ADT initiated based on a PSA rise to a predetermined threshold (i.e., 10–20) and the use of intermittent therapy (preplanned breaks in ADT) for men who obtain an excellent PSA decline with initial ADT after 6–12 months. In this nonmetastatic setting, intermittent ADT appears equivalent to continuous ADT and may reduce CV mortality.

Treatment outcomes

The prognosis of early prostate cancer is excellent, with median survival times >10 years for patients treated by either radical prostatectomy or radiotherapy.

Although disease progression as measured by rising PSA occurs in ~30%–40% of locally treated patients, the natural history of recurrent disease may be very slow. United States data indicate that the median time from PSA rise postprostatectomy to the development of metastatic disease may be as long as 8 years.

The median time from PSA rise after radical radiotherapy until metastatic disease is shorter, approximately 5 years, almost certainly reflecting the more advanced stages of disease treated with this modality.

- For metastatic disease, the median duration of response to hormone therapy is 18–24 months.
- The median survival time after development of hormone-refractory disease is 12 months.

Metastatic disease

Although distant spread of prostate cancer is incurable, most patients can have excellent palliation of their symptoms and a survival time of at least 2 years with appropriate hormone therapy, and some men go on with only this therapy for decades.

The growth of prostate cancer is androgen dependent, and a number of hormone treatment options are effective. Most patients (>80%) have an excellent response to hormonal therapy and have dramatic drops in PSA levels.

In patients who relapse after primary therapies for local prostate cancer, the timing of when to start androgen deprivation therapy remains controversial. Hormonal therapy is not proven to be curative and some argue that waiting until clear progression (not PSA alone) is the ideal time to initiate hormonal therapy.

Early hormonal therapy may improve prostate cancer outcomes and survival when combined with radiation therapy, when used in lymph node-positive men after surgery, and for men with metastatic disease. Intermittent ADT is not recommended for men with metastatic disease based on the lack of noninferiority in randomized trials in this setting.

- Men with rapid PSA doubling times (<6 months) are also likely to need hormonal therapy earlier in the disease course, although this remains unproven.
- For men with relatively slow PSA doubling times (>12–15 months), deferred treatment remains a reasonable standard of care to prevent the adverse effects of androgen deprivation, including fracture, cardiovascular risk, diabetes, weight gain, and symptomatic hot flashes.
- For men with intermediate-risk disease (PSADT 6–12 months), the timing of ADT remains controversial and is individualized in most patients on the basis of patient preference, cardiovascular risk, and other risk factors for metastatic disease progression, such as time from surgery to recurrence, Gleason sum, and disease symptoms.

Randomized trials in this population of early versus deferred ADT are clearly needed but difficult to carry out because of the prolonged disease process.

Surgical castration
- Achieves permanent reduction in circulating androgens
- Inexpensive
- Major toxicities include impotence and loss of libido, fatigue, mood disturbance, hot flashes, weight gain, diabetes risk, cardiovascular risk, and muscle weakness.
  - In long-term survivors it causes osteoporosis and fractures.
  - It may not be acceptable to the patient.

Medical castration
- LHRH agonist, e.g., goserelin (Zoladex), leuprolide acetate (Lupron), triptorelin (Trelstar) OR LHRH antagonist, e.g., degarelix acetate (Firmagon)
- Administered as either a subcutaneous or intramuscular injection monthly or every 3–6 months

Medical castration has the flowing features:
- Treatment with LHRH agonists cause an initial flare with a rise in testosterone followed by a fall to castrate level. Therefore, concurrent anti-androgen therapy is recommended for 2 weeks after the first injection (e.g., bicalutamide [Casodex], flutamide [Eulexin], or nilutamide [Nilandron]).
- It has similar toxicities to those of surgical castration.
- There is concern about potential increased cardiovascular risk for patients on these therapies for a prolonged period of time, and clinicians need to be aware of underlying cardiovascular risk before offering and continuing this therapy.
- The effects are reversible, but it may take many months for the testosterone level to recover after withdrawal of the LHRH agonist.

Androgen blockade
This carried out with nonsteroidal agents, e.g., bicalutamide (Casodex), flutamide (Eulexin), or Nilutamide (Nilandron).
- Anticancer effects are less, but may preserve libido and sexual potency
- May cause gynecomastia
- Major side effects include GI disturbances, elevated liver function tests, hot flashes, and fatigue. Nilutamide may lead to visual disturbances.

Combined androgen blockade
Combined androgen blockade (CAB) is a combination of surgical or medical castration plus androgen blockade. It is a very controversial topic and recent guidelines indicate that combined therapy should be "considered."

There is no clear evidence of superior outcomes over those with castration alone, but there is evidence from meta-analyses to support a 15%–20% relative benefit and an absolute 3%–5% long-term survival benefit with CAB compared with GnRH agonist therapy alone. Studies clearly show that a combined approach leads to increased toxicities compared with monotherapy with medical castration alone.

Most centers in the United States use medical castration as the initial therapy for patients with metastatic prostate cancer.

Castration-resistant metastatic disease

After a median of 2–4 years of androgen deprivation, patients with metastatic prostate cancer demonstrate evidence of hormone-refractory or castration-resistant disease. Introduction of an androgen blocker, e.g., bicalutamide, in combination with surgical or medical castration leads to PSA response in >20%, with duration of response is 2–6 months. Patients who respond to maximal androgen blockade and then have PSA rise may respond to withdrawal of the oral antiandrogen because of the paradoxical agonist properties of these agents at the androgen receptor in select patients. Inevitably, however, additional therapies will be needed. Initially, men are asymptomatic with rising PSA, but they may eventually develop symptomatic progression of disease, most commonly painful bone metastases. There are increasing treatment options for men with progressive castration-resistant prostate cancer (CRPC).

Hormonal therapies

One option is to block the release of testosterone from the adrenal glands, where approximately 10% of the circulating testosterone is produced. The drugs commonly used for this purpose, ketoconazole and the newer agent abiraterone acetate (Zytiga), are administered in conjunction with steroids to avoid the side effects from blocking the normal function of the adrenal glands. Abiraterone acetate with low-dose prednisone prolongs progression-free survival and is U.S. FDA-approved for men with CRPC when given either before or after chemotherapy. This agent prolonged overall survival in the postdocetaxel setting by 4–5 months, and in the predocetaxel setting has been demonstrated to delay clinical and radiographic progression by 15–18 months, with the majority of men attaining a PSA decline. Although abiraterone acetate is generally well tolerated, side effects may include fatigue, high blood pressure, leg swelling, and electrolyte or liver abnormalities, and patients need to be monitored regularly.

In August 2012, the FDA approved enzalutamide (Xtandi) for the treatment of men with CRPC and disease progression after chemotherapy. Similar to but more effective than the antiandrogens, enzalutamide blocks the androgen receptor. Approval was based on the results of the AFFIRM randomized, phase 3, placebo-controlled trial in which both survival and quality of life were improved with enzalutamide treatment. Side effects are mild but include fatigue, diarrhea, hot flushes, headache, and very rarely seizures (<1%) due to cross-reactivity at the GABA receptor. Enzalutamide treatment does not require concurrent steroid therapy and is a new treatment option for men in the postchemotherapy CRPC setting. The PREVAIL study and other ongoing investigations may provide evidence to support the use of enzalutamide earlier in the disease course.

In these trials, bone scans flares or healing reactions are commonly observed on the initial reassessment bone scan posttreatment, indicated by new or brighter existing bone lesions. Prostate Cancer Working Group 2 guidelines call for the continuation of therapy until a confirmation bone scan indicating additional new lesions to prevent premature discontinuation of an effective systemic agent. However, if PSA is rising and pain is progressing with radiographic progression, bone scan flare is less likely and consideration of alternative therapies is needed.

Immunotherapy

Therapeutic vaccines stimulate the immune system to fight prostate cancer by recognizing proteins that are specific to cancer cells. One such vaccine, sipuleucel-T (Provenge), is U.S. FDA-approved for men with CRPC with minimal to no symptoms. Treatment involves filtering out a patient's immune cells by leukopheresis, then stimulating the cells in a laboratory with a prostate cancer specific protein known as prostatic acid phosphatase (PAP) and boosting with GM-CSF. These cells are then returned to the patient intravenously. This process is repeated every 2 weeks for a total of 3 treatments, with the goal of stimulating the patient's own immune system to fight the cancer cells. Although sipuleucel-T therapy does not lower PSA or delay disease progression, this treatment does prolong survival by approximately 20%, with some suggestion of a greater benefit in men with lower disease burden (PSA <20). Ongoing studies are attempting to clarify the mechanisms behind this. There are other promising immunotherapies for prostate cancer on the horizon including prostvac and immune checkpoint blockade agents (CTLA4).

Bone-targeted therapy

Treatment with bisphosphonates or denosumab can help prevent complications related to bone metastases, like fractures. Bone-targeted therapy is designed to reset the balance between bone growth and destruction. Zoledronic acid (Zometa) is an intravenous bisphosphonate that can delay the onset of complications associated with bony metastases and also relieve pain. Denosumab (Xgeva), given as a subcutaneous injection, is a monoclonal antibody against RANK ligand, which is a protein important for osteoclast function. Both classes of bone-targeted agents have a risk of causing osteonecrosis of the jaw and should be taken with daily calcium and vitamin D supplementation. Although these agents do not have a proven overall survival benefit, they are very effective at reducing clinically important skeletal-related events such as fractures, cord compression, and need for palliative surgery or radiation.

Palliative external beam radiotherapy has been used successfully for many years to alleviate symptoms from metastatic prostate cancer. Painful bony metastases can often be treated with 1-2 weeks of daily radiation therapy with successful relief of symptoms.

Patients with diffuse painful bony metastases may be treated with radiopharmaceuticals, which are radioactive isotopes that home to and kill the cancer cells in the bone. Radioactive strontium-89 and samarium-153 can be administered systemically to provide targeted irradiation to multiple bone metastases. These treatments can provide adequate pain relief and are generally well tolerated, although can cause significant myelosuppression.

A new radiopharmaceutical called alpharadin (Xofigo) is more effective and less toxic and has recently been U.S. FDA-approved for men with advanced CRPC and painful bony metastases without visceral metastases. The ALSYMPCA trial showed that alpharadin treatment improves both symptoms and incidence of new metastases relative to placebo, and most importantly, also prolongs overall survival. This randomized trial of best supportive care with or without monthly injections of radium-223 led to a 3–4 month improvement in survival, accompanied by pain palliation and reductions in bone marker turnover and a reduced risk of skeletal events including spinal cord compression and fracture over time. Whether this agent can be safely combined with newer hormonal or chemotherapy agents remains to be studied.

Chemotherapy for metastatic disease

In the past, chemotherapy was viewed as inappropriate for most patients, due to the limited number of active agents, the age and frailty of these patients, and marrow compromise by metastatic disease and radiotherapy. One of the first regimens to show improvement in quality of life, yet no overall survival benefit, was mitoxantrone with prednisone.

In 2004, two landmark randomized, controlled, multicenter, prospective trials of docetaxel given every 3 weeks with daily prednisone showed for the first time a survival benefit for men with CRPC.

The current indications for systemic chemotherapy are clinical or radiographic progression in the face of castrate-levels of testosterone.

- Symptomatic disease is not necessary, given that the survival advantage was seen in men with or without baseline pain, and men who are pain-free may be better able to tolerate a full 30-week course of docetaxel.
- Progression of pain or delay in onset of symptomatic disease is a reasonable goal of therapy, particularly in men at risk of rapid progression.

Recent studies have shown that patients who had a PSA decline of >30% within 3 months of therapy with docetaxel had the highest degree of surrogacy for overall survival. This may be a useful guide at 3 months for determining benefit to a patient with this regimen.

- Docetaxel and prednisone (DP) 75 mg/m^2 every 3 weeks has been shown to improve median survival time 2–3 months compared with mitoxantrone and prednisone, with accompanying improvements in pain palliation, quality of life, and rates of PSA decline. Adverse effects of this therapy include fatigue, nausea, hair loss, infection, neutropenia, neuropathy, swelling, tearing, and nail disorders.
- Weekly docetaxel 30 mg/m^2 for 5 of 6 weeks or docetaxel 50 mg/m^2 every 2 weeks are also reasonable palliative regimens. The every 2 week regimen has been shown to have similar efficacy but less neutropenia compared with the standard 3 weekly docetaxel.
- Treatment generally is given until clinical progression, rather than PSA progression alone, because PSA "blips" occur in a minority of patients (<20%) within the first 3–4 months of therapy and should

not be reason for discontinuation of chemotherapy before clinical or radiographic progression.

In the TAX327 study, overall survival was improved from 16.3 with mitoxantrone to 19.2 months with docetaxel given every 3 weeks. Weekly docetaxel had an intermediate survival of 17.8 months, but similar rates of PSA declines and pain palliation.

In 2010, another taxane chemotherapy, cabazitaxel (Jevtana) given with prednisone, was FDA-approved for treatment of CRPC that progressed after docetaxel treatment. Like docetaxel, cabazitaxel prolongs life and improves symptoms in men with advanced CRPC; however, side effects including fatigue, diarrhea, and myelosuppression somewhat limit the use of this agent. Survival is improved by 2–3 months in this setting with cabazitaxel dosed at 25 mg/m^2 every 3 weeks with prednisone.

Other palliative regimens include docetaxel with estramustine, docetaxel with carboplatin, vinorelbine, paclitaxel, etoposide, oral cyclophoshamide, and corticosteroids. Clinical trials are highly recommended in this disease state for the study of novel agents.

Future directions

Although many new agents with varying mechanisms of action are available to patients, conferring incremental survival benefits, patients with CRPC are not cured. The best way to sequence these therapies as well as optimal combination therapies are active areas of investigation. Clinical trial participation is thus essential.

New insight into the molecular pathogenesis of prostate cancer has led the way for the potential development of targeted therapies in patients with CRPC. Agents currently being studied include ARN-509 and TOK-001 (androgen receptor antagonists), orteronel (androgen synthesis inhibitor), cabozantinib (VEGFR2 and MET tyrosine kinase inhibitor), immunotherapies (Prostvac), ipilimumab (CTLA4 blockade), anticlusterin (OGX-011) strategies and others.

Further reading

Armstrong AJ, Garrett-Mayer E, Ou Yang YC, et al. (2007). Prostate-specific antigen and pain surrogacy analysis in metastatic hormone-refractory prostate cancer. *J Clin Oncol* 25:3965–3970.

Armstrong AJ, Garrett-Mayer ES, Yang YC, et al. (2007). A contemporary prognostic nomogram for men with hormone-refractory metastatic prostate cancer: a TAX327 study analysis. *Clin Cancer Res* 13:6396–6403.

Boustead G, Edwards SJ (2007). Systematic review of early vs deferred hormonal treatment of locally advanced prostate cancer: a meta-analysis of randomized controlled trials. *BJU Int* 99:1383–1389.

D'Amico AV, Manola J, Loffredo M, et al. (2004). 6-month androgen suppression plus radiation therapy vs radiation therapy alone for patients with clinically localized prostate cancer: a randomized controlled trial. *JAMA* 292:821–827.

De Bono JS, Oudard S, Ozguroglu M, et al. (2010). Prednisone plus cabazitaxel or mitoxantrone for metastatic castration-resistant prostate cancer progressing after docetaxel treatment: a randomised open-label trial. *Lancet* 376:1147–1154.

De Bono JS, Logothetis CJ, Molina A, et al. (2011). Abiraterone and increased survival in metastatic prostate cancer. *N Engl J Med* 364:1995–2005.

DeVita VT, Hellman S, Rosenberg SA. (2005). *Cancer: Principles & Practice of Oncology* (7th ed.). Philadelphia: Lippincott Williams & Wilkins.

Freedland SJ, Humphreys EB, Mangold LA, et al. (2005). Risk of prostate cancer-specific mortality following biochemical recurrence after radical prostatectomy. *JAMA* 294:433–439.

Freedland SJ, Partin AW (2006). Prostate-specific antigen: update 2006. *Urology* 67:458–460.

Govindan R (2008). *The Washington Manual of Oncology* (2nd ed.). Philadelphia: Lippincott Williams & Wilkins.

Greene FL (2002). American Joint Committee on Cancer. American Cancer Society. *AJCC Cancer Staging Manual* (6th ed.). New York: Springer-Verlag.

Halabi S, Small EJ, Kantoff PW, et al. (2003). Prognostic model for predicting survival in men with hormone-refractory metastatic prostate cancer. *J Clin Oncol* 21:1232–1237.

Jemal A, Siegel R, Ward E, et al. (2007). Cancer statistics, 2007. *CA Cancer J Clin* 57:43–66.

Kantoff PW, Higano CS, Shore ND, et al. (2010). Sipuleucel-T immunotherapy for castration-resistant prostate cancer. *N Engl J Med* 363:411–422.

Klotz L (2005). Active surveillance for prostate cancer: for whom? *J Clin Oncol* 23:8165–8169.

Loblaw DA, Virgo KS, Nam R, et al. (2007). Initial hormonal management of androgen-sensitive, metastatic, recurrent, or progressive prostate cancer: 2006 update of an American Society of Clinical Oncology practice guideline. *J Clin Oncol* 25:1596–1605.

Prostate Cancer Trialists' Collaborative Group (2000). Maximum androgen blockade in advanced prostate cancer: an overview of the randomised trials. *Lancet* 355:1491–1498.

Mendiratta P, Armstrong AJ, George DJ (2007). Current standard and investigational approaches to the management of hormone-refractory prostate cancer. *Rev Urol* 9(Suppl 1):S9–S19.

NCCN Clinical Practice Guidelines in Oncology: Prostate Cancer. V.2. 2007. National Comprehensive Cancer Network. 2007.

Petrylak DP, Tangen CM, Hussain MH, et al. (2004). Docetaxel and estramustine compared with mitoxantrone and prednisone for advanced refractory prostate cancer. *N Engl J Med* 351:1513–1520.

Ryan CJ, Smith MR, de Bono JS, et al. (2013). Abiraterone in metastatic prostate cancer without previous chemotherapy. *N Engl J Med* 368:138–148.

Scher HI, Fizazi K, Saad F, et al. (2012). Increased survival with enzalutamide in prostate cancer after chemotherapy. *N Engl J Med* 367:1187–1197.

Stephenson AJ, Kattan MW (2006). Nomograms for prostate cancer. *BJU Int* 98:39–46.

Tannock IF, de Wit R, Berry WR, et al. (2004). Docetaxel plus prednisone or mitoxantrone plus prednisone for advanced prostate cancer. *N Engl J Med* 351:1502–1512.

Wilt TJ, Brawer MK, Jones KM, et al. (2012). Radical prostatectomy versus observation for localized prostate cancer. *N Engl J Med* 367:203-13.

Walsh PC, DeWeese TL, Eisenberger MA (2007). Clinical practice. Localized prostate cancer. *N Engl J Med* 357:2696–2705.

Zietman AL, DeSilvio ML, Slater JD, et al. (2005). Comparison of conventional-dose vs high-dose conformal radiation therapy in clinically localized adenocarcinoma of the prostate: a randomized controlled trial. *JAMA* 294:1233–1239.

Chapter 35

Genitourinary cancers III: testicular cancer

Prateek Mendiratta
Andrew J. Armstrong

Testicular cancer *590*
Management of testicular cancer *598*
Follow-up *603*
Further reading *604*

Testicular cancer

The treatment of advanced testicular cancer represents one of the great successes of medical oncology in the last 20 years. This is one of the few solid tumors for which the majority of patients with metastatic disease can expect to be cured (>95%).

Some of the reasons for these improved outcomes include early detection and awareness, the excellent response to cisplatin-based chemotherapy, better staging, multimodality therapy, and awareness and reduction of the long-term toxicities of these therapies.

Epidemiology and etiology

The majority (95%) of testicular tumors are of germ cell origin. In the United States, there are roughly 8000 new cases annually with 400 expected deaths yearly. However, testicular tumors are the most common cancer in men aged 15–35 years, and their incidence has doubled over the last 30 years. The reason for this increase is not clear.

Nonseminoma most commonly presents in the third decade whereas the seminomas are most commonly seen in the fourth and fifth decades. The age distribution is dependent on pathology.

Seminoma is the most frequent pathology (55%):
- Peak incidence at age 30–40 years
- Occasionally seen at 60–70 years

Nonseminoma (45%) peak incidence is at age 20–30 years.

Increased risk of testicular cancer is observed in men with the following:
- History of undescended testis (risk is 5- to 50-fold higher)
- Previous testicular cancer (relative risk 25x)
- Testicular carcinoma in situ
- Family history of testicular cancer
- Klinefelter's syndrome (usually extragonadal)
- Atrophic testis and infertility
- In utero exposure to estrogens

It is believed that both environmental and genetic factors combine to give rise to testicular dysgenesis, manifested as either Leydig cell malfunction with failure of normal testicular descent or impaired germ cell differentiation with poor sperm production and/or malignant change.

Further work is being done to investigate biological and molecular alterations that lead to the development and progression of testicular cancer. Some work has shown that underlying defects in *p53* may increase risk and the potential development of isochromosome 12p as a genetic marker.

Screening

There is no evidence to support population screening for this disease; however, some centers recommend that young males and their physicians perform manual bilateral testicular examination yearly to detect new lumps or masses.

Pathology

Germ cell tumors are classified into two major groups: seminomas and nonseminomas. *Nonseminomas* include teratoma, choriocarcinoma, yolk sac, and embryonal carcinomas.

Some tumors have components of both seminoma and nonseminoma and are usually treated like nonseminomatous germ cell tumors (NSGCT). These tumors arise from germinal epithelium, and seminomas and NSGCT are thought to arise from preexisting carcinoma in situ.

The natural histories of seminoma and NSGCT differ, and these differences dictate the variation in management between the two pathologies.

Most *seminomas* (75%) present with disease confined to the testis. Spread tends to be predictable, to the para-aortic lymph nodes and, subsequently, to the supradiaphragmatic lymph nodes and other metastatic sites. Tumor growth can be very slow, thus untreated microscopic metastatic disease may take up to 10 years to become clinically apparent.

Only approximately half of testicular NSGCT present with localized disease. Blood-borne and lymphatic spread occurs earlier than with seminoma. In addition, NSGCT produce markers in the form of the human chorionic gonadotrophin (hCG) and/or α-fetoprotein (AFP) in 75% of cases.

Seminomas, by contrast, have no reliable tumor marker to monitor disease, although the hCG may be moderately elevated in ~25% of cases.

Lactate dehydrogenase (LDH) may be raised in both tumors and is useful for defining a prognostic group, correlating with tumor bulk. But it is not a reliable marker for monitoring response to treatment or subsequent relapse.

The rest of testicular tumors are not of germ cell origin or due to metastatic disease. Possible etiologies include the following:
- Lymphomas
- Leydig cell tumors
- Sertoli cell tumors
- Sarcomas
- Paratesticular tumors

Serum tumor markers

The three most common markers used to diagnose, provide prognostic information for, and follow patients with germ cell tumors are LDH, hCG, and AFP.

LDH has a serum half-life of approximately 24 hours, and is nonspecific yet more commonly elevated in seminomas. LDH is not as good at following response as the other two markers, yet LDH has been shown to be an independent prognostic variable.

hCG has a serum half-life of 24–36 hours and is elevated in 60% of nonseminomas and 20% of seminomas. If still inappropriately elevated (according to expected rate of decline) after surgery, it usually means there is metastatic disease.

AFP is elevated in 50% of germ cell tumors and has a half-life of 5–7 days. This is usually seen in patients with nonseminomas. Elevations are rarely seen in patients with pure seminomas. A patient who presents with an elevated AFP and a mediastinal mass should raise concern for an extragonadal germ cell tumor.

Presentation

Most patients commonly present with a testicular lump, which may be painless or may be mistaken for epididymorchitis. Patients with testicular symptoms that persist despite one course of antibiotics should be referred to a urology clinic for assessment including ultrasound examination of the testes.

Differential diagnosis includes hernia, hydrocele, spermatocele, and testicular torsion.

Pain is present is less than one third of patients.

Men with tumors producing high levels of hCG may develop gynecomastia, which resolves with treatment of the cancer.

Metastatic disease may present with the following:
- Lumbar back pain associated with bulky (>5 cm) para-aortic lymphadenopathy
- Cough and dyspnea with multiple lung metastases
- SVC syndrome or obstruction with mediastinal lymphadenopathy
- CNS symptoms or symptoms consistent with brain metastasis

Many patients with relapsed disease are diagnosed with asymptomatic spread of disease picked up on routine monitoring of serum markers, chest X-ray, or CT scan.

Investigation of testicular germ cell tumors

Initial studies include the following:
- Ultrasound, of both testes
- Chest X-ray
- Tumor markers (AFP, hCG, LDH)
- Renal function panel
- CT scan of the abdomen or pelvis with contrast, once patients are diagnosed with testicular cancer, for staging purposes
- Have a low threshold for evaluation of CNS metastases for patients who have symptoms of headaches or mental-status changes.
- Pulmonary function testing with diffusion capacity for those men who are to receive bleomycin

When the patient has obvious and widespread metastases or a mediastinal primary tumor, immediate referral for chemotherapy may be necessary, but for the majority the initial management will be inguinal orchiectomy.
- Tumor biopsy or even tumor marker levels may be the diagnostic confirmation if no testicular primary tumor is identified.
- The most common approach is an inguinal approach. A transscrotal approach is contraindicated due to the possibility of tumor seeding.
- A biopsy of the contralateral testis should be considered when there is a high risk of carcinoma in situ. Patients at risk include those with a history of maldescent or who have a small testis (<12 mL), and patients aged <30 years.

Further staging investigations will usually be performed postoperatively.

Staging investigations and prognostic grouping

For all patients staging investigations will include a CT scan of the thorax, abdomen, and pelvis. In patients with high hCG (>10,000 IU/L) or bulky mediastinal disease or symptoms and signs of CNS disease, a brain scan is advisable.

Postoperative tumor markers should be serially checked, if raised, to assess whether they are falling with an appropriate half-life (4–6 days for AFP, 24 hours for hCG). Other investigations such as a bone scan may be necessary if clinically indicated.

Staging is based on serum tumor markers in combination with the TNM staging system (see Table 35.1).

The International Germ Cell Consensus Classification (IGCCC) prognostic grouping (see Table 35.2) is applicable for all patients.

Each individual stage has prognostic implications for overall survival, with 5-year survival for good prognosis being >90%, intermediate prognosis 80%, and poor prognosis 48%.

Sperm storage

Sperm count and storage should be considered at an early stage when patients are likely to require further therapy.

- It should be remembered that up to 50% of patients with testicular germ cell tumors may be subfertile at presentation.

Baseline analysis should include serum LH, FSH, testosterone, and semen analysis.

Oligo- or azospermia is relatively common even before administration of chemotherapy in these patients. Cisplatin-based chemotherapy may reduce sperm count and function in a dose-related fashion.

Table 35.1 TNM staging for testicular cancer

Primary tumor	
pTx	Primary tumor cannot be assessed
pT0	No evidence of primary tumor
pTis	Intratubular germ cell neoplasia (carcinoma in situ)
pT1	Tumor limited to the testis and epididymis and no vascular or lymphatic invasion; tumor may invade the tunica albuginea, but not the tunica vaginalis
pT2	Tumor limited to the testis and epididymis with vascular or lymphatic invasion or tumor extending throughout the tunica albuginea with involvement of tunica vaginalis
pT3	Tumor invades the spermatic cord with or without vascular or lymphatic invasion
pT4	Tumor invades the scrotum with or without vascular or lymphatic invasion
Regional lymph nodes	
Clinical	
Nx	Regional lymph nodes cannot be assessed
N0	No regional lymph node metastasis
N1	Lymph node mass <2 cm in greatest dimension; or multiple lymph node masses, none >2 cm greatest dimension
N2	Lymph node mass >2 cm, but <5 cm in greatest dimension; or multiple lymph node masses, any one masses >2 cm, but <5 cm in greatest dimension
N3	Lymph node mass >5 cm in greatest dimension
Pathological	
pN0	No evidence of tumor in lymph node
pN1	Lymph node mass <2 cm in greatest dimension and <5 nodes positive, none 2 cm in greatest dimension
pN2	Lymph node mass >2 cm, but <5 cm in greatest dimension; >5 nodes positive, none >5 cm; evidence of extranodal extension of tumor
pN3	Lymph node mass >5 cm in greatest dimension; >5 nodes positive, none >5 cm; evidence of extranodal extension of tumor
pN3	Lymph node mass >5 cm in greatest dimension
Distant metastasis	
M0	No evidence of distant metastases
M1	Nonregional nodal or pulmonary metastases
M2	Lymph node mass >5 cm in greatest dimension

Table 35.1 (Cont.)

Serum marker	LDH	hCG (mIU/mL)	AFP (ng/mL)
SX	Not assessed	Not assessed	Not assessed
S0	<Normal	<Normal	<Normal
S1	<1.5 × N	>5000	<1000
S2	1.5–10 × N	5000–50,000	1000–10,000
S3	>10 × N	>50,000	>10,000
Stage group			
Stage 0	pTisN0M0S0		
Stage I	T1–T4N0M0SX		
Stage IA	T1N0M0S0		
Stage IB	T2–T4N0M0		
Stage IS	Any TN0M0S1–S3		
Stage II	Any T any N M0SX		
Stage IIA	Any TN1M0S0–S1		
Stage IIB	AnyTN2M0S0–S1		
Stage IIC	AnyTN3M0S0–S1		
Stage III	Any T any N M1 SX		
Stage IIIA	Any T any N M1 S0–S1		
Stage IIIB	Any T any N M0–M1 S2		
Stage IIIC	Any T any N M0–M1a S3		
Stage IIIC	Any T any N M1b any S		

Table 35.2 IGCCC prognostic grouping for metastatic germ-cell tumors

Nonseminoma germ cell tumor (NSGCT)	Seminoma
Good prognosis with all of:	
Testis/retroperitoneal primary	Any primary site
No nonpulmonary visceral metastases	No nonpulmonary visceral metastases
AFP <1000 ng/mL	Normal AFP
hCG <5000 IU/mL	Any hCG
LDH 1.5 upper limit of normal	Any LDH
56% of NSGCT: 5-year survival 92%	90% of seminomas; 5-year survival 86%
Intermediate progress with any of:	
Testis/retroperitoneal primary	Any primary site
No nonpulmonary visceral metastases	Nonpulmonary visceral metastases
AFP >1000 and <10,000 ng/mL	Normal AFP
hCG >5000 and <50,000 IU/mL	Any hCG
LDH >1.5 × normal <10 normal	Any LDH
28% of teratomas: 5-year survival 80%	10% of seminomas: 5-year survival 73%
Poor prognosis with any of:	
Mediastinal primary	No patients in this group
Nonpulmonary visceral metastases	
AFP >10,000 ng/mL	
hCG >50,000 IU/mL	
LDH >10 × normal	
16% of teratomas: 5-year survival 48%	

Management of testicular cancer

The management of seminoma and NSGCT depends on the stage of disease and involves all three major modalities for the treatment of cancer: surgery, radiotherapy, and chemotherapy.

Carcinoma in situ

Germ cell carcinoma in situ may progress to invasive cancer, either seminoma or NSGCT, with 50% producing invasive tumors 5 years from diagnosis. Once this diagnosis is made, treatment should be offered, although this may not need to be given immediately. Carcinoma in situ can be eradicated by low-dose radiotherapy to the testis (20 Gy in 10 fractions).

The advantage of this treatment is that, in most cases, it will avoid orchiectomy and not affect Leydig cell function, and long-term hormone therapy should not be necessary.

Stage I seminoma

Radical orchiectomy through a groin incision must be radical and the incision must be in the groin to avoid scrotal skin tumor seedlings. Recommend rechecking serum tumor markers (LDH, B-hCG, and AFP) if elevated preoperatively, until normalized.

Despite a negative staging CT scan, 20% of these patients develop recurrent seminoma after orchiectomy; 90% of relapses are in para-aortic nodes, but some of these are late, up to 10 years after orchiectomy.

Relapse is more common after orchiectomy for testicular tumors >4 cm diameter and invasion into the rete testis, but it is usually marker negative and only detectable on CT scan.

The prognosis is excellent, because almost all patients with relapsed disease are cured by salvage therapy.

Treatment options

Adjuvant radiotherapy to the para-aortic nodes and para-caval nodes, T11–L5 (20–30 Gy in 10 fractions) reduces the relapse rate to 4%.

- It is well tolerated, but there is increased risk of second malignancy.
- Most patients who relapse after radiation, relapse with disease outside the radiation field and can be salvaged with systemic chemotherapy.
- Side effects include secondary malignancies in the radiation field, cardiovascular risk (depending on treated field), and urinary symptoms.

Surveillance is another option in the compliant patient and includes every 3–4 months CT scanning of the abdomen and pelvis, monitoring of tumor markers (β-hCG and LDH each visit), and chest X-ray. Given that long-term survival rates remain in excess of 95% with initial surveillance, this remains a preferred option for men at low risk of recurrence.

Surveillance can be strongly considered for men who wish to avoid the risks of radiotherapy, who have a horseshoe kidney, or who have contraindications to radiotherapy, such as inflammatory bowel disease or prior radiation exposure.

Adjuvant chemotherapy comprises one cycle of carboplatin chemotherapy (AUC 7).
- Recent results suggest a similar reduction in relapse rate to that with radiotherapy to retroperitoneal lymph nodes, although long-term (>10 years) data are lacking.
- Side effects of 1–2 doses of carboplatin are short term in general, with no significant reports of secondary malignancies or cardiovascular disease, although there are reports of a higher risk for bladder cancer in platinum-treated patients.

Stage IIA and IIB seminoma

These patients are best treated with radiotherapy to the para-aortic and ipsilateral iliac lymph nodes.
- IIA: 35–40 Gy in 15 fractions leads to 95% disease-free survival after 5 years.
- IIB: 35–40 Gy in 18 fractions leads to 90% disease-free survival after 5 years. Four cycles of EP chemotherapy is a reasonable alternative for select patients with IIb disease.

Stage I NSGCT

After orchiectomy alone the relapse rate is ~30%, with most relapses occurring in the first 2 years. Many are detected by a rise in tumor markers with only low-volume disease in the para-aortic nodes or lungs. As a result, the outcome of treatment for relapsed stage I disease is excellent, with cure rates >95%.

The best predictor of relapse is the presence of vascular invasion in the tumor: 50% of these men develop metastatic disease if given no adjuvant therapy.

Treatment options
- Surveillance (for compliant patients) including frequent clinic visits, chest X-ray, tumor marker monitoring, and regular CT scans, particularly in the first 2 years but extending to 5 years
- For high-risk patients (T2–T4 disease and/or lymphovascular invasion), options include nerve-sparing retroperitoneal lymph node dissection (RPLND), adjuvant chemotherapy with 1–2 cycles of bleomycin-etoposide-cisplatin (BEP) chemotherapy, and surveillance followed by salvage chemotherapy.
- Each of these options results generally in >95% long-term disease-free survival.

Stage IIc–Stage III Seminoma

Chemotherapy is the mainstay of treatment for all these stages of testicular cancer and has been the key to the improvement in prognosis for this disease over the last 20 years. For the vast majority of patients, treatment is based on the BEP regimen.

All patients should be assigned an International Germ Cell Consensus Classification prognostic group.

Good-prognosis disease

Standard treatment comprises 3 cycles of BEP chemotherapy, monitoring tumor markers weekly, and restaging by CT scan at the end of chemotherapy.

In patients in whom bleomycin is unsafe (older patients with poor lung function), an alternative regimen with equivalent results is 4 cycles of EP chemotherapy or 3–4 cycles of VIP (etoposide, infusional ifosfamide, and cisplatin) chemotherapy.

The toxicities of this chemotherapy include the following:
- Nausea and vomiting (largely prevented with appropriate antiemetics including $5HT_3$ antagonist and dexamethasone)
- Febrile neutropenia
  - Dose delays and reductions should be avoided.
  - G-CSF may be used as secondary prophylaxis after one episode of febrile neutropenia but should not be used with concurrent bleomycin given risks of pulmonary toxicity.
- Neuropathy (cisplatin causes sensory peripheral neuropathy and high-tone hearing loss)
  - Cisplatin causes a fall in glomular filtration rate (GFR) and tubular damage is often associated with hypomagnesemia.
  - Best managed by prevention (pre- and posthydration, diuretic, e.g., furosemide and mannitol, IV magnesium supplements)
  - Vascular damage includes Raynaud's phenomenon and elevated cardiovascular risk.
  - Secondary malignancies (leukemia, myelodysplasia, bladder cancer, melanoma, among others) occur rarely.
- Pulmonary fibrosis
  - The risk relates to the cumulative dose of bleomycin >400 IU.
  - This toxicity can be fatal and should be monitored with serial pulmonary function tests with DL_{CO} measures.
  - Concomitant use of GCSF growth factor support may increase this risk.

Residual tumor masses postchemotherapy

After completion of chemotherapy, a CT scan may show persistent masses at the site of the original metastatic disease.

For patients with seminoma, such masses are managed expectantly unless they are >3 cm or PET positive, or biopsy-confirmed viable tumor is present, and the majority are seen to slowly regress on serial scans. Thus, PET scanning is indicated for residual mass evaluation in this setting. However, for patients with NSGCT in whom residual tumor (>1–2 cm) is apparent, surgical resection should be performed.

PET scanning is less clinically useful to rule out viable tumor in NSGCT. The majority of these will be in the retroperitoneum, and extensive and difficult surgery is often necessary for a complete resection. The residual masses may contain
- Necrotic tumor (50%);
- Mature teratoma (35%); although histologically benign, excision is important as this tissue can give rise to malignancy if left in situ;
- Viable tumor—15% may require additional or alternative chemotherapy.

Surgery should usually only be undertaken when markers have normalized.
- Persistently elevated tumor markers may be causes for nontumor-related etiologies, such as hypogonadism (LH/FSH may cross-react with hCG assay) or cirrhosis or hepatitis C (AFP).
- Residual pulmonary masses should also be resected where possible.
- The problems of surgical technique and anesthetic risk, particularly as most patients will have been exposed to bleomycin, demand that patients be operated on in a center experienced in this surgery.
- Retroperitoneal node dissection can be performed laparoscopically in experienced centers.

Intermediate- and poor-prognosis disease
Although no chemotherapy regimen has been proven to be superior to 4 cycles of BEP chemotherapy for these groups of patients, the outcomes of treatment are significantly poorer, with 5-year survival:
- Intermediate-prognosis group: 80%
- Poor-prognosis group 48%.

All such patients should be considered for clinical trials exploring novel or more intensive treatment options.

Randomized studies of first-line autologous bone marrow transplantation in poor-risk patients have not demonstrated an overall survival advantage and cannot be currently recommended. However, in the subset of men with inadequate tumor marker decline following initial chemotherapy, there was a suggestion of benefit to transplantation.

Patients with primary mediastinal NSGCT have a particularly poor prognosis (<40% long-term survival) and should be considered for aggressive strategies and clinical trials.

Relapsed disease

Patients with NSGCT who, after initial therapy, have persistently elevated tumor markers are deemed to have an incomplete response. Current salvage regimens include VeIP (vinblastine, ifosfamide, and cisplatin) or TIP (paclitaxel, ifosfamide, and cisplatin). See Table 35.3.

Some patients may need surgical management of residual disease.

High-dose systemic chemotherapy with autologous stem cell transplant is an option as salvage therapy and is being done in experienced high-volume centers.

Most patients with relapsed, refractory disease should be enrolled in clinical trials. Further research is needed in developing new agents and combinations for this population.

Complications of therapy

- Potential surgery complications are usually from RPLND and include impotence and retrograde ejaculation.
- Recent studies have looked at long-term complications of radiation and chemotherapy.
- Each individual chemotherapy has its own side effect; yet, the most concerning is pulmonary fibrosis, which can be seen in up to 5% of patients treated with bleomycin.
- Radiotherapy and chemotherapy have been shown to increase the risk of developing secondary malignancies (including leukemia, bladder, gastric, and colon) and cardiovascular disease to a similar extent due to smoking.

Follow-up

After primary management of metastatic disease, regular follow-up is necessary as, in those patients who relapse, salvage therapy can be effective in 725% of cases.

Contralateral testicular cancer may be present in 3%–5% of patients over the subsequent 5 years and should be monitored through physical examinations over time.

Complications of survivorship are essential to monitor, including secondary malignancies, cardiovascular risk, and depression.

Nongerm cell testicular tumors

These represent a very small proportion of testicular tumors. Stromal tumors such as those arising from Leydig cells are generally benign, but metastases have been reported in approximately 10% of cases.

Testicular lymphomas are the most common testicular cancer in elderly men and should be treated along the same principles as lymphomas arising at other sites.

Table 35.3 Examples of chemotherapy regimens for testicular cancer

BEP			
Bleomycin	30 mg	d1, 8, 15	
Etoposide	100 mg/m^2	d1–5	q3 weeks
Cisplatin	20 mg/m^2	d1–5	
EP			
Etoposide	100 mg/m^2	d1–5	q3 weeks
Cisplatin	20 mg/m^2	d1–5	
VIP			
Etoposide	75 mg/m^2	d1–5	
Ifosfamide	1.2 g/m^2	d1–5	q3 weeks
Cisplatin	20 mg/m^2	d1–5	
VeIP			
Vinblastine	0.11 mg/kg	d1–2	
Ifosfamide	1200 mg/m^2	d1–5	q3 weeks
Cisplatin	20 mg/m^2	d1–5	
TIP			
Paclitaxel	250 mg/m^2	d1 (24 hours)	
Ifosfamide	1500 mg/m^2	d2–5 w/Mesna	q3 weeks
Cisplatin	25 mg/m^2	d2–5	

Further reading

Albers P, Albrecht W, Algaba F, et al. (2005). Guidelines on testicular cancer. *Eur Urol* 48:885–894.

DeVita VT, Hellman S, Rosenberg SA (2005). *Cancer: Principles & Practice of Oncology* (7th ed.). Philadelphia: Lippincott Williams & Wilkins.

de Wit R, Fizazi K (2006). Controversies in the management of clinical stage I testis cancer. *J Clin Oncol* 24:5482–5492.

Einhorn LH (2007). Role of the urologist in metastatic testicular cancer. *J Clin Oncol* 25:1024–1025.

Einhorn LH, Brames MJ, Juliar B, Williams SD (2007). Phase II study of paclitaxel plus gemcitabine salvage chemotherapy for germ cell tumors after progression following high-dose chemotherapy with tandem transplant. *J Clin Oncol* 25:513–516.

Einhorn LH, Williams SD, Chamness A, et al. (2007). High-dose chemotherapy and stem-cell rescue for metastatic germ-cell tumors. *N Engl J Med* 357:340–348.

Govindan R (2008). *The Washington Manual of Oncology* (2nd ed.). Philadelphia: Lippincott Williams & Wilkins.

Greene FL (2002). American Joint Committee on Cancer. American Cancer Society, *AJCC Cancer Staging Manual* (6th ed.). New York: Springer-Verlag.

Hinton S, Catalano PJ, Einhorn LH, et al. (2003). Cisplatin, etoposide and either bleomycin or ifosfamide in the treatment of disseminated germ cell tumors: final analysis of an intergroup trial. *Cancer* 97:1869–1875.

International Germ Cell Consensus Classification: a prognostic factor-based staging system for metastatic germ cell cancers. International Germ Cell Cancer Collaborative Group (1997). *J Clin Oncol* 15:594–603.

Jemal A, Siegel R, Ward E, et al. (2007). Cancer statistics, 2007. *CA Cancer J Clin* 57:43–66.

Kondagunta GV, Bacik J, Bajorin D, et al. (2005). Etoposide and cisplatin chemotherapy for metastatic good-risk germ cell tumors. *J Clin Oncol* 23:9290–9294.

Kondagunta GV, Bacik J, Donadio A, et al. (2005). Combination of paclitaxel, ifosfamide, and cisplatin is an effective second-line therapy for patients with relapsed testicular germ cell tumors. *J Clin Oncol* 23:6549–6555.

Loehrer PJ Sr, Gonin R, Nichols CR, et al. (1998). Vinblastine plus ifosfamide plus cisplatin as initial salvage therapy in recurrent germ cell tumor. *J Clin Oncol* 16:2500–2504.

Motzer RJ, Nichols CJ, Margolin KA, et al. (2007). Phase III randomized trial of conventional-dose chemotherapy with or without high-dose chemotherapy and autologous hematopoietic stem-cell rescue as first-line treatment for patients with poor-prognosis metastatic germ cell tumors. *J Clin Oncol* 25:247–256.

Motzer RJ, Sheinfeld J, Mazumdar M, et al. (1995). Etoposide and cisplatin adjuvant therapy for patients with pathologic stage II germ cell tumors. *J Clin Oncol* 13:2700–2704.

National Comprehensive Cancer Network (2007). NCCN Clinical Practice Guidelines in Oncology: Testicular Cancer V.2.2008.

Nichols CR, Catalano PJ, Crawford ED, et al. (1998). Randomized comparison of cisplatin and etoposide and either bleomycin or ifosfamide in treatment of advanced disseminated germ cell tumors: an Eastern Cooperative Oncology Group, Southwest Oncology Group, and Cancer and Leukemia Group B Study. *J Clin Oncol* 16:1287–1293.

van den Belt-Dusebout AW, de Wit R, Gietema JA, et al. (2007). Treatment-specific risks of second malignancies and cardiovascular disease in 5-year survivors of testicular cancer. *J Clin Oncol* 25:4370–4378.

Williams SD, Birch R, Einhorn LH, et al. (1987). Treatment of disseminated germ-cell tumors with cisplatin, bleomycin, and either vinblastine or etoposide. *N Engl J Med* 316:1435–1440.

Zon RT, Nichols C, Einhorn LH (1998). Management strategies and outcomes of germ cell tumor patients with very high human chorionic gonadotropin levels. *J Clin Oncol* 16:1294–1297.

Chapter 36

Gynecological cancer

Jason Cory Barnett
Andrew Berchuck

Ovarian cancer *606*
Cancer of the uterine corpus *610*
Cancer of the cervix *614*
Vulvar and vaginal cancer *618*

Ovarian cancer

- Ovarian cancer is the sixth most common cancer in U.S. women, with 22,000 new cases diagnosed per year.
- It is the most common cause of death from gynecologic malignancy, and the fifth most common cause of cancer-related death overall (15,500 deaths/year).
- One in 70 American women is affected; it is more common in whites.

Etiology and risk factors

"Incessant ovulation" is a major contributor to increased risk of ovarian cancer.

- Risk rises with increasing number of ovulatory cycles in a woman's lifetime (e.g., nulliparity, infertility).
- Factors that decrease the number of ovulatory cycles are protective (e.g., parity, oral contraceptive use, breastfeeding).

Endometriosis increases risk, as some cases may arise in endometriosis implants.

Heritable syndromes (i.e., BRCA1, BRCA2, HNPCC) account for approximately 10% of epithelial ovarian cancers. Prophylactic bilateral salpingoophorectomy is recommended in mutation carriers who have completed childbearing.

Pathology

Most (90%) ovarian cancers are epithelial and resemble one or more mullerian cell type; serous cystadenocarcinoma is the most common.

Other types include mucinous, endometrioid, clear cell, and transitional cell carcinomas. Nonepithelial cases include germ cell, sex cord-stromal tumors, or metastases (GI tract and breast cancer metastases are most common).

Presentation

Vague symptoms and lack of a screening test contribute to the propensity for ovarian cancer to present at a late stage. Common presenting symptoms are nonspecific and include bloating, pelvic or abdominal pain, early satiety, and urinary urgency or frequency.

Ultrasound or CT scan is the best modality for imaging; surgical pathology is required for diagnosis.

Some 80%–85% of epithelial ovarian cancers have elevated serum CA-125 levels at diagnosis. CA-125 is also used to monitor treatment response and to detect recurrence. It is not used as a screening test because it lacks specificity. Elevation is also associated with many benign conditions (e.g., endometriosis, fibroids, peritoneal irritation, liver or renal failure).

Granulosa cell tumors (sex cord-stromal tumors) may present with abnormal vaginal bleeding or precocious puberty secondary to estrogen secretion. Alternatively, Leydig cell tumors can present with virilization secondary to androgen secretion.

Serum levels of β-hCG and/or AFP may be elevated in some germ cell tumors (see Table 36.1) and assist in diagnosis and treatment monitoring in these patients. LDH is often a marker for dysgerminomas.

Table 36.1 Germ cell markers

	hCG	AFP
Dysgerminoma	±	–
Endodermal sinus tumor	–	+
Choriocarcinoma	+	–
Immature teratoma	–	±
Embryonal carcinoma	+	±
Polyembryoma	+	±
Mixed germ-cell tumor	±	±–

Table 36.2 Prognosis for advanced stage disease

Stage	Presentation	5-year survival
I	23%	60%–90%
II	13%	65%–80%
III	47%	30%–50%
IV	16%	13%

Treatment

Standard treatment of epithelial cancers involves surgical staging and tumor cytoreduction followed by systemic chemotherapy.
- The most important prognostic factors are stage, residual disease after surgery, and grade.
- Advanced-stage disease confers poor prognosis (see Table 36.2).
- Neoadjuvant chemotherapy with interval surgical cytoreduction may be used in patients who are poor surgical candidates or who have a low likelihood of achieving optimal debulking.

Surgery and staging

Ovarian cancer is surgically staged (see Table 36.3). Approximately 30% of cases that appear confined to the ovary have occult metastatic disease that will be detected if surgical staging is performed.

Surgical staging can be performed by laparoscopy or laparotomy and involves the following:
- Cytologic washings
- Total abdominal hysterectomy
- Bilateral salpingoophorectomy
- Omentectomy
- Multiple peritoneal biopsies
- Pelvic and aortic lymph node sampling

In early-stage cases, the uterus and contralateral ovary may be retained if fertility is desired. In advanced-stage cases, the amount of residual disease at the conclusion of surgery is designated optimal if all residual tumor implants are ≤1 cm in diameter, or suboptimal if residual nodules are >1 cm. Optimal cytoreduction is associated with improved survival.

Table 36.3 International Federation for Gynecology and Obstetrics (FIGO) staging for ovarian cancer

Stage	Description
I	Growth limited to the ovaries
IA	Growth limited to one ovary; no ascites containing malignant cells. No tumor on the external surface; capsule intact
IB	Growth limited to both ovaries; no ascites containing malignant cells. No tumor on the external surface; capsule intact
IC	Tumor either stage IA or IB but with tumor on the surface of one or both ovaries; or with capsule ruptured; or with ascites present containing malignant cells or with positive peritoneal washings
II	Growth involving one or both ovaries with pelvic extension
IIA	Extension and/or metastases to the uterus and/or tubes
IIB	Extension to other pelvic tissues
IIC	Tumor either stage IIa or IIb, but with tumor on the surface of one or both ovaries; or with capsule(s) ruptured; or with ascites present containing malignant cells or with positive peritoneal washings
III	Tumor involving one or both ovaries with peritoneal implants outside the pelvis and/or positive retroperitoneal or inguinal nodes. Superficial liver metastasis equals stage III. Tumor is limited to the true pelvis, but with histologically proven malignant extension to small bowel or omentum.
IIIA	Tumor grossly limited to the true pelvis with negative nodes but with histologically confirmed microscopic seeding of abdominal peritoneal surfaces
IIIB	Tumor of one or both ovaries with histologically confirmed implants of abdominal peritoneal surfaces, none exceeding 2 cm in diameter. Nodes are negative.
IIIC	Abdominal implants >2 cm in diameter and/or positive retroperitoneal or inguinal nodes
IV	Growth involving one or both ovaries with distant metastasis. If pleural effusion is present, there must be positive cytologic test results to allot a case to stage IV. Parenchymal liver metastasis equals stage IV.

Primary chemotherapy

Patients with metastatic disease and high-risk early-stage disease receive chemotherapy after surgery.

Several trials have demonstrated superior survival using a platinum-based chemotherapy regimen, with the addition of paclitaxel providing further improvement. The most common regimen is carboplatin AUC 5–7.5 and paclitaxel 135–175 mg/m^2 every 3 weeks for 6 cycles.

There is some evidence that optimally cytoreduced patients may benefit from administration of combined intravenous and intraperitoneal cisplatin and paclitaxel. The intraperitoneal approach is more toxic and is best suited to patients who do not have significant medical comorbidities.

Recurrent disease

The response rate for primary platinum-based combination chemotherapy approaches 90%, with 70% of patients achieving a complete response.
- The likelihood of relapse for advanced-stage disease is over 75%.
- Length of disease-free interval is predictive of response to secondary treatment; longer intervals show better response to retreatment.
- Advanced stage and suboptimal cytoreduction at initial surgery are the strongest risk factors for relapse.
- Recurrence can be determined by examination, imaging, or serum markers (i.e., rising CA-125 level).

Chemotherapy is the primary treatment modality for recurrent disease; surgery is reserved for select patients with recurrences thought to be completely resectable. Disease-free interval from primary treatment is considered in determining the type of salvage chemotherapy. Disease is defined as platinum sensitive if >6 months has elapsed from completion of initial treatment to recurrence vs. platinum resistant if <6 months.

A platinum-based chemotherapy regimen is usually used in platinum-sensitive recurrent disease.

There are numerous salvage regimens. Agents such as topotecan, liposomal doxorubicin, and gemcitabine are used in platinum-resistant disease and have response rates of 15%–20%.

Treatment of germ cell and sex cord tumors

Unilateral salpingoophorectomy is appropriate for stage I disease in women desiring fertility.

Bleomycin-etoposide-platinum (BEP) adjuvant chemotherapy is used in most germ cell tumors except IA dysgerminoma and stage I well differentiated immature teratoma. Overall, germ cell tumors have an excellent prognosis. Even those that have metastasized are usually cured with surgery and chemotherapy.

Surgery alone is acceptable treatment for stage I stromal tumors (most present as stage I disease). Platinum-based chemotherapy is used for metastatic disease, but efficacy is much less than in germ cell tumors.

New approaches

Investigation of novel agents for treatment of ovarian cancer is an active area of research. Examples include drugs targeting angiogenesis and upregulated biological pathways as well as immunological approaches.

Cancer of the uterine corpus

The vast majority of uterine cancers are adenocarcinomas. Sarcomas represent less than 5% of uterine cancers.

Endometrial cancer

- Endometrial cancer is the most common gynecologic malignancy and the fourth most common cancer in women overall, with 47,000 new cases and over 7500 deaths per year.
- Women have a 2.6% lifetime risk of developing endometrial cancer.
- Overall it has an excellent prognosis due to diagnosis at an early stage, with a 70%–95% 5-year survival for stage I disease.
- Although primarily a disease of postmenopausal women, 5% of cases occur in women younger than 40.

Etiology and risk factors

Most (80%) endometrial cancers are related to chronic exposure of the endometrium to unopposed estrogen, often related to one or more of the following risk factors:
- Obesity
- Nulliparity
- Early menarche and late menopause
- Chronic anovulation
- Exogenous estrogen in the form of hormonal therapy
- Tamoxifen

Diabetes and hypertension also increase risk.

Cancers originating independent of estrogen stimulation confer a worst prognosis and are associated with more aggressive histologic subtypes (serous, clear cell) and advanced stage.

Endometrial cancer is the second most common malignancy in the HNPCC hereditary nonpolyposis colorectal cancer syndrome. These cases account for 3% of all endometrial cancers and typically occur in younger women.

Pathology

The most common histologic subtype is endometrioid adenocarcinoma (75%–80%). Atypical endometrial hyperplasia, now called endometrial intraepithelial neoplasia (EIN), is a precursor lesion to this subtype of endometrial cancer, which is most often well differentiated and has a favorable prognosis. Grade and depth of invasion into the myometrium are strong prognostic factors.

Serous and clear cell histology is associated with more virulent behavior, and these cancers commonly present at an advanced stage and have a high mortality rate.

Presentation

Most patients present with postmenopausal vaginal bleeding. Premenopausal women may present with abnormal, irregular menses.

Tissue sampling with endometrial biopsy or uterine curettage is diagnostic.

Surgery and staging
Endometrial cancer is often surgically staged, which includes assessment of the regional lymph nodes (see Table 36.4).

Hysterectomy and bilateral salpingoophorectomy are almost always performed. Pelvic ± aortic lymph node sampling is performed in most early-stage cases to identify occult metastatic disease.

A laparoscopic approach provides comparable results to those with open surgical techniques.

Table 36.4 Revised FIGO staging for endometrial cancer

Stage	Definition
IA	Invasion to <1/2 myometrium
IB	Invasion to >1/2 myometrium
II	Cervical stromal invasion
IIIA	Tumor invades serosa and/or
IIIB	Vaginal or parametrial metastasis
IIIC1	Metastases to pelvic lymph nodes
IIIC2	Metastases to para-aortic lymph nodes
IVA	Tumor invasion of bladder and/or bowel mucosa
IVB	Distant metastases including intra-abdominal and/or inguinal lymph nodes

Surgery
Surgery is the mainstay of treatment, although primary radiation and progestin hormonal therapy are options for poor surgical candidates. Prognosis is primarily dependent on pathologic findings and stage (see Table 36.5).

Patients with endometrial intraepithelial neoplasia or well differentiated invasive disease who desire preservation of fertility can be treated with progestins. Close follow-up with repeat endometrial biopsy is indicated.

Table 36.5 Poor prognostic factors for endometrial cancer

Advanced stage
Clear cell or serous cell type
Advanced grade
Deep myometrial invasion (>50%)
Occult cervical tumor extension
Lymphvascular space invasion

*5-year survival by FIGO stage	
IA	91.1%
IB	89.7%
IC	81.3%
IIA	78.7%
IIB	71.4%
IIIA	60.4%
IIIB	30.2%
IIIC	52.1%
IVA	14.6%
IVB	17.0%

Modified with permission granted by the International Federation of Gynecology and Obstetrics (FIGO) from: Creasman WT, Odicino F, Maisonneuve P, Beller U, Benedet JL, Heintz AP, et al. (2003) Carcinoma of the corpus uteri. *Int J Gynecol Obstet* 83(Suppl 1):79–118.

Adjuvant radiation

Radiation therapy is the mainstay of adjuvant therapy for endometrial cancer. It decreases local pelvic recurrences, but it has not definitively been shown to improve survival.

Adjuvant radiation may be considered for patients with early-stage disease who have a high risk of recurrence or for patients with demonstrated locoregional metastatic disease in the pelvis or lymph nodes.

External beam radiation may be used to treat the pelvis and/or aortic nodal areas. Vaginal brachytherapy is sometimes used to prevent vaginal cuff recurrence.

Chemotherapy

There is no evidence to date that adjuvant chemotherapy after primary surgery reduces recurrence.

Patients with high-risk histologic subtypes (serous, clear cell) are sometimes treated with chemotherapy after surgery, instead of or in combination with, radiation.

Patients with intraperitoneal or distant metastases are treated with chemotherapy, but outcome is very poor.

Sarcoma

Sarcomas are rare forms of uterine cancer that generally have a poor prognosis. Surgical evaluation and staging are similar to that of endometrial carcinomas.

There are three main types of uterine sarcomas.
- **Mixed mullerian tumors** (carcinosarcomas) are most common and have both malignant glandular and stromal elements. They tend to grow rapidly by local extension in the pelvis and spread to regional lymph nodes.
- **Leiomyosarcomas** arise in the myometrium or in a myoma. They are graded based on cellular atypia, necrosis and mitotic counts: those with >10 mitoses per 10 high-powered fields are almost uniformly fatal. They spread hematogenously and have the worst prognosis.
- **Endometrial stromal sarcomas** are the least common and arise from the specialized stroma between endometrial glands.

Adjuvant radiation may reduce local recurrence in early stage disease, but does not improve overall survival.

Chemotherapy has minimal activity; regimens used include adriamycin, gemcitabine-docetaxel, and ifosphamide-cisplatin.

Cancer of the cervix

- There are 12,700 new cases and 4,300 deaths in the United States per year.
- Cervical cancer is a global epidemic with approximately 530,000 new cases per year. It is the leading cause of female cancer-related death in developing countries.
- Mean age at diagnosis is 47 years old.

Etiology and HPV

Human papilloma virus (HPV) infection is central to the development of cervical dysplasia and cancer. There are multiple HPV subtypes, but certain high-risk, oncogenic types cause most cases (e.g., HPV types 16, 18, 31, 45).

Behaviors that increase the risk for acquiring HPV and conditions or behaviors that impede clearance of infection contribute to the development of cervical cancer, including the following:
- Multiple male sexual partners
- Early onset of sexual intercourse
- Nonbarrier contraceptive methods
- Immunosuppression (e.g., HIV, immunosuppressive drugs used after organ transplantation)
- Tobacco use

Preinvasive disease

Cervical cancer screening is highly effective and is responsible for the lower incidence in developed countries.

Preinvasive disease can be detected through screening with Papanicolou smears and/or HPV testing and confirmed with colposcopic-directed biopsies. Treatment of preinvasive disease through laser or cryoablation or excision of the lesion using a conization or loop electrosurgical excision procedure (LEEP) is usually curative.

HPV immunization

A recent major advance in the prevention of cervical cancer is the FDA approval of vaccinations in women ages 9–26 for high-risk HPV types. A quadrivalent (HPV 6/11/16/18) vaccine is available and has proven to be almost completely effective in prevention of cervical neoplasia caused by these subtypes.

Although this advance holds great promise in the prevention of cervical cancer, it does not preclude the need to have regular screening exams, since not all high-risk HPV subtypes are covered.

Pathology

- 80% squamous cell carcinoma
- 15% adenocarcinoma
- 3%–5% adenosquamous carcinoma
- 1% neuroendocrine or small cell carcinomas

Presentation
- Vaginal discharge
- Postcoital bleeding
- Pelvic pain and pressure
- Intermenstrual or postmenopausal bleeding
- The above are symptoms of invasive cancer: patients with preinvasive cervical dysplasia are usually asymptomatic

Staging
Staging is clinical (see Table 36.6) and primarily based on the extent of disease palpated in the cervix and surrounding tissues. This system is used to standardize staging worldwide, since more expensive diagnostic modalities like CT scans are not usually available in underdeveloped countries.

Tests used in the FIGO staging system for cervical cancer include the following:
- Physical and pelvic exam
- Colposcopy, biopsy and conization of the cervix
- Cystoscopy
- Proctoscopy
- Intravenous pyleogram
- Chest X-ray

Although FIGO staging is primarily clinical, surgical findings or other imaging modalities (e.g., CT, PET scan) are often used to determine a treatment plan.

Prognosis
Stage is most predictive for 5-year survival. Survival by stage at 5 years:
- IA: 100%
- IB: 70%–90%
- II: 50%–70%
- III: 25%–60%
- IV: 10%–20%

Table 36.6 FIGO cervical cancer staging

Stage	Description
I	Cervical carcinoma confined to uterus (extension to corpus should be disregarded)
IA	Invasive carcinoma diagnosed only by microscopy; stromal invasion with a maximal depth of 5.0 mm measured from the base of the epithelium and a horizontal spread of 7.0 mm or less
IA1	Measured stromal invasion 3 mm or less in depth and 7 mm or less in lateral spread
IA2	Measured stromal invasion >3.0 mm and not >5.0 mm with a horizontal spread 7.0 mm or less
IB	Clinically visible lesion confined to the cervix or microscopic lesion greater than IA2
IB1	Clinically visible lesion 4.0 cm or less in greatest dimension
IB2	Clinically visible lesion >4.0 cm
II	Cervical carcinoma invades beyond the uterus but not to the pelvic wall or to the lower third of the vagina
IIA	Tumor without parametrial invasion
IIB	Tumor with parametrial invasion
III	Tumor extends to the pelvic wall, and/or involves the lower third of the vagina, and/or causes hydronephrosis or nonfunctioning kidney
IIIA	Tumor involves lower third of the vagina, no extension to the pelvic wall
IIIB	Tumor extends to the pelvic wall and/or causes hydronephrosis or nonfunctioning kidney
IV	Cervical carcinoma has extended beyond the true pelvis or has involved (biopsy proven) the bladder mucosa or rectal mucosa. Bullous edema does not qualify as a criterion for stage IV disease.
IVA	Spread to adjacent organs (bladder, rectum, or both)
IVB	Distant metastasis

Management

Treatment of cervical cancer is based on stage of disease, size of tumor, the patient's age and fertility desires, and coexistent medical comorbidities.

Treatment is either surgical or chemoradiation in early-stage disease, whereas more advanced stages require primary chemoradiation. Surgery is most often used in younger, healthy patients who are the best candidates for surgery and in whom conservation of ovarian and vaginal function is beneficial.

Prospective randomized trials have shown that addition of weekly cisplatin to radiation treatments improve response and overall survival.

Chemoradiation involves the following:
- Weekly cisplatin administration (40 mg/m^2)
- External beam radiation followed by brachytherapy

There is a 5%–10% risk of late sequelae. Risk increases if radiation is given after primary surgical treatment.

Risks related to radiation include the following:
- Colitis or cystitis
- Chronic nonhealing tissue ulceration
- Intestinal obstruction
- Gastrointestinal or urinary tract fistulas
- Vaginal shortening and/or narrowing

Treatment options based on stage

Microinvasive disease (IA1)
- Cervical conization (fertility sparing) *or*
- Simple hysterectomy

Early disease (IA2, IB1, IB2, and non-bulky IIA)
- Radical hysterectomy with pelvic ± aortic lymph node dissection *or*
- Radical trachelectomy and laparoscopic pelvic lymph node dissection (fertility sparing for IA2 to IB1) *or*
- Chemoradiation therapy

Advanced-stage disease
- Primary chemoradiation

Adjuvant treatment
Adjuvant chemoradiation is often administered after radical hysterectomy to patients at the highest risk of recurrence based on deep invasion, positive margins, lymph node metastases, vascular invasion, or poor differentiation.

Chemotherapy
- Chemotherapy is used to treat patients with distant metastases (lung, liver, bone, lymph nodes) or recurrent disease.
- Cisplatin is considered the most active agent for treatment.
- Multiagent regimens combining agents such as topotecan with cisplatin show minimal gains in efficacy with increased toxicity.

Recurrent disease
- Most recurrences occur within 2 years after treatment, and these may be local in the pelvis or vagina.
- Local recurrences may be salvaged with pelvic exenteration and/or radiation.
- Distant recurrences are almost uniformly fatal.

Vulvar and vaginal cancer

Vaginal cancer
- Primary vaginal cancer is relatively rare.
- There are 2140 cases with 790 deaths annually.
- Metastatic disease in the vagina from cervix, endometrium, vulva, rectum, and a variety of other malignancies is not uncommon.

Etiology
Preinvasive and invasive squamous disease is associated with high-risk HPV types and has the same risk factors as cervical cancer, although vaginal epithileum is more resistant to malignant transformation.

A high percentage of women with vaginal squamous cell carcinoma have been previously treated for anogenital dysplasia or cancer in other areas.

Pathology
Primary vaginal cancer consists of a variety of histological types:
- 90% squamous cell carcinoma
- 5% adenocarcinoma
  - Most common vaginal cancers in women younger than 20 years
  - Clear cell carcinoma is associated with in utero exposure to diethylstilbestrol (DES).
- Sarcoma, melanoma, lymphoma, and other cell types may occur, but are exceedingly rare.
- Rhabdomyosarcoma (sarcoma botryoides) is a virulent form of vaginal cancer that occurs in infants.

Presentation
- Most cases present with either postmenopausal or postcoital vaginal bleeding.
- Abnormal vaginal discharge and urinary symptoms are also common.
- 20% are asymptomatic and are detected during PAP screening for cervical cancer.
- Tumors most commonly originate in the upper third of the vagina on the posterior vaginal wall.

Staging
Vaginal cancer is clinically staged. Physical examination, cystoscopy, proctoscopy, and chest X-ray are used for staging.

Stage is based on the extent of local disease and presence or absence of metastatic disease.

Treatment
Vaginal cancer can be difficult to treat because of its anatomical location. Proximity to the bladder, urethra, and rectum render surgical excision with adequate margins difficult in most cases. Although the proximity of these organs also poses risks with radiation, this is generally the treatment of choice for most vaginal cancers.

- Small (<2 cm) upper vaginal stage I cancers can be treated with wide excision or radical hysterectomy including upper vaginectomy and lymph node dissection.
- External beam radiation + brachytherapy is used for larger stage I cancers or for more advanced-stage disease.
- Recurrent disease may be amenable to pelvic exenteration in some cases.

Significant morbidity is associated with treatment; 10%–15% of patients have complications such as fistulas, cystitis, colitis, and/or vaginal stenosis or necrosis.

Prognosis
Outcomes associated with vaginal cancer are primarily related to stage of disease at presentation, with survival of 67%, 39%, 33%, and 19% for stage I–IV disease, respectively.

Vulvar cancer
- There are 3490 cases and 880 deaths per year in the United States.
- This is most common in postmenopausal women, with a median age of 65 at diagnosis.

Etiology
Squamous cell carcinoma is the most common histologic type. Risk factors are similar to those for cervical cancer.

Oncogenic HPV subtypes contribute to the disease, along with tobacco use and immunosuppression.

Vulvar lichen sclerosis increases the risk of non-HPV-mediated vulvar cancer, and as many as 15% of women with vulvar cancer have a history of lichen sclerosis.

Pathology
- >90% are squamous carcinomas.
- Melanoma and basal cell carcinoma represent 5% and 2% of cases, respectively.
- Extramammary Paget's disease is an intraepithelial lesion in the vulva that rarely may be associated with underlying adenocarcinoma.
- Bartholin's gland adenocarcinoma may also occur in the vulva.

Presentation
- Puritus and pain are the most common presenting symptoms.
- Labia majora is the most common site of disease; biopsy of lesion is essential for diagnosis.
- Thorough evaluation of the vulva is necessary (this may require colposcopy); multifocal disease is not uncommon.

Staging
Staging is surgical; biopsy of the lesion and inguinofemoral lymph node dissection are necessary for staging and treatment planning (see Table 36.7).

There is a growing trend to use sentinel lymph node biopsy techniques to determine the presence of lymph node metastases and need for full lymphadenectomy.

Treatment
Both surgery and radiation are treatment modalities used for vulvar cancer. Treatment is based on the stage of disease.
- Stage IA disease can be managed with wide local excision (at least 1 cm margin, 2 cm ideal). Lymphadenectomy is unnecessary secondary to a low incidence of metastases (<1%).
- Stage IB/II disease requires radical local excision with ipsilateral inguinofemoral lymphadenectomy for lateral lesions and bilateral lymphadenectomy for central lesions.
- Inguinofemoral lymph node metastases usually require adjuvant radiation.
- Radiation is most commonly used to treat stage III or IV disease.

Local recurrence is managed surgically; lymph node or distant recurrence is managed by either radiation and/or chemotherapy.

Prognosis
Advanced age, large tumor size, and lymph node involvement are most predictive of poor survival. Table 36.8 outlines stage-specific survival.

Trophoblastic tumors
This is a unique form of tumor that develops from aberrant proliferation of placental (nonmaternal) trophoblastic tissue.

Most trophoblastic disease arises from a molar pregnancy, but the antecedent pregnancy may be a spontaneous abortion, term pregnancy, or ectopic pregnancy.

There are several distinct subtypes. All share β-hCG as a common tumor marker.
- Hydatidiform mole (complete or partial)
- Malignant gestational trophoblastic disease (GTD)
  - Invasive molar disease
  - Choriocarcinoma
  - Placental site trophoblastic tumors

Hydatidiform moles (molar pregnancy)
- 1 of 1500 pregnancies in the United States
- Comprises 80% of trophoblastic disease
- 20% of moles develop malignant sequelae necessitating chemotherapy.

Classification
Hydatidiform moles are classified as complete or partial, based on cytogenetic, pathologic, and clinical characteristics (see Table 36.9).

Table 36.7 FIGO staging for vulvar cancer

Stage	Findings
0	Carcinoma in situ
IA	Tumor confined to perineum, ≤2 cm, (−) nodes, invasion <1 mm
IB	Tumor confined to perineum, ≤2 cm, (−) nodes, invasion >1 mm
II	Tumor confined to perineum, >2 cm, (−) nodes
III	Tumor of any size with spread to lower urethra or anus and/or unilateral groin lymph node metastasis
IVA	Tumor spread to lower urethra, bladder or rectal mucosa, pelvic bone, or bilateral groin lymph node metastasis
IVB	Distant metastasis including pelvic lymph nodes

Table 36.8 Vulvar cancer survival by stage

Stage	5-year survival
I	97.9%
II	87.4%
III	74.8%
IV	29%

Table 36.9 Classification of molar pregnancies

Feature	Partial mole	Complete mole
Karyotype	Most commonly 69, XXX or 69, XXY	Most commonly 46, XX or 46, XY
Pathology		
Fetus	Often present	Absent
Amnion, fetal red cells	Usually present	Absent
Villous edema	Variable, focal	Diffuse
Trophoblastic proliferation	Focal, slight to moderate	Diffuse, slight to severe
Clinical presentation		
Diagnosis	Missed abortion	Molar gestation
Uterine size	Small for gestational age	50% larger for gestational age
Theca-lutein cysts	Rare	15%–25%
Medical complications	Rare	<25%
Malignant sequelae	<5%	6%–32%

Modified from Soper JT, Lewis JL Jr, Hammond CB. (1997). Gestational trophoblastic disease. In: Hoskins WJ, Perez CA, Young RC (eds.). *Principles and practice of gynecologic oncology*, 2nd ed. Philadelphia: Lippincott-Raven, p. 1040. Reprinted with permission.

Presentation
- Most commonly diagnosed in first trimester of pregnancy
- Abnormal vaginal bleeding is common.
- May find size of uterus greater than dates, hyperemesis gravidarum, preeclampsia before 20 weeks gestation, or thyrotoxicosis
- Complete moles are often associated with extremely high levels of β-hCG.
- Ultrasound shows the uterus filled with irregular tissue ("snow flake" pattern) and absence of a fetus.

Management

Uterine evacuation via suction curettage is required for diagnosis and treatment. β-hCG levels are followed to normal values after evacuation; a plateau, rise, or persistent value likely indicates persistent disease requiring chemotherapy.

Reliable contraception during surveillance should be implemented to ensure that any elevation in β-hCG is not due to new pregnancy.

Malignant GTD

Invasive GTD has several subtypes.
- Invasive molar disease
  - Chorionic villi with diffuse edema; trophoblastic proliferation with myometrial invasion
  - Most common malignant GTD
- Choriocarcinoma
  - Syncytiotrophoblastic and cytotrophoblastic neoplasia
  - No chorionic villi
  - Early metastatic disease in lungs is common.
- Placental site trophoblastic tumor
  - Most rare GTD
  - Lower β-hCG levels
  - Least sensitive to chemotherapy; histologic diagnosis is important (intermediate trophoblasts, no chorionic villi)
  - Hysterectomy is primary treatment.

Diagnosis

Diagnosis of malignant GTD is usually made clinically. This is most often determined during routine surveillance of β-hCG levels following evacuation of a molar pregnancy.

Diagnosis after other types of pregnancies is more difficult; signs and symptoms are subtle and a high index of suspicion is necessary. Criteria for diagnosis of malignant GTD include the following:
- Plateau, rise, or persistent β-hCG after molar pregnancy
- Pathologic diagnosis of invasive mole, choriocarcinoma, or placental-site trophoblastic tumor determined from uterine evacuation, uterine specimen, or metastatic biopsy

Clinical or radiographic evidence of metastatic disease with elevated β-hCG requires management.

Management

Treatment strategies are based on risk stratification using one of a number of systems (FIGO, WHO, NIH). Table 36.10 illustrates the FIGO staging and scoring strategy. A score ≥7 signifies high-risk disease.

Single-agent chemotherapy can be used for low-risk disease, whereas multiagent therapy is often required for high-risk disease. Complete evaluation for metastatic disease is necessary once the diagnosis is made (full-body MRI, CT scans).

Methotrexate is the most common single-agent therapy (30–50 mg/m^2 IM weekly). Actinomycin D is also a commonly used single agent. EMA/CO is the most often used multiagent regimen.

β-hCG levels are followed to monitor treatment. A plateau or rise in levels indicates need to switch agents or implement multiagent treatment.

Hysterectomy does not increase the success rate, but it does shorten time to resolution and the amount of chemotherapy needed in nonmetastatic disease; it has little role in metastatic disease. An exception to this is placental-site trophoblastic tumor, which is a relatively chemoresistant tumor, and hysterectomy is considered first-line therapy.

Prognosis

Almost all patients with malignant GTD are cured with chemotherapy, but there are exceptions. Patients with high-risk disease are best treated in centers with special expertise.

Few women who obtain a normal β-hCG level will relapse. Of those who relapse, 85%–95% relapse within 18 months with only a 1% recurrence rate after 1 year.

Periodic evaluation of β-hCG for 12 months after remission is essential to discover these recurrences. Most recurrences are curable.

Table 36.10 FIGO (2000) staging for gestational trophoblastic neoplasia (GTN)

Stage I	Disease confined to the uterus
Stage II	GTN extends outside of the uterus, but is limited to the genital structures (adnexa, vagina, broad ligament)
Stage III	GTN extends to the lungs, with or without known genital tract involvement
Stage IV	All other metastatic sites

FIGO scoring stratification

Scoring	1	2	3	4
Age (years)	<40	≥40	—	—
Antecedent pregnancy	Mole	Abortion	Term	—
Interval months from index pregnancy	<4	4–7	7–13	≥13
Pretreatment serum hCG (IU/L)	<10^3	10^3–10^4	10^4–10^5	≥10^5
Largest tumor size (cm) (including uterus)	<3	3–5	≥5	—
Site of metastasis	Lung	Spleen, kidney	GI	Brain, liver
Number of metastasis	—	1–4	5–8	>8
Previous failed chemotherapy	—	—	Single drug	2 or more drugs

Chapter 37

Tumors of the central nervous system

Annick Desjardins
James Vredenburgh

Primary brain tumors *626*
Primary central nervous system lymphoma *636*
Brain metastases *638*
Further reading *641*

Primary brain tumors

Epidemiology
The incidence worldwide is very uniform, with a few exceptions such as a higher incidence of pineal tumors in Japan and central nervous system (CNS) lymphoma in AIDS populations. Recent reports suggest that the incidence of glioma and (non-AIDS) lymphoma is increasing in developed countries. In the United States:
- Incidence is ~22,000 per year
- Deaths ~13,000 per year
- Approximately 2% of all malignancies
- Brain metastases are at least 10x more common than primary tumor.
- Bimodal age distribution
  - In children they are the most common solid tumor, predominantly arising in the posterior fossa.
  - There is a second peak in (late) middle age, with largely supra-tentorial tumors.

Etiology
- The majority of primary brain tumors are sporadic.
- Gliomas and meningiomas may be induced by radiation.
- There is an association between primary CNS lymphoma and immunosuppression, including HIV infection.
- There is increased incidence of meningiomas in patients with breast cancer.
- Other candidate etiological agents remain controversial and unproven, e.g., industrial and agricultural chemicals, electromagnetic fields, viruses, and trauma.
- A number of rare familial syndromes are associated with CNS tumors (see Table 37.1).

Pathology
Primary brain tumor pathology is extremely varied, reflecting diverse histogenesis. The most widely used classification system is the WHO 2000 scheme (see Table 37.2).

In general, primary brain malignant tumors are highly infiltrative, with a tendency to spread along white matter tracts to more distant regions of the brain. This feature contributes to their resistance to curative treatment, e.g., by surgery or radiotherapy. They rarely metastasize outside the CNS.

Spread through cerebrospinal fluid (CSF) to remote areas of the neuraxis is a feature of germ cell tumors, medulloblastoma (20%–25%), and other primitive neuroectodermal tumors.

Gliomas are the most common tumors, accounting for approximately half of primary brain tumors. Their behavior and prognosis are strongly linked to histological grade:
- Grade I tumors are slow growing and may be cured by surgical excision.
- Grade II tumors are slow growing but infiltrative, recurring after surgery.

- Grade III and IV tumors show typical features of malignancy with mitotic activity, nuclear atypia, invasion of adjacent normal brain, and occasionally distant spread.
- Grade IV tumors are differentiated from grade III tumors by the presence of vascular proliferation or necrosis.

Table 37.1 Hereditary syndromes associated with primary brain tumors

Predisposing syndrome	Tumor
Neurofibromatosis type 1	Glioma, meningioma, nerve sheath tumors
Neurofibromatosis type 2	Nerve sheath tumors, optic glioma, meningioma
Li-Fraumeni syndrome	Glioma
Von Hippel-Lindau syndrome	Hemangioblastoma
Familial glioma	Glioma
Tuberose sclerosis	Ependymoma, subependymal giant cell astrocytoma, ganglioneuroma

Table 37.2 Abbreviated WHO (2000) classification of intracranial tumors

Subgroup	Grade or type	Prognosis
Astrocytoma	I, Pilocytic	Excellent
	II, Low grade	Good
	III, Anaplastic	Poor
	IV, Glioblastoma	Very poor
Oligodendroglioma	Low grade	Good
	Anaplastic	Poor
Ependymoma	Low grade	Good
	Anaplastic	Poor
Pineal tumors	Variable	
Embryonal tumors	Medulloblastoma and PNET	Good
Pituitary tumors	Usually benign	Good
Germ-cell tumors	Germinoma or teratoma	Good
Lymphomas	High grade	Poor
Meningioma	Usually benign	Good
Schwannoma	Benign	Good

Benign tumors (e.g., meningiomas) are not uncommon (30%).

Some malignant nonglial tumors carry a good prognosis (medulloblastoma, pineal germinoma).

Precise histological identification is essential to appropriate management.

Investigations and staging

The dominant prognostic features for most brain tumors are usually a combination of histological type and clinical features such as age and performance status. Spread to regional lymph nodes and blood-borne spread to distant sites are rare in most pathologies. Therefore, staging systems commonly used for other tumor types are rarely used for brain tumors.

Investigation is dominated by brain imaging.

- **CT**: Contrast-enhanced CT of the brain is readily available and frequently adequate to demonstrate CNS tumors.
- **MRI**: Full-sequence scanning with gadolinium enhancement provides maximal tumor resolution in structural imaging. It is the preferred imaging method.
- **Functional imaging** with SPECT, PET, and MRS are gaining importance both in diagnosis and assessment of response to treatment.
  - Imaging agents thallium-201 and ^{123}I-tyrosine in SPECT scanning and ^{18}FDG glucose in PET give important insights into the functional activity of the tumor.
  - Functional imaging can aid differentiation between high- or low-grade neoplasms and treatment-induced necrosis.
- Tumors that spread via CSF pathways require whole neuraxis MRI.

Histological confirmation of the diagnosis should ideally be obtained in all cases by

- stereotactic biopsy or
- craniotomy and excision or debulking of tumor.

Presentation

Brain tumors present with either neurological dysfunction or symptoms and signs of raised intracranial pressure. Presentation with epilepsy or with slow onset of symptoms carries a relatively favorable prognosis (lower grade tumors). High-grade gliomas are typically associated with considerable edema in the surrounding normal brain, and this contributes significantly to elevated intracranial pressure symptoms (see Table 37.3).

Symptom relief may be obtained through reduction of cerebral edema by the introduction of steroids, e.g., dexamethasone with proton pump inhibitor (PPI) gastroprotection, before biopsy or craniotomy. Maintenance of symptom control can often be achieved with a reduced dexamethasone dose. The dexamethasone dosage can be adjusted according to the patient's status.

Table 37.3 Presenting symptom in patients with intracranial glioma

Symptom	Frequency as principal presenting symptom (%)	Overall frequency at presentation (%)
Epilepsy	30	53
Headache	25	71
Cognitive distance	12	52
Motor disturbance	8	43
Speech disturbance	5	27
Clouding of consciousness	4	25
Visual disturbance	4	25
Sensory change	2	14
Miscellaneous	10	

Management of gliomas

Multidisciplinary management

Patients with brain tumors suffer a wide variety of related physical, cognitive, and emotional problems. Prominent are the following:
- Movement disorders
- Tumor-associated epilepsy
- Pain (headache)
- Speech disorders
- Cognitive decline

These are best managed jointly by the primary care physician and a hospital neuro-oncology group, including a neurosurgeon, neuro-oncologist, radiation oncologist, neurologist, nurse specialist, and rehabilitation team, whose intentions are to maximize the quality of life and deliver optimal therapy to improve survival.

Early involvement of the specialist palliative care team can be valuable for patients with high-grade glioma.

Medical management

Low-grade astrocytoma presenting with epilepsy alone with no mass effect on imaging may be managed for years with anticonvulsants only.

Regular review and repeat scanning are required. Because of the slow growth of those tumors, any new MRI should be compared to the MRI obtained at the time of diagnosis.

Intervention, e.g., surgery, may be indicated if new neurological symptoms develop or there is radiological evidence of mass effect, tumor growth, or transformation to high-grade tumor.

Surgery

Biopsy before extensive surgery for histology is usually required using stereotactic frame, CT, or MRI to target.

Surgery is often covered with steroids (except in lymphoma) to reduce cerebral edema. Surgery is also often covered with anticonvulsants (depending on the neurosurgeon preferences) to prevent the risk of seizure during the procedure.

Surgery alone, guided by MRI, is the treatment of choice for resectable low-grade gliomas, e.g., cerebellar pilocytic astrocytoma in children.

Suspected high-grade glioma is treated initially by craniotomy and debulking of tumor when possible.

Limits of resection can be guided with the patient awake (under local anesthetic) to map speech, motor, and sensory areas.

Surgery may rapidly improve elevated intracranial pressure symptoms. It may not be feasible, however, as poor performance status, or the site or size of tumor carries a high risk of postoperative neurological deficit.

Surgery may be appropriate in relapsed disease (the vast majority [80%] of tumor recurrences occur at the original primary site).

Radiotherapy

Low-grade gliomas

- **Adults**: Postoperative radiotherapy (54 Gy/30 fractions) delays recurrence but has no impact on overall survival, and is often reserved for treatment of recurrent disease, postponing potential radiation-associated toxicity.
- **Children**: Optic nerve or brainstem gliomas may be treated expectantly, but unresectable symptomatic tumors may require radiotherapy.

High-grade gliomas

- Postoperative radiotherapy is commonly given, except in elderly and poor-performance status patients, where prognosis is dismal irrespective of treatment.
- Volume irradiated is limited to tumor-bearing brain.
- A dose of 30–60 Gy is given over 2–6 weeks, depending on prognosis. The standard is a dose of 59.4 Gy over 6 weeks.

Chemotherapy

Brain tumors are traditionally viewed as a chemoresistant tumor, with the blood-brain barrier providing a further obstacle limiting drug access to the tumor, except for lipophilic agents. However, the blood-brain barrier is disrupted in many CNS malignant tumors. Areas of gadolinium enhancement represent areas of blood-brain barrier disruption (see Table 37.4).

Chemotherapy adds little benefit in the setting of first-line therapy for glioma. Active agents include temozolomide, nitrosoureas (BCNU, CCNU), procarbazine, and platinum complexes.

Objective response rates are 15%–40%. There are better results with grade 3 than grade 4 gliomas.

A positive result was reported in glioblastoma patients randomized to receive radiotherapy alone or radiotherapy plus concomitant temozolomide, followed by temozolomide 150–200 mg/m^2 days 1–5 every 28 days for six cycles (median survival improved from 12 months to 14.6 months with chemotherapy).

There is also current interest in the initial treatment of low-grade tumors.

Treatment outcomes and prognostic factors

Tumor grade is the most important predictor. Low-grade gliomas have a relatively good prognosis, with median survival times in excess of 5 years. However, the results of treatment of high-grade gliomas remain poor. Median survival times are as follows.

Anaplastic astrocytoma
- Surgery only: 1 year
- Surgery plus radiotherapy: 3 years

Glioblastoma
- Surgery only: 3 months
- Surgery plus radiotherapy: 10 months
- Surgery plus radiotherapy plus temozolomide: 14.6 months

Other predictors of outcome
- Extent of surgical excision
- Age (worse survival >50 years)
- Performance status
- Mini-mental score (see Table 37.5)
- Pineocytoma and pineoblastoma treated by surgery and local radiotherapy
- Germinoma: Craniospinal radiotherapy results in 95% 5-year survival.
- Chemotherapy may allow a reduction in radiotherapy dose.

Table 37.4 Examples of chemotherapy regimens for CNS tumors

Glioma

Temozolomide 200 mg/m^2 oral d1–5 q 28 days
CCNU 110 mg/m^2 oral d1 q 42 days
VP-16 50 mg/m2 oral d1–21 q 28 days
CPT-11 125 mg/m^2 IV d1, 8, 22 and 29 q 42 days

Medulloblastoma/PNET

Alternating 3-week cycles of:

Vincristine 1.5 mg/m^2 (max 2 mg) IV d1, 8, 15
Etoposide 100 mg/m^2 IV d1–3
Carboplatin 500 mg/m^2 IV d1, 2

And

Vincristine 1.5 mg/m^2 (max 2 mg) IV d1, 8, 15
Etoposide 100 mg/m^2 IV d1–3
Cyclophosphamide 1.5 g/m^2 IV d1

Table 37.5 Mini-mental test

Maximum score	Patient's Score	Questions
5		What is the date? Day, month, year?
5		Where are we now?
3		Examiner names three unrelated objects and asks the patient to repeat these
5		Subtract serial 7's from 100
3		Ask patient to recall the same three objects
2		Ask patient to name two simple objects, e.g., watch and pen
1		Ask patient to repeat "no ifs, ands, or buts"
3		Give patient a piece of paper and ask them to take the paper in their right hand, fold it in half, and put it on the floor
1		Give patient written instruction, e.g., "close your eyes"
1		Ask patient to make up and write one sentence
1		Ask patient to copy a picture
30		Total

Impairment: score 10–20 moderate; 0–10 severe.

Management of other central nervous system tumors

Medulloblastoma
- Hydrocephalus due to blockage of fourth ventricle is common (60%).
- Surgical excision or debulking
- Staging within 1–2 weeks following surgery (MRI of the spine, CSF cytology)
- Postoperative craniospinal radiotherapy
  - Whole neuraxis 35 Gy/21 fractions
  - Posterior fossa boost 20 Gy/12 fractions (posterior fossa, localization of 50%–70% of recurrences)
- When possible, delay radiotherapy for children younger than 3 years of age to allow continuous development of the central nervous system.
- Postoperative chemotherapy improves disease-free survival.
  - Localized disease: 70% 5-year survival
  - M1: 57% 5-year survival
  - M2, M3, M4: 40% 5-year survival

Ependymoma
- Low-grade tumors are treated by surgery and radiotherapy.
- Anaplastic tumors require craniospinal radiotherapy.
- Safe resection of all tumor is the goal. Residual tumor carries a poor prognosis.

Pineal tumors
- Pineocytoma is treated by surgery with or without radiotherapy.
- Pineoblastoma requires craniospinal radiotherapy and chemotherapy.
- Pineal germinoma is treated by local radiotherapy or craniospinal radiotherapy for advanced disease (>90% 5-year survival).
- Nongerminoma germ-cell tumors are treated by chemotherapy (e.g., BEP) followed by craniospinal radiotherapy (~60% 5-year survival).

Meningioma
- These are benign, but complete excision may be difficult as some are in inaccessible areas and surgery involves much brain retraction.
- Some are very vascular.
- Long-term recurrence is significant (30% at 15 years) even after complete removal.
- Surgery is the mainstay of treatment.
- Postoperative radiotherapy and/or chemotherapy are administered after subtotal excision and for malignant meningiomas.

Pituitary tumors
- Trans-sphenoidal excision of macroadenoma is performed to decompress visual pathways.
- Endoscopic trans-sphenoidal approaches are being evaluated.
- Radiotherapy after subtotal resection
- Medical therapy
  - Bromocriptine is usually first-line therapy for prolactinoma.
  - Octreotide is for refractory growth-hormone-secreting adenoma.

Recent advances and future treatments

Neuronavigation

In surgical neuronavigation, recently acquired images of the patient's brain are projected intraoperatively onto the operating field. This facilitates accurate laser or ultrasound resection of tumor.

Intraoperative therapy

This involves use of photoactivated cytotoxic compounds or postresection application to the cavity of sustained-release chemotherapy (BCNU coated wafers-Gliadel).

Radiotherapy

Improved accuracy and dose escalation are feasible with stereotactic localization, although results are disappointing in high-grade glioma.

Gene therapy

Much attention has focused on the HSVtk/acyclovir suicide gene system. Other therapeutic strategies are possible, but the lack of effective vectors currently limits the applicability of this approach. Use of adenovirus or herpes simplex virus might overcome the limitations inherent in the current retroviral approaches.

Antiangiogenic therapy
Growth of all tumors is dependent on angiogenesis, the formation of new blood vessels from preexisting vasculature. VEGF is a paramount common denominator required for tumor angiogenesis and pathogenesis. Increased VEGF expression predicts glioma aggressiveness and poorer outcome.

Specifically, the regimen of bevacizumab (BV), a humanized anti-VEGF monoclonal antibody, plus irinotecan achieved a 10-fold improvement in radiographic response as well as a near doubling of both progression-free and overall survival among recurrent glioblastoma (GBM) patients.

Other VEGF-directed therapies include the following:
- VEGF receptor tyrosine kinase inhibitors: Vatalanib (PTK787/ZK222584) and cediranib (AZD2171), a potent, oral pan-VEGFR, PDGFR, and c-kit inhibitor
- Decoy-ligand: VEGF-Trap

Other therapies
Other therapies are under investigation at this time, including targeted therapies, vaccine, and convection-enhanced delivery.

Primary central nervous system lymphoma

Epidemiology and etiology
Primary central nervous system lymphoma (PCNSL) affects at least 2%–6% of HIV-positive individuals, with autopsy series suggesting the incidence may be greater.

It accounts for 15% of non-Hodgkin's lymphomas (NHLs) in HIV-infected patients, in contrast to 1% in the general population. It is usually a late manifestation of AIDS (CD4 ≤50 μ/L), and patients often have other serious opportunistic infections.

Presenting symptoms
- Focal, e.g., hemiparesis, aphasia, focal seizures
- Nonfocal, e.g., confusion, lethargy, headaches
- Constitutional, "B" symptoms are identified in ~80% of cases.

Pathology
The histology is similar to that of AIDS-related NHL except that almost all cases are associated with Epstein-Barr virus (EBV). This is very different from primary CNS lymphoma in seronegative patients, which is not associated with EBV.

Investigations
MRI is the investigation of choice. Typical appearance is of a well defined enhancing focal lesion, which may be indistinguishable from cerebral toxoplasmosis.
- CSF cytology ± amplification of EBV DNA in CSF sample
- Toxoplasmosis serological testing
- Brain biopsy is occasionally necessary.
- Single-photon emission computed tomography (SPECT) scanning, e.g., using thallium-201. This is under investigation as a means of noninvasively differentiating between PCNSL and toxoplasmosis.

Management
The use of steroids should ideally be delayed until after investigations have been completed, because they may affect tumor size, radiological enhancement after contrast injection, and diagnostic yield at biopsy.

The standard first-line treatment for AIDS-associated PCNSL is whole-brain radiotherapy in combination with corticosteroids. Complete response rates as high as 50% have been reported.

Intrathecal chemotherapy is occasionally used but there is little evidence to support the use of systemic chemotherapy.

Entry into clinical trials should be offered wherever possible.

Treatment should be combined with appropriate highly active antiretroviral therapy (HAART). Multidrug resistance is common in the group of patients whose immunosuppression puts them at greatest risk of developing PCNSL.

Median survival from diagnosis remains just 2–4 months. This is largely due to the context of severe immunocompromise in which PCNSL typically develops: death is usually due to opportunistic infections. A good performance status at diagnosis is associated with longer survival, and palliation for up to 18 months may sometimes be possible.

Chemotherapy followed by whole-brain radiotherapy results in 5-year survival of approximately 30% in HIV-negative patients. Prognosis is better if <60 years of age. In AIDS patients, antiretroviral therapy and cranial radiotherapy may improve an otherwise dismal prognosis.

Brain metastases

Epidemiology

Metastasis to the brain from an extracranial primary site is common. Brain metastases represent significantly more than one-half of all brain tumors.

Symptomatic metastases have an incidence of ~6 per 100,000, but autopsy studies have revealed an overall occurrence in 24% of patients with known cancer. They can be found in 40% of patients with systemic cancer. There is a slight male preponderance and the incidence increases with age.

While brain metastases may arise from any primary site, the most common are from the following:
- Lung cancer (16%–20%, 64% autopsy)
- Breast cancer (5%, 21% autopsy)
- Melanoma (7%)
- Renal cancer (7%–10%)
- GI cancer (1%–2%)
- Approximately 10%, primary site is unknown

Some cancers that commonly metastasize to other organs rarely involve the brain, e.g., prostate, bladder, cervix, and ovary. The reason for this is not known.

Rare tumors that have a predilection for the brain include choriocarcinoma and malignant testicular teratoma with trophoblast elements.

Carcinomatous meningitis is less common but may occur in
- Lung cancer
- Breast cancer
- Leukemia and lymphoma

Pathology

The histology reflects the original primary tumor. Vascular proliferation and tumor necrosis are common features. There is often demarcation from adjacent brain.
- 30% single
- 80% cerebral hemispheres, 15% posterior fossa
- Usually surrounded by edema adding to their mass effect

Presentation

The presentation of brain metastases is similar to that of primary brain tumors:
- Headache (40%–50%, higher frequency with posterior fossa metastasis)
- Focal weakness (20%–40%)
- Altered mental status (30%–35%)
- Seizures (10%–20%)
- Ataxia

The patient may be unwell with systemic disease involving other organs.

Investigation

Imaging is most commonly with contrast-enhanced CT of the brain, because of its availability. However, the most sensitive investigation is high-resolution contrast enhanced MR scan:
- Metastases most frequently appear as multiple, discrete, well demarcated lesions localized at the junction of the gray-white matter.
- Hypointense on T1
- Hyperintense on T2
- Marked gadolinium enhancement
- Often copious surrounding vasogenic edema compared with the size of the lesion
- Up to 20% of lesions revealed on MRI are not seen on CT.

Management

Initial management requires control of the presenting symptoms, with anticonvulsants, analgesics, and other medication as appropriate.
- Dexamethasone is indicated in the majority of patients.
- It frequently produces a reversal of symptoms and neurological deficit.
- PPI gastroprotection must also be initiated.
- Improvement can often be maintained with lower doses.
- Failure of a response to dexamethasone may be an argument against further therapy in poor-performance patients.

For patients with multiple brain metastases whose condition is good at presentation or improved after dexamethasone, treatment with radiotherapy can be offered with the following aims:
- Temporary tumor control
- Modest improvement in survival time
- To allow reduction in the steroid dose without deterioration in symptoms (reducing problems of candidiasis, proximal myopathy, Cushingoid appearance)

Typically, the whole brain is irradiated: a dose of 30 Gy in 10 fractions has been shown to be as effective as any of the more protracted fractionation schemes.

Solitary brain metastasis

This is defined as metastatic disease within the brain in the absence of demonstrable malignancy elsewhere in the body. A biopsy may be required, especially when there is no history of previous cancer.

Surgical excision of a single metastasis should be considered in patients with good performance status and no evidence of disease elsewhere. Postoperative whole-brain radiotherapy is given (20 Gy in 5 fractions or 30 Gy in 10 fractions) with or without a local boost.

An alternative to surgery is stereotactic radiosurgery (20 Gy in a single fraction), again followed by whole-brain irradiation.

Chemotherapy

In general, the CNS is considered a sanctuary site; the majority of cytotoxics do not cross the blood-brain barrier. However, the blood-brain barrier is disrupted in many metastases.

Chemotherapy may be useful in patients with brain metastases from sensitive primaries, e.g., small-cell lung cancer. It is used as first-line therapy (or after resection) in metastatic germ cell tumors, and as second-line treatment in, e.g., breast cancer.

Because the outcome for patients with multiple adverse prognostic factors is very poor irrespective of treatment, it is reasonable to manage those individuals with steroids and symptom control alone.

Outcome

Overall, the prognosis is poor for patients with brain metastases from the common cancers. For patients with poor prognostic features, the median survival may be only 6–8 weeks, irrespective of treatment.

At the opposite end of the spectrum, patients with "good" prognosis, solitary metastases that are treated with surgery and radiotherapy, enjoy a better outlook, with median survival of approximately 10 months (see Table 37.6).

Table 37.6 Prognostic factors for patients with brain metastases

Factor	Description	Influence
Age	Increasing age (>50)	Adverse
Performance status	Poor general condition	Adverse
	Fixed neurological deficit	Adverse
Histology	Adenocarcinoma	Favorable
	Squamous (especially lung)	Adverse
	Germ cell	Very favorable
Number	Solitary	Favorable
	Multiple	Adverse
Size	Small	Favorable
	Large	Unfavorable
Operability	Resectable	Favorable

Further reading

Henry RG, Berman JI, Nagarajan SS, et al. (2004). Subcortical pathways serving cortical language sites: initial experience with diffusion tensor imaging fiber tracking combined with intraoperative language mapping. *Neuroimage* 21:616–622.

Stupp R, Mason WP, van den Bent MJ, et al. (2005). Radiotherapy plus concomitant and adjuvant temozolomide for glioblastoma. *N Engl J Med* 352:987–996.

Vredenburgh JJ, Desjardins A, Herndon JE 2nd, et al. (2007). Bevacizumab plus irinotecan in recurrent glioblastoma multiforme. *J Clin Oncol* 25:4722–4729.

Chapter 38

Head and neck cancers

Neal Ready

Introduction 644
Etiology 646
Epidemiology 648
Screening and prevention 649
Pathology 650
Presentation 652
Investigations 654
Staging 656
Management 657
Prognosis and follow-up 662
Rehabilitation 663
Intraocular tumors 664
Further reading 665

Head and neck cancers

Introduction

Malignancy of the head and neck cancer is the fifth most common cancer worldwide and the most common in central Asia. It encompasses a range of neoplasms arising from different anatomical sites:
- The larynx: including the supraglottic, glottic, and subglottic regions
- The oral cavity: including the lips, gums, anterior tongue, floor of the mouth, hard palate, and buccal mucosa
- The pharynx: including the nasopharynx, oropharynx, and hypopharynx
- The nasal cavity and paranasal sinuses: maxillary, frontal, ethmoid, and sphenoid
- The salivary glands

In the United States, the incidence of cancer at each separate anatomical site is relatively low. However, as a group, these patients account for approximately 50,000 new diagnoses per year.

Although the term *head and neck cancer* includes many different diseases, most of the skills required to assess and manage these patients are broadly similar.

Etiology

Smoking and alcohol
Smoking and alcohol use remain the major modifiable risk factors in the Western world and together are believed to account for >75% of cases of head and neck cancer.
- The effect on the risk of malignancy is synergistic (multiplicative).
- Cigarette smoking is associated with >10 times greater risk of all head and neck cancers.
- Heavy smoking combined with excess alcohol consumption results in >35 times the risk of oral cancer of a person who does neither.
- Chewing tobacco and pipe smoking are particularly associated with oral cancer.
- These carcinogens do not have a significant role in the development of cancers of the nasal cavity, paranasal sinuses, or salivary glands.

Diet
Low risk is associated with a well balanced diet rich in vegetables and fruit. Increased risk accompanies a poor diet, particularly deficient in vitamins A and C. Nitrosamines in salted fish are implicated in a Chinese diet.

Infections
Human papillomavirus (HPV) infection is a risk factor for cancer of the larynx, pharynx, and oral cavity. Recent data suggest that up to 40%–50% of squamous cell carcinomas of the oropharynx are HPV related. The strains of HPV that have been reported in squamous cell carcinoma of the head and neck are the same high-risk strains that cause cervical cancer.

Virally induced cancers may have a better prognosis than those attributable to smoking and alcohol use. Herpes simplex viruses 1 (HSV-1) and 2 (HSV-2) are associated with oral cancer.

Epstein-Barr virus (EBV) infection is associated with the undifferentiated form of nasopharyngeal cancer. Analyses of tissue from these tumors confirm that all are EBV positive with monoclonal viral copies identified within malignant cells. The precise role of EBV in malignant transformation remains to be established. EBV is also implicated in some salivary gland tumors.

Chronic syphilis infection is implicated in cancer of the oral cavity, in particular the tongue.

Genetic susceptibility
There is believed to be a genetic susceptibility to some of the head and neck cancers. Germline mutations in *p53* have been associated with oral cancer.

Certain major histocompatibility complex profiles are associated with nasopharyngeal cancer.

Other environmental agents
- Formaldehyde: Cancers of the pharynx and oral cavity
- Hardwood dust: Adenocarcinoma of the ethmoids—woodworkers have a 70 times greater relative risk.
- Softwood dust: Squamous cell carcinoma of the nasal cavity and paranasal sinuses
- Radiation exposure: Salivary gland tumors.

Epidemiology

Laryngeal cancer
- This is the second most common of the head and neck cancers, although it comprises <2% of all carcinomas in men.
- Annual incidence is 3–10 per 100,000.
- It is a predominantly male disease, as are most head and neck cancers.
- Typically age of incidence is 40–80 years.
- There is a higher incidence in urban than rural areas.

Cancer of the oral cavity
Worldwide, oral cancer has the highest incidence of the head and neck cancers.

Patients of South Asian origin are at increased risk. It is more common in men than in women.

Some 10%–30% of patients with cancer of the oral cavity subsequently develop a second head and neck primary cancer. The incidence of lung and bladder tumors is also increased in this population.

Cancer of the pharynx
Orophraynx squamous cell cancer is one of the sites associated with high-risk HPV strains.

Nasopharyngeal cancer is rare in the United States but more frequent in individuals of southern Chinese and South East Asian origin, reflecting a combination of differing genetic, dietary, and viral etiological factors.

Cancer of the nasal cavity and paranasal sinuses
Sinonasal malignancy is rare, <3% of head and neck cancer. Global figures suggest an incidence of <1/100,000 people per year in most countries.

Occupational factors produce regional differences.

The male-to-female ratio is approximately 2:1. Most cases present between the age of 50 and 70 years.

Cancer of the salivary glands
- 3%–6% of all head and neck neoplasms
- Incidence of 1–3 per 100,000/year
- Cancerous tumors present at a mean age of 60 years; benign disease is more common in a younger age group.

Screening and prevention

There is currently no national screening program for this group of cancers.

In the United States, the emphasis is on public health education to tackle the major modifiable risk factors of tobacco and alcohol use and to raise awareness of these cancers and their presenting symptoms. These efforts are to reduce the number of patients presenting with advanced-stage disease.

Pathology

Squamous cell carcinoma

Over 90% of cancers of the head and neck are squamous cell carcinomas, particularly those involving the larynx and oral cavity. These are categorized as well, moderately, or poorly differentiated depending on the degree of keratinization.

Typically they invade adjacent structures, depending on the site of origin, and spread via lymphatics to regional lymph nodes in the cervical chain, in preference to blood-borne spread. Distant metastases are usually associated with advanced or recurrent primary tumor and may include mediastinal lymph nodes, lung, liver, and bone spread.

There is an association between squamous cell malignancy of the head and neck and several pathological diagnoses believed to represent premalignant conditions.

- **Leukoplakia** is a nonspecific, descriptive term; the important issue is whether dysplasia or carcinoma in situ is present.
- **Leukoplakia**: Hyperparakeratosis ± underlying epithelial hyperplasia. If this is an isolated abnormality there is believed to be ≤5% chance of subsequent malignant change.
- **Erythroplakia**: Superficial red patches adjacent to normal mucosa. It is frequently associated with epithelial dysplasia. It is associated with carcinoma in situ or invasive disease in up to 40% of cases.
- **Dysplasia**: or carcinoma in situ (if it involves the full mucosal thickness). Progression to invasive disease is believed to occur in 15%–30% of cases.
- A **verrucous tumor** (also named Ackerman's tumor) is a variant of well differentiated squamous cell carcinoma presenting as a whitish, cauliflower-like growth. Histology confirms a pushing margin with a marked surrounding inflammatory cell response. Lymphatic spread is rare. Spindle cell carcinomas behave as squamous cell carcinomas.

Other pathologies

- Adenocarcinomas arising from salivary tissue, e.g., in the oral cavity
- Melanoma
- Sarcoma, e.g., rhabdomyosarcoma

Patients with head and neck squamous cancer are more likely to develop second primary cancers than any other group of patients with malignancies. These may be

- **Synchronous**: occurring at or near the same time as the original tumor.
- **Metachronous**: >6 months later
- **Second tumors** are often clonally distinct and therefore not felt to represent locoregional recurrence or metastatic spread from the original primary tumor.

This high risk of multiple primaries reflects the carcinogenic effects of prolonged exposure to tobacco and alcohol over the whole of the aerodigestive tract and urothelium ("field effect").

Tumors of the salivary glands

These represent a very different spectrum of diseases compared with the more common head and neck tumors.

The most common location of a salivary gland tumor is the parotid gland (70%–85%). Most parotid tumors are benign (>75%).

Tumors of the minor salivary glands represent only 5%–8% of salivary gland disease but >80% of these are cancerous.

The most frequent salivary gland tumor is the pleomorphic adenoma (also known as the mixed parotid tumor), a benign epithelial tumor that only rarely undergoes malignant transformation. Local recurrence after enucleation is common and treatment is most commonly with formal parotidectomy.

Malignant tumors that occur in the salivary glands include the following:
- Mucoepidermoid carcinoma
- Adenocarcinoma
- Squamous carcinoma
- Adenoid cystic carcinoma
- Undifferentiated carcinoma
- Metastasis from other primary sites, e.g., breast or lung cancer
- Lymphoma

Presentation

Characteristic local symptoms depend on the site and size of the primary lesion. Malignancy of the head and neck may not uncommonly present with painless cervical lymphadenopathy.

Laryngeal cancer

A hoarse voice is typical if the cancer is affecting the glottis (the most common site of laryngeal cancer in the United States).

A persistent, irritating cough and dysphagia or odynophagia (painful swallowing) are characteristic of supraglottic carcinoma, which typically presents with advanced disease, often including a palpable neck mass.

Dyspnea and stridor can be caused by subglottic cancers that grow circumferentially. These are rare (<5%).
- ± Referred pain in the ear
- ± Hemoptysis

Cancer of the oral cavity

This cancer presents with persistent mouth ulcers, painful ulcerative lesion on lip, or exophytic growth.
- White or red patches on tongue, gums, or lining of mouth
- Dental problems, e.g., loose teeth, dentures no longer fitting
- Dysphagia, odynophagia
- Referred pain in the ear.
- Dysarthria if there is involvement of the tongue
- Weight loss

Tumors commonly extend to involve >1 region within the oral cavity:
- Tongue, 60%
- Floor of mouth, 15%
- Alveolar ridge or retromolar trigone, 10%
- Buccal mucosa, 10%
- Hard palate, 5%

Cancer of the pharynx

The pattern of symptoms tends to differ according to the primary site of disease.

Nasopharyngeal cancer
- Nasal symptoms: bleeding, obstruction, or discharge
- Unilateral hearing loss (secondary to eustachian tube blockage) ± tinnitus
- Cervical lymphadenopathy
- Headache
- Cranial nerve palsies due to base of skull invasion

Oropharyngeal cancer
- Sore throat or lump in the throat
- Pain referred to ear

Hypopharyngeal cancer
- Dysphagia and lump in the throat
- Odynophagia
- Pain referred to ear
- Hoarse voice

Cancer of the nasal cavity and paranasal sinuses
- Epistaxis
- Unilateral nasal obstruction ± serosanguinous or purulent discharge
- Pain and paraesthesia
- Proptosis, diplopia, chemosis ± visual loss if there is involvement of the orbit with displacement of the globe

Tumors of the salivary glands
There is a painless lump within the substance of a salivary gland, as opposed to enlargement of the whole gland.

Differentiation between an enlarged gland and a lump in the gland is often difficult. Benign and malignant salivary gland tumors may be indistinguishable clinically.

Features highly suggestive of malignancy include
- Infiltration of surrounding structures
- Facial nerve palsy

Investigations

The aims of investigations include the following:
- Identifying the primary tumor site and extent, including cytological or histological confirmation of the diagnosis
- Detecting any other synchronous primaries, which are not uncommon in this group of patients
- Staging the disease
- Assessing the general fitness of patients. Significant comorbidities such as ischemic heart disease and obstructive airways disease are common in patients with head and neck cancer, primarily because these conditions share etiological risk factors.

Physical examination
- Inspection of the region including mirror examination
- This has largely been superseded by flexible fiberoptic endoscopy, to allow visualization of the nasopharynx, hypopharynx, base of tongue, larynx, and vocal cord mobility.
- Bimanual examination of the oral cavity
- Palpation of regional lymph nodes. Cervical lymph node spread is an important determinant of prognosis.
- Clinical examination should be combined with appropriate imaging because of the high false-negative rate (15%–30% for cervical lymph nodes) and false-positive rate (30%–40% for cervical nodes) from |clinical examination alone.
- General physical examination, as a clinical assessment of potential metastatic disease (which is commonly asymptomatic)
- ± Examination and biopsy under anesthesia

Bloods
- CBC, electrolytes, and creatinine
- Liver function tests and coagulation screen are commonly abnormal because of concomitant alcohol excess.

Imaging
The extent of imaging will depend on the site and size of the primary tumor, e.g., early laryngeal cancer has a very low risk of distant spread and requires only locoregional cross-sectional imaging.

CT scanning is used to determine the extent of local tumor infiltration, particularly invasion of bone or cartilage (T4 disease), radiological evidence of regional nodal involvement, or the presence of distant metastases. The most common sites of dissemination are the lungs, then liver, then bones.

An MRI of head and neck may provide better soft-tissue definition, especially if the tumor involves the sinuses or skull base.

Obtain a bone scan if bone metastases are suspected.

Positron emission tomography (PET) is used for staging or to identify primary tumor in metastatic squamous carcinoma of the head and neck with unknown primary tumor.

Histology

Obtain a biopsy if the primary tumor is identified and accessible. The exception is salivary gland tumors, for which fine needle aspiration (FNA) is preferred to biopsy to minimize the risk of tumor seeding.

FNA is also used for a metastatic lymph node mass. It is nondiagnostic in up to 15% of cases, although this figure improves with the use of ultrasound guidance.

Staging

Staging systems for head and neck cancers are based on the TNM system and are broadly similar for each of the anatomical sites of origin.

Details that differ between staging systems typically take into account whether involvement of particular local structures will affect the efficacy of radical treatment and hence the effect on overall prognosis.

- T—extent of primary tumor
  - Generally reflects the size of the tumor ± involvement of bone or cartilage (T4)
  - For some sites T4 tumors are further divided into potentially resectable (T4a) or unresectable (T4b).
- N—involvement of regional lymph nodes
- M—absence (0) or presence (1) of distant metastases or inability to assess for their presence (X)

Management

Premalignant lesions

Premalignant lesions require specialist management for two reasons.
- They may subsequently develop into frank carcinoma.
- Patients with premalignant lesions are at high risk of other primary malignant neoplasms, especially within the upper aerodigestive tract and lungs.

Treatment is usually by excision followed by examination by an experienced pathologist. Classification should be based on grade of dysplasia, as this has a bearing on prognosis.

Radiotherapy may be appropriate for frequently recurring or diffuse lesions, e.g., on the vocal cords.

Malignant lesions

Investigation and management should be coordinated by a multi-disciplinary team with expertise in the complex medical, psychological, and functional issues that affect patients with head and neck cancers. Coexisting socioeconomic deprivation can complicate management and compliance may be problematic.

The aim of treatment is to combine optimal rates of cure with the best functional results. When cure is not feasible, every attempt should be made to provide locoregional disease control.

Before beginning treatment it is important to do the following:
- Establish nutritional status, including baseline weight and risk of malnutrition during therapy (elective insertion of a nasogastric or enterostomy feeding tube may be appropriate). A specialist dietician should be involved whenever possible.
- Refer for dental assessment, including completion of any necessary dental treatment. Ongoing mouth-care advice will be needed during and after treatment.
- Correct anemia: Hb must be maintained at ≥12 g/dL throughout treatment for optimal results from radiotherapy. However, erythropoietin therapy is not appropriate because clinical trials showed no benefit in this setting.
- Undertake a speech and language assessment.

There are few randomized trials comparing treatment modalities—the evidence is mainly at level III (i.e., based largely on retrospective case series). This is partly due to the relative rarity of tumors arising from each anatomical site.

Most head and neck cancers are treated with surgery, radiotherapy, or a combination of the two.

Generally, T1–2, N0, M0 disease can be treated with single-modality treatment and retrospective data suggest that the results achieved by surgery or radiotherapy alone are equivalent.

The modality of therapy that will give the best long-term quality of life should be chosen for stage I and II cancers. In more advanced disease, combined-modality regimes are frequently adopted, depending on the primary site.

Management of early stage disease

Some 30%–40% of patients with head and neck cancer present with stage I or II disease, with an overall prognosis of 60%–98% depending on the site of primary cancer.

Surgery alone

Potential advantages of surgery alone include the following:
- It provides complete pathological staging of the disease.
- It provides quick local clearance of disease.
- Newer surgical techniques, e.g., for early laryngeal cancer, may conserve the voice.
- Treatment of metachronous head and neck tumors is not compromised.
- It avoids the toxicity of radiotherapy, including the risk of radiotherapy-induced second malignancies.
- For salivary gland tumors, preoperative biopsy may be avoided (risk of tumor seeding). Primary excision can be used as a simultaneous diagnostic and therapeutic procedure.

Radiotherapy alone

A typical radiotherapy regime might comprise 60–70 Gy administered to the primary site over 6–7 weeks. Treatment may be with external photon beams alone or with photons followed by an electron boost or by interstitial therapy, e.g., using iridium wire. Intensity-modulated radiation therapy (IMRT) is an advanced form of conformal radiation therapy frequently used for head and neck cancer, in which a large number of treatment fields are used to maximize conformal radiation to the tumor and spare surrounding normal structures.

Advantages of primary radiotherapy include the following:
- Avoidance of operative mortality in patients who have significant comorbidities
- Surgical clearance may be difficult or impossible.
- Organ conservation is more likely, including preservation of the voice and swallowing.
- The option of elective radiotherapy treatment of clinically occult regional lymph node disease has relatively little extra morbidity (compared with elective neck dissection).
- Surgery remains an option as salvage therapy in the event of treatment failure. However, subsequent surgery is likely to be associated with greater morbidity, e.g., total laryngectomy is usually required after failure of primary radiotherapy for laryngeal cancer.
- Radiotherapy enables treatment of multiple synchronous primaries.

Toxicity of radiotherapy includes the following:
- Mucositis and a dry mouth that may persist depending on the amount of salivary tissue spared from irradiation
- Chronic ulceration of the mucosa and osteonecrosis are risks, particularly with locally advanced tumors involving the mandible.
- The radiation dose to the eyes, brain, and spinal cord must be kept within tolerance to minimize risks of dry eye or cataract, pituitary dysfunction, and CNS necrosis. Conformal techniques and CT planning allow reduction in the dosage to normal tissue.

Surgery versus radiotherapy?

Cure rates with primary radiotherapy are generally believed to be equivalent to those for surgery for early-stage disease of many head and neck tumors.

However, in certain clinical situations, radiotherapy is clearly the first-line treatment of choice, e.g., in nasopharyngeal carcinoma when the use of surgery is limited to staging, and in the elective dissection of neck nodes that have not regressed 3 months after radiotherapy.

In other clinical situations, surgery is the first choice if at all possible, e.g., tumors of the nasal cavity and paranasal sinuses. Surgery is the treatment of choice when the tumor is clearly invading into bone such as the mandible, if complete surgical resection is feasible.

Combined surgery and radiotherapy

Bulky tumors are generally best treated by a combination of surgery and radiotherapy. The aim of using both modalities is to minimize the risk of locoregional disease recurrence.

The most important risk factors for prediction of recurrence and the need for postoperative radiotherapy are the following:
- Positive resection margins
- Extracapsular lymph node spread
- T3–4 primary tumor
- Perineural or vascular invasion
- Poorly differentiated tumor
- ≥N2 disease

Management of involved neck nodes

Options include the following:
- Therapeutic radiotherapy is appropriate for N1 disease, particularly if radiotherapy is also being used to treat the primary cancer. A dose of 60–65 Gy administered over 6 weeks will control 90% of N1 nodes.
- Therapeutic neck dissection should be considered for patients with more advanced nodal disease (N2–3) and an operable primary. There are no prospective trials to support subsequent adjuvant radiotherapy, but retrospective series suggest it has a role if there is a high risk of local relapse.
- Radical neck dissection removes the superficial and deep cervical fascia with the enclosed lymph nodes (level I to V) along with sternomastoid muscle, omohyoid muscle, internal and external jugular veins, accessory nerve, and submandibular gland.
- A modified neck dissection preserves vital structures such as the accessory nerve (functional dissection).

Complications after neck dissection include hematoma, seroma, lymphoedema, infection, damage to VII, X, XI, XII cranial nerves, and carotid rupture.

For postirradiation neck dissection, surgery may be planned electively after radiotherapy (e.g., 50 Gy) for advanced nodal disease, or more commonly used to salvage regional relapse after radiotherapy.

The role of sentinel node biopsy and the management of micrometastases are uncertain.

Postoperative chemoradiotherapy
Results published in 2004 from two large randomized trials support the use of postoperative chemoradiotherapy in selected high-risk, fit patients with resected squamous cell head and neck cancers.

The indications for adding chemotherapy to radiotherapy would include the presence of lymph nodes with extracapsular tumor spread and/or bulky lymph node metastases.

Radiotherapy with concurrent administration of cisplatin has been associated with fewer locoregional relapses and improvements in disease-free survival. An improvement in overall survival has not been consistently demonstrated.

In addition, the incidence of significant acute toxicity in the patients receiving both cisplatin and radiotherapy was over double the incidence in patients receiving radiotherapy alone.

Treatment of locally advanced unresectable disease

Chemoradiotherapy
>60% of squamous cell head and neck cancers have advanced locoregional disease at presentation (stage III/IV M0). In some cases, surgery remains an option and can result in 5-year survival rates of 20%–50% if combined with radiotherapy.

However, in many cases surgery is either technically not possible or would be associated with unacceptable morbidity, e.g., base of tongue cancer requiring glossectomy and consequent loss of normal voice and swallow. Alternatively, significant comorbidity may mean that operative risk is deemed too great.

Primary radiotherapy for unresectable stage III or IV head and neck cancer is associated with a 5-year survival of only 10%–30%. In such cases, the use of radiotherapy with concurrent chemotherapy has been demonstrated to be associated with a survival advantage over treatment with radiotherapy alone. Meta-analysis of all phase III trials shows a 4%–8% increase in 5-year survival.

Phase III trials comparing definitive radiotherapy with or without full-dose cisplatin in oropharynx cancer have shown a 20%–30% increase in local control and 10%–20% increase in survival at 5 years.

Although combined-modality therapy is associated with increased acute toxicity compared with radiation alone, concurrent full-dose platinum-based chemotherapy with radiation should be considered standard therapy to optimize the chance for organ preservation, locoregional control and survival in patients with good performance status, and relatively few comorbidities.

Distant metastatic disease is now a significant clinical concern after concurrent chemoradiotherapy for locally advanced head and neck cancer.

Two important ongoing phase III trials (DeCIDE and PARADIGM) are investigating whether induction chemotherapy improves survival when added to concurrent chemoradiotherapy.

Biological therapies

Cetuximab (Erbitux) is an intravenously administered human/mouse chimeric monoclonal antibody that binds to the epidermal growth factor receptor (see p. 178). This receptor is overexpressed in many head and neck cancers.

A recent randomized trial compared radiotherapy alone to the combination of radiotherapy and concurrent weekly cetuximab in patients with locally advanced squamous cell carcinoma of the head and neck.

The use of cetuximab was associated with significant improvements:
- Median survival (54 vs. 28 months)
- 2-year survival (62% vs. 55%)
- There was no increase in mucositis, although significant skin toxicity was more frequent in the group receiving combined-modality treatment.

Management of metastatic disease

Chemotherapy

Certain chemotherapy agents, e.g., cisplatin, docetaxel, 5-fluorouracil, methotrexate, and bleomycin, have been shown to be active in advanced squamous cell carcinoma. The highest response rates appear to be achieved by combination regimes, although a survival advantage with this approach has not consistently been demonstrated.

Nasopharyngeal carcinomas seem particularly chemosensitive, with response rates of up to 70% reported in advanced disease.

Chemotherapy can also be used in disseminated or unresectable salivary gland tumors, which are typically chemosensitive. Response rates of up to 50% are reported, although the duration of response is usually only a few months. The regime chosen can be tailored to the histology of the disease.

Cetuximab also has activity in advanced squamous cell carcinoma. A recent large phase III trial showed an improvement in median survival from 7 to 10 months when cetuximab was added to platinum and 5-fluorouracil chemotherapy.

Prognosis and follow-up

Follow-up is important in patients treated with curative intent for head and neck cancer. The aims of surveillance include the following:
- Early detection of locoregional recurrence: early detection will improve the chances of successful salvage therapy.
- Detection of new primaries: the incidence of new primary cancers is 3%–4% per year (10%–15% overall).
- Management of the late effects of treatment

Laryngeal cancer
- 90% of recurrences occur within 3 years.
- There is a high risk of second primary malignancies (12%–20%).
- Patients with supraglottic laryngeal cancer are at particular risk of subsequent primary lung cancer. A chest X-ray and even bronchoscopy may be considered in regular follow-up. Spiral CT may also have a role.

Cancer of the oral cavity
- >80% 5-year survival for those presenting with early-stage, localized disease
- >40% 5-year survival for patients with locoregional nodal involvement
- <20% 5-year survival for those with distant metastases

Cancer of the pharynx

Reported 5-year survival rates for nasopharyngeal carcinoma range from >80% for stage I disease to <30% for patients presenting with advanced tumors.

Follow-up after treatment for early-stage disease should be most intensive in the first 3 years, when the majority of recurrences occur.

Prognosis is less good for localized oropharyngeal cancers, with a 5-year survival of 50% for those presenting with stage I disease, although survival with advanced disease is similar to that with metastatic nasopharyngeal cancer.

Tonsillar cancer, in general, has better prognosis, with survival of >80% at 5 years, even for stage III disease.

Cancer of the nasal cavity and paranasal sinuses

Presentation is most commonly with locally advanced tumors that remain potentially curable with radical surgery and radiotherapy.

Regional metastases are infrequent, occurring in <20% of patients at presentation.

Cancer of the salivary glands

Five-year survival is 75%–85% for those presenting with early-stage, localized (stage I) malignant disease of the salivary glands but falls to 30% for patients presenting with disseminated disease (stage IV).

More than one fifth of recurrences occur over 5 years after treatment for the primary disease.

Rehabilitation

The treatment of many head and neck cancers has significant associated long-term morbidity. Patients may have to adjust to huge changes in both appearance and function.

A high level of specialist support from many different disciplines in the months and years following their treatment can significantly improve quality of life.

Physical therapy can help with maintaining range of motion in the neck and minimizing treatment-related edema.

Specific difficulties

Difficulties that require ongoing input include the following.

Speech

The greatest handicap for patients after a total laryngectomy is the loss of voice. Options include the following:
- 40% of patients acquire socially useful esophageal speech.
- Some patients successfully use an artificial larynx device.
- Fistula operations with insertion of speech valvulas are increasingly performed and well tolerated.
- Specialist speech and language therapists should be involved throughout the patient's care.
- Some patients find support groups or Web-based information sites helpful, e.g., http://www.theial.com/ial/.

Airway management

Patients may have to adjust to breathing through a stoma. If the airway has been separated from the gullet they will have to learn to manage their airway secretions.

Heat and moisture exchangers are commonly used to lower the risk of respiratory problems and can be positioned in front of the stoma.

Dentistry

Specialist dentists should be involved in follow-up for the specific problems that occur after, e.g., radiotherapy to the mouth. These include frequent dental caries, poor healing after tooth extraction, and the potential for late osteonecrosis.

Nutrition

Late effects from radiotherapy and surgery may affect nutritional intake in the long term. Factors to address include any alterations in the normal swallow mechanism, altered salivary production, and altered taste.

Input from a dietician with expertise in patients treated for head and neck cancers is vital.

Other difficulties

Patients may need to be helped to cope with disfigurement and altered body image.

Strenuous efforts must also be made to encourage patients to stop smoking and to cut back on their alcohol intake.

Intraocular tumors

Melanoma

- Melanoma can affect the uveal tract.
- The most frequent location is the choroid.
- Biopsies should not be performed.
- Diagnosis should be made by an ophthalmologist with experience in this field.
- Treatment may be observation, radioactive eye plaque (ruthenium or iodine), local resection, charged particles (proton beam), or enucleation.
- See Chapter 39.

Retinoblastoma

This is a rare intraocular tumor arising in young children, usually in the first 2 years of life. The incidence is 1 in 20,000. The disease is hereditary (autosomal dominant) and often bilateral.

Patients should be managed in combined clinics by ophthalmologists experienced in management of retinoblastoma. Biopsy should not be performed.

Management

- Small tumors not adjacent to the macula or optic disc: photocoagulation
- Small or moderate tumors: radioactive plaques (iodine, ruthenium plaques, 40 Gy)
- Large or multiple tumors: external radiotherapy
- May need to radiate the whole eye (40 Gy, 20 fractions over 4 weeks); try to maintain vision
- Occasionally enucleation is required, if tumor fills the whole globe.

The tumor is also chemosensitive:
- Platinum
- Etoposide
- Vincristine
- Doxorubicin
- Cyclophosphamide

Chemotherapy is useful if the tumor has a bad prognosis or in a neoadjuvant setting.

Prognosis is 90% survival; 80% of patients can have the eye preserved.

Metastatic disease

Metastatic disease involving the eye is usually associated with choroidal metastases. The most common tumors implicated are lung and breast.

This is an oncological emergency if vision is threatened.

Usually treatment is with radiotherapy.

Further reading

American Joint Committee on Cancer (2003). *AJCC Cancer staging Manual.*, 6th ed. New York: Springer-Verlag.

Andry G, Hamoir M, Leemans CR (2005). The evolving role of surgery in the management of head and neck tumours. *Curr Opin Oncol* 17:241–248.

Cooper JS, Pajak TF, Forastiere AA, et al. (2004). Postoperative radiotherapy and chemotherapy for high-risk squamous-cell carcinoma of the head and neck. *N Engl J Med* 350:1937–1944.

Guidance on cancer services—improving outcomes in head and neck cancers, November 2004. NICE, London.

Salama JK, Seiwert TY, Vokes EE (2007). Chemoradiotherapy for locally advanced head and neck cancer. *J Clin Oncol* 25:4118–4126.

Chapter 39

Cutaneous malignancies

April K. S. Salama

Malignant melanoma *668*
Management of malignant melanoma *672*
Intraocular melanoma *678*
Nonmelanoma skin cancer *680*
Merkel cell carcinoma *684*
Further reading *685*

Malignant melanoma

Primary cutaneous malignant melanoma arises from the melanocytes found in the basal layer of skin. These cells produce melanin pigment and are responsible for the tanning response observed after exposure to ultraviolet (UV) radiation.

Epidemiology and etiology

Incidence rates are rising faster than for any other cancer worldwide. In 2013, an estimated 76,690 new cases and 9480 deaths are anticipated in the United States.

The lifetime risk is currently estimated at >1:80 for Caucasians, but as low as 1:1200 among those with pigmented skin. Rates in Australia are the highest in the world and continue to double each decade.

The incidence among women is at least comparable to the incidence in men, although death from melanoma is more common in men.

Sunlight is the main environmental cause of melanoma. Excess exposure to UV radiation, particularly in early life, is strongly associated with subsequent risk of developing melanoma. A history of severe sunburn or intense, intermittent exposure may be particularly relevant.

Genetic risk plays a role, with ~10% of cases having a strong family history of melanoma. A melanoma susceptibility gene *CDKN2A* on chromosome 9 has been identified as a tumor suppressor gene. Germline mutations are implicated in up to 40% of patients with familial melanoma and may have a role in sporadic cases.

Benign pigmented nevi (see Fig. 39.1 and Fig. 39.2) may be precursor lesions to malignant disease, but more frequently these are markers of a more general increased risk within the individual.

Immunosuppression, as occurs in patients after organ transplantation, appears to be associated with an increased risk of developing melanoma (see Fig. 39.3 and Fig. 39.4). Currently, there is no evidence that melanoma is more prevalent in the HIV-positive population.

MALIGNANT MELANOMA

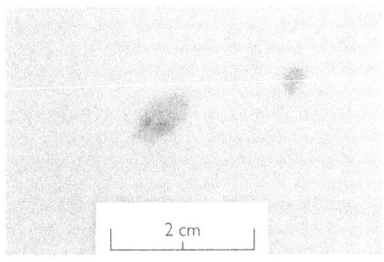

Figure 39.1 Benign pigmented lesion (see Plate 3 for a full color version).

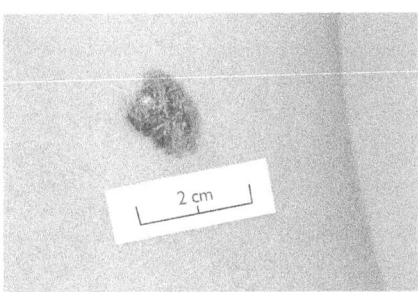

Figure 39.2 Benign nevus close-up (see Plate 3 for a full color version).

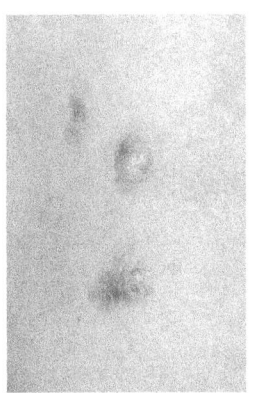

Figure 39.3 Malignant melanoma close-up (see Plate 4 for a full color version).

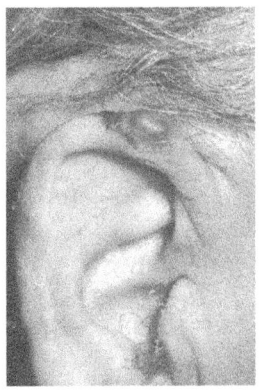

Figure 39.4 Malignant melanoma close-up (see Plate 5 for a full color version).

Screening and prevention

Strenuous efforts must be made to minimize the occurrence of melanoma and to maximize the chances of early diagnosis where curative treatment is possible.

Exposure to sunlight has been identified as the major modifiable risk factor. This has led to public health drives to promote sun avoidance:
- The Australian "Slip (on a shirt), Slap (on a hat), Slop (on sunscreen)" campaign
- Promotion of artificial tanning products as an acceptable cosmetic alternative to UV exposure
- Sun hats as part of the uniform in some schools

Screening may be an appropriate option for patients deemed at particular risk for the disease, e.g., those with a strong family history of melanoma or with a personal history of any skin cancer or of blistering sunburn in early life.

Serial photographs can be useful in patients with a high mole burden, as can inspection via a magnifying dermatoscope.

Clinical presentation

Common
- Alteration in a preexisting pigmented mole on the skin
- A new pigmented lesion: This is particularly relevant if the patient is ≥40 years old, when the acquisition of new moles is uncommon.
- Irregular brown or black pigmentation of a lesion.
- Irregular border or new asymmetry of a lesion
- Oozing, crusting, itching, or bleeding
- Differential diagnosis: (1) benign melanocytic nevi; (2) seborrheic keratoses (older ages).

Less common
- Palpable regional lymphadenopathy
- Metastatic disease to viscera (primary lesion may not be identified)

Investigations

A full clinical examination includes the following:
- Skin
- Regional and distant lymph nodes
- Palpation of the abdomen
- Neurological examination if indicated

Excisional biopsy is required for any pigmented lesion of concern. Complete excision with normal skin margins is optimal.

Shave biopsy should be avoided to minimize the risk of incomplete excision; appropriate staging requires depth measurement.
- Chest X-ray
- Serum biochemistry including LDH, once diagnosis of melanoma has been confirmed
- Further imaging
  - CT chest/abdomen
  - High false-positive rate

Pathology
- Confirms neoplastic melanocytic cells invading beneath the basement membrane into the underlying dermis
- Histological subtype
  - Superficial spreading
  - Nodular
  - Acral lentiginous melanoma
  - Lentigo maligna
- Tumor thickness (Breslow depth) in millimeters
  - From the epidermal granular layer to the base of the tumor at its thickest point
- Invasion of dermal blood vessels and lymphatics
- Presence or absence of ulceration
- Margins—whether involved or width of normal tissue surrounding melanoma
- Any microsatellites of melanoma

Staging
In 2009, the American Joint Committee on Cancer (AJCC) produced a revised, validated staging system based on tumor thickness, presence of ulceration, and identification of metastases to provide guidance for management decisions and likely prognosis.

Management of malignant melanoma

Surgical management

Surgery at the primary site
The treatment for primary malignant melanoma is complete excision of the lesion. The recommended margin of excision of normal skin varies according to the thickness of the tumor.
- In situ disease only: 0.5 cm
- ≤1.0 mm: 1.0 cm
- >1.0–2.0 mm: 1.0–2 cm
- >2.0–4.0 mm thick: at least 2.0 cm
- >4.0 mm: 2.0 cm margin recommended

Margins may be modified according to anatomic location and patient situation. Excision must be adequate in depth as well as laterally.

Unusual sites of disease, e.g., foot sole, nail bed, require tailored surgical techniques.

Most patients with primary melanoma have the defect closed directly. A small number may require a flap or a graft to achieve closure.

Surgery for the regional lymph nodes
One in five patients who are clinically node negative will have metastatic deposits. Regional lymph node dissection is indicated in patients with clinical evidence of lymph node involvement.

Therapeutic lymphadenectomy of palpable or histologically proven metastatic lymph nodes may be curative, e.g., 10-year disease-free survival of ~25% for all node-positive patients treated surgically. Lymph node dissection also minimizes the risk of local ulceration or fungation.

Complications after surgery are common and include infection and seroma formation in the short term and lymphedema in the longer term.

Elective lymph node dissection in patients without definite evidence of regional nodal involvement has not yet shown to improve survival in patients with tumors that are <1 mm or ≥4 mm thick. There is suggestion of a survival benefit in younger patients with tumors of intermediate depth.

The main benefit of establishing the status of regional lymph nodes is for accurate staging, provided this will affect options for subsequent adjuvant therapy.

Sentinel lymph node biopsy
- Blue dye and/or a radiolabeled tracer
- Identifies patients with definite lymph node metastasis who can then proceed to full regional nodal dissection
- Represents a staging investigation rather than a therapeutic intervention

Early studies suggested that the sentinel node can be identified in up to 90% of cases and the false-negative rate may be as low as 2%. In 30%–50% of patients the sentinel node is the only positive node identified.

The risk of detecting malignant deposits in the sentinel node increases with primary tumor thickness (see Table 39.1). If the sentinel node is

Table 39.1 Risk of identifying a metastatic deposit in a sentinel lymph node according to primary tumor thickness

Tumor thickness	Risk of metastatic deposit in sentinel node
Breslow depth <0.75 mm	1%
≥0.75 Breslow depth <1.5 mm	8%
≥1.50 Breslow depth <4.0 mm	23%
Breslow depth ≥4.0 mm	36%

negative for tumor deposit a full nodal dissection is generally not performed, avoiding the associated morbidity.

The results of several large-scale trials that should help clarify whether this approach compromises long-term survival are awaited.

Prognosis and risk of relapse

For most patients who present with stage I to IIA disease appropriate surgery is curative in 70%–90% of cases.

Relapse rates escalate rapidly with advancing stage:
- Stage IIB disease has a risk of recurrence of 40% after local excision.
- Stage III disease, which includes regional node involvement, is associated with relapse rates of >80%.
- Stage IV disease is generally associated with a median survival of <9 months

Cerebral metastases are relatively common in long-term survivors from melanoma. Leptomenigeal involvement is associated with median survivals of 5–16 weeks.

Chemotherapy, immunotherapy, and radiotherapy

Adjuvant therapy

Patients with malignant melanoma should be managed by a multidisciplinary team including a dermatologist, dermatopathologist, plastic or general surgeon, medical oncologist, and the primary care physician. The role of adjunctive therapy in patients with resected malignant melanoma continues to evolve.

Patients should be encouraged to enroll in controlled clinical trials of adjuvant therapy.

For stage IA–IIB melanoma, options include no further therapy or a clinical trial.

For stage IIC–III melanoma the options include the following:
- Clinical trial
- No treatment
- High-dose intravenous interferon-α (HDI): Several large trials have produced conflicting results and comparison of the outcomes is complex.
- Pegylated interferon-α: A large randomized trial demonstrated a small reduction in risk of recurrence.

Interferon α-2B in intermediate- and high-risk patients may be associated with modest improvement in relapse-free survival, although the impact on overall survival is less clear. Side effects include flu-like symptoms, myelosuppression, fatigue, and depression. There is no consensus on the optimal regime.

Locoregionally advanced disease

Locoregional metastases include recurrence at the site of the resected primary disease, in-transit and satellite metastases, and regional lymph node metastases.

If there is no evidence of disseminated disease, further resection should be considered, as this approach can sometimes produce long-term survivors. Alternative approaches for local control of unresectable disease include hyperthermic isolated limb perfusion or isolated limb infusion with melphalan and occasionally radiotherapy.

Stage IIIC patients with multiple positive nodes or extranodal extension, particularly with a head and neck primary cancer, may be considered for adjuvant radiation therapy to the nodal bed. A recent analysis showed that although adjuvant RT can reduce local recurrence rates, there is no significant impact on relapse free or overall survival, and thus should only be considered in selected patients at high risk of recurrence.

Management of metastatic disease

Although metastatic disease remains incurable for the majority of patients, new developments in systemic therapies are rapidly expanding the number of available treatment options.

Surgery

Procedures to debulk the tumor and optimize local control are occasionally appropriate.

Resection of limited residual disease after adjuvant therapy or removal of solitary sites of visceral metastases in selected patients is sometimes offered.

Immunotherapy

High-dose interleukin-2

Although U.S. FDA-approved, interleukin-2 (IL-2) yields response rates of <20%, although there is the potential for durable complete remissions in 5%–7% of patients. Multiorgan toxicity including arrhythmias, hypotension, and capillary leak syndrome limit this approach for many patients.

Ipilimumab

Ipilimumab is a CTLA-4 antibody that was FDA approved in 2011.
- Has demonstrated an overall survival benefit in a randomized phase III trial
- Has the potential to induce durable disease control in some patients, with responses lasting more than 2–3 years
- CTLA-4 directed therapy is associated with a unique side effect profile, including the development of immune related adverse events (irAEs)
- The most common irAEs include rash, colitis, hepatitis, and endocrinopathies

Targeted agents
The discovery that MAPK pathway alterations, specifically BRAF V600 gene mutations, are a major driver of oncogenesis in approximately half of all melanomas has led to the development of a number of novel targeted therapies.

BRAF inhibitors
- Vemurafenib and dabrafenib
- Vemurafenib and dabrafenib are selective $BRAF^{V600}$
- inhibitors recently approved by the FDA.
  - Both have demonstrated clinical benefit when compared with standard chemotherapy in randomized phase III trials.
  - Response rates are approximately 50%, with the potential for rapid symptomatic improvement
  - The median duration of response in most studies is 6–7 months.

MEK inhibitors
Trametinib recently received FDA approval in 2013 based on results from randomized phase III trial demonstrating a survival benefit in patients with $BRAF^{V600}$ mutated metastatic melanoma when compared with standard chemotherapy.
- Response rates appear to be lower than that of BRAF inhibitor monotherapy, at approximately 20%.
- Median duration of response is 5–6 months.
- Trametinib is not indicated for patients who have progressed on a BRAF inhibitor

Chemotherapy
- **Dacarbazine (DTIC)**: Response rates of 7%–20% are documented in the literature with a median duration of response of 4–6 months.
  - Treatment is generally well tolerated.
  - Data demonstrating a survival advantage are still lacking from randomized controlled clinical trials.
  - Combining DTIC with either tamoxifen or IFN-A has produced no compelling evidence of benefit.
- **Temozolomide** is an oral analogue of DTIC with phase III data to support its equivalent activity in metastatic melanoma and with the potential advantage of greater CNS penetration.
- Combination regimens of cisplatin, carboplatin, vinblastine, and others with DTIC or paclitaxel do not provide consistent evidence to support superiority over single-agent DTIC, and toxicity is significantly greater.

Radiotherapy
Palliation can be achieved for pain from skeletal metastases.

Symptomatic cerebral metastases should be treated with corticosteroids and cranial irradiation should be considered. Controversy exists at to whether to treat asymptomatic cerebral disease.

Future directions

The landscape of available treatment options for melanoma is rapidly changing. Ipilimumab was the first agent to demonstrate an overall survival benefit for metastatic melanoma in a phase III trial. Novel immunomodulators, including those that target PD-1 and PD-L1, among others, are at various stages of development and have shown promise. In addition, early data from phase I/II studies suggests that the combination of a BRAF + MEK inhibitor results in an improved response rate and PFS when compared with BRAF inhibitor monotherapy. The results of phase III studies to confirm this are currently pending. Future work centers on novel combination strategies, and participation in clinical trials remains critical.

Intraocular melanoma

Epidemiology and etiology
This is a rare malignancy affecting the uveal tract, most frequently involving the choroid. Risk factors include UV exposure, light iris color, inability to tan, and previous personal or family history of melanoma.

Presentation
Often it presents as an incidental finding at a routine visit to the optician in an asymptomatic individual. Alternatively, patients may present with visual loss.

Investigation
Biopsies should not be performed. Diagnosis should be made by an ophthalmologist with experience in this field.

Management
Ideally, treatment is carried out in a combined ophthalmic–oncology clinic. Options include the following:
- Observation
- Brachytherapy with radioactive eye plaques (e.g., ruthenium-106 or iodine-125) charged-particle irradiation
- Local resection
- Enucleation.

Prognosis
Generally prognosis is poor, with death from metastatic disease in >50% of affected patients.

Dissemination is hematogenous with hepatic involvement in 90% of those with metastatic disease.

Nonmelanoma skin cancer

The two main forms of primary skin cancer in this group are
- Squamous cell carcinoma (SCC)
- Basal cell carcinoma (BCC), i.e., keratinocyte skin cancers

Malignant skin lesions may also represent metastases, e.g., from breast, lung, or gastrointestinal primary cancers.

There are also several uncommon skin cancers beyond the scope of this chapter, e.g., Kaposi's sarcoma and cutaneous angiosarcoma.

Epidemiology and etiology

These cancers are the most common malignancy in the United States and most Western populations, occurring particularly in fair-skinned Caucasians.

Risk factors include the following:
- UV radiation: Sunlight remains the principal environmental cause of the keratinocyte skin cancers.
- Ionizing radiation
- Chronic inflammation
- Human papilloma virus (HPV)
- Immunosuppression, e.g., after organ-transplant
- Hereditary conditions, e.g., 0.5% of BCCs occur in patients with the autosomal dominant basal cell nevus syndrome.

Presentation

Squamous cell carcinomas
See Fig. 39.5
- Represent ~20% of nonmelanoma skin cancers
- Arise on sun-exposed sites or at sites of chronic inflammation
- Rapidly growing, red papule or nonhealing skin lesion
- Often background of actinic keratosis
- Ulceration and bleeding may occur.

Some 5%–10% of SCC metastasize, initially to regional lymph nodes. Risk factors for metastasis include the following:
- Recurrent disease
- Large size
- Deep invasion
- Chronic scars, sinus tracts
- Certain anatomical sites, e.g., lip

Locoregional disease is associated with a 5-year survival of ≤65%. Disseminated disease has a very poor prognosis.

Basal cell carcinomas
See Fig. 39.6
- Represent 75% of nonmelanoma skin cancers
- Lesions arise on sun-exposed areas, e.g., face, ears, scalp.
- Normally confined to hair-bearing skin
- Slow-growing, pink papule with telangiectasia
- Typically they are indolent, although they can be locally invasive, causing significant disfigurement.
- Metastases are rare (0.1%).

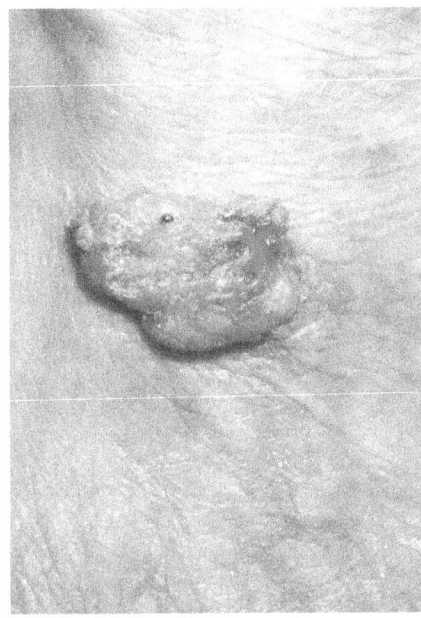

Figure 39.5 Squamous cell carcinoma (see Plate 6 for a full color version).

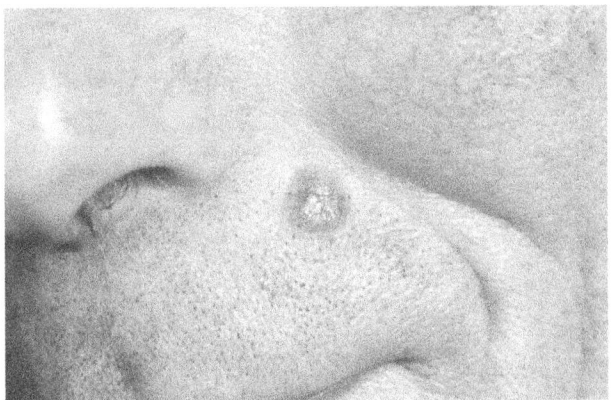

Figure 39.6 Basal cell carcinoma (see Plate 7 for a full color version).

Management

Squamous cell carcinoma

The most common treatment is surgical excision of the primary disease ± locoregional lymph node dissection of any clinically evident lymph node metastases. This allows histological assessment of the adequacy of the margin of excision.

A 5-year cure rate of >90% is reported for excision of localized primary disease. The potential role for sentinel lymph node biopsy awaits further study.

Cryotherapy or electrosurgery can be used for in situ disease or for small, low-risk lesions. Both techniques do not permit confirmation of clear margins.

Radiotherapy is most useful for small, well localized lesions. The reported 5-year cure rate is approximately 90%. It can also be used as adjuvant treatment after incomplete surgical excision or in patients with nodal involvement.

Platinum-based chemotherapy is sometimes used for disseminated disease.

Ongoing Surveillance

- 95% of relapses will occur within 5 years.
- 50% of patients will also develop a new nonmelanoma skin cancer within the same period.

Basal cell carcinoma

More than 90% of BCC are curable, although certain factors predict a higher risk of local recurrence:

- Sclerosing, micronodular, or mixed growth pattern
- Perineural invasion
- Basosquamous differentiation

Despite low metastatic potential, early definitive treatment is important, as local invasion can be associated with significant morbidity. Surgical excision allows assessment of histological features and adequacy of resection margin.

Cryotherapy, e.g., using pressurized liquid nitrogen, is sometimes used for low-risk lesions.

Radiotherapy is appropriate for recurrent disease, particularly in elderly patients. Avoid its use in those <50 years old because of the long-term risk of secondary cutaneous malignancies within the radiation field. It yields 5-year cure rates of >90% for previously untreated lesions.

Radiotherapy may be useful around the eyelids, nose, and lips when the cosmetic result is likely to be superior to that with surgical techniques. It is contraindicated in patients with the hereditary basal cell nevus syndrome.

Chemotherapy, e.g., with topical 5-FU, may achieve cure rates of >90% in selected patients with low-risk BCC.

Ongoing surveillance
- 80% of recurrences will occur within the first 5 years.
- Approximately 40% of patients will develop a new primary BCC within the same period.
- Patients are also at risk of other cutaneous malignancies.

Prevention and future directions
Any patient with a nonmelanoma skin cancer should be advised about the importance of sun avoidance to minimize future risk.

Merkel cell carcinoma

These rare, malignant skin tumors arise most commonly in the head and neck area or the limbs. They have a propensity for local recurrence and regional and distant spread.

These tumors have neuroendocrine features. Clinically, they commonly present with a red or purple nodule with shiny overlying epithelium.

Staging requires a chest X-ray and assessment of regional lymph nodes, by CT or MRI scan. Sentinel node biopsy is sometimes used.

At presentation:
- 40% are localized
- 50% have regional spread
- <10% are metastatic disease

The optimal management of these tumors remains controversial. Patients with operable disease are best managed by surgery. Adjuvant radiotherapy and chemotherapy, e.g., platinum and etoposide, may be considered for patients with regional spread.

Treatment outcome depends on the stage at presentation:
- Localized node-negative disease has an >90% 5-year survival.
- Positive lymph nodes indicate a 50%–60% 5-year survival.
- Metastatic disease has 9-month median survival.

Further reading

Balch CM, Gershenwald JE, Soong SJ, et al. (2009). Final version of the American Joint Committee on Cancer staging system for cutaneous melanoma. *J Clin Oncol* 27:6199–6206.

Balch CM, Soong SJ, Gershenwald J, et al. (2001). Prognostic factors analysis of 17,600 melanoma patients: validation of the new AJCC melanoma staging system. *J Clin Oncol* 19:3622–3634.

Shivers SC, Wang X, Li W, et al. (1998). Molecular staging of malignant melanoma: correlation with outcome. *JAMA* 280:1410–1415.

Thompson JF, Scolyer RA, Kefford RF (2005). Cutaneous melanoma. *Lancet* 365:687–701.

Chapter 40

Soft tissue and bone sarcomas

Richard F. Riedel

General overview *688*
Soft tissue sarcomas *694*
   Gastrointestinal stromal tumor (GIST) *694*
   Rhabdomyosarcoma *696*
Kaposi sarcoma *700*
Other soft tissue sarcomas *704*
Bone sarcomas *706*
   Osteosarcoma *706*
   Ewing's sarcoma *708*
Other primary bone sarcomas *712*
Giant Cell Tumor of Bone *713*
Surveillance *714*
Suggested reading *715*

General overview

Sarcomas are a rare, heterogeneous group of tumors, largely of mesenchymal origin, that can occur anywhere in the body.

There are over 50 histological subtypes with variable degrees of aggressiveness and responsiveness to therapy. In general, they can be divided into
- Soft tissue sarcomas
- Bone sarcomas

Epidemiology
- U.S. incidence (2012)
  - 11,280 cases of soft tissue sarcoma (STS)
  - 2890 cases of bone sarcoma
- U.S. deaths (2012)
  - 3900 deaths from STS
  - 1410 deaths from bone sarcoma
- STS represents 1% of adult malignancies and 6% of childhood cancers.
- Primary bone cancers are <0.2% of all cancer.
- The most common site of metastasis is the lung.

Lymph node involvement is rare except for the following:
- Synovial sarcoma
- Clear cell sarcoma
- Angiosarcoma
- Rhabdomyosarcoma
- Epitheliod sarcoma

Etiology

There is no clear etiology. Sarcomas may be associated with trauma (with no causal relationship). Prior radiation therapy increases risk. Osteosarcoma is the most common radiation-induced sarcoma.

Genetic predisposition to developing sarcomas:
- Neurofibromatosis (*NF-1*)
- Retinoblastoma (*Rb-1*)
- Li-Fraumeni syndrome (*p53*)
- Gardner's syndrome (*APC*)

Chronic lymphedema after breast irradiation is associated with the development of angiosarcomas (Stewart-Treves). Rarely, chemical exposure (vinyl chloride, herbicides, dioxins) may be implicated.

Presenting symptoms and signs include the following:
- Development of a mass
- STS location
  - 50% extremities
  - 20%–25% gastrointestinal
  - 15%–20% retroperitoneal
  - 10% head and neck
- Painless or painful
- Increasing size
- May have erythema and tenderness

Pathology
- Spindle-cell neoplasms
- Named for normal tissue they mimic
- Mesenchymal in origin
  - Muscle (rhabdomyosarcoma, leiomyosarcoma)
  - Bone (osteosarcoma)
  - Cartilage (chondrosarcoma)
  - Fat (liposarcoma)
  - Fibrous tissue (fibrosarcoma)
  - Blood vessels (angiosarcoma)
  - Nerves (MPNST, malignant peripheral nerve sheath tumor)
- >50 histological subtypes of sarcoma
- Vascular invasion is common
- Characteristic chromosomal changes in some (see Table 40.1)

Diagnosis and staging studies
- Referral to a multidisciplinary team
- Carefully planned biopsy
  - Ideally by surgeon who will perform resection
  - Establish grade, histology, cytogenetics
- MRI or CT scan of primary tumor Chest imaging to rule out metastases
- Bone scan (for bone sarcomas)
- PET is investigational
- Consider CT of the abdomen and pelvis for myxoid/round cell liposarcoma, epitheliod sarcoma, angiosarcoma, and leiomyosarcoma (NCCN 2013 guidelines).

Table 40.1 Select cytogenetic abnormalities in soft tissue and bone sarcomas

Tumor	Translocation	Involved gene
Alveolar rhabdomyosarcoma	t(2;13)	PAX3-FKHR
Clear cell sarcoma	t(12;22)	EWS-ATF1
Dermatofibrosarcoma protuberans (DFSP)	t(17;22)	COL1A1-PDGFB
Ewing's sarcoma	t(11;22)	EWS-FLI1
Malignant fibrous histiocytoma (MFH)	Complex	
Myxoid/round cell Liposarcoma	t(12;16)	TLS (FUS)-CHOP
Synovial sarcoma	t(X;18)	SYT-SSX1 SYT-SSX2

Staging system

Soft tissue sarcoma. See Table 40.2.
- Tumor size and location
  - T1 <5 cm
  - T2 >5 cm
  - a: superficial
  - b: deep
- Absence (N0) or presence (M1) of lymph node metastases
- Absence (M0) or presence (M1) of metastases
- Grade (Low: G1, Intermediate: G2, High: G3)

Bone sarcoma

See Table 40.3
- Tumor size: T1 ≤8 cm; T2 >8 cm; T3: discontinuous tumors in primary site
- Lymph node status: N1 is stage IVB
- Distant metastasis: M1a: lung metastasis; M1b: other distant metastasis

Surgery

Surgical excision is the only curative therapy. Involvement of a surgical or orthopedic oncologist is key.

Potential tumor contamination of tissue planes and compartments can occur at the time of biopsy. Remove biopsy tract en bloc during definitive resection.

Limb-sparing surgery is possible in most patients. The amputation rate is <5%.

Types of surgery include the following:
- **Intralesional or intracapsular**: Excision passes through the tumor with involved margins. The risk of local recurrence approaches 100%.
- **Marginal**: Tumor is shelled out through the pseudocapsule. The recurrence rate is 20%–70%.
- **Wide excision**: A wide margin of local tissue is removed along with tumor. This is adequate for low-grade sarcoma but has a recurrence rate of up to 30% with high-grade disease.
- **Radical excision** is carried out by en bloc dissection of tumor and muscular compartment. There is a low risk of local recurrence, but the procedure may lead to an unacceptable loss of function.
- Patients who relapse with pulmonary-only metastasis may be cured by metastatectomy.

Radiotherapy

Adjuvant radiation therapy improves local control when combined with limb-sparing surgery, compared to surgery alone.

There is no difference in disease-free (DFS) or overall (OS) survival when limb-sparing surgery combined with radiation is compared with amputation.

Radiotherapy may be administered as neoadjuvant or adjuvant therapy.

Neoadjuvant therapy involves a smaller dose (~50 Gy) and field, but increased lower-extremity wound complications. Intraoperative radiation or boost can be given to positive margins.

Table 40.2 AJCC staging of soft tissue sarcomas (Adapted from 7th edition)

Stage	Primary tumor	Tumor grade	Lymph node	Metastasis
IA	T1a,1b	Low: G1	N0	M0
IB	T2a,2b	Low: G1	N0	M0
IIA	T1a,1b	Int/High: G2,3	N0	M0
IIB	T2a,2b	Int: G2	N0	M0
III	T2a,2b	High: G3	N0	M0
	Any	Any	N1	M0
IV	Any	Any	Any	M1

Table 40.3 AJCC staging of bone sarcomas (Adapted from 7th edition)

Stage	Primary tumor	Tumor grade	Lymph node	Metastasis
IA	T1	Low: G1,2	N0	M0
IB	T2	Low: G1,2	N0	M0
	T3	Low: G1,2	N0	M0
IIA	T1	High: G3,4	N0	M0
IIB	T2	High: G3,4	N0	M0
III	T3	High: G3,4	N0	M0
IVA	Any	Any	N0	M1a
IVB	Any	Any	N1	Any
	Any	Any	N0	M1b

Note: Extraskeletal osteosarcoma and extraskeletal myxoid chondrosarcoma are staged as soft tissue sarcomas. Adjuvant therapy involves a larger dose (~66–70 Gy) and field to include the tumor bed, scar, drain sites, and adequate margins. Complications include fibrosis, joint stiffness, and edema.

Radiotherapy may be used for palliative treatment of bone metastases.

Chemotherapy

Soft tissue sarcomas

Traditionally, chemotherapy is reserved for the advanced setting. Neoadjuvant or adjuvant strategies may be considered in the localized setting (large, high-grade tumors) but remains controversial.

Active chemotherapy agents include the following:
- Doxorubicin (A): Response rates 10%–30%
- Ifosfamide with mesna (I): Response rates 10%–30%
- Dacarbazine (D)
- Gemcitabine-docetaxel combination
- Trabectedin (not approved in the United States)

Of note, pazopanib, a multitargeted tyrosine kinase inhibitor, was approved in 2012 as the first targeted therapy for the treatment of non-GIST, nonadipocytic, metastatic soft tissue sarcoma.

Combination regimens (i.e., adriamycin, ifosfamide, mesna [AIM], mesna, adriamycin, ifosfamide, dacarbazine [MAID]) improve response rates but have increased toxicity and no statistically significant improvement in overall survival. The Sarcoma Meta-Analysis Collaboration (SMAC) reviewed adjuvant chemotherapy data from 14 trials with >1500 patients and found that it reduces the risk of disease recurrence (by 10% at 10 years). No significant survival benefit has been demonstrated. Additional trials since 1997 have failed to show a consistent improvement in overall survival, including a large multicenter randomized controlled trial which showed no improvement in relapse-free or overall survival (Lancet Oncol, 2012)

Bone sarcomas

Neoadjuvant and adjuvant chemotherapy plays an important role in the management of primary bone sarcomas.
- Ewing's
- Osteosarcoma

Active agents in Ewing's sarcoma include the following:
- Ifosfamide and/or cyclophosphamide
- Etoposide
- Doxorubicin
- Vincristine

Active agents in osteosarcoma:
- Doxorubicin
- Cisplatin
- Ifosfamide
- Methotrexate

There is no current role for chemotherapy in the treatment of conventional chondrosarcoma. There is some data to support the treatment of dedifferentiated chondrosarcomas and mesenchymal chondrosarcomas with osteosarcoma and Ewing's sarcoma regimens, respectively. Consider clinical-trial enrollment for these patients.

Soft tissue sarcomas

Classification

Although the histological classification is complex, staging and management are similar for most sarcoma subtypes. A representative sampling is shown in Box 40.1, with specific tumor types highlighted in the following pages.

Gastrointestinal stromal tumor (GIST)

GIST is the most common sarcoma of the GI tract. Incidence is estimated at 3000–5000 cases/year. GIST arises from the interstitial cells of Cajal (gut pacemaker cells). It is characterized by gain-of-function mutation in *KIT* (CD 117).

GIST occurs in the following locations:
- Gastric: 70%
- Small bowel: 20%
- Esophagus, colorectal and retroperitoneum: 10%

For assessment of risk in localized GIST see Table 40.4.

Advanced disease

Traditionally, GIST is unresponsive to conventional chemotherapy. Tyrosine kinase inhibition (TKI) is the treatment paradigm for advanced or inoperable disease.

Imatinib became U.S. FDA approved in 2002 for treatment of unresectable and/or metastatic GIST. Sunitinib was approved by the FDA in 2006 for imatinib-refractory GIST. Regorafenib was approved by the FDA in 2013 for imatinib- and sunitinib-refractory GIST.

Responsiveness to imatinib is dependent on mutational status:
- Exon 11: Response rates of 85% (70%)
- Exon 9 and others: Less responsive to standard dosing (400 mg/day). Exon 9 mutations may benefit from increased imatinib dosing

Recently, succinyl dehydrogenase (SDH) mutations have been identified in KIT-mutant negative GISTs.

Imatinib interruption is not recommended for patients with advanced disease. According to the French Sarcoma Group, compared with continuous dosing, interruption results in rapid progression in most patients with advanced GIST.

Common mild or moderate toxicities to TKI include the following:
- Imatinib: Edema (periorbital), anemia, nausea, lethargy, diarrhea, skin rash
- Sunitinib: Diarrhea, hand–foot syndrome, asthenia, altered taste, hypertension, hypothyroidism, decrease in left ventricular ejection fraction (LVEF)

RECIST criteria are less accurate in predicting survival for GIST compared with other solid tumors.

Localized disease

The mainstay of treatment for localized disease is surgery. The North American Intergroup phase III trial ACOSOG Z9001 (*Lancet*, 2009) reported improved 1-year recurrence-free survival for patients

Box 40.1 Pathological classification of soft tissue sarcomas

- Alveolar soft part sarcoma (ASPS)
- Angiosarcoma
- Clear cell sarcoma
- Dermatofibrosarcoma protuberans
- Desmoplastic small cell tumor
- Epitheliod sarcoma
- Extraosseous Ewing's tumor
- Extraskeletal chondrosarcoma
- Extraskeletal osteosarcoma
- Fibrosarcoma
- Gastrointestinal stromal tumor (GIST)
- Kaposi sarcoma
- Leiomyosarcoma
- Liposarcoma
- Malignant fibrous histiocytoma (MFH)
- Malignant giant cell tumor of tendon sheath
- Malignant hemangiopericytoma
- Malignant peripheral nerve sheath tumor (MPNST)
- Malignant solitary fibrous tumor
- Rhabdomyosarcoma (RMS)
- Synovial sarcoma

Table 40.4 Risk of metastases or disease-related death in GIST based on tumor size, number of mitoses, and location

Tumor Size	Number of Mitoses (per 50 hpf)	Gastric	Duodenum	Jejunum/Ileum	Rectum
≤2 cm	≤5	None seen	None seen	None seen	None seen
>2 to ≤5 cm	≤5	Very low	Low	Low	Low
>5 to ≤10 cm	≤5	Low	Moderate	N/A	N/A
>10 cm	≤5	Moderate	High	High	High
≤2 cm	>5	None	High	N/A	High
>2 to ≤5 cm	>5	Moderate	High	High	High
>5 to ≤10 cm	>5	High	High	N/A	N/A
>10 cm	>5	High	High	High	High

Adapted from Miettinen M and Lasota J. (2006) "Gastrointestinal Stromal Tumors: Pathology and Prognosis at different sites." *Semin Diagn Pathol* 23(2):70–83. With permission of Elsevier.

who received adjuvant imatinib therapy for 1 year after resection (tumor size >3 cm). Data on overall survival were immature.

More recently, data from SSGXVII were reported (*JAMA*, 2012) revealing improvements in both relapse-free and overall survival for 36 months of adjuvant imatinib compared to 12 months of therapy in a patient population with high risk of recurrence.

The optimal duration of adjuvant imatinib in unknown.

Rhabdomyosarcoma

Rhabdomyosarcoma (RMS) is the most common soft tissue tumor in childhood and adolescence, with 350 cases per year reported in the United States. More than 50% occur in children under 10 years of age; RMS is rare in adults over 40.

RMS arises from primitive mesenchymal cells with the capacity for rhabdomyoblastic development. The most common sites of origin are the following:
- Head and neck
- Genitourinary tract
- Retroperitoneum
- Extremities

Disease is locally invasive (e.g., spreads from the orbit to the meninges and central nervous system). It disseminates to the lymph nodes, lungs, bones, marrow, and brain.

Outlook depends on the disease site and histological subtype:
- Good prognosis: Botryoid, spindle cell
- Intermediate: Embryonal
- Poor prognosis: Alveolar and undifferentiated

Embryonal RMS

- Approximately 60% of cases
- Occurs mainly in children under 15
- Occurs in the head and neck (including orbit), genitourinary tract, and retroperitoneum
- Spectrum of cells involved, from primitive round cells to rhabdomyoblasts
- Lymph nodes are involved in 12%–14% of patients.

Botryoid RMS is a subtype characterized by polypoid growth, like a "bunch of grapes," usually found in hollow organs (e.g., vagina, bladder, and nasopharyngeal sinuses).

Alveolar rhabdomyosarcoma

Poorly differentiated round or oval cells form irregular spaces and are separated by fibrous septae, giving the appearance of "alveoli." Sometimes this appearance is absent, but the uniform appearance of the cells is distinct from that of the embryonal variety.

Diagnosis may be confirmed by the presence of a t(2;13)(q35;q14 PAX3-FKHR) or variant t(1;13) (p36;q14 PAX 7-FKHR) chromosomal translocation. PAX7 has a better prognosis than PAX3 in the metastatic setting. The alveolar type has significantly worse prognosis than that of the embryonal type.

Pleomorphic rhabdomyosarcoma

- Rare adult soft tissue tumor
- Behaves similarly to other adult soft tissue sarcomas
- May be curable if localized, with surgery and radiotherapy
- Poor prognosis for locally advanced or metastatic disease

Staging

See Table 40.5 and Table 40.6
Note: Bone marrow aspirate and biopsy should be included.

Determine group (postoperatively)

- Group I: Localized disease completely resected and N0
- Group IIA: Localized disease resected with microscopic residual disease and N0
- Group IIB: Locoregional disease with lymph node involvement (N1) completely excised without residual disease
- Group IIC: Locoregional disease with lymph node involvement and residual disease at primary site.
- Group III: Localized gross residual disease
- Group IV: Distant metastasis

Determine stage (STS-COG)

- **Favorable sites**: Orbit; nonparameningeal head and neck; genitourinary nonbladder/prostate; biliary tract
- **Unfavorable sites**: Any site is not considered favorable.

Management

Treatment is tailored according to the prognosis, balancing the need for effective local and systemic treatment against the late morbidity particularly of radiotherapy and chemotherapy.

Table 40.5 STS-COG Staging

Stage	Primary site	Tumor size	Regional lymph nodes	Distant metastasis
1	Favorable	Any	Any	M0
2	Unfavorable	T1a–2a	N0 or Nx	M0
3	Unfavorable	T1a–2a	N1	M0
	Unfavorable	T1b–2b	Any	M0
4	Any	Any	Any	M1

Table 40.6 Risk group classification (IRSG)

Risk group	Histology	Stage	Group
Low risk	Embryonal	1	I, II, III
	Embryonal	2, 3	I, II
Intermediate risk	Embryonal	2, 3	III
	Alveolar	1, 2, 3	I, II, III
Poor risk	Any	4	IV

Chemotherapy
- Often given before definitive local surgery.
- Vincristine (V) and actinomycin D (A) are for good-prognosis disease.
- Other drugs are added to VA for worse-prognosis disease (e.g., cyclophosphamide [C] or ifosfamide [I], doxorubicin [adr]).
- Irinotecan and high-dose chemotherapy may have a role in metastatic disease.

Local treatment

Local treatment is with surgery, ideally with complete removal of all local disease and lymph node sampling (15% have positive LN). N1 is stage III, in contrast to stage IV in other soft tissue sarcomas. Surgery may not be feasible because of tumor extent or may lead to unacceptable mutilation or loss of function.

RMS is highly sensitive to radiotherapy.
- Give concomitant with chemotherapy.
- Doses of 40–50 Gy will achieve local disease control.
- Adjuvant radiation is often advocated if margins are <2 cm or the primary tumor is >5 cm.
- In upper extremity RMS, neoadjuvant radiation therapy is preferred to decrease fibrosis and edema.

Radiotherapy may safely be omitted from treatment for infants and children with localized, favorable-prognosis disease, e.g., embryonal RMS of the orbit. Extremity tumors, alveolar histology, and parameningeal tumors require radiotherapy.

Metastatectomy is usually not useful in stage IV RMS.

Intergroup Rhabdomyosarcoma Study Group

Intergroup Rhabdomyosarcoma Study I
- No advantage for adjuvant radiotherapy in Group I patients
- No advantage for addition of low-dose cyclophosphamide in Group II patients
- No advantage for addition of adriamycin in Group III and IV patients

Intergroup Rhabdomyosarcoma Study II
- Removal of cyclophosphamide from Group I or Group II patients did not have an effect on overall or disease-free survival.
- Addition of adriamycin to VAC did not affect the outcome of Group III or Group IV patients.
- Pulsed monthly chemotherapy with VAC improved outcomes in Group III/IV patients (Intergroup Rhabdomyosarcoma Study [IRS]-II vs. IRS-I)

Intergroup Rhabdomyosarcoma Study III
- Group I (favorable histology): VA treatment for 1 year was as effective as a more intensive VAC regimen.
- Group II (favorable histology): Addition of adriamycin to VA + radiation therapy did not alter outcome.
- Intensification of therapy provided most benefit for Group III patients

Intergroup Rhabdomyosarcoma Study IV
- Assessment of response to induction therapy had no influence on failure-free survival

Kaposi sarcoma

- Most common malignancy seen in patients with AIDS
- Incurable multifocal soft tissue sarcoma of vascular origin
- Highly variable clinical course
- Cutaneous involvement is characteristic.
- Disease progression may be slow but it can behave aggressively.
- May affect visceral sites causing significant morbidity and mortality

Epidemiology and etiology
Four clinical settings are recognized.

Classical form
- This form affects predominantly the extremities of elderly men of Mediterranean, Middle Eastern, or Eastern European origin.
- It often follows an indolent course.

Endemic African variant
- Predates HIV
- Male predominance
- May be indolent or aggressive.

Iatrogenic
- This is seen in patients receiving immunosuppressive therapy, e.g., in organ transplant recipients, typically 1–2 years after transplant.
- Male predominance
- Tumor may regress when this treatment is reduced.

Epidemic AIDS-related form
- Most common form in developing world
- Associated with HHV-8 infection

Presentation

Cutaneous
- Multiple nonpainful, red-purple lesions
- Flat l plaques l nodules with edema
- Typically affect upper body, face, and legs.
- Kaposi sarcoma in the oral cavity is present in one third of patients and seen in 80% of autopsies without skin involvement.

Systemic
- Pulmonary: Cough, breathlessness, occasionally hemoptysis
- GI (~40% at diagnosis): Weight loss, pain, obstruction, bleeding

Pathology
All forms demonstrate similar features:
- Angiogenesis
- Microhemorrhages
- Hemosiderin deposition
- Proliferation of spindle cells
- Inflammatory infiltrate

A diagnostic feature is the intradermal proliferation of abnormal vascular structures lined with large, spindle-shaped endothelial cells.

Staging

The Aids Clinical Trials Group (ACTG) has developed a staging classification designed to assist with prognosis (see Table 40.7). Poor tumor and systemic risk factors have been shown to correlate with prognosis in the highly active antiretroviral therapy (HAART) era.

Table 40.7 ACTG guidelines

	Good prognosis—all of	Poor prognosis—any of
Tumor	Skin only ± lymph nodes and/or minimal oral disease	Edema/ulceration, extensive oral disease, visceral KS
Immunological	CD4 >200	CD4 <200
Symptoms	Nil, Karnofsky >70	Opportunistic infection or thrush, B symptoms, Karnofsky <70, other HIV-related illness

Management

Treatment is palliative
- Poor risk: Start chemotherapy with HAART
- Good risk: Treat initially with HAART alone.
- Note: Approximately 7% of patients can develop immune reconstitution syndrome with worsening of the lesions after starting HAART.

Local therapy
- Cryotherapy and laser, especially if lesions are <1 cm
- 9-cis retinoic acid (alitretinoin). Local response after 4–8 weeks. Patient-administered therapy with low toxicity (local irritation)
- Intralesional chemotherapy, e.g., with vinblastine. Injection into the KS lesion can produce short-term regression in approximately 75% of cases. Mean duration of palliation is typically 3–4 months.
- Radiotherapy. A response rate equal to intralesional chemotherapy can be achieved with single-fraction doses of 8 Gy. This can be repeated if there is recurrence or insufficient regression. Palatal lesions can also be irradiated using iridium wire moulds.
- Photodynamic therapy is under investigation.

Systemic therapy

This is usually indicated if there are >20 lesions, symptomatic edema, oral lesions, and flare due to immune reconstitution.

Chemotherapy

Liposomal anthracyclines (e.g., pegylated liposomal doxorubicin) are the first-line choice. Response rates of 30%–60% have been observed and may be greater if given in combination with HAART. Treatment is usually well tolerated, and cardiotoxicity with the new liposomal preparations is less than that with conventional anthracyclines.

Paclitaxel can be used for second-line treatment in selected patients. Decreasing the dexamethasone premedication to 10 mg 12 and 6 hours prior to paclitaxel may be considered, because there is theoretical concern of HHV-8 reactivation with steroids.

Paclitaxel can also interact with HAART, because it is metabolized through P450.

Biological therapies

Interferon-α is most effective if disease is nonvisceral and the CD4 count is >200 µ/L. Response rates of 20%–40% have been observed. Potential toxicity includes flu-like symptoms, marrow suppression, and depression. IFN requires approximately 4 months for response, thus is not appropriate for visceral disease.

Antiangiogenic agents are being used in small clinical trials only. For thalidomide treatment response rates up to 40% have been reported.

Imatinib, mTOR inhibitors, and matrix metalloproteinase inhibitors are under study.

Other soft tissue sarcomas

Angiosarcoma
- Usually in scalp, face, or irradiated fields
- Lymphedema may predispose (Stewart-Treves)
- Treatment is with surgery and radiation.
- Paclitaxel and liposomal doxorubicin are effective.

Dermatofibrosarcoma protuberans
- Characterized by t(17;22) COL1A1-PDGFB
- Most commonly in the trunk, then limbs, then head and neck
- Spindle cells CD34$^+$
- The fibrosarcomatous variant is more aggressive.

Treatment is with wide surgical excision. Radiation therapy may have a role in unresectable or close margins.

There have been good responses to imatinib as neoadjuvant therapy and in the surgically relapsed or refractory setting. Sunitinib may have a role in the imatinib-refractory setting.

Desmoid
Also known as aggressive fibromatosis, desmoid tumors are characterized by mesenchymal cell proliferation that infiltrates but lacks metastatic potential. It is associated with Gardner's syndrome (intestinal polyposis, osteomas, fibromas, sebaceous and epidermal cysts) or familial adenomatous polyposis (FAP) syndrome. Gardner's is now considered a subtype of FAP.

Desmoid tumors usually occur in the extremities or superficial trunk, but they can appear in the head and neck or visceral areas. Size >5 cm is more common in visceral areas.

Traditionally, surgery was considered the mainstay of treatment. More recently, nonsurgical options, including medical therapy, radiation therapy and even observation (for select cases), may be considered if significant morbidity or functional consequences exist for surgery. Resectability depends on morbidity.

Margin positivity as a marker for local recurrence is still debated, and acceptable if having negative margins would result in unacceptable morbidity. Local recurrence is ~20%–30%.

Tamoxifen and sulindac have response rates of between 15% and 20%. Spontaneous regressions have been seen.

Due to PDGFR mutation, imatinib has been tried in inoperable disease with some success.

Chemotherapy with adriamycin, dacarbazine, and ifosfamide has also been associated with good responses. Low-dose weekly methotrexate and vinblastine have been studied as well.

Liposarcomas

These account for 20% of soft tissue sarcomas in the United States. There are four subtypes: well differentiated, dedifferentiated, myxoid/round cell (30%–35%), and pleomorphic. Myxoid/round cell is characterized by t(12;16) or t(12;22).

Aggressiveness depends on the component of round cells within the tumor. The myxoid variant is unique, because it spreads to serosal membranes and metastasizes to distant soft tissues and bones in the absence of lung metastasis.

Despite surgery and radiation there is a 40% relapse rate.

Chemotherapy is reserved for relapses and advanced cases. Anthracyclines, ifosfamide and taxanes have reported responses. Recently, Trabectedin (ET 743) has shown response rates from 17% to 50% in previously treated patients.

Leiomyosarcomas

Leiomyosarcomas (LMS) is a highly aneuploid karyotype. Uterine leiomyosarcomas are more sensitive to gemcitabine than other histologies (and other sites of LMS as well).

Gemcitabine and docetaxel have shown response rates as high as 50%, particularly in uterine leiomyosarcomas. Pulmonary toxicity, refractory pulmonary edema, and myelosuppression are the main toxicities.

Synovial sarcomas

These are monophasic (pure spindle cells) and biphasic (spindle and epitheliod cells). The majority (90%) have t(X;18)-SS18-SSX1.

These sarcomas are sensitive to ifosfamide-containing regimens.

Bone sarcomas

Osteosarcoma

Epidemiology and etiology

Osteosarcoma (OS) has bimodal distribution, with 75% of patients being <20 years of age, and a second peak >65 years.

OS occurs predominantly in adolescence. A peak incidence coincides with the growth spurt, usually where the greatest increase of bone length and bone growth occurs (metaphysis).

Cases occurring over the age of 40 years are usually associated with a recognized predisposing lesion:
- Paget's disease
- Irradiated bone (4–40 years after exposure)
- Multiple hereditary exostoses
- Polyostotic fibrous dysplasia

The male-to-female ratio is 1.6:1. Sixty percent of cases arise around the knee (distal femur more than proximal tibia).

Pathology

There are 11 variants, composed of malignant spindle cells and osteoblasts that produce osteoid or immature bone.

The "classic" subtype is a central medullary tumor. Rarer types with a better prognosis include parosteal, periosteal, and low-grade intra-osseous osteosarcoma. Small cell, telangiectatic, multifocal, and MFH subtypes are potentially worse

Local invasion is into the medulla and through the bony cortex, with 20% of patients having occult or overt metastatic disease at presentation.

Genetics

Occasionally OS is associated with Li-Fraumeni syndrome (germline mutation of $p53$), Rothmund-Thompson syndrome, or hereditary retinoblastoma. A history of Paget's disease is associated with loss of heterozygosity (LOH) 18.

Radiographic appearance

Plain X-rays of the affected area are often sufficient to suggest the diagnosis of osteosarcoma.

The classic radiological features of osteosarcoma include the following:
- Poorly delineated or absent margins around the bone lesion
- Periosteal reaction, usually noncontinuous and thin, with multiple laminations
- New bone formation with calcification of the matrix
- Bone destruction

There are no specific tumor markers, but serum alkaline phosphatase is elevated in 50% of cases (it may correlate with tumor burden).

Note. Histological confirmation of the radiological diagnosis of a primary bone tumor must be deferred until the patient is assessed by a surgeon with expertise in the management of bone malignancies.

Management
- Multimodality therapy is key.
- OS is chemoresponsive.
- Amputation has mostly been replaced by limb-sparing surgery.

Chemotherapy
The most active agents are the following:
- Doxorubicin
- Cisplatin (carboplatin is inferior)
- High-dose methotrexate
- Ifosfamide
- Etoposide

Chemotherapy is commonly given pre- and postoperatively. This has several potential benefits:
- Treatment starts without delay (production of a customized endoprosthesis takes several weeks).
- Tumor volume may be reduced, making surgery easier.
- It allows the pathological assessment of response to chemotherapy in the resected tumor. Over 90% necrosis is a favorable prognostic factor (75% 5-year OS vs. 55% if <90% necrosis).

Typically, 2–3 cycles of chemotherapy are delivered, followed by surgery, followed by a further 3–4 cycles of chemotherapy. Dose intensity has not been found to correlate to prognosis in the COSS study group.

Alternating chemotherapy based on response to neoadjuvant treatment has *not* proven to improve outcome.

Radiotherapy
Osteosarcomas are relatively radioresistant. Radiotherapy is rarely used in the primary treatment of this disease. Its use is limited to high-dose palliative treatment for patients who refuse surgery or for axial osteosarcomas that are not resectable;

Metastatic osteosarcoma

At presentation, 15% of OS cases are metastatic. With combination chemotherapy, followed by resection of the primary and, when feasible, of metastatic disease, long-term survival can be achieved in 20%–30% of patients. Most patients who relapse have pulmonary metastases.

Up to 40% 5-year survival can be achieved by surgical resection of the metastases. Metastasectomy may be considered for multiple and bilateral lung deposits and on more than one occasion.

Local recurrences are managed by surgical resection (usually amputation) or palliative irradiation.

Treatment outcomes and prognostic factors
- Operable localized disease: 60%–70% 5-year survival
- Metastatic disease: 10%–30% 5-year survival
- There is better prognosis with limb than with axial primary disease.
- Good response of >95% cell kill in resected specimen conveys 80% 5-year survival and is seen in ~60% patients with current regimens.
- Poor response to chemotherapy conveys 40%–50% 5-year survival.

Recent developments
- Maintenance interferon (IFN) after MAP (high-dose methotrexate, doxorubicin, cisplatin) chemotherapy is under investigation
- Chemotherapy intensification with addition of ifosfamide and etoposide in poorly responding tumors after surgery in the EURAMOS1 trial. Adjuvant IFN is currently under study in the ongoing EURAMOS 1 trial.
- New targeted agents such as mTOR inhibitors and antiangiogenic drugs are becoming areas of intense research.

Ewing's sarcoma

When compared with osteosarcoma there are three main differences:
- Ewing's sarcoma (ES) is radiosensitive, whereas OS is not.
- ES occurs in younger populations, hence there is concern for long-term development of radiation-induced secondary malignancies.
- ES occurs in diaphysis in contrast to metaphysis (OS).

Epidemiology and etiology
- Annual incidence is 0.1 per 100,000.
- Comprises 6%–10% of all primary bone tumors
- Less common in non-Caucasians
- Peak age is 10–20 years.
- Etiology is unknown.
- ES is not associated with cancer family syndromes.
- It may affect any bone; 55% of cases arise in the axial skeleton.
- It may also arise in soft tissue.

Pathology
The Ewing's sarcoma family of tumors includes the following:
- Ewing's tumor of bone
- Peripheral primitive neuroectodermal tumor (PNET)
- Askin tumor (arising on chest wall)

ES is believed to arise from neural crest cells.
Microscopy shows small, round, blue cells with rosette formation and positive staining for
- *MIC2* gene (CD99)
- Neural markers (NSE, S100)
- Glycogen (PAS)

Typically, they arise in the diaphysis of long bones or in flat bones, e.g., pelvis, invade through the medulla, but also extend through the cortex to form a significant soft-tissue extraosseous mass in at least 50%.

Blood-borne spread to the lung and bone is common, and 20%–25% of patients have overt metastases at presentation. Microscopic systemic disease is present in the majority of patients with radiologically localized disease.

Genetics
- >95% have reciprocal rearrangement, usually t(11;22).
- Multiple gene fusions have been described, and studies are underway to correlate molecular heterogeneity with prognosis.
- Del 1p and mutations of *p53* have been associated with poor outcome.

Radiographic appearance
- Plain X-ray typically shows a destructive, osteolytic lesion, with periosteal elevation ("onion skinning"), although 25% have a sclerotic component.
- MRI scan demonstrates both osseous and extraosseous disease extent.

Staging (see general overview)
- Bone marrow aspirate and biopsy from sites distant from known disease should be included.

Management
- Initial chemotherapy, e.g., alternating induction chemotherapy (1 course of vincristine, doxorubicin, cyclophosphamide [VAC] followed by 1 cycle with ifosfamide and etoposide [IE]), repeat to complete 4 total cycles (~10–12 weeks of therapy)
- Local therapy to the primary tumor at week 12, e.g., surgery, radiotherapy, or both (chemotherapy continues concomitant with radiotherapy)
- Further chemotherapy (VAC alternating with IE) to complete ~12 months of total therapy
- Recent results from AEWS0031 have suggested that interval-compressed chemotherapy (chemotherapy with growth factor support every 2 weeks) is more effective than standard 3-week chemotherapy, with a similar toxicity profile. Extrapolation to an adult population is limited due to number of adult patients enrolled.

Local therapy of the primary tumor
- Local control with surgery, radiation, or both
- Choice depends on functionality postsurgery vs. risk of secondary malignancy (radiation-induced)
- If tumor is potentially resectable, surgery should be strongly considered.
- Radiation therapy postsurgery for marginal excision

Management of metastatic disease

Patients presenting with metastatic disease are managed initially with induction chemotherapy followed by local therapy to the primary tumor.

Patients with lung metastases may then be treated with conventional chemotherapy and whole-lung irradiation (18 Gy in 10 fractions) or high-dose chemotherapy, e.g., busulphan and melphalan with peripheral blood stem cell support.

Patients with bone or marrow metastases have a poorer prognosis, and high-dose chemotherapy with autologous stem cell transplant may be considered.

Treatment outcomes and prognostic factors
5-year survival:
- Localized disease: 55%–65%
- Metastatic disease: 10%–20%
- Lung-only metastases: 30%

The major prognostic factors are the following:
- Metastases at presentation
- Site and volume of the primary
  - Tumor <100 mL in a long bone: 80% 5-year survival
  - Tumor diameter >8–10 cm
- Pelvic tumor: 30% 5-year survival
- Pathological response to chemotherapy
- Local therapy (suggested in retrospective studies that surgery is better)
- Short telomeres predict worse outcome.

Other primary bone sarcomas

Primary malignant spindle cell sarcoma of bone
- Most often malignant fibrous histiocytoma
- All are rare, <1% of all bone tumors.
- Arise in any bone (usually the metaphysis of a long bone)
- Occur mainly in middle age
- Can occur after a previous insult to the bone, e.g., ionizing radiation, bone infarct, or fibrous dysplasia
- Usually treated similar to osteosarcoma

Chondrosarcoma
- Cartilage-forming malignancy
- Tumors of middle to late age
- Second most common primary bone tumor (~30%)
- Intramedullary (conventional, clear cell, dedifferentiated, mesenchymal) or juxtacortical
- Typically presents with painful, enlarging mass in the pelvis, proximal femur, humerus, or ribs; unusual in distal bones
- Treatment is surgical resection with limb conservation, if possible.
- Traditionally both chemotherapy and radiation resistant
- No proven role for adjuvant chemotherapy
- Dedifferentiated high-grade lesions are treated as osteosarcomas.
- Mesenchymal condrosarcomas are treated as Ewing's sarcoma.
- Consider clinical-trial enrollment

Chordoma
- Slow-growing tumor that arises from notochord remnants
- Accounts for 2%–4% primary bone tumors
- Sited in the sacrum/coccyx (50%), skull base/clivus (35%), or upper cervical vertebrae.
- Presents in middle age with persistent pain
- Often only discovered on CT or MRI after "normal" plain X-rays of the bone
- Metastases are rare (lung or bone)
- Survival is determined by the success or failure of local control.
- Surgery is the treatment of choice but may not be feasible or may cause significant morbidity because of the tumor site.
- Radiotherapy (55–60 Gy) after incomplete resection or as palliation
- Particle therapy with protons has shown some promise.
- 30%–50% 5-year survival, but late recurrences are possible
- Phase II data suggest a role for imatinib in advanced PDGFR-positive disease.

Giant Cell Tumor of Bone

- Primary osteolytic bone tumor composed of osteoclast-like giant cells
- Low metastatic potential although metastases can occur
- Occurs in skeletally mature individuals
- Surgery is definitive therapy
- Tumor cells express RANK and adjacent stromal cells express RANKL
- Denosumab is a fully human monoclonal antibody that inhibits RANKL
- Denosumab induced tumor reduction and bone formation in patients with giant-cell tumor of bone
- Denosumab was U.S. FDA approved for treatment of giant cell tumor (GCT) of bone in 2013.

Surveillance

Follow-up varies according to the type and stage of tumor. General principles for follow-up after curative approach include the following:
- Chest imaging every 3–4 months x 2–3 years, then every 6 months to complete 5 years, then annually thereafter
- The primary site should also be imaged, depending on location (www.nccn.com).

Patients who are long-term survivors from sarcomas are at high risk of developing secondary malignancies.

Guidelines have been published by the Children's Oncology Group for long-term survivors and are available at: www.survivorshipguidelines.org.

Suggested reading

Benjamin RS, Choi H, Macapinlac HA, et al. (2007). We should desist using RECIST, at least in GIST. *J Clin Oncol* 25:1760–1764.

Blay JY, Le Cesne A, Ray-Coquard I, et al. (2007). Prospective multicentric randomized phase III study of imatinib in patients with advanced gastrointestinal stromal tumors comparing interruption versus continuation of treatment beyond 1 year: the French Sarcoma Group. *J Clin Oncol* 25:1107–1113.

Branstetter DG, Nelson SD, Manivel JC, et al. (2012). Denosumab induces tumor reduction and bone formation in patients with giant-cell tumor of bone. *Clin Cancer Res* 18:4415–4424.

Chugh R, Tawbi H, Lucas DR, et al. (2007). Chordoma: the nonsarcoma primary bone tumor. *Oncologist* 12:1344–1350.

Delattre O, Zucman J, Merlot T, et al. (1994). The Ewing family of tumors—a subgroup of small-round-cell tumors defined by specific chimeric transcripts. *N Engl J Med* 331:294–299.

Dematteo RP, Ballman KV, Antonescu CR, et al. (2009). American College of Surgeons Oncology Group (ACOSOG) Intergroup Adjuvant GIST Study Team. Adjuvant imatinib mesylate after resection of localised, primary gastrointestinal stromal tumour: a randomised, double-blind, placebo-controlled trial. *Lancet* 373:1097–1104.

Demetri GD, Benjamin RS, Blanke CD, et al. (2007). NCCN Task Force. NCCN Task Force report: management of patients with gastrointestinal stromal tumor (GIST)—update of the NCCN clinical practice guidelines. *J Natl Compr Cancer Netw* 5(Suppl 2):S1–S29.

Demetri GD, Reichardt P, Kang YK, et al. (2013). Efficacy and safety of regorafenib for advanced gastrointestinal stromal tumours after failure of imatinib and sunitinib (GRID): an international, multicentre, randomised, placebo-controlled, phase 3 trial. GRID study investigators. *Lancet* 381:295–302.

Demetri GD, von Mehren M, Blanke CD, et al. (2002). Efficacy and safety of imatinib mesylate in advanced gastrointestinal stromal tumors. *N Engl J Med* 347:472–480.

Demetri GD, van Oosterom AT, Garrett CR, et al. (2006). Efficacy and safety of sunitinib in patients with advanced gastrointestinal stromal tumour after failure of imatinib: a randomised controlled trial. *Lancet* 368:1329–1338.

Di Lorenzo G, Konstantinopoulos PA, Pantanowitz L, et al. (2007). Management of AIDS-related Kaposi's sarcoma. *Lancet Oncol* 8:167–176.

Eilber FC, Brennan MF, Eilber FR, et al. (2007). Chemotherapy is associated with improved survival in adult patients with primary extremity synovial sarcoma. *Ann Surg* 246:105–113.

Fata F, O'Reilly E, Ilson D, et al. (1999). Paclitaxel in the treatment of patients with angiosarcoma of the scalp or face. *Cancer* 86:2034–2037.

Fayette J, Coquard IR, Alberti L, et al. (2005). ET-743: a novel agent with activity in soft tissue sarcomas. *Oncologist* 10:827–832.

Garcia-Carbonero R, Supko JG, Maki RG, et al. (2005). Ecteinascidin-743 (ET-743) for chemotherapy-naive patients with advanced soft tissue sarcomas: multicenter phase II and pharmacokinetic study. *J Clin Oncol* 23:5484–5492.

Grier HE, Krailo MD, Tarbell NJ, et al. (2003). Addition of ifosfamide and etoposide to standard chemotherapy for Ewing's sarcoma and primitive neuroectodermal tumor of bone. *N Engl J Med* 348:694–701.

Heinrich MC, Corless CL, Demetri GD, et al. (2003). Kinase mutations and imatinib response in patients with metastatic gastrointestinal stromal tumor. *J Clin Oncol* 21:4342–4349.

Janeway KA, Kim SY, Lodish M, et al. (2011). Defects in succinate dehydrogenase in gastrointestinal stromal tumors lacking KIT and PDGFRA mutations. *Proc Natl Acad Sci U S A* 108:314–318.

Lev D, Kotilingam D, Wei C, et al. (2007). Optimizing treatment of desmoid tumors. *J Clin Oncol* 25:1785–1791.

Maki RG (2007). Gemcitabine and docetaxel in metastatic sarcoma: past, present, and future. *Oncologist* 12:999–1006.

Maki RG, Wathen JK, Patel SR, et al. (2007). Randomized phase II study of gemcitabine and docetaxel compared with gemcitabine alone in patients with metastatic soft tissue sarcomas: results of sarcoma alliance for research through collaboration study 002. *J Clin Oncol* 25:2755–2763.

Miettinen M, Lasota J (2006). Gastrointestinal stromal tumors: pathology and prognosis at different sites. *Semin Diagn Pathol* 23:70–83.

O'Sullivan B, Davis AM, Turcotte R, et al. (2002). Preoperative versus postoperative radiotherapy in soft-tissue sarcoma of the limbs: a randomised trial. *Lancet* 359:2235–2241.

Raney RB, Maurer HM, Anderson JR, et al. (2001). The Intergroup Rhabdomyosarcoma Study Group (IRSG): major lessons from the IRS-1 through IRS-IV studies as background for the current IRS-V treatment protocols. *Sarcoma* 5:9–15.

Sarcoma Meta-analysis Collaboration (1997). Adjuvant chemotherapy for localised resectable soft-tissue sarcoma of adults: meta-analysis of individual data. *Lancet* 350:1647–1654.

Siegel R, Naishadham D, Jemal A (2013). Cancer statistics, 2013. *CA Cancer J Clin* 63:11–30.

Stacchiotti S, Longhi A, Ferraresi V, et al. (2012). Phase II study of imatinib in advanced chordoma. *J Clin Oncol* 30:914–920.

Thomas D, Henshaw R, Skubitz K, et al. (2012). Denosumab in patients with giant-cell tumour of bone: an open-label, phase 2 study. *Lancet Oncol* 11:275–280.

van der Graaf WT, Blay JY, Chawla SP, et al. (2012). Pazopanib for metastatic soft-tissue sarcoma (PALETTE): a randomised, double-blind, placebo-controlled phase 3 trial. *Lancet* 379:1879–1886.

Woll PJ, Reichardt P, Le Cesne A, et al. (2012). EORTC Soft Tissue and Bone Sarcoma Group and the NCIC Clinical Trials Group Sarcoma Disease Site Committee. Adjuvant chemotherapy with doxorubicin, ifosfamide, and lenograstim for resected soft-tissue sarcoma (EORTC 62931): a multicentre randomised controlled trial. *Lancet Oncol* 13:1045–1054.

Womer RB, West DC, Krailo MD, et al. (2012). Randomized controlled trial of interval-compressed chemotherapy for the treatment of localized Ewing sarcoma: a report from the Children's Oncology Group. *J Clin Oncol* 30:4148–4154.

NCCN Guidelines

Soft tissue sarcoma

- http://www.nccn.org/professionals/physician_gls/PDF/sarcoma.pdf

Bone cancer

- http://www.nccn.org/professionals/physician_gls/PDF/bone.pdf

Chapter 41

Acute leukemia

Acute myeloid leukemia *718*
Acute lymphoblastic leukemia *724*

Acute myeloid leukemia

Jacob Laubach
Joseph Moore

Epidemiology

Incidence

The incidence of acute myeloid leukemia (AML) is 1.5–4 cases per 100,000. AML affects individuals of all ages, but the incidence of the disease is highest in the elderly.

The median age at diagnosis is 67 years. AML causes 80% of acute leukemia cases in adults.

Etiology

In most individuals with AML, the cause is unknown.

Environmental factors have been associated with the development of AML, including the following:
- Ionizing radiation
- Benzene
- Chemotherapeutic drugs
- Tobacco

Various acquired disorders involving myeloid and nonmyeloid cells can evolve into AML:
- Myeloproliferative disorders
  - Chronic myelogenous leukemia
  - Primary myelofibrosis
  - Essential thrombocytosis
  - Polycythemia vera
- Paroxysmal nocturnal hemglobinuria
- Aplastic anemia

A number of inherited conditions are associated with AML. These include the following:
- Bloom syndrome
- Diamond-Blackfan syndrome
- Down syndrome
- Fanconi anemia
- Neurofibromatosis
- Noonan syndrome.

Pathology

AML is characterized by clonal proliferation of myeloid precursor cells with reduced capacity to differentiate into mature myeloid cells.

Because a clonal population of cells can develop at any point in myeloid differentiation, AML is a heterogeneous disease, described by the French American British (FAB) classification system as follows:
- Myeloblastic ($M_{0,1,2}$)
- Promyelocytic (M_3)
- Myelomonocytic (M_4)
- Monoblastic (M_5)
- Erythroblastic (M_6)
- Megakaryoblastic (M_7)

In all subgroups, immature leukemic cells infiltrate the bone marrow and impair production of normal, mature blood cells.

Clinical presentation

Symptoms and signs are related to dysregulated hematopoiesis that occurs as a result of the underlying leukemia, which can develop acutely or insidiously.

Symptoms
- Fatigue
- Generalized weakness
- Dizziness
- Dyspnea
- Bone pain
- Easy bruising and bleeding events such as epistaxis or conjunctival hemorrhage occur in some patients.

Physical findings
- Conjunctival hemorrhage.
- Manifestations of extramedullary disease such as skin lesions, gingival infiltration, and lymphadenopathy
- Central nervous system involvement is rare, but can occur.
- Altered mental status may develop in the setting of hyperleukocytosis.

Diagnosis and classification

In many instances, diagnosis of AML is made by the primary care provider.

Anemia with a low or normal reticulocyte count, thrombocytopenia, and leukopenia are commonly found on examination of peripheral blood. Less frequently, leukocytosis is present at diagnosis.

Although myeloblasts are present in the peripheral blood, their identification requires careful evaluation in patients with leukopenia. By contrast, myeloblasts are readily identified in the bone marrow, where they represent between 20% and 95% of marrow cells in AML.

The diagnosis of AML relies on specimens from bone marrow and peripheral blood:
- Cell morphology
- Cytochemistry
- Cytogenetic findings
- Immunophenotype

Submicroscopic genetic aberrations in specific genes such as *FLT3* and *NPM1*, which are not detected by traditional cytogenetics, have assumed an important role in the diagnosis of AML.

Various systems have been developed to classify AML.
- The FAB system categorizes AML based on the distinctive subgroups described under Pathology (see p. 703).
- The WHO classification of AML is based on molecular characteristics of the disease defined at the time of diagnosis and a patient's clinical history (see Box 41.1).

Box 41.1 WHO classification of acute myeloid leukemia
- Acute myeloid leukemia with recurrent genetic abnormalities, including t(8;21), inv(16), and t(15;17)
- Acute myeloid leukemia with multilineage dysplasia
- Acute myeloid leukemia and myelodysplastic syndromes, therapy related
- Acute myeloid leukemia not otherwise categorized

Prognosis

The prognosis of an individual patient with AML can be estimated on the basis of various disease characteristics.

Cytogenetic abnormalities, classified as good, standard, or poor risk, are an important prognostic determinant.

Good-risk cytogenetic findings include t(15;17), t(8;21), and inv(16)/t(16;16), all of which involve chromosomal regions coding for core-binding factor.

Poor-risk cytogenetic findings include monosomy chromosome 5 or 7, del(5q), and complex karyotype.

A normal karyotype and other karyotypes not classified as either good or poor risk are categorized as standard risk.

Specific gene mutations also carry prognostic significance. Mutation of the *FLT3* gene, for example, is associated with decreased survival whereas *NPM1* gene mutation is associated with improved survival.

Poor prognostic factors include the following:
- Age
- Obesity
- Performance status
- Bone marrow blast count ≥75%
- Serum lactate dehydrogenase (LDH) >2.9 times the upper limit of normal
- Elevated white blood cell count (>100,000/mm^3)
- Systemic infection at diagnosis
- Treatment-induced AML or history of myelodysplastic syndrome
- Expression of multidrug resistance gene product P-glycoprotein
- Incomplete response to induction chemotherapy

Treatment

Supportive care

Supportive care is a vital component of therapy for AML. Before initiating therapy, the patient typically undergoes placement of a tunneled venous catheter, which provides access to the circulation for chemotherapy delivery, intravenous fluids, antibiotics and frequent laboratory studies.

An echocardiogram is obtained to assess cardiac function prior to chemotherapy, as anthracycline agents used in treatment of AML can be cardiotoxic.

If the white blood cell count is >100,000/mm^3, cytoreduction with hydroxyurea to minimize complications of hyperleukocytosis may be achieved.

Allopurinol should be administered to treat or prevent hyperuricemia if the uric acid level is elevated or there are a high percentage of blasts in the bone marrow or peripheral blood.

Finally, effective antiemetic therapy has been an important advance in the care patients with AML.

Induction chemotherapy

The goal of AML treatment is to eradicate the malignant cell population, allowing normal stem cells to repopulate the bone marrow.

The standard induction regimen used to achieve remission in AML—the so-called 7 and 3 regimen—includes cytarabine for 7 days and daunorubicin for 3 days. The anthracycline idarubicin or anthraquinone mitoxantrone can be substituted for daunorubicin.

A complete remission with <2% marrow blasts, neutrophil count >1000/mm^3, and platelet count >100,000/mm^3 is the goal of induction therapy. If a patient harbors residual leukemia after induction therapy, a second course of chemotherapy similar to the first is given.

Consolidation chemotherapy

If complete remission is achieved, postremission, or consolidation, chemotherapy is administered.

Postremission therapy consists of either stem cell transplantation for appropriately selected patients (see Stem cell transplantation in AML, p. 706) or high-dose cytarabine.

Patients with t(8;21) are particularly responsive to high-dose cytarabine. Patients who receive high-dose cytarabine receive corticosteroid eye drops to prevent conjunctivitis and are monitored for cerebellar toxicity.

No consistent role for maintenance chemotherapy in AML has been defined.

A general scheme for treatment of AML
Induction Rx Consolidation Rx ? Role of Maintenance Rx
Diagnosis → Remission → Long-term remission/Cure

Stem cell transplantation in acute myeloid leukemia

Stem cell transplantation represents an important treatment modality in the management of patients with AML. It can be used during first remission in patients considered at high risk for relapse, based on prognostic features.

Stem cell transplantation is also an option for patients in second remission after disease relapse.

Autologous transplantation

In autologous transplantation, stem cells are collected from the patient in remission, and reinfused after high-dose chemotherapy and/or radiotherapy. Residual leukemia cells can be purged from the stem cell harvest, although this technique has not yielded improvements in survival to date.

A 3-year disease-free survival period of 40% has been reported with autologous stem cell transplantation.

Allogeneic transplantation

In allogeneic transplantation, stem cells collected from a compatible donor are infused in a patient who has undergone preparative therapy.

An HLA-matched sibling represents the ideal donor, but in only 10%–20% of cases is such a match available. Other potential donors include HLA-matched unrelated donors and HLA-mismatched family members.

Patients deemed too old or frail for *myeloablative* regimens are candidates for *nonmyeloablative* transplantation, a technique that relies primarily on the graft-versus-leukemia effect of donor cells.

Treatment of acute promyelocytic leukemia

The management of acute promyelocytic leukemia (APL) warrants additional discussion because it differs from that of other forms of AML.

With current therapy, APL is associated with high rates of response and survival. t(15;17), which results in formation of the PML/RAR-A fusion gene, is the genetic hallmark of APL.

With regard to clinical features of the disease, the presence of disseminated intravascular coagulation (DIC) at diagnosis distinguishes APL from other forms of acute leukemia. DIC places the patient at risk for severe, life-threatening hemorrhage and thus is managed as a medical emergency.

Induction chemotherapy regimens for APL combine all-*trans* retinoic acid (ATRA), which targets the PML/RAR-A fusion product, with daunorubicin and cytarabine. Patients who respond to induction then receive daunorubicin and cytarabine as postremission therapy, followed by maintenance ATRA for up to 1 year.

Recent evidence suggests arsenic trioxide has activity against APL in the induction and postremission settings.

ACUTE MYELOID LEUKEMIA

Emerging therapies in acute myeloid leukemia

With further characterization of genetic events underlying AML, novel therapies for the disease are emerging.

Gemtuzumab ozogamicin (GO), a humanized anti-CD33 monoclonal antibody, is now approved for use as monotherapy in patients 60 years of age or older with relapsed AML who are not considered candidates for cytotoxic chemotherapy.

Ongoing research seeks to define the therapeutic role of multidrug resistance modulators:
- Farnesyltransferase inhibitors
- FLT-3 inhibitors
- Histone deacetylase inhibitors
- Inhibitors of vascular endothelial growth factor

Tailored to the unique biology of AML, these therapies provide reason for optimism that further improvement in the care of patients with the disease can occur.

Acute lymphoblastic leukemia

Phuong L. Doan
Jon Gockerman

Epidemiology
- Incidence: 4000 cases per year in United States
  - 60% of these cases were diagnosed in patients <20 years old.
- Most common cancer in children and adolescents
- Overall cure rate is more favorable in children than in adults.

Clinical features
Signs and symptoms at presentation represent the degree of bone marrow failure and the extent of extramedullary spread.

Symptoms
- Fever, fatigue, lethargy
- Pallor, petechiae, ecchymosis
- The elderly may have anemia-associated dyspnea, angina, and dizziness.

Signs
- Hepatosplenomegaly and lymphadenopathy
- Thymic mass that can cause superior vena cava syndrome or superior mediastinal syndrome associated with neck and facial swelling
- Children may have a limp or arthralgia due to marrow leukemic infiltration.
-ABnormal laboratory values are marked leukocytosis, pancytopenia, elevated lactate dehydrogenase, and mild coagulopathy.

Diagnosis
Bone marrow
Bone marrow examination enables morphologic, flow analysis cytochemical, and genetic analysis.

Lymphoblasts are small cells with light-blue cytoplasm, a round or slightly indented nucleus, and fine to coarse chromatin, and may they contain nucleoli.

Cytochemical stains with Sudan black stain and stains for myeloperoxidase and esterases can differentiate acute lymphoblastic leukemia (ALL) from AML. Lymphoblasts will not react with these stains.

Immunophenotyping is always needed in diagnosis, because lymphoblasts may lack characteristic morphology and cytochemical features.

Immunophenotyping
There are six immunophenotype classifications, but the only subtypes of therapeutic significance are as follows.

Precursor B-cell acute lymphoblastic leukemia
This type is associated with favorable prognosis in children with low leukocyte count and hyperploidy. Approximately 80% of precursor B-cell ALL will express CD10 and generally has a favorable prognosis.

T-cell acute lymphoblastic leukemia

T-cell ALL is associated with a standard risk of relapse and the following:
- Male predominance
- Hyperleukocytosis at diagnosis
- Older age
- Mediastinal mass
- Extramedullary disease

Mature B-cell acute lymphoblastic leukemia

This is also called Burkitt cell leukemia. It is associated with male predominance and bulky extramedullary disease, and often presents with CNS leukemia.

Some patients with mature B-cell ALL will have a translocation (8;14) creating the *MYC* oncogene. If this translocation is present, patients have a favorable prognosis with intensive chemotherapy.

Estimated event-free survival in this subtype, with rearranged *MYC*, for adults is 55% at 4 years.

Lumbar puncture should be performed at diagnosis to evaluate for CNS disease.

Genetic analysis

Normal karyotype has neither good nor poor prognostic significance.

Favorable cytogenetics
- Hyperploidy (>50 chromosomes per leukemia cell)
- Translocation (12;21) with *TEL-AML1* fusion gene

Adverse cytogenetics
- Hypoploidy (<45 chromosomes per leukemia cell)
- Translocation (4;11) with *MLL-AF4* fusion gene
- Translocation (9;22) with *BCR-ABL* fusion: frequency increases with age, from 3% in children to 20% in adults to >50% in adults older than 50 years.

Less than 10% of adults with BCR-ABL translocation will have an event-free survival at 3 years.

Risk assessment

Adults are divided into standard-risk and high-risk groups.

Standard risk
- Age at diagnosis <35 years
- Favorable cytogenetics
- Leukocyte count less than 30×10^9 per liter for B-cell ALL
- Less than 100×10^9 per liter for T-cell ALL
- Absence of CNS disease at diagnosis
- B-cell phenotype versus T-cell phenotype

High risk

Adults are high risk if they do not meet the above criteria.

Supportive care

Metabolic complications of hyperuricemia and hyperphosphatemia with secondary hypocalcemia may be present at diagnosis. Treat with hydration, oral phosphate binders, and inhibition of purine synthesis with allopurinol or rasburicase, a recombinant urate oxidase.

Treat hyperleukocytosis with leukopheresis or exchange transfusion to prevent leukostasis.

Control infection with broad-spectrum antibiotics in febrile ALL patients until the infection is excluded. All patients should receive prophylaxis for *Pneumocystic jiroveci* pneumonia.

Transfusion of blood products should be given to prevent bleeding complications from severe thrombocytopenia and anemia. All blood products should be irradiated to prevent graft-versus-host disease.

Antileukemic therapy

Treatment is directed according to risk assessment. Treatment regimens vary in relative minor aspects and emphasize the following:
- Induction therapy
- Intensification therapy
- Maintenance treatment to eradicate residual disease
- Treatment directed to the central nervous system

Early response to treatment

Response to therapy is the most accurate prognostic indicator, as it reflects the genetics of the leukemia cells and patient pharmacodynamics and pharmacogenetics.
- Flow cytometry or polymerase chain reaction (PCR) allows for accurate measurement of minimal residual disease.
- Patients with measurable disease at >1% at the end of induction therapy have a very high risk of relapse should receive intensified therapy.

Induction therapy

Treatment goals are to reduce tumor burden by >99% and restore normal hematopoiesis. There is no single best induction regimen.

Induction regimens often contain L-asparaginase or anthracyclines. Children with high-risk ALL and most young adults receive a four-drug regimen that includes glucocorticoids, vincristine, asparaginase, or anthracycline.

Imatinib, an oral tyrosine kinase inhibitor, is effective for inducing and consolidating remissions in BCR-ABL-positive patients. Complete remission rates can be achieved in 98% of children and >90% of adults with standard risk.

Induction mortality is 5%, with opportunistic infections being the major cause of death due to prolonged myelosuppression.

Consolidation therapy

In children, options for intensification include regimens containing high-dose methotrexate, L-asparaginase given over an extended period of time, and reinduction therapy. Randomized trials have failed to show a benefit of this intensification regimen in adults.

Adults with high-risk disease should be offered high-dose chemotherapy with stem cell transplant in the first complete remission.

High-dose chemotherapy with allogeneic hematopoietic stem cell transplantation offers long-term disease-free survival of 45%–75%, compared with 40%–30% with chemotherapy alone.
- This is an option for children with very high risk ALL.
- This is an option for adults with BCR-ABL translocation, or poor initial response to induction therapy, or relapse after short response.

Patients with the best outcome from standard chemotherapy have the greatest benefit from stem cell transplantation.

Maintenance therapy

Patients require prolonged continuation therapy for 2 years or more. Efforts to shorten duration have yielded poorer outcomes in children and adults.

Most regimens consist of weekly methotrexate and daily mercaptopurine.

Novel therapies

Monoclonal antibodies
- CD20 and CD22 are expressed on most B-cell ALL. CD33 and CD52 are present on many T- and B-cell ALL.
- Rituximab is anti-CD20 and has antiproliferative effects.
- Epratuzumab is anti-CD22 and has immunomodulatory effects and is in clinical trials.
- Gemtuzumab is anti-CD33 and has efficacy in some case reports.
- Alemtuzumab is anti-CD52 and will be studied in patients with newly diagnosed ALL.

Chemotherapy formulations

Advances in chemotherapy formulations with liposomal vincristine and intrathecal liposomal cytarabine may offer less neurotoxicity and prolonged action, respectively.

Kinase inhibitors desatinib and nilotinib are in phase I–II clinical trials and may be beneficial in patients with the BCR-ABL translocation.

Further reading

Armstrong SA, Look AT (2005). Molecular genetics of acute lymphoblastic leukemia. *J Clin Oncol* 23:6306–6315.

Pui CH, Evans WE (2006). Treatment of acute lymphoblastic leukemia. *N Engl J Med* 354:166–178.

Rowe JM, Goldstone AH (2007). How I treat acute lymphocytic leukemia in adults. *Blood* 110:2268–2275.

Chapter 42

Chronic leukemias and myelodysplastic syndromes

Chronic myeloid leukemia *730*
Myelodysplastic syndromes *736*
Chronic lymphoid leukemias *742*

Chronic myeloid leukemia

Carling Ursem
Arati V. Rao

Epidemiology

Chronic myeloid leukemia (CML) constitutes 15%–20% of all leukemias in adults. The disease most commonly presents between the ages of 40 and 60 years with equal incidence in both sexes. There is an association with exposure to ionizing radiation, for example, in atomic-bomb survivors.

Pathophysiology

CML is one of the myeloproliferative disorders. It develops from a mutated hematopoietic, pluripotent stem cell that leads to a clonal population of cells that replace the normal bone marrow. Unlike the acute leukemias, the cells retain their ability to differentiate during the chronic phase of the disease.

Philadelphia chromosome

In 97.5% of cases of CML, there is a reciprocal translocation between chromosomes 9 and 22, t(9;22), which is recognized as the Philadelphia chromosome.

This leads to part of the *BCR* (breakpoint cluster region) gene from chromosome 22 (region q11) to be fused with part of the *ABL* (Abelson) gene on chromosome 9 (region q34) to form a new fusion gene called *BCR-ABL*.

- The resultant bcr-abl transcript is constitutively active
- It has tyrosine kinase activity
- It causes downstream activation of proteins that control the cell cycle, speeding up cell division.

The bcr-abl protein also inhibits DNA repair, leading to
- Genomic instability and
- Cells being more susceptible to developing further genetic abnormalities

Clinical features and phases

Clinical phases

CML has three phases: chronic, accelerated, and blast crisis.

Eighty-five percent of patients present in the *chronic phase*, which can last for several years.
- Approximately 20%–50% of patients are asymptomatic at diagnosis.
- Presenting symptoms, when present, include anemia, weight loss, fatigue, malaise, and splenomegaly.
- Patients can develop gouty arthritis.
- Rarely, extreme leukocytosis can lead to hyperviscosity, which can cause altered consciousness, blurred vision, and cardiorespiratory failure.

Patients may then progress to an *accelerated phase*, during which leukocytosis becomes more difficult to control and there is decreased neutrophil differentiation.

Some patients eventually progress to *"blast crisis,"* which resembles an acute leukemia with elevated myeloid or lymphoid blasts in the bone marrow and peripheral blood. This can occur 3–5 years after the initial diagnosis of CML and 18 months after onset of the accelerated phase.

Investigations
- Complete blood count
- Peripheral blood film
- Bone marrow aspiration and biopsy for morphology and flow cytometry
- Cytogenetics
- Fluorescent in situ hybridization (FISH) for bcr-abl
- Quantitative Reverse transcription polymerase chain reaction (RT-PCR) for the *BCR-ABL* fusion gene transcript

Leukocytosis
Leukocytosis is a uniform feature, and white cell counts can be in excess of 300×10^9/L. This can be differentiated from a leukemoid reaction by the leukocyte alkaline phosphatase (LAP) score:
- Typically low in CML
- Normal to elevated in leukemoid reactions

Patients typically may have basophilia and eosinophilia. A normochromic anemia may be present and platelets are increased (sometimes over 1000×10^9/L). The bone marrow is hypercellular with predominant granulocytopoiesis.

In accelerated phase there is an increase in blasts to 10%–19% in blood and bone marrow. This progresses to ≥20% blasts, with worsening anemia and thrombocytopenia, in blast crisis.

Cytogenetics
Approximately 95% of patients have the Philadelphia chromosome on bone marrow cytogenetic testing and a further 2.5% will have an occult t(9;22) translocation identified by a positive RT-PCR for the bcr-abl transcript.

Approximately 2.5% patients are negative for the t(9;22) translocation; this condition is termed atypical Philadelphia-negative CML. These patients usually have a poorer prognosis, are older and more anemic, and have extreme leukocytosis.

Differential diagnosis for CML
- Juvenile myelomonocytic leukemia
- Chronic myelomonocytic leukemia
- Chronic eosinophilic leukemia
- Leukemoid reaction
- Myelodysplastic syndrome
- Chronic neutrophilic leukemia

Management

Chronic phase-chronic myeloid leukemia

There has been tremendous progress in the treatment of chronic phase-chronic myeloid leukemia (CP-CML) based on the discovery of the BCR-ABL fusion gene, such that the median survival in chronic phase is now 25–30 years. This progress is due to the introduction of a series of increasingly effective tyrosine kinase inhibitors (TKIs). All of these oral medications work by binding to the BCR-ABL fusion product and inhibiting its activity. TKIs are now the standard of care for all phases of CML.

Imatinib: This was the first TKI developed for use in CML. The landmark IRIS trial led to approval of Imatinib at 400 mg daily Thus far, the 6-year overall survival (OS) and progression free survival (PFS) rates are 85% and 92%, respectively.

Dasatinib and Nilotinib: These drugs represent the second-generation of TKIs and are now approved for frontline therapy. The DASISION trial evaluated dasatinib 100 mg daily compared with imatinib 400 mg daily, whereas the ENESTnd trial compared nilotinib 300 mg or 400 mg daily to imatinib 400 mg daily. In both trials, there was a deeper and faster hematologic, cytogenetic, and molecular remission with the second-generation agents compared with Imatinib. However, at 3-years there was no difference in OS.

Bosutinib and Ponatinib: These two agents represent the third generation of TKIs approved for use only in patients who are intolerant of, or refractory/resistant to therapy with imatinib, dasatinib, or nilotinib. One reason for resistance is the emergence of new mutations in the BCR-ABL gene. In particular, the T315I mutation is present in up to 20% of patients with resistance to TKIs, and Ponatinib was specifically designed so that its chemical structure is not blocked by the T315I mutation and is thus very active in this group of patients.

Omacetaxine: This is a protein translation inhibitor and was previously known as homoharringatonine. It is approved only for use in patients with resistance/intolerance to ≥2 TKIs.

Response criteria

There are three separate elements of monitoring the response to TKI therapy.

Hematologic response: Complete normalization of peripheral blood counts with leukocyte count $<10 \times 10^9/L$, platelet count $<450 \times 10^9/L$ with no immature cells, such as myelocytes, promyelocytes, or blasts in peripheral blood and no signs and symptoms of disease with disappearance of palpable splenomegaly

Cytogenetic response: Chromosomal cytogenetics, more commonly with FISH, are performed on a bone marrow biopsy specimen to determine the percentage of bone marrow cells carrying the Philadelphia chromosome. Complete Cytogenetic response (CCy):No Ph-positive metaphases; Partial: 1%–35% Ph-positive metaphases; Major: 0%–35% Ph-positive metaphases (complete + partial) and finally Minor: presence of >35% Ph-positive metaphases

Molecular response: Quantitative RT-PCR of peripheral blood is performed to determine the number of circulating cells that harbor the

BCR-ABL fusion gene. A complete molecular response is no detectable BCR-ABL mRNA by quantitative RT-PCR (International scale) using an assay with a sensitivity of at least 4.5 logs below the standardized baseline. A Major molecular response (MMR) is a ≥3-log reduction in BCR-ABL mRNA transcripts.

Monitoring

Although achievement of MMR is not predictive of survival, the best predictor for long-term response is in fact short-term response. Recent studies have confirmed that the BCR-ABL transcript level at 3 months is the strongest predictor of outcome. Patients with a good molecular response early in their treatment course, characterized by low numbers of circulating BCR-ABL transcripts, have the best OS and PFS. For this reason, early monitoring of BCR-ABL transcript level is crucial in the decision to consider alternate therapy. After initiating TKI therapy monitoring should consist of:

RT-PCR every 3 months if the patient is responding to the TKI

If BCR-ABL transcripts increase by 1 log or more, RT-PCR should be performed every 1–3 months

If CCyR is sustained for 3 years, RT-PCR can be performed every 3–6 months

Side effects of tyrosine kinase inhibitors

Although each of the TKIs has a unique side effect profile, they are all generally well tolerated and most side effects can be overcome by adjunctive measures without interrupting therapy. The most common side effects universal to most TKIs includes cytopenias, elevated transaminases, bilirubin, amylase and lipase. Imatinib can cause nausea, diarrhea, fluid retention, arthralgias, and cytopenias especially anemia. Dasatinib causes pancytopenia, fluid retention including pleural effusions requiring thoracentesis, diarrhea, headaches and very rarely pulmonary arterial hypertension. Nilotinib causes pancytopenia and prolongation on the QTc and thus should be administered with caution if patients are on other QT-prolonging drugs. It can also cause hyperglycemia, rash, and pancreatitis. Bosutinib mainly has GI side effects diarrhea, nausea, vomiting, and abdominal pain as common side effects. Finally, Ponatinib can cause pancytopenia, and GI side-effects but carries a black-box warning for its effect on the cardiovascular system and these include: hypertension, myocardial infarction, congestive heart failure, and arterial ischemias. There are very clear guidelines on how to manage these toxicities, including holding therapy and dose reduction.

Resistance to tyrosine kinase inhibitors

This is unfortunately a common occurrence in CP-AML and it is thus recommended that patients who receive Imatinib as first line therapy and do not achieve a MMR by 3 months or a CCyR at 12–18 months should be tested for BCR-ABL kinase domain mutation analysis before switching to another TKI. Patients who received Dasatinib or Nilotinib as initial therapy and either have not achieved CCyR, or initially achieved CCyR and have now relapsed, should first be evaluated for medication adherence followed by BCR-ABL kinase domain mutation analysis for consideration of changing to a different TKI. This testing is also recommended in patients who progress to accelerated phase or blast crisis.

Accelerated phase chronic myeloid leukemia
With the use of TKIs, progression to accelerated phase chronic myeloid leukemia (AP-CML) has decreased to 1%–1.5% per year, compared to greater than 20% per year before their use. Based on the clinical trials conducted thus far, the second generation TKIs are better than Imatinib in preventing the conversion from chronic phase to accelerated phase CML. The goal of therapy here is to eliminate the BCR-ABL gene and try to revert back to CP-AML. The starting dose of Imatinib with AP-CML is higher i.e., 600-800 mg daily. Progression to accelerated phase is generally treated the same as resistance to TKIs, including mutational analysis and changing to an alternative TKI.

Blast phase chronic myeloid leukemia
It is critical for the pathologist to perform flow cytometry to evaluate for myeloid vs. lymphoid blast crisis. The overall goal of therapy in blast phase (BP) is a return to chronic phase followed by an allogeneic stem cell transplant. Typically, the treatment of choice is high dose combination chemotherapy based on the phenotype of the blasts. ALL-type chemotherapy regimens are associated with higher response rates than AML-type regimens. Several studies have now added a TKI to chemotherapy and the choice of TKI depends on which agents the patient has previously received as well as the mutation profile. The dose of the TKI is usually higher than that used in CP-AML.

Allogeneic stem cell transplant
Allogeneic stem cell transplant (SCT) is a potentially curative treatment for patients with CML, but the excellent results with TKI therapy have changed this and very few patients are now even considered for allogeneic SCT as first-line therapy. It is important to note that pretransplant Imatinib or other TKI does not compromise the outcome of a subsequent allogeneic SCT. Allogeneic HSCT is recommended for patients with T315I mutation who do not respond to any of the TKIs. It can also be considered for patients with disease progression to accelerated or BP on TKI therapy. The risks including the high treatment-related mortality and a good risk-benefit assessment must be performed and discussed with the patient.

Myelodysplastic syndromes

Lindsay A. M. Rein
Carlos M. deCastro

Myelodysplastic syndromes (MDS) are a group of neoplastic disorders of the bone marrow, characterized by dysplastic hematopoiesis and peripheral blood cytopenias including anemia, thrombocytopenia, and leukopenia. It belongs to the family of myeloid neoplasms and has a tendency and risk to progress to acute myeloid leukemia.

Epidemiology

Incidence and risk factors

The incidence of MDS ranges from 4 to 12 per 100,000 per year, with a peak incidence of >20 per 100,000 in those over age 80. The median age for development of MDS is in excess of 65 years.

Risk factors for developing MDS include exposure to previous chemotherapy, especially alkylating agents, radiation, and benzene.

Pathology

Bone marrow evaluation

Hallmarks of these diseases are as follows:
- Hypercellular bone marrow with dysplastic cell morphology
- Paradoxical peripheral blood cytopenias.

The paradox may result from apoptosis of dysplastic bone marrow progenitor cells, leading to ineffective production of differentiated cells for release into the blood.

Specific genetic mutations have been discovered and may contain prognostic information. Common mutations include *TET2*, *ASXL1*, *RUNX1*, *TP53*, and *EZH2*. Mutations in the spliceosome gene *SF3B1* have been found in the majority of patients with ringed sideroblasts.

Disease subtypes are classified according to WHO criteria based on the following:
- Number of lineages involved
- Presence of ring sideroblasts
- Blast count
- Presence of specific cytogenetic abnormalities (see Table 42.1 and Box 42.1)

Clinical features

Symptoms and signs

Symptomatic anemia is the most common presentation. Patients may also present with bleeding from thrombocytopenia or with recurrent infections owing to neutropenia.

Patients with chronic myelomonocytic leukemia (CMML) may have hepatosplenomegaly or other evidence of tissue infiltration by leukemic cells.

Table 42.1 WHO classification of myelodysplastic syndromes

Refractory anemia

Refractory anemia with ring sideroblasts (RARS)

Refractory cytopenia with multilineage dysplasia (RCMD)

Refractory cytopenia with multilineage dysplasia and ringed sideroblasts (RCMD-RS)

Refractory anemia with excess blasts-1 (RAEB-1; 5%–10% blasts)

Refractory anemia with excess blasts-2 (RAEB-2; 11%–20% blasts)

Myelodysplastic syndrome unclassified (MDS-U)

MDS associated with isolated del(5q)

Reprinted with permission from WHO.

Box 42.1 WHO classification of myelodysplastic and myeloproliferative syndromes

Chronic myelomonocytic leukemia (CMML)

Atypical chronic myelomonocytic leukemia (aCMML)

Juvenile myelomonocytic leukemia (JMML)

Reprinted with permission from WHO.

Work up
- CBC
- Blood film
- Bone marrow biopsy
- Cytogenetics
- Flow cytometry

CBC
Macrocytic anemia is usual. Neutropenia, thrombocytopenia, and monocytosis may also be evident.

Peripheral blood smear
The peripheral blood film should show evidence of dysplasia:
- Misshapen, large red blood cells
- Agranular neutrophils
- Circulating blast cells

Bone marrow aspirate
- The bone marrow is usually hypercellular.
- Dysplasia is present in one or more cell lines.
- Ring sideroblasts may be present.
- The blast count may be increased to 5%–20%.
- A clonal cytogenetic abnormality is often present which is of prognostic importance.

Management

The ultimate goals of therapy in MDS are to control symptoms, improve quality of life, and decrease progression to acute myeloid leukemia.

Blood and platelet transfusion

Traditionally, management has been focused on supportive care with blood and platelet transfusions as required. Iron chelation therapy may be required for excessive iron loading with repeated transfusions in patients with a good overall prognosis.

Erythropoietin and colony-stimulating factors

Treatment with hematopoietic growth factors, including erythropoietin (EPO) and granulocyte colony-stimulating factor (G-CSF), can improve anemia and neutropenia and potentially reduce both fatigue and the risk of infection.

Patients are more likely to respond to EPO if they have mild anemia, no or minimal transfusion requirements (<2 units per month), and a low endogenous EPO level.

Patients with ring sideroblasts are more likely to respond to the combination of EPO and G-CSF than to EPO alone.

Chemotherapy

Several agents are approved for the treatment of MDS.

New agents

- **Lenalidomide**: Lenalidomide (Revlimid), an immune modulator, has recently been shown to alleviate anemia in a high proportion of MDS patients with the cytogenetic abnormality deletion 5q(31–33) or 5q- syndrome.
- **Hypomethylating agents**: 5-azacytidine and decitabine produce hematologic improvement and remissions in patients with increased numbers of blasts and have been shown to have a survival advantage or delay the progression to leukemia when compared with best supportive care.
- **Immunosuppressive therapy**: Antilymphocyte globulin (ALG) can result in transfusion independence in approximately one third of patients with MDS.

Selected patients with increased blast cells may achieve temporary remission with AML-type chemotherapy. This is most useful as a way of achieving remission before allogeneic transplantation. Patients with MDS seldom tolerate more than one or two courses of combination chemotherapy.

Allogeneic stem cell transplantation

Allogeneic stem cell transplantation is currently the only treatment for MDS with curative potential. Conventional myeloablative stem cell transplants are reserved for young patients, but recent use of highly immunosuppressive, reduced-intensity conditioning regimens—"mini allografts"—in older patients up to 65 years is encouraging.

Clinical trials

Several clinical trials using combinations of hypomethylating agents with either lenalidomide or HDAC inhibitors are ongoing. Newer agents are also undergoing investigation.

Prognosis

International prognostic scoring system

The International Prognostic Scoring System (IPSS) (see Table 42.2) predicts prognosis based on the following:
- Number of cytopenias (anemia, neutropenia, and thrombocytopenia)
- Blast cell percentage
- Cytogenetic abnormalities (good risk, intermediate risk, or poor risk)

Prognosis ranges from a few months (patients with excess blasts) to several years (refractory anemia with ring sideroblasts).

Patients die from either transformation to acute myeloid leukemia or from the effects of bone marrow failure and associated treatment.

The WHO-based prognostic scoring system combines the IPSS with the WHO classification system and with transfusion dependency to produce a dynamic prognostic scoring system.[1]

More recently, IPSS-R (revised) was published. The IPSS-R incorporates more recent cytogenetic data, depth of cytopenias, and a small factor for age. It still lacks inclusion of factors such as patient co-morbidities, transfusion requirements, or specific genetic mutations.

Table 42.2 IPSS-R Prognostic Score Values

Prognostic Variable	0	0.5	1.0	1.5	2.0	3.0	4.0
Cytogenetics	Very good	—	Good	—	Intermediate	Poor	Very Poor
BM Blast, %	≤2	—	>2–<5	—	5–10	>10	—
Hemoglobin	≥10	—	8–<10	<8	—	—	—
Platelets	≥100	50–<100	<50	—	—	—	—
ANC	≥0.8	<0.8	—	—	—	—	—

Risk Category	Risk Score
Very low	≤1.5
Low	>1.5–3
Intermediate	>3–4.5
High	>4.5–6
Very high	>6.0

---

1 Malcovati L, Germing U, Kuendgen A, et al. (2007). Time-dependent prognostic scoring system for predicting survival and leukemic evolution in myelodysplastic syndromes. *J Clin Oncol* 25:3503–3510.

References

1. Bejar R, Stevenson K, Abdel-Wahab O, et al. (2011). Clinical effect of point mutations in myelodysplastic syndromes. *N Eng J Med* 364:2496–2506.
2. Papemmanuil E, Cazzola M, Boultwood J, et al. (2011). Somatic SF3B1 mutation in myelodysplasia with ring sideroblasts. *N Eng J Med* 365:1384–1395.
3. Greenberg PL, Tuechler H, Schanz J, et al. (2012). Revised international prognostic scoring system for myelodysplastic syndromes. *Blood* 120:2454–2465.

Chronic lymphoid leukemias

Mark C. Lanasa
J. Brice Weinberg

Introduction

The chronic lymphoid leukemias are a heterogeneous group of lymphoproliferative disorders associated with accumulation of mature lymphoid cells in the peripheral blood. They are classified by
- Morphology
- Surface immunophenotype
- Cytogenetics
- Molecular markers

Some lymphomas may present with lymphadenopathy and bone marrow infiltration in addition to leukemia. The present WHO classification of mature lymphoid leukemia is shown in Box 42.2.

The remainder of this chapter will focus on B-CLL.

Epidemiology

Incidence and prevalence

Chronic lymphoid leukemia (CLL) is the most prevalent leukemia in the United States and Europe; an estimated 85,000 Americans are living with CLL in 2008.

The age-adjusted annual incidence in the United States is 4.0 per 100,000, and the lifetime risk of developing CLL is 1 in 221 (0.45%).

Risk factors

It predominantly affects older individuals, with a median age at diagnosis of 72. A male predominance is observed, with a male-to-female incidence ratio of 2:1.

Genetic factors likely contribute to the development of CLL. The relative risk of CLL conferred to first-degree relatives of patients with CLL is estimated at between 4.5 and 7.0. This is among the highest inherited relative risks of any type of malignancy. Approximately 8% of CLL cases have a family history of CLL.

The widely divergent incident rates of CLL among different ethnic groups also support an inherited predisposition.

Pathology and pathophysiology

Pathogenesis

CLL is characterized by the accumulation of small, mature B lymphocytes in the peripheral blood, bone marrow, and lymphatic tissues.

Although CLL has historically been considered a disorder of ineffective apoptosis, recent research shows that CLL lymphocytes also have significant proliferative capacity. Moreover, interactions between the CLL lymphocytes and the tumor microenvironment, including T cells, stromal elements, and cytokines, potentiate cell survival.

These tumor-host interactions may contribute to leukemic cell accumulation more than an inherent apoptotic defect in CLL lymphocytes. The gradual accumulation of small lymphocytes causes progressive enlargement of the lymph nodes and infiltration of spleen and bone marrow.

It has been proposed that the proliferative compartment of CLL is in the bone marrow and lymphoid tissues, rather than in the peripheral blood.

Subtypes

Two related subtypes of B-CLL have been characterized on the basis of presence or absence of somatic mutations in the immunoglobulin heavy chain. Both arise from antigen-experienced B cells, but these subtypes generally follow very different clinical courses.

Patients with immunoglobulin unmutated CLL show shortened time to treatment and overall survival. Other features include the following:
- Approximately 15% have a positive direct Coombs' test, with clinical autoimmune hemolytic anemia in a subset of these patients.
- Idiopathic thrombocytopenic purpura (ITP)
- Hypogammaglobulinemia
- Disorders of T-lymphocyte function

Box 42.2 Mature lymphoid leukemia as classified by WHO

B cell

B-cell chronic lymphocytic leukemia/small lymphocytic lymphoma (B-CLL/SLL)
B-cell prolymphocytic leukemia (B-PLL)
Hairy-cell leukemia and variants
Splenic marginal zone lymphoma with circulating villous lymphocytes (SLVL)
Leukemic phase of mantle cell lymphoma
Leukemic phase of follicle center cell lymphoma
Leukemic phase of lymphoplasmacytoid lymphoma

T cell

T-cell prolymphocytic leukemia (T-PLL)
T-cell large granular lymphocytic leukemia (T-LGL)
NK-cell leukemia
Adult T-cell leukemia/lymphoma
Leukemic phase of mycosis fungoides/Sézary syndrome

Reprinted with permission from WHO.

Clinical presentation

Symptoms and signs

Asymptomatic
Approximately 75% of CLL diagnoses are made in patients with asymptomatic, early-stage leukemia.

These cases are typically identified by a complete blood count obtained as part of an unrelated medical evaluation.

Symptomatic
The remaining 25% present with lymphadenopathy, anemia, or atypical infection. Constitutional symptoms are restricted to patients with advanced-stage disease and include fatigue, night sweats, and weight loss.

In advanced disease there is bone marrow failure due to diffuse marrow infiltration with resultant anemia, thrombocytopenia, and neutropenia. Organomegaly is also common in advanced disease.

Lymphadenopathy may be asymmetric, and can involve any lymph node group.

Splenomegaly is now uncommon at presentation, and hepatomegaly is even less frequent.

Involvement of other organs is rarely observed.

Diagnostic evaluation
- Complete blood count
- Blood film
- Bone marrow aspirate and biopsy
- Lymphocyte immunophenotyping
- Interphase cytogenetics (FISH) for loci with somatic abnormalities of prognostic significance

Chronic lymphoid leukemia diagnostic criteria
The 1996 NCI working group criteria for the diagnosis of CLL have been updated by the International Workshop on CLL Working Group (2007 iwCLL; see Box 42.3).

The B-lymphocyte count is elevated and the blood film shows small lymphocytes with disrupted "smudge cells."

Surface antigen immunophenotyping is essential to exclude reactive causes and other lymphoproliferative disorders. CLL lymphocytes express surface CD19, CD5, and CD23, and weakly express CD20, CD79b, and surface IgM.

Interphase cytogenetics (FISH) shows abnormalities in 80% of cases. Deletion of 17p13 predicts chemotherapy resistance and inferior prognosis.

Bone marrow examination is not required, but helpful in cases with unexplained cytopenias.

Management

Therapeutic criteria
CLL generally follows an indolent clinical course.

There is no evidence that treatment of patients with early-stage disease (uncomplicated lymphocytosis or lymphadenopathy) prolongs survival. Systemic therapy is only indicated for advanced or symptomatic disease.

The iwCLL Working Group guidelines (2007) for initiating treatment are as follows; only one criterion is required:
- Anemia with hemoglobin <10 g/dL
- Thrombocytopenia with platelet count <100 x 10^9/L
- Symptomatic or massive lymphadenopathy (>10 cm)
- Symptomatic or massive splenomegaly (>6 cm below costal margin)
- Constitutional symptoms referable to CLL (weight loss >10% in 6 months, fatigue with performance score 2 or worse, unexplained fever, night sweats)
- Lymphocyte doubling time (LDT) <6 months or a 50% increase in lymphocyte count in 2 months or less
- Autoimmune cytopenias refractory to corticosteroids

Response assessment (per iwCLL WG)
- *Complete response (CR)*: Normalization of lymphocyte count; resolution of lymphadenopathy and organomegaly; normalization of hemoglobin, platelet, and neurtrophil counts for at least 3 months
- *Partial response (PR)*: >50% reduction in lymphocyte count, lymphadenopathy, and organomegaly; >50% improvement in hemoglobin, platelet, and neutrophil counts if abnormal before initiation of therapy
- *Progressive disease (PD)*: >50% increase in lymphocyte count, lymphadenopathy, or organomegaly; Richter's transformation
- *Stable disease (SD)*: Does meet criteria for CR, PR, or PD

Box 42.3 iwCLL Working Group revised criteria for diagnosis of CLL

Peripheral blood lymphocytosis (required)
1. Absolute B-lymphocyte count >5 x 10^9/L
2. Morphologically mature appearing lymphocytes, "smudge" cells may be present

Immunophenotype (required)
1. Expansion of B lymphocytes: Coexpress CD5, CD19, CD23, and dim CD20, CD79b
2. Light-chain restriction, i.e., monoclonal κ or λ expression
3. Low-density surface immunoglobulin (sIgM) expression

Molecular genetics (not required)
1. Interphase cytogenetics (FISH):
   del 13q14.3, trisomy 12, del 11q22-23, del 6q21, del 17p13

Bone marrow examination (not required)
1. >30% lymphocytes in bone marrow aspirate
   Diffuse marrow infiltration on trephine biopsy is a poor prognostic marker

First-line therapy

Cytotoxic chemotherapy

- *Chlorambucil*: The alkylating agent chlorambucil (Chl) was the first widely used systemic agent in CLL. Chl rarely produces a CR, and yields a PR in approximately 50% of patients.
- *Fludarabine*: A phase III study showed single-agent fludarabine (F) to be superior to Chl with higher CR (20% vs. 4%) and progression-free survival (PFS).
  - Randomized studies have also shown that F yields a higher overall response (ORR) and PFS than cyclophosphamide, adriamycin, and prednisolone (CAP); cyclophosphamide, vincristine, and prednisolone (CVP); or cyclophosphamide, adriamycin, vincristine, and prednisolone (CHOP).
  - However, no study has shown a statistically significant improvement in overall survival for patients receiving F as first-line therapy.
  - F can precipitate autoimmune hemolysis and should be used with caution in DAT-positive patients.

More recently, the randomized U.S. Intergroup trial E2997 showed that the combination of cyclophosphamide and fludarabine (FC) yielded superior CR, OR, and PFS (32 vs. 19 months) compared with that with F alone.

Similarly, the recently completed LRF CLL4 trial also demonstrated the superiority of FC over F or Chl.

Neither trial showed improved overall survival in the FC arm.

Chemoimmunotherapy

- *Rituximab*: The utility of the anti-CD20 monoclonal antibody rituximab (R) has not been evaluated in randomized trials. However, a retrospective comparison of two phase II trials, CALGB 9712 and CALGB 9011, showed FR to be superior to F alone.

Cross-trial comparisons should always be made with caution; nonetheless, the eligibility criteria and study participants were virtually identical.

The FC combination showed significant improvement over F alone in both 2-year PFS (67% vs. 45%) and OS (93% vs. 81%). A subsequent study of FCR showed an unprecedented CR rate of 70%. R has minimal activity as a single agent in CLL.

Randomized studies comparing chemoimmunotherapy to chemotherapy alone are underway.

- *Alemtuzumab*: Alemtuzumab (A) is a chimeric anti-CD52 antibody. CD52 is expressed on a wide range of lymphocytes including CLL cells.

A phase III study comparing A to Chl showed A to have superior PFS and ORR. Impressive response rates were observed among patients with del11q (97%) and del 17p (64%).

A appears to be more effective at clearing disease in the blood and marrow than bulky lymph nodes.

It is profoundly immunosuppressive and is associated with an increased risk of viral infections, specifically reactivation of CMV.

Second-line and subsequent therapy

Chemotherapy

Treatment decisions in CLL depend on the following:
- Patient characteristics: age, performance status
- Disease characteristics: response to first line therapy, duration of response, and adverse risk cytogenetics

Chlorambucil: Patients relapsing after an initial response to Chl may be retreated with Chl, especially if the first response was relatively durable.

Fludarabine: Patients refractory to low-dose Chl should be treated with an F-containing regimen.

Alternate nucleoside analog: Patients with a good initial response to F may be retreated with an alternate nucleoside analog (*pentostatin or cladribine*) with R.

Chemoimmunotherapy

Patients with good performance status who develop progressive disease within 1 year of previous F-containing regimen should be treated with a combination chemoimmunotherapy.

FCR, PCR, and CFAR all have very good ORR in previously treated patients, of 73%, 75%, and 65%, respectively.

Alemtuzumab

A is also approved for the treatment of F-treated CLL. A should be strongly considered in patients with del 17p or del 11q.

Patients who are F refractory have a poor prognosis.

All patients should be considered for clinical trials.

Stem cell transplantation

Myeloablative allogeneic transplantation has been carried out in CLL. It is associated with a high transplant-related mortality predominantly relating to the age of the patients and the immune dysfunction associated with prior chemotherapy.

There likely exists a graft-versus-leukemia effect for CLL, and use of reduced-intensity conditioning regimes is being explored.

However, to date, there are no data to support autologous bone marrow transplantation (auto-BMT) over other conventional first- and second-line therapies. A European Group for Bone Marrow Transplantation (EBMT) randomized trial evaluating consolidation auto-BMT after induction therapy is underway. Auto-BMT should be considered experimental.

Radiotherapy

Radiotherapy is an effective local salvage modality for lymph nodes compromising vital organ function.

Splenic irradiation is effective for painful splenomegaly, although splenectomy is better for massive splenomegaly if the patient is fit for surgery.

Splenectomy

Splenectomy can be considered in fit patients with the following:
- Massive splenomegaly
- Symptomatic splenomegaly
- Cytopenias due to hypersplenism
- Immune cytopenias refractory to corticosteroids

Before splenectomy the patient requires pneumococcal, meningococcal, and *Hemophilus* vaccination.

Prognosis

Good prognosis

Patients with immunoglobulin (Ig) heavy-chain mutated CLL have a long time to first treatment and median survival of approximately 25 years.

Poorer prognosis

Patients with CLL containing unmutated Ig genes have a shorter median survival, of the order of 8 years.

The expression of cell surface CD38 and intracellular ZAP-70 are associated with a poorer prognosis.

Genetic abnormalities including del 11q and del 17p and resistance to fludarabine are associated with poor prognosis.

U.S. Intergroup trial E2997 (FC vs. F) prospectively evaluated a comprehensive panel of molecular prognostic factors. Using a multivariate regression model, only del 17p and del 11q were associated with shortened PFS.

Future directions

It is increasingly recognized that the quality of the response in CLL correlates with the length of remission.

Data from treatment with combination chemoimmunotherapy emphasizes the importance of achieving a complete response using sensitive techniques, such as four-color flow cytometry, to detect minimal residual disease.

Further attempts to reduce minimal residual disease burden and effect a cure may involve the following:
- Alemtuzumab consolidation after chemoimmunotherapy induction
- Combinations of antibodies, e.g., alemtuzumab and rituximab
- Maintenance antibody/chemotherapy
- Reduced-intensity allogeneic transplantation in selected cases

Promising therapeutics in development include the following:
- Flavopiridol: A synthetic flavone that inhibits cyclin-dependent kinases. Response rates of >40% have been observed among heavily pretreated patients. Responses are observed in patients with del 17p and del 11q.
- Lenalidomide: An immunomodulatory analog of thalidomide. A recent phase II trial of lenalidomide showed a 9% CR and 47% ORR among previously treated patients.
- Lumiliximab: A chimeric anti-CD23 monoclonal antibody. A randomized phase II trial studying FCR with and without lumiliximab is currently underway.

Chapter 43

Multiple myeloma

Kathleen Lambert
Christina Gasparetto

Introduction 750
Epidemiology and risk factors 750
Pathogenesis 751
Clinical features 752
Diagnosis 754
Staging and prognosis 756
Treatment 758
Further reading 765

Multiple myeloma

Introduction

Multiple myeloma (MM) is a B-cell lymphoproliferative disorder characterized by the following:
- Bone marrow infiltration with an excessive number of malignant plasma cells
- Increased production of intact monoclonal immunoglobulin (IgA, IgG, IgE, IgD) or free monoclonal κ or λ light chains (Bence-Jones protein)
- Bone destruction

Epidemiology and risk factors

Incidence and mortality

Multiple myeloma accounts for 1%–2% of all malignancies and 10%–15% of hematologic tumors, representing the second most frequently occurring hematologic malignancy in the United States.

The overall incidence rate is approximately 5.6 per 100,000 persons. Nearly 19,000 individuals were diagnosed with MM in the United States in 2007, and more than 11,000 die of this disease every year. The overall 5-year survival is approximately 33%.

Rick factors

Risk factors include increasing age, male sex, and black race. Diagnosis is rare under the age of 40, with a median age at presentation of 65 years.

The cause of multiple myeloma is unknown, but a number of factors increase risk:
- Ionizing radiation
- Environmental toxins
- Viruses
- Genetic factors

Pathogenesis

The pathogenesis of multiple myeloma occurs by a multistep process that originates from a somatically mutated and isotype-switched follicle center B cell.

Virtually all myeloma cells have chromosomal aberrations. Hypodiploid tumors are associated with a poorer prognosis than that of hyperdiploid tumors. The most frequently observed chromosomal abnormality in multiple myeloma involves somatic hypermutations in the Ig heavy-chain gene locus.

During the evolution of multiple myeloma, additional mutations take place, such as
- Loss of chromosome 13
- Secondary myc translocations
- Activating mutations in N-ras, K-ras, or fibroblast growth factor receptor3 (FGFR3)

Once developed, myeloma cells home to the bone marrow where the microenvironment sustains survival, growth, and resistance to apoptosis.

Clinical features

Anemia
Anemia of variable severity affects more than two thirds of patients with myeloma.

Symptoms associated with anemia, such as weakness and fatigue, occur in approximately half the patients. Pallor is the most frequent physical finding.

Most patients have an inappropriate erythropoietin response for the degree of anemia, which is further exacerbated in the presence of renal failure.

Bone pain
Bone pain, particularly in the back and chest, is present in more than two thirds of patients at diagnosis. Pain is often aggravated by movement and frequently results from vertebral compression fractures or lytic lesions.

Localized pain can also be induced by regional tumor growth or amyloid deposition at various anatomic sites, including the spinal cord and nerve roots.

Renal insufficiency
Renal insufficiency occurs in approximately one-third of patients with MM. This is often due to "myeloma kidney," in which the tubular absorptive capacity for light chains is exhausted, resulting in interstitial nephritis from laminated light-chain casts, consisting mainly of Bence-Jones proteins.

Hypercalcemia is also a common, preventable cause of renal insufficiency. Other less common causes of renal insufficiency include primary (AL) amyloidosis and light-chain deposition disease (LCDD); both these disorders typically present with nephrotic syndrome.

Infections
Patients with multiple myeloma have a defective cellular immune function as well as an impaired humoral immune response to antigen. As a result, myeloma patients have increased susceptibility to bacterial infections, particularly pneumococcal pneumonia.

The incidence of gram-negative infections and herpes zoster is also increased in myeloma patients.

Neuropathy
Neurologic involvement in myeloma most commonly results in radiculopathy, particularly in the thoracic and lumbar areas. This usually occurs from nerve compression by a paravertebral plasmacytoma but can also occur from the collapsed bone itself.

Peripheral neuropathy is uncommon except in association with amyloidosis and osteosclerotic myeloma or POEMS (Polyneuropathy, Organomegaly, Endocrinopathy, Monoclonal gammopathy, and Skin changes) syndrome.

Spinal cord compression or cauda equina syndrome occurs in approximately 5% of patients.

Leptomeningeal infiltration by myeloma cells occurs infrequently.

Hyperviscosity

Hyperviscosity occurs in <10% of patients with myeloma. Symptoms of hyperviscosity result from circulatory problems leading to renal, pulmonary, cerebral, and other organ dysfunction.

Patients with IgA and IgM (Waldenstrom macroglobulinemia) myeloma are particularly prone to hyperviscosity syndrome.

Bleeding and thrombosis

Bleeding may occur due to the following:
- Anoxia and thrombosis in the capillary circulation
- Acquired coagulopathy such as factor X deficiency
- Rarely, thrombocytopenia

Thromboembolic disease has also been linked to the use of thalidomide and lenalidomide. Risk is increased with these agents when combined with chemotherapy and/or dexamethasone.

Prophylaxis with a low-molecular-weight heparin or adjusted-dose warfarin (INR ~1.5) is recommended

Extramedullary disease

Extramedullary plasmacytomas are more common in the late stages of disease. They can occur in any organ but most commonly affect
- The upper respiratory tract
- Lymph nodes
- Liver
- Kidney
- Skin
- The central nervous system

Secondary plasma cell leukemia can develop in 5% of patients, usually as a terminal-disease manifestation.

Diagnosis

Laboratory studies
- CBC, differential
- BUN/creatinine, electrolytes
- Calcium, albumin
- Quantitative immunoglobulins
- Serum protein electrophoresis and immunofixation
- β_2 microglobulin (β_2M), C-reactive protein
- Lactate dehydrogenase (LDH)
- Serum free light-chain assay
- 24-hour urine protein electrophoresis and immunofixation
- Skeletal survey (X-rays, CT, MRI, PET scans as indicated)
- Bone marrow aspirate and biopsy
- Cytogenetics and FISH analysis for 17p (p53), t(4;14), t(14;16), t(11;14)

Consider the following under special circumstances
- Plasma cell labeling index (PCLI)
- Fat pad biopsy for amyloid
- Tissue biopsy for plasmacytoma
- Serum viscosity level

International myeloma working group classification

Box 43.1 summarizes the simplified criteria for classification of myeloma, issued by the International Myeloma Working Group. All three criteria are required for diagnosis.

The most important determinant of symptomatic disease, and hence initiation of therapy, is evidence of organ or tissue impairment manifested by the following (CRAB):
- Hypercalcemia
- Renal failure
- Anemia
- Bone lesions

Table 43.1 summarizes categories of multiple myeloma including indications for treatment.

Box 43.1 Criteria for diagnosis of multiple myeloma

1. Monoclonal plasma cells in bone marrow >10% and/or presence of biopsy-proven plasmacytoma
2. Monoclonal protein present in serum and/or urine
3. Myeloma-related organ dysfunction (1 or more):
   C Calcium elevation in blood (serum calcium >10.5 mg/L or >2 mg above upper limit of normal)
   R Renal insufficiency (SCr >2 mg/dL)
   A Anemia (Hg <10 g/dL or 2 g< below lower limit of normal)
   B Lytic bone lesions or osteoporosis

Other: symptomatic hyperviscosity, amyloidosis, recurrent bacterial infections (>2 episodes in 12 months)

Table 43.1 Categories of multiple myeloma

Classification	Characteristics	Management
Monoclonal gammopathy of undetermined significance (MGUS)	<ul><li>Serum M protein <3 g/dL</li><li>Bone marrow plasma cells <10%</li><li>Absence of anemia, renal failure, hypercalcemia, lytic bone lesions</li></ul>	Observation, with treatment beginning at disease progression
Smoldering multiple myeloma	<ul><li>Serum M protein <3 g/dL and/or bone marrow plasma cells <10%</li><li>Absence of anemia, renal failure, hypercalcemia, lytic bone lesions</li></ul>	Observation, with treatment beginning at disease progression
Indolent multiple myeloma	<ul><li>Presence of serum/urine M protein</li><li>Bone marrow plasmacytosis</li><li>Mild anemia or few small lytic lesions</li><li>Absence of symptoms</li></ul>	Monitoring every 3 months, with treatment beginning at disease progression
Symptomatic multiple myeloma	<ul><li>Presence of serum/urine M protein</li><li>Bone marrow plasmacytosis</li><li>Anemia, renal failure, hypercalcemia, lytic bone lesions</li></ul>	Immediate treatment

Staging and prognosis

Durie-Salmon staging system
The Durie-Salmon staging system for patients with previously untreated MM was introduced in 1975. It separates patients mainly by tumor burden and renal function without taking into account any prognostic indicators. It has now been supplanted by the International Staging System (ISS) (see Table 43.2).

The ISS incorporates serum albumin and serum concentration of $\beta_2 M$, resulting in low-, intermediate-, and high-risk patients. High serum concentration of $\beta_2 M$ and low serum albumin are poor prognostic factors recognized in the ISS.

Other recognized poor prognostic factors include the following:
- IgA subtype
- Elevated LDH
- Increased number of circulating plasma cells in the peripheral blood
- Extramedullary disease
- Older age
- Chromosome abnormalities including deletion 13 detected by standard cytogenetics, and t(4;14), t(14;16) or 17p (p53) detected by FISH analysis.

Table 43.2 International Staging System for multiple myeloma

Stage	Criteria	Median survival
I	Serum $\beta_2 M$ <3.5 mg/dL Serum albumin ≥3.5mg/dL	62 months
II	Serum $\beta_2 M$ <3.5 mg/dL Serum albumin ≤3.5mg/dL OR Serum $\beta_2 M$ 3.5 mg/dL to ≤5.5 mg/dL	44 months
III	Serum $\beta_2 M$ ≥5.5 mg/dL	29 months

Treatment

Indications for treatment
- Symptomatic disease
- Evidence of organ impairment
  - Anemia
  - Hypercalcemia
  - Lytic bone lesions
  - Renal failure
  - Demonstration of disease progression.

Patients with stage I and smoldering or indolent multiple myeloma should not be treated until progressive disease is evident.

Because multiple myeloma is considered incurable, the goals of treatment are relief of symptoms, prolongation of a good quality of life, and attempts to reduce the burden of malignant plasma cells.

Systemic therapy

Systemic therapy is the preferred initial therapy for symptomatic multiple myeloma. Table 43.3 lists the most commonly used chemotherapy agents in nontransplant and transplant candidates and in relapsed or refractory myeloma, based on the 2007 National Comprehensive Cancer Network (NCCN) guidelines.

In general, older chemotherapy regimens have been supplanted by novel agents (thalidomide, lenalidomide, bortezomib) and should be used in the first-line setting, if appropriate. Table 43.4 lists selected chemotherapy regimens, including dosing and schedule.

Local radiation should be reserved for patients with disabling pain not responsive to systemic therapy.

If a patient is found to have high-risk prognostic factors (deletion 17p, translocations 4;14 or 4;16, deletion 13q, hypodiploidy, PCLI ≥3%), then novel treatment programs or clinical trials should be considered, as these patients do not usually respond to standard treatments.

Table 43.3 Chemotherapy

Primary therapy in nontransplant candidates	Primary therapy for transplant candidates†	Treatment for relapsed or refractory multiple myeloma‡
• Melphalan–Prednisone–Thalidomide (MPT)* • Melphalan–Prednisone–Bortezomib (MPV)* • Doxil–Vincristine–Dexamethasone (DVD)* • Thalidomide–Dexamethasone • Dexamethasone • Melphalan–Prednisone (MP) • Vincristine–Doxorubicin–Dexamethasone (VAD)	• Lenalidomide–Dexamethasone* • Bortezomib–Dexamethasone* • Bortezomib–Doxorubicin–Dexamethasone* • Bortezomib–Thalidomide–Dexamethasone* • Vincristine–Doxorubicin–Dexamethasone (VAD) • Thalidomide–Dexamethasone • Doxil–Vincristine–Dexamethasone (DVD) • Dexamethasone	• Bortezomib–Doxil* • Bortezomib* • Bortezomib–Dexamethasone • Lenalidomide–Dexamethasone • Lenalidomide • Thalidomide–Dexamethasone • Thalidomide • Dexamethasone • Cyclophosphamide VAD • High-dose Cyclophosphamide • Dexamethasone, Thalidomide, Cisplatin, Doxorubicin, Cyclophosphamide, Etoposide (DT-PACE) • Dexamethasone, Cyclophosphamide, Etoposide, Cisplatin (DCEP)

*Preferred first-line regimens, based on available evidence.

†Exposure to alkylating agents should be avoided in patients who are transplant candidates.

‡In general, patients may be treated with the same primary induction regimen if relapse occurs at >6 months of the initial therapy.

Table 43.4 Selected chemotherapy regimens

Regimen	Dose and schedule	Reference
MP	Melphalan 0.15 mg/kg po qd d1–7 q6 weeks × 12 cycles Prednisone 20 mg po tid d1–7 q6 weeks × 12 cycles OR Melphalan 0.25 mg/kg po qd d1–4 q6 weeks × 12 cycles Prednisone 2 mg/kg po qd d1–4 q6 weeks × 12 cycles	Facon T et al., *Blood* 2006; 107:1292
MPT	Melphalan 0.25 mg/kg po qd d1–4 q6 weeks × 12 cycles Prednisone 2mg/kg po qd d1–4 q6 weeks × 12 cycles Thalidomide 100–400 mg po qd OR Melphalan 4 mg/m² po qd d1–7 q4 weeks × 6 cycles Prednisone 40 mg/m² po qd d1–7 q4 weeks × 6 cycles Thalidomide 100 mg po qd until disease progression	Facon et al., *Lancet* 2007; 370:1209; Palumbo A et al., *Lancet* 2006; 367:825
MPB	Melphalan 9 mg/m² po qd d1–4 q6 weeks × 4 cycles followed by maintenance phase of q5 weeks × 5 cycles Prednisone 60 mg/m² po qd d1–4 q6 weeks × 4 cycles followed by maintenance phase of q5 weeks × 5 cycles Bortezomib 1 or 1.3 mg/m² IV d1, 4, 8, 11, 22, 25, 29, 32 q6weeks × 4 cycles followed by maintenance phase of 1 or 1.3 mg/m² IV d1, 8, 15, 22 q5weeks × 5 cycles	Mateos MN et al., *Blood* 2006; 108: 2165–2172
VAD	Vincristine 0.4 mg IV qd d1–4 q4 weeks × 4 cycles Doxorubicin 9 mg/m² IV qd d1–4 q4 weeks × 4 cycles Dexamethasone 40 mg po qd d1–4, 9–12, 17–20 q4 weeks (during odd cycles only)	Segeren CM et al., *Br J Haematol* 1999; 105:127
Dexamethasone	Dexamethasone 40 mg po qd d1–4, 9–12, 17–20 q35 days OR Dexamethasone 20 mg/m2 po qd d1–4, 9–12, 17–20 q35 days	Alexanian R et al., *Blood* 1992; 80:887

Table 43.4 (Cont.)

Regimen	Dose and schedule	Reference
Thalidomide–Dexamethasone	Thalidomide 100–200 mg po qd Dexamethasone 40 mg po qd d1–4, 9–12, 17–20 for odd cycles and d1–4 only for even cycles q4weeks	Rajkumar SV et al. *J Clin Oncol* 2003; 21:16
DVD	Liposomal doxorubicin (Doxil) 40 mg/m2 IV d1 q4 weeks Vincristine 2 mg IV d1 q4 weeks Dexamethasone 40 mg po qd d1–4 q4 weeks	Hussein MA et al. *Cancer* 2002; 95:2160
Lenalidomide–Dexamethasone (low dose)	Lenalidomide 25 mg po qd d1–21 Dexamethasone 40 mg po qd d1, 8, 15, 22 q4 weeks	Rajkumar SV et al. 2007 ASCO annual meeting, LBA8025
Bortezomib ± Dexamethasone	Bortezomib 1.3 mg/m2 IV d1, 4, 8, 11 q3 weeks In patients with disease progression after 2 cycles or with stable disease after 4 cycles, add: Dexamethasone 20 mg po qd d1, 2, 4, 8, 9, 11, 12 q3 weeks	Richardson PG et al. *N Engl J Med* 2003; 348: 2609–2617
Bortezomib + liposomal Doxorubicin	Bortezomib 1.3 mg/m2 IV d1, 4, 8, and 11 q3 weeks Liposomal doxorubicin 30 mg/m2 IV d1 q3 weeks	Orlowski RZ et al. *J Clin Oncol* 2007; 25:3892
DT-PACE	Dexamethasone 40 mg po qd d1–4 q4–6 weeks Thalidomide 400 mg po qd continuously Cisplatin 10mg/m2 IV qd d1–4 q4–6 weeks Cyclophosphamide 400 mg/m2 qd d1–4 q4–6 weeks Etoposide 40 mg/m2 IV qd d1–4 q4–6 weeks Doxorubicin 10mg/m2 qd d1–4 q4–6 weeks	Lee CK et al. *J Clin Oncol* 2003; 21: 2732–2739

Hematopoietic stem cell transplant

Autologous

In 1996, the first randomized trial by the French Myeloma Group comparing high-dose chemotherapy followed by autologous hematopoietic stem cell transplant (HSCT) with conventional chemotherapy demonstrated a statistically significant higher response rate, event-free, and overall survival favoring the transplant group.

Similar results have been confirmed in other randomized trials, whereas others have failed to report similar results. Discrepancies may be related to the different regimens used in the trials.

In most patients with newly diagnosed myeloma, the advantages and disadvantages of an autologous HSCT should be discussed before chemotherapy is given.

Contraindications include the following:
- Multiple comorbidities
- Organ failure
- Poor performance status
- Age alone is NOT a contraindication.

Hematopoietic stem cells should be collected before the patient is exposed to alkylating agents. The overall mortality from autologous HSCT is 1%–2%.

There is controversy concerning the need for double (tandem) autologous HSCT.

Overall, randomized trials have not found a survival benefit for planned tandem transplant except in patients who did not achieve a complete response (CR) or a very good partial response (VGPR) after the first transplant.

Allogeneic

Regarding allogeneic stem cell transplantation, the major advantages are that the graft contains no tumor cells and the transplant can produce a graft-versus-myeloma effect. However, the high treatment-related mortality and inability to find a suitable donor have limited this approach.

Efforts to reduce the mortality rate with a nonmyeloablative ("mini") transplant may result in lower mortality, and studies are currently underway to address this issue.

Until more data are available, however, conventional and "mini" allogeneic HSCT are not recommended in myeloma patients outside the setting of a clinical trial.

Supportive therapy

Myeloma causes a variety of medical problems that can be treated with supportive therapy in addition to therapy directed at the disease itself.

These problems and their associated treatments are summarized in Table 43.5.

Table 43.5 Supportive therapy

Bone disease • Lytic lesions • Osteopenia	1. Bisphosphonates • Pamidronate 90 mg IV monthly* • Zoledronic Acid 4 mg IV monthly* *Dental evaluation prior to bisphosphonate therapy is recommended due to high incidence of osteonecrosis of the jaw
Bone pain	2. Palliative low-dose involved field radiation therapy (10–30 Gy) 3. Pain management: opioids
Bone fractures	1. Spinal compression fractures: vertebroplasty, kyphoplasty 2. Spinal cord compression: high-dose dexamethasone; immediate referral for radiotherapy or surgery 3. Nonweight-bearing bones: radiotherapy 4. Fractures of long bones of arms and legs: surgical fixation
Anemia	Erythropoietin (not recommended in patients on thalidomide or lenalidomide therapy due to increase risk of blood clots)
Hypercalcemia	1. Hydration/furosemide 2. Bisphosphonates 3. Steroids 4. Calcitonin
Renal disease	1. Hydration 2. Plasmapheresis 3. Renal replacement therapy 4. Avoid IV contrast, NSAIDs, nephrotoxins
Hyperviscosity	1. Plasmapheresis
Infections	1. Vaccination: Pneumovax and influenza 2. Herpes Zoster prophylaxis in patients on Bortezomib 3. PCP and fungal prophylaxis: consider in patients on high-dose steroids 4. Intravenous monthly immunoglobulin for recurrent life-threatening infections

Table 43.5 (Cont.)

Coagulopathy/thrombosis	1. Anticoagulation prophylaxis is recommended in patients on thalidomide-based therapy • Therapeutic dose warfarin • Lovenox 40 mg2/day 2. Full anticoagulation therapy is recommended in patients on lenalidomide + pulse dose dexamethasone (high-dose dexamethasone), or in patients at high risk of developing a blood clot. Daily aspirin is recommended in patients on lenalidomide 9 weekly dexamethasone (low-dose dexamethasone)
Peripheral neuropathy	1. Discontinuation or dose reduction of drugs causing peripheral neuropathy • Thalidomide • Bortezomib • Cisplatin • Vincristine 2. Pain medications • Opioids • Antidepressants • Antiepileptics • Vitamin B complex, folic acid, magnesium tablets • Local anesthetic injections 3. Transcutaneous electric nerve stimulation (TENS)

Further reading

Attal M, Harousseau JL, Stoppa AM, et al. (1996). A prospective, randomized trial of autologous bone marrow transplantation and chemotherapy in multiple myeloma: Intergroupe Français du Myelome. *N Engl J Med* 335:91–97.

Barlogie B, Shaughnessy J, Epstein J, et al. (2006). Plasma cell myeloma. In Lichtman MA (ed.). *Williams Hematology*. 7th ed. New York: McGraw-Hill, pp. 1501–1533.

International Myeloma Working Group (2003). Criteria for the diagnosis of monoclonal gammopathies, multiple myeloma and related disorders: a report of the International Myeloma Working Group. *Br J Haematol* 121:749–757.

Greipp PR, San Miguel J, Durie B, et al. (2005). International staging system for multiple myeloma. *J Clin Oncol* 23:3412–3420.

NCCN Clinical Practice Guidelines in Oncology V.1.2008.

Chapter 44

Malignant lymphoma

Anne W. Beaven
Louis F. Diehl

Hodgkin lymphoma (HL) 768
Non-Hodgkin lymphomas (NHL) 774
Non-Hodgkin lymphomas and acquired
    immunodeficiency disorder 786

Hodgkin lymphoma (HL)

Epidemiology
Hodgkin lymphoma has a bimodal age distribution with a peak at ages 15–34 and over 60. The incidence varies with age and gender. The incidence rates per 100,000 population per year are 2.81 for males and 2.39 for females ages 15–34, and 3.34 for males and 2.90 for females age >60. In developing countries there is a higher frequency of childhood cases.

Risk factors
HL is clearly associated with EBV and HIV. Other associations, except for higher income and education level, are controversial (see Table 44.1).

Pathology
Traditionally, Hodgkin lymphoma has been divided into four subtypes (see Box 44.1). Recent biological and clinical evidence has refined this into two distinct subgroups:
- Classical Hodgkin lymphoma (nodular sclerosis, mixed cellularity, lymphocyte-rich classic HL, lymphocyte depleted)
- Nodular lymphocyte-predominant Hodgkin lymphoma (NLPHL)

The differences between the two types are listed in Table 44.2.

Table 44.1 Possible associations with HL

Seasonality	February, March
Clusters	Equivocal
Socioeconomic status	Better educated, higher income
Epstein-Barr virus	3-fold increase in young adults with seropositive infectious mononucleosis
Human immunodeficiency virus	Increase varies, 2.5- to 39-fold
Human herpes virus 6	Controversial
Occupation (teachers, woodworkers)	Controversial
Exposures (benzene, herbicides, pesticides)	Controversial
Familial	Aggregation HLA A1, B5, B18

Box 44.1 WHO classification of HL

Classical Hodgkin lymphoma
Nodular sclerosis classical HL (NSCHL) (50%)
Mixed cellularity classical HL (MCHL) (30%–40%)
Lymphocyte-rich classical HL (LRCHL)
Lymphocyte-depleted classical HL (LDHL) (rare)

Table 44.2 Differences between NLPHL and classical Hodgkin lymphoma

	Nodular lymphocyte-predominant Hodgkin lymphoma	Classical Hodgkin lymphoma
Reed-Sternberg cell	L & H cells (large cells, one large nucleus, scant cytoplasm)	Large cells, abundant cytoplasm, two large nuclei, one nucleolus
Background	Small lymphocytes, histiocytes	Lymphocytes, plasma cells, eosinophils, sclerosing bands
CD30	(−)	(+)
CD15	(−)	(+/−)
CD45	(+)	(−)
CD20	(+)	(−/+)

Staging

Traditionally, complete staging of HL involved an exploratory laparotomy with splenectomy plus liver and lymph node biopsy. Due to the complications associated with surgery, the improved radiographic imaging modalities available, and the increased use of chemotherapy, surgical staging is now rarely performed. Currently, the evaluation and staging of HL is identical to that used in non-Hodgkin lymphoma (Box 44.2).

Box 44.2 Ann Arbor staging system for HL and NHL

Stage	Feature
I	Disease in a single lymph node region
II	Disease in two or more regions on the same side of the diaphragm
III	Disease in two or more regions on both sides of the diaphragm
IV	Diffuse or disseminated disease in extralymphatic sites including liver and bone marrow

Various suffixes are added to each anatomical stage:

- A: No systemic symptoms
- B: Systemic symptoms present
- E: Extranodal disease

Clinical subtypes

Nodular lymphocyte-predominant Hodgkin lymphoma is a distinct clinical and pathological entity that is usually limited stage and has a longer survival than classical HL. It typically behaves in a more indolent fashion with relapses that can occur many years later.

Patients with classical Hodgkin lymphoma usually present with asymptomatic lymph node enlargement confined to one to two lymph node areas. Symptoms occur in 40%. Mediastinal masses, possibly quite large, occur predominantly in nodular sclerosis. Abdominal involvement is slightly more common with mixed cellularity.

The hallmark of Hodgkin lymphoma is that it systematically spreads from one lymph node group to the adjacent lymph node group. The differences between the clinical presentation of classical HL and NLPHL are depicted in Table 44.3.

Table 44.3 Differences between classical Hodgkin lymphoma and NLPHL

	Classic Hodgkin lymphoma		NLPHL
	Early stage	Advanced stage	All stages
Age >50	23%	21%	18%
Male	61%	61%	74%
Stage I	12%		53%
Stage II	46%		28%
Stage III	29%		14%
Stage IV	13%		6%
B symptoms	26%	71%	10%
Mediastinal mass	70%	67%	7%
Bulky disease	21%	22%	13%
Spleen	0	57%	8%
Liver	0	12%	3%
Bone marrow	0	13%	1%
Lung	0	14%	1%

Prognosis

Overall survival for early-stage patients

The 10-year overall survival for patients with stage I or II Hodgkin lymphoma is over 85%. Patients are considered high risk if they have elevated ESR, large mediastinal mass, involvement of >3 nodal areas, or extranodal disease. Male gender, age >50 and B symptoms have also been associated with a worse prognosis.

Overall survival for advanced-stage patients

International prognostic score

For patients with advanced (stage IIB to IVB) disease, seven prognostic factors have been identified in an analysis of over 5000 patients treated conventionally (see Box 44.3).

Malignant lymphoma

> **Box 44.3 International Prognostic Score for advanced HL**
> Albumin <4.0 g/dL
> Hemoglobin <10.5 g/L
> Male gender
> Age > 45 years
> Lymphocyte count <0.6 x 10^9/L or 8% of WCC
> White cell count (WCC) > 15 x 10^9/L
> Stage IV
>
> In the absence of any adverse factors, the 5-year failure-free survival (FFS) rate is 84%. The presence of each of these factors reduces the expected 5-year FFS by ~7%. Having three or more factors is generally considered a poor prognostic group.

The 5-year freedom from progression ranges from 84% in patients with no risk factors to only 42% for patients with ≥5 factors.

Management

Early stage (IA and IIA)

The standard treatment of stage I or II classical Hodgkin lymphoma involves chemotherapy plus involved field (IF) radiation therapy. Most patients with good prognosis early-stage HL treated outside a clinical trial are offered 2 courses of standard ABVD (adriamycin, bleomycin, vinblastine, dacarbazine) chemotherapy, followed by IF radiotherapy. Patients with poor prognosis early-stage HL usually receive 4 cycles of ABVD followed by higher doses of radiotherapy.

Patients with very favorable stage IA NLPHL or NSCHL involving the high cervical region and a low ESR are at very low risk of occult subdiaphragmatic disease and may be treated with IF radiotherapy alone. Patients with early-stage disease but poor prognostic features would be treated like those with advanced disease in many centers.

Advanced stage

Advanced-stage disease is treated with chemotherapy alone or with the addition of radiation in patients with bulky disease at diagnosis or areas of residual disease after chemotherapy.

ABVD is the chemotherapy regimen most frequently used in the United States, but many other regimens are available:
- MOPP (nitrogen mustard, vincristine, procarbazine, and prednisone)
- BEACOPP (bleomycin, etoposide, doxorubicin, cyclophosphamide, vincristine, procarbazine, and prednisolone)
- Stanford V (nitrogen mustard, doxorubicin, vinblastine, prednisone, vincristine, bleomycin, and etoposide combined with radiation)

Lymphocyte-predominant HL

Advanced stage LPHL is typically treated with ABVD, sometimes with the addition of rituximab. For limited stage disease acceptable treatment options include observation in fully resected disease, radiation, rituximab or chemotherapy.

Salvage therapy

At the time of relapse, patients with limited disease or an initial remission lasting >12 months may be treated with radiation and a different chemotherapy regimen than that used initially.

In higher-risk patients or those in second relapse, autologous stem cell transplantation can lead to long-term survival in over 50% of patients.

Late effects

Given the young age of the typical HL patient at diagnosis, the long overall survival, and use of radiation fields often involving the mediastinum, patients are at risk of developing long-term sequelae from therapy:
- Coronary artery disease
- Congestive heart failure
- Secondary malignancies
- Hypothyroidism

Intercurrent deaths (disease other than HL) are significantly higher than for an age-matched population, indicating that the treatment of HL results in an increase in heart disease and second malignancies.

Analysis of late effects after HL shows that at 30-year follow-up, twice as many patients have died from second cancers and heart disease as from relapsed HL. Careful screening for these complications should begin 5–10 years after therapy. The alkylating agents are associated with secondary myelodysplasia, AML, and NHL, as well as infertility.

Recognition of long-term toxicity associated with prior radiation therapy, particularly to the mediastinum (second malignancies, including lung and breast cancer; pulmonary fibrosis; coronary artery disease), has led to a major reevaluation of the use of extensive radiotherapy. In recent years, research has demonstrated that lower doses of radiation are equally effective and it is likely that this will lead to decreased long-term treatment related morbidity and mortality.

The ultimate aim must be to maintain high cure rates but reduce long-term toxicity, especially in early-stage disease.

Non-hodgkin lymphomas (NHL)

The non-Hodgkin lymphomas (NHL) are a diverse group of diseases, all arising from the lymphoid arm of the immune system, ranging from relatively benign diseases with more than a 20-year survival to diseases from which the majority of patients die within 6 months.

Incidence

There are approximately 70,000 new cases of NHL diagnosed in the United States each year.

The incidence has doubled in the last three decades, and currently occurs at a rate of 19 cases per 100,000 population per year.

- 50% higher in males than females
- 35% higher in whites than African Americans
- 40% higher in urban counties than in rural counties.

Risk factors

Figure 44.1 depicts the incidence with age of the common NHL subtypes.

Although the pathogenesis of most of NHL is unknown, identified risk factors can be divided into the five categories depicted in Table 44.4.

Classification of non-hodgkin lymphomas

The pathologic classification of the non-Hodgkin lymphomas has evolved from two subcategories in the Gall-Mallory (1941) classification to more than 40 separate categories in the WHO classification.

Today's classifications depend on morphology, clinical aspects, flow cytometry, cytogenetics, and molecular studies. The pathological classification presently used is the WHO classification (see Box 44.4).

Table 44.5 presents the most common forms according to immunophenotype and cytogenetics.

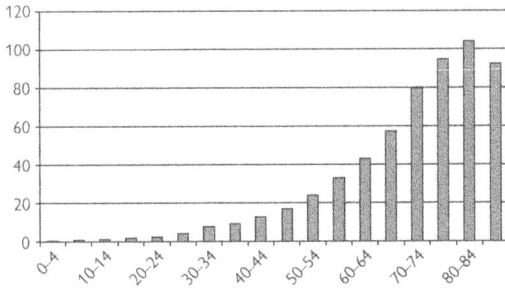

Figure 44.1 Incidence of NHL, by age. Adapted from SEER data.

Table 44.4 Five categories of risk factors for NHL

Chemical agents	Immune stimulation	Immuno-suppression	Infectious agents	Contro-versial
• Pesticide (organophosphates, phenoxyacetic acid, chlorophenols) • Solvents (benzene, butadiene, carbon tetrachloride) • Wood preservatives (creosote, pentachlorophenol) • Drugs (alkylating agents)	• Rheumatoid arthritis • Sjögren's syndrome • Systemic lupus erythematosis	• Organ transplant • HIV/AIDS	• EBV • HTLV-I • *Helicobacter pylori* • *Chlamydia psittacosis* • *Campylobacter jejuni* • Hepatitis C	• Diet high in animal protein • Cigarette smoking • Hair-coloring products

Box 44.4 WHO classification of NHL

B-cell lymphoma
Precursor B-cell neoplasms
Precursor B-lymphoblastic leukemia/lymphoma

Mature B-NHL
Small lymphocytic lymphoma (lymphomatous manifestation of chronic lymphocytic leukemia)
Lymphoplasmacytic lymphoma
Splenic marginal zone lymphoma
Extranodal marginal zone lymphoma of mucosa-associated lymphoid tissue (MALT-lymphoma)
Nodal marginal zone lymphoma
Follicular lymphoma
Mantle cell lymphoma
Diffuse large B-cell lymphoma
Mediastinal (thymic) large B-cell lymphoma
Intravascular large B-cell lymphoma
Primary effusion lymphoma
Burkitt lymphoma/leukemia

T-cell and NK-cell lymphoma
Precursor T-cell neoplasm
Precursor T-lymphoblastic lymphoma/leukemia

Mature T-cell and NK-cell neoplasm

Cutaneous
Mycosis fungoides
Sézary syndrome
Primary cutaneous anaplastic large cell lymphoma
Lymphomatoid papulosis

Extranodal
Extranodal NK/T-cell lymphoma, nasal type
Enteropathy-associated T-cell lymphoma
Hepatosplenic T-cell lymphoma
Subcutaneous panniculitis-like T-cell lymphoma

Nodal
Angioimmunoblastic T-cell lymphoma
Anaplastic large T-cell lymphoma
Peripheral T-cell lymphoma, unspecified

Leukemic
T-cell prolymphocytic leukemia
T-cell large granular lymphocytic leukemia
Aggressive NK-cell leukemia
Adult T-cell leukemia/lymphoma

Table 44.5 Most common forms of NHL by immunophenotype and cytogenetics

Disease	TdT	CD20	CD10	CD5	CD23	SIg	CD2 CD7	CD4 CD8	Cytogenetic	Gene express
Burkitt	–	+	+	–	–	+	–	–	t(8;14) t(2;8) t(8;22)	c-myc
LBL B-cell	+	+	+	–	–	CIg+	–	–	t(4;11) t(9;22)	Ph1 AF4/MLL
LBL T-cell	+	–	–	–	–	–	+ +	+/–	14q 7q	T-cell receptor
DLC B-cell	–	+	+/–	–	–	50%	–	–	–	–
Anaplastic large cell	–	–	–	–	–	–	–	+	t(2;5)	ALK
Peripheral T-cell	–	–	–	–	–	–	+ +/–	+ 17%	–	–
Follicular	–	+	+	–	–(+)	+	–	–	t(14;18)	Bcl-2

Table 44.5 (Cont.)

Disease	Immunophenotype							Cytogenetic	Gene express
	TdT	CD 20	CD 10	CD 5	CD 23	SIg	CD2 CD7	CD4 CD8		
SLL	–	+	–	+	+	Dim	–	–	Trisomy 12 Del 13	–
Mantle cell	–	+	–	+	–	+	–	–	t(11;14)	bcl-1
Marginal zone	–	+	–	–	–	+	–	–		
MALT	–	+	–	–	–	CIg+	–	–	t(1;14) t(11;18)	bcl-10 API-2
Lymphoplasmacytic	–	–	–	–	–	–	+ +/–	+ 17%	t(9;14)	PAX-5

LBL, lymphoblastic lymphoma; DLCBC, diffuse large cell B cell; SLL, small lymphocytic lymphoma; MALT, mucosa associated lymphoid tissue lymphoma; sIg, surface Ig; cIg, cytoplasmic Ig.

Clinical features and staging of non-hodgkin lymphomas

Clinical features
See Table 44.6

The majority of adult patients (60%–70%) present with nodal disease, whereas most children present with extranodal disease.

Critical elements of the history include the following:
- Drenching night sweats in the past month
- Recurrent fevers >38°
- Weight loss >10% over the prior 6 months

Eastern Cooperative Oncology Group Performance Status (ECOG PS)
- 0 = full activity
- 1 = restricted in physically strenuous activity but able to do light work
- 2 = ambulatory and able to do self-care but cannot do any work activities for >50% of waking hours
- 3 = limited self-care and 50% of waking hours in bed
- 4 = completely disabled, no self-care, confined to bed or chair.

For clinical management and treatment decision-making, the NHL can be divided into three types:
- Aggressive
- Intermediate
- Indolent

Malignant lymphoma

Table 44.6 Clinical aspects of major NHL diseases

	Disease	Median age	B symptoms	Stage				Extra nodal		
				I	II	III	IV	Any	BM	GI
Aggressive	Burkitt's	31	22	37	25	0	38	78	33	11
	LBL	28	21	0	11	14	75	82	50	4
Intermediate	DLC B-cell	64	33	25	29	13	33	71	16	118
	Anaplastic large cell	34	53	19	32	10	39	59	13	9
	Peripheral T-cell	61	50	8	12	15	61	82	36	15
Indolent	Follicular	59	28	18	15	16	51	64	42	4
	SLL	65	33	4	5	8	83	80	72	3
	Mantle cell	63	28	13	7	9	71	81	64	9
	MALT	60	19%	39	28	2	31	98	14	50
	Marginal zone, nodal	58	37%	13	13	34	40	47	32	5
	Lymphoplasmacytic	63	13%	7	13	7	73	100	73	7

Staging

See Table 44.7

Once a pathological diagnosis of lymphoma has been made through biopsy of a lymph node or an involved extranodal site, a thorough evaluation is undertaken. The physical examination should pay particular attention to lymphadenopathy and splenomegaly.

Laboratory tests include a complete blood count (CBC) with differential, creatinine, bilirubin, alkaline phosphatase, AST, ALT, calcium, uric acid, B_2-microglobulin, and serum lactate dehydrogenase (LDH).

A bone marrow biopsy is necessary for staging.

A lumbar puncture is sent for protein, glucose, cell count, cytology, and flow cytometry for patients with neurologic symptoms, patients with intermediate-grade NHL with risk factors (sinus, testicular, or bone marrow involvement) or with high-grade lymphoma such as Burkitt or lymphoblastic lymphoma.

Radiographic studies include CT scan of the chest, abdomen, and pelvis and a PET scan.

Medical emergencies associated with NHL include the following:
- Mediastinal obstruction
- Obstructive nephropathy
- Spinal cord compression
- Hypercalcemia
- Other metabolic derangements

Patients may develop bone marrow failure from lymphomatous involvement, and low-grade NHL can cause immune-mediated hemolysis or thrombocytopenia.

Table 44.7 International Prognostic Index for NHL

Diffuse large cell B-cell lymphoma					
Pre-rituximab				Revised IPI in rituximab era	
All ages		Age ≤ 60		All ages	
Risk factors	5-year OS	Risk factors	5-year OS	Risk factors	4-year OS
0–1	73%	0	83%	0	94%
2	52%	1	69%	1–2	79%
3	43%	2	46%	3–5	55%
4–5	26%	3	32%		

Prognosis

International prognostic index (high-grade non-hodgkin lymphomas)
The International Prognostic Index (IPI) provides prognostic information on patients based on the presence or absence of five risk factors:
- Age >60 years
- Stage III or IV
- Number of extranodal sites >1
- Elevated LDH
- ECOG performance status ≥2

While the initial IPI was created prior to the use of rituximab, it still appears to offer valuable prognostic information (see Table 44.7).

Follicular lymphoma international prognostic index

Similar to the IPI for aggressive lymphomas, five prognostic risk factors have been identified for follicular lymphoma (follicular lymphoma IPI, or FLIPI) (see Table 44.8):
- Age >60 years
- Stage III or IV
- Elevated LDH
- Hemoglobin <12.0 g/dL
- Involvement of >4 nodal areas

Outcomes have improved with the addition of rituximab and a second generation FLIPI2 score was developed (see Table 44.8). The five prognostic factors for the post rituximab era are as follows:
- β_2 microglobulin > upper limits of normal
- Hemoglobin <12
- Age >60
- Largest Lymph node diameter >6 cm
- + Bone marrow involvement

Table 44.8 International Prognostic Index for follicular lymphoma

Follicular lymphoma				
FLIPI (Pre-rituximab)			FLIPI2 (rituximab era)	
Risk factors	5-year OS	10 year OS	Risk Factors	5-year OS
0–1	90.6%	70.7%	0	98%
2	77.6%	50.9%	1–2	88%
3–5	52.5%	35.5%	>3	77%

Gene expression profiling

Although the IPI and FLIPI provide useful prognostic information, even within different risk groups, there is significant clinical heterogeneity, with some good-risk patients progressing rapidly and poor-risk patients living for many years.

Recently, the use of microarrays to develop gene-expression profiles has provided additional prognostic information for follicular lymphoma and DLBCL. Through gene expression profiling, DLBCL can be subclassified into "activated" and "germinal-center" B-cell types. Patients with the germinal-center B-cell type of DLBCL have a significantly superior overall survival.

In follicular lymphomas different molecular features of nonmalignant tumor infiltrating cells correlate with length of survival.

These and other tests still under development are coming into increasing use and will eventually have an important role in directing patient care.

Management strategies

Low-grade non-hodgkin lymphoma

Despite recent advances, such as the addition of rituximab to therapeutic regimens, there is no known cure for low-grade lymphomas. Early intervention does not provide a survival advantage.

Treatment is typically delayed until the following occur:
- Rapidly progressive disease
- Organ impairment
- Disease-related symptoms

The only exception to this rule is for the small number of patients with stage I disease for whom involved field radiotherapy may offer the chance of prolonged disease free survival.

Initial treatment

Once treatment is instituted, the mainstay of therapy is a combination of chemotherapy and the monoclonal anti-CD20 antibody rituximab (R).

Younger patients or those with many symptoms may begin treatment with a multiagent regimen such as R-bendamustine, R-CHOP or R-CVP (rituximab, cyclophosphamide, vincristine, prednisone, doxorubicin,) and occasionally R-FC (rituximab, fludarabine, cyclophosphamide); there is no known advantage of one regimen over the other.

Older patients or those with few symptoms may begin treatment with single-agent rituximab.

Maintenance rituximab is well tolerated and improves the progression free survival, so this is occasionally administered every 2-3 months for 2 years after completing chemotherapy. Consolidation with radioimmunotherapy is an alternative approach.

Treatment of relapsed disease

At the time of relapse, depending on the length of the first remission, treatment may consist of the following:
- Retreatment with the initial chemotherapy
- A new regimen may be used if the first duration was short.
- The patient may move toward a form of stem cell transplantation.

Other treatment options include the following:
- Other purine analogues
- 2-chlorodeoxyadenosine (2-CdA)
- Pentostatin
- Radiolabeled anti-CD20 antibodies
- Retreatment with rituximab
- Lenalidomide

When possible, patients with relapsed low-grade lymphoma should be enrolled in clinical trials.

Important questions that still need to be answered include:
- Long-term benefit of maintenance rituximab therapy versus re-treatment
- Potential of cure with allogeneic stem cell transplantation

Aggressive lymphomas (diffuse large B-cell lymphoma)

Initial treatment

Initial therapy for DLBCL requires 6–8 cycles of chemotherapy with the R-CHOP regimen given every 14-21 days.

Patients with limited disease may be treated with fewer cycles of R-CHOP (usually 3 cycles) followed by involved field radiation therapy.

Maintenance therapy with rituximab has no demonstrated benefit in the management of DLBCL.

Treatment of relapsed disease

Patients with relapsed DLBCL should be treated with a salvage chemotherapy regimen followed by high-dose chemotherapy and autologous stem cell transplantation.

There is no proven role for transplantation outside of the relapsed setting.

Highly aggressive lymphomas (Burkitt lymphoma, lymphoblastic lymphoma)

Burkitt lymphoma, endemic
- Endemic in equatorial Africa
- 90% associated with EBV infection.
- Young adults and children, present with head and neck tumors

Burkitt lymphoma, nonendemic
- NHL is associated with EBV in approximately 20%.
- Abdominal disease is more common.
- Associated with HIV infection

Lymphoblastic lymphoma
- Presents with or without leukemia
- More common in children than adults
- Most often T-cell type, typically featuring a mediastinal mass and pleural effusion

Treatment

Highly aggressive lymphomas such as Burkitt lymphoma and lymphoblastic lymphoma are treated with intensive chemotherapy regimens similar to those used in the treatment of acute lymphoblastic leukemia. Due to the high risk of CNS involvement, CNS prophylaxis with intrathecal chemotherapy is an important part of therapy.

Although not required in the treatment of Burkitt lymphoma, maintenance therapy with 6-mercaptopurine, methotrexate, vincristine, and dexamethasone is required for several years after completion of chemotherapy for lymphoblastic lymphoma.

Non-hodgkin lymphoma and acquired immunodeficiency disorder

Non-Hodgkin lymphoma is the second most common malignancy to affect those with AIDS.

Epidemiology and etiology

The risk of a person with HIV developing lymphoma is 60–160 times greater than in the seronegative population. The incidence of systemic NHL increases with worsening immunosuppression.

Almost half of patients will previously have had an AIDS-defining illness. NHL also has a higher incidence among individuals who are immunocompromised for other reasons.

There is a close association between the development of NHL in AIDS and infection with EBV. EBV proteins can be demonstrated in ≥50% of lymphomas, particularly immunoblastic and large cell lymphomas.

It is thought that the proliferation of EBV-infected cells in the immune-deficient host may proceed unchecked.

Oncogenic mutations have also been identified, e.g., in the *p53* tumor suppressor gene and *c-myc* gene.

Presentation

- Typically seen in advanced HIV infection (CD4 ≤100 μ/L)
- Frequently involves extranodal sites
- Approximately 80% have stage IV disease at presentation, e.g., involving the GI tract, bone marrow, CNS, liver, or recurrent effusions.
- Constitutional "B" symptoms are common.

Pathology

- ~80% of AIDS-associated NHL is high grade.
- ≥90% of cases are diffuse large B-cell (immunoblastic subtype) or Burkitt-like lymphoma.

Poor prognostic factors

- Prior AIDS-defining diagnosis or CD4 count <100 μ/L
- Karnofsky performance score <70
- Age >35 years
- Extranodal disease including bone marrow involvement
- Elevated LDH
- Immunoblastic subtype

Management

Management should be coordinated in a center with both HIV and hematology/oncology expertise. Concomitant HAART reduces the incidence of opportunistic infections and may improve survival.

Although, potentially curative local treatments can be considered for patients presenting with stage I or II NHL, the vast majority of patients with AIDS-associated NHL present with stage IV disease and require systemic therapy.

Treatment is with combination chemotherapy (see Non-Hodgkin lymphoma, Treatment, p. 770). However, more intensive chemotherapy regimens tend to be poorly tolerated, partly due to baseline immunodeficiency and reduced bone marrow reserve.

The role of rituximab has not been fully defined in this population, with no phase III data yet supporting its use, and evidence to suggest it may decrease CD4 counts, increase viral load, and increase infectious deaths.

Leptomeningeal involvement requires intrathecal chemotherapy usually with methotrexate and cytarabine. Intrathecal prophylaxis should be considered in those at high risk of meningeal involvement (e.g., patients with Burkitt lymphoma, paraspinal or paranasal disease, or bone marrow infiltration) or patients with EBV detected in their CSF.

Response rates to treatment and time to progression are less in patients with AIDS than in seronegative patients treated for lymphomas of similar histology.

Chapter 45

Cancer of unknown primary

Gary H. Lyman

Clinical presentation 790
Initial workup 791
Metastases to lymph nodes and peritoneum 792
Metastases to other sites 794
Malignant pleural effusion 795
Etiology, pathology, and clinical presentation of cancer of unknown primary 796
Management of cancer of unknown primary 798

Clinical presentation

Cancer of unknown primary (CUP) is a common problem in oncology, representing up to 10% of all new diagnoses.

The priority is to
- Exclude potentially curable malignancies, e.g., germ cells, lymphomas, thyroid cancer
- Identify specific clinical syndromes that predict responsiveness to therapy, e.g., squamous cell carcinoma metastatic to cervical lymph nodes treated as advanced head and neck cancer
- Perform investigations that will change management

Initial workup

Initial evaluation
Before accepting the diagnosis of cancer of unknown primary, it is important that every patient undergo the following:
- A thorough history, including detailed family history
- Full physical examination, including pelvic, breast, and rectal examination
- Appropriate additional investigations, including, at a minimum:
  - CBC
  - Serum biochemistry including liver function tests (LFTs)
  - Chest X-ray
  - Ultrasound or CT of the abdomen

Further investigations, including tumor markers, will depend on the clinical scenario. Common tumor markers, e.g., CA 125, CA 15–3, CEA, and CA 19–9, have only a limited role in diagnosis and prognosis.

Immunohistochemistry
Immunohistochemical analysis is essential when germ cells or lymphoma are possibilities. The initial panel of stains is likely to use antibodies to the following:
- Carcinoembryonic antigen (CEA)
- Prostate-specific antigen (PSA)
- Cytokeratin
- Vimentin
- Common leukocyte antigen (CLA): carcinoma vs. lymphoma (see Table 45.1).

ER/PR staining should be requested if presentation is compatible with metastatic breast cancer.

Electron microscopy
This is useful for distinguishing lymphoma from carcinoma. It can sometimes assist in identifying neuroendocrine tumors, melanomas, and poorly differentiated sarcomas.

Table 45.1 Site-specific immunohistochemical stains

Stain	Tumor
Common leukocyte antigen (CLA)	Lymphoma
B- & T-cell gene rearrangement	Non-Hodgkin's lymphoma
Prostate-specific antigen (PSA)	Prostate
Thyroglobulin	Thyroid

Metastases to lymph nodes and peritoneum

Metastases to lymph nodes are more common than presentation with visceral or bony metastases.

Axillary lymph nodes in women
Metastatic adenocarcinoma in axillary lymph nodes may indicate an occult breast cancer, even with a negative mammogram. MRI of the breasts should be considered if the mammogram is normal.
- ER/PR staining should be performed on the biopsy sample.
- In the absence of distant metastatic disease, locoregional therapy with surgical excision and radiation and chemotherapy should be given.
- Such patients are potentially curable.

Cervical lymph nodes
Squamous or undifferentiated carcinoma in cervical lymph nodes must be referred for full ENT examination under anesthesia with biopsy of the naso-, oro-, and hypopharynx. PET scanning may also have a role.
- Radical locoregional radiotherapy can result in median survivals of several years, particularly when the nodes are high in the neck.
- Thyroid cancer can be excluded by staining for thyroglobulin.
- Supraclavicular lymph node metastases are usually associated with widespread malignancy and have a poor prognosis.

Inguinal lymph nodes
Careful examination of most patients with squamous cell carcinoma in inguinal nodes will demonstrate a detectable primary site in the anorectal or genital region.
- Digital rectal examination, proctoscopy, and examination of the penis or vulva, vagina, or cervix should be performed.
- Small anal cancers remain potentially curable despite local lymph node involvement. Treatment often includes inguinal node dissection and combined-modality treatment with chemoradiotherapy.
- Primary skin cancer should also be considered.

Retroperitoneal or mediastinal lymph nodes in men
Elevated serum human chorionic gonadotropin (hCG) and α-fetoprotein (AFP) may suggest a germ cell origin.
- Poorly differentiated adenocarcinoma with feature of extragonadal germ cell malignancy is treated as non-seminomatous extragonadal germ cell malignancy with curative intent.
- Platinum-based chemotherapy should be considered and is often associated with an excellent response, even in the absence of histological confirmation of germ cell cancer or elevated serum tumor markers.

Peritoneal carcinomatosis in women

Adenocarcinoma with diffuse peritoneal disease has a gynecological origin in 55% of cases, most likely from ovaries. Other possibilities include primary peritoneal disease (which occurs more commonly in women with *BRCA1* mutations), the GI tract (particularly if mucin-secreting), and breast.
- Serum CA 125 and pelvic ultrasound may be useful but are not specific.
- A trial of platinum-based chemotherapy with palliative intent may be pragmatic and good responses can be achieved.
- Debulking surgery should be considered if disease is large volume.
- Malignant ascites in women, even without evidence of solid disease, is treated as advanced ovarian cancer, often with long-term survival.

Metastases to other sites

Lung
Primary disease commonly metastasizing to the lung includes head and neck squamous cell carcinoma, and breast, kidney, and large bowel cancer. These are identified on chest X-ray or CT of the thorax.

Bronchoscopy is used for central lesions with brushings, and biopsy for visible tumor or washings if tumor is not visible. Lymph nodes may be accessible by transbronchial needle aspiration.

Perform CT- or ultrasound-guided percutaneous biopsy for peripheral lesions. Sputum cytology provides a low yield.

Immunohistochemistry may help identify primary disease:
- CK-7: lung or breast
- CK-20: colorectal
- TTF-1: lung (surfactant apoprotein)
- CK-7 *and* TTP-1 positive are 94% specific for lung primary

PET may be useful for staging particularly if a lung primary is suspected or if the primary is not identified on CT.

Resection of solitary metastases occasionally produces long-term survivors, e.g., from colorectal/renal primaries.

Liver
Common primary sites include the GI tract and breast. They are usually identified on ultrasound or CT scan.

Completion of staging investigations is required to determine the extent of disease and any obvious primary disease.

Biopsy under image guidance after correction of coagulation is usually needed if treatment is to be considered.

Liver resection, often with preoperative chemotherapy, can sometimes be considered for solitary or limited adjacent hepatic metastases with a resectable colorectal primary in the absence of disease elsewhere.

If the patient appears disproportionately well for the volume of liver disease, consider atypical diagnoses such as neuroendocrine tumors, e.g., carcinoid.

Bone
If adenocarcinoma appears on biopsy, common primary sites include lung, prostate, breast, and, less frequently, kidney and thyroid.

Measure PSA in men with metastases predominantly affecting bone. Biopsy tissue may also stain for PSA in stage IV prostate cancer.

Brain
Metastases are the most common form of intracranial tumor. Common potential primary sites include lung, breast, and melanoma.

Prognosis is often dictated by the extent of extracranial disease.

Malignant pleural effusion

Etiology

If the effusion is a transudate, other diagnoses to consider include congestive cardiac failure, constrictive pericarditis, hypoalbuminemia, and nephrotic syndrome.

The differential diagnosis of an undiagnosed exudative effusion includes the following:
- Infection, e.g., bacterial pneumonia, tuberculosis
- Pulmonary embolism
- Inflammatory disorders, e.g., sarcoidosis, pancreatitis
- Metabolic causes, e.g., hypothyroidism

Malignancy is more likely to be the cause if
- The patient is older.
- There are other risk factors, e.g., smoking, past history of asbestos exposure.
- Effusion is an exudate.

Malignant causes include the following:
- Metastatic carcinoma, e.g., breast or lung primary
- Lymphoma
- Mesothelioma
- Leukemia
- Chylothorax
- Meigs' syndrome (ovarian fibroma, ascites, pleural effusion)
- Paraproteinemia, e.g., multiple myeloma

Evaluation

- CT chest to assess for thoracic lymphadenopathy, pulmonary or pleural primary, or metastatic disease.
- Fluid for cytology
- Percutaneous pleural biopsy via image guidance under local anesthesia
  - Low sensitivity for malignant mesothelioma
- Thoracoscopy is more sensitive, particularly for malignant causes of effusions.
- Open pleural biopsy is occasionally necessary.
- Bronchoscopy is rarely helpful unless the patient has imaging to suggest a parenchymal lesion or symptoms suggestive of intrabronchial pathology, e.g., hemoptysis.

Etiology, pathology, and clinical presentation of cancer of unknown primary

Etiology and pathology

An undetected primary site is most likely due to metastatic potential of the tumor. Occasionally there has been regression of the primary, e.g., as well recognized in melanoma. Primary disease may remain undetected even after postmortem examination (25%).

The pattern of metastatic disease is often very different from cases in which the primary site is known, e.g., lung cancer causes bone metastases 10 times more often when the primary site is known than when the lung cancer is occult.

Mean age at diagnosis is 60 years. CUP is a common cancer presentation in those ≥70 years old; it is rare in patients ≤40 years old.

A median survival of 4 months is seen in most series. However, some clinical scenarios are associated with much longer survival and it is these that are important to identify.

The diagnosis encompasses tumors from many primary sites with varying biology.

Five broad groups can be identified by light microscopy, which guides further investigation:
- Adenocarcinoma (60%–70%)
- Poorly differentiated carcinoma (20%–30%) can be confused with seminoma, amelanotic melanoma, and epidermal carcinoma.
- Undifferentiated malignancy (<5%) requires further staining to exclude lymphoma.
- Squamous carcinoma (<5%)
- Neuroendocrine carcinoma is uncommon. Most patients with metastatic small-cell anaplastic carcinoma have a bronchial primary identified either via CT thorax or on bronchoscopy.

Favorable prognostic factors
- Female sex
- Fewer sites of metastatic disease, especially lymph node or soft tissue rather than liver or bone.
- Good performance status
- Normal serum Lactic Acid Dehydrogenase (LDH)

Clinical presentation

Symptoms usually arise from the site of metastasis.

Management of cancer of unknown primary

The priority is to identify curable malignancies or clinical syndromes that respond well to specific therapy (see Fig. 45.1).

Select appropriate patients who may benefit from chemotherapy with palliative intent. This depends on specific tumor characteristics, including chemoresponsiveness and patient characteristics such as organ function and performance status.

There are relatively few randomized trials of chemotherapy in CUP.

Local treatment for symptomatic metastases should be considered, e.g., radiotherapy for painful bone metastases or for brain metastases.

Occasionally, only a single metastatic site of disease is identified despite full staging investigations. In most instances, other metastases become clinically evident within a short time. If no further disease is identified, resection should be considered, which can occasionally produce long disease-free intervals.

Empiric systemic therapy for unresponsive histologies and likely primary disease sites rarely yields net benefit to the patient.

Involvement of palliative care services is usually appropriate for all patients.

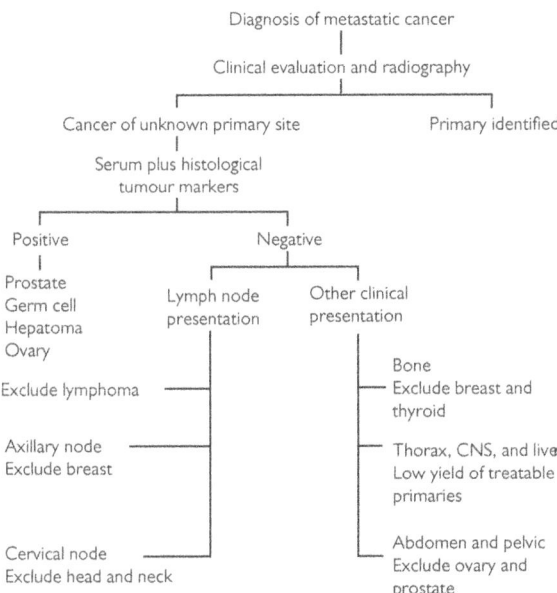

Figure 45.1 Identification of treatable cancer of unknown primary site. Reproduced with permission from Cassidy J, Bissett D, Spence RAJ (1995). *Oxford TextBook of Oncology*, 1st ed. Oxford: Oxford University Press.

Appendix

Karnofsky performance status

Box A.1 Karnofsky Performance Status

(%)	Performance
100	Normal, no evidence of disease
90	Able to carry on normal activity, minor signs or symptoms of disease
80	Normal activity with effort, some signs or symptoms of disease
70	Unable to perform normal activity, cares for self
60	Requires occasional assistance
50	Requires considerable assistance and frequent medical care
40	Disabled, requires special care and assistance
30	Severely disabled, hospitalization may be required
20	Hospitalization necessary for support, very sick
10	Moribund, rapid progression of disease
0	Dead

WHO performance criteria

Box A.2 WHO Performance Criteria

0 Normal activity
1 Symptoms but nearly fully ambulatory
2 Some bed time but needs to be in bed <50% of normal daytime
3 Needs to be in bed >50% of normal daytime
4 Unable to get out of bed

BSA nomogram

Nomogram for determination of body surface from height and mass

Nomogram for determination of body surface area. *Geigy Scientific Tables* (8th edn.) (ed. Lentner, C.) Ceiba Geigy Switzerland, 1981. Copyright © Novartis AG. Used by permission.

Dose adjustment of chemotherapeutic agents in hepatic failure

Table A.1 Dose adjustments of commonly used chemotherapeutic agents in hepatic failure

Drug	Dose modification (percentage reduction)	Bilirubin (mg/dL)	SGOT (mg/dL)	Alkaline phosphatase
Alemtuzumab	None	—	—	—
Amifostine	None	—	—	—
Arsenic trioxide	None 7	—	—	—
x-Asparaginase	Use caution	—	—	—
Bevacizumab	None	—	—	—
Bleomycin	None	—	—	—
Bortezomib	Use caution	—	—	—
Busulfan	None	—	—	—
Carboplatin	None	—	—	—
Carmustine	Use caution	—	—	—
Cisplatin	None	—	—	—
Cetuximab	None	—	—	—
Cladribine	None	—	—	—
Cyclophosphamide	25%	3.0–5.0	>180	—
Cyclophosphamide	Hold dose	>5.0	—	—
Cytarabine	Use caution	—	—	—
Dacarbazine	Use caution	—	—	—
Dactinomycin	50%	>3.0	—	—
Daunorubicin	25%	1.2–3.0	60–80	—
Daunorubicin	50%	>3.0	>180	—
Daunorubicin	Hold dose	>5.0	—	—
Docetaxel	Hold dose	>1.5	>60	>2.5 times ULN
Doxorubicin	50%	1.2–3.0	60–80	—
Doxorubicin	75%	3.1–5.0	>180	—
Doxorubicin	Hold dose	>5.0	—	—
Doxorubicin liposomal	50%	1.2–3.0	—	—

Table A.1 (Cont.)

Drug	Dose modification (percentage reduction)	Bilirubin (mg/dL)	SGOT (mg/dL)	Alkaline phosphatase
Doxorubicin liposomal	75%	3.1–5.0	—	—
Doxorubicin liposomal	Hold dose	>5.0	—	—
Epirubicin	50%	1.2–3.0	2–4 times ULN	—
Epirubicin	75%	>3.0	>4 times ULN	—
Etoposide	50%	1.5–3.0	60–180	—
Etoposide	Hold dose	>3.0	>180	—
Etoposide phosphate	50%	1.5–3.0	60–180	—
Etoposide phosphate	Hold dose	>3.0	>180	—
Fludarabine	None	—	—	—
5-Fluorouracil	Hold dose	>5.0	—	—
Gemcitabine	None	—	—	—
Idarubicin	25%	1.5–3.0	60–180	—
Idarubicin	50%	3.1–5.0	>180	—
Idarubicin	Hold dose	>5.0	—	—
Ifosfamide	Use caution	—	—	—
Irinotecan	Hold dose	>2.0	>3 times ULN	—
Mechlorethamine	None	—	—	—
Mesna	None	—	—	—
Methotrexate	25%	3.1–5.0	>180	—
Methotrexate	Hold dose	>5.0	—	—
Mitomycin	None	—	—	—
Mitoxantrone	25%	>3.0	—	—
Oxaliplatin	None	—	—	—
Paclitaxel	Hold dose	>5.0	>180 or 1.5 times ULN	—

Table A.1 (Cont.)

Drug	Dose modification (percentage reduction)	Bilirubin (mg/dL)	SGOT (mg/dL)	Alkaline phosphatase
Pemetrexed	Use caution	—	—	
Pentostatin	None	—		
Rituximab	None	—	—	
Streptozocin	Use caution	—	—	
Topotecan	None	—	—	
Trastuzumab	None	—		
Vinblastine	50%	>3.0	>180	
Vincristine	50%	1.5–3.0	60–180	
Vincristine	Hold dose	>3.0	>180	
Vinorelbine	50%	2.1–3.0	—	
Vinorelbine	75%	3.1–5.0	—	
Vinorelbine	Hold dose	>5.0	—	—

Govindan, Ramaswamy. The Washington Manual of Oncology 2nd ed. Lippincott, Williams and Wilkins, Philadelphia, 2007. Reprinted with permission.

Dose adjustment of chemotherapeutic agents in renal failure

Table A.2 Dose adjustments of commonly used chemotherapeutic agents in renal failure

Drug	Dose modification (percentage reduction)	Creatinine clearance (CrCl)
Amifostine	None	—
Arsenic trioxide	Use caution	—
L-asparaginase	Hold dose	<60 mL/min
Bevacizumab	Hold for severe proteinuria	—
Bleomycin	25%	10–50 mL/min
Bleomycin	50%	<10 mL/min
Bortezomib	None	—
Carboplatin	AUC dose based on CrCl	—
Carmustine	Hold dose	<60 mL/min
Cetuximab	None	—
Cisplatin	50%	30–60 mL/min
Cisplatin	Hold dose	<30 mL/min
Cladribine	Use caution	—
Cyclophosphamide	25%	10–50 mL/min
Cyclophosphamide	50%	<10 mL/min
Cytarabine	Use caution	—
Dacarbazine	Use caution	—
Dactinomycin	None	—
Daunorubicin	50%	S.Cr. >3.0 mg/dL
Docetaxel	None	—
Doxorubicin	25%	<10 mL/min
Doxorubicin liposomal	25%	<10 mL/min
Epirubicin	Use caution	—
Etoposide	25%	10–50 mL/min
Etoposide	50%	<10 mL/min
Etoposide phosphate	25%	10–50 mL/min
Etoposide phosphate	50%	<10 mL/min

Table A.2 (Cont.)

Drug	Dose modification (percentage reduction)	Creatinine clearance (CrCl)
Fludarabine	Use caution	—
5-Fluorouracil	None	—
Gemcitabine	Use caution	—
Idarubicin	Use caution	—
Ifosfamide	25%–50%	S.Cr. = 2.1–3.0 mg/dL
Ifosfamide	Hold dose	S.Cr. >3.0 mg/dL
Irinotecan	None	—
Mechlorethamine	None	—
Mesna	None	—
Methotrexate	50%	10–50 mL/min
Methotrexate	Hold dose	<10 mL/min
Mitomycin	25%	<10 mL/min
Mitomycin	Hold dose	S.Cr. > 1.7 mg/dL
Mitoxantrone	None	—
Oxaliplatin	None	—
Paclitaxel	None	
Pemetrexed	Dose adjust/hold	<45 mL/min
Pentostatin	Dose adjust	30–60 mL/min
Rituximab	None	—
Streptozocin	Hold dose	<60 mL/min
Topotecan	50%	20–39 mL/min
Topotecan	Hold dose	<20 mL/min
Trastuzumab	None	—
Vinblastine	None	—
Vincristine	None	—
Vinorelbine	None	—

Govindan, Ramaswamy. The Washington Manual of Oncology 2nd ed. Lippincott, Williams and Wilkins, Philadelphia, 2007. Reprinted with permission.

Table A.3 Response Evaluation Criteria in Solid Tumors (RECIST)

Table A.3 Evaluation of target and nontarget lesions

Target lesions	
Complete response (CR)	Disappearance of all target lesions
Partial response (PR)	At least a 30% decrease in the sum of the LD of target lesions, taking as reference the baseline sum LD
Progressive disease (PD)	At least a 20% increase in the sum of the LD of target lesions, taking as reference the smallest sum LD recorded since the treatment started or the appearance of one or more new lesions
Stable disease (SD)	Neither sufficient shrinkage to qualify for PR nor sufficient increase to qualify for PD, taking as reference the smallest sum LD since the treatment started
Non-target lesions	
Complete response (CR)	Disappearance of all nontarget lesions and normalization of tumor marker level
Incomplete response/stable disease (SD)	Persistence of one or more nontarget lesion(s) and/or maintenance of tumor marker level above the normal limits
Progressive disease (PD)	Appearance of one or more new lesions and/or unequivocal progression of existing nontarget lesions

Target lesions	Nontarget lesions	New lesions	Overall response	Target lesions
CR	CR	No	CR	CR
CR	Incomplete response/SD	No	PR	CR
PR	Non-PD	No	PR	PR
SD	Non-PD	No	SD	SD
PD	Any	Yes or no	PD	PD

Table A.4 Drug, dose, and schedule recommendations for antiemetic regimens

Table A.4 Chemotherapy induced carmustine, cisplatin, cyclophosphamide >1500 mg/m^2, dacarbazine, dactinomycin, mechlorethamine, streptozotocin

Day 1	Day 2	Day 3	Day 4
5-HT$_3$ serotonin receptor antagonist	Dexamethasone (8 Aprepitant (80 mg)	Dexamethasone (8 Aprepitant (80 mg)	Dexamethasone (8 mg)
Dolasetron (oral: 100 mg; IV: 100 mg or 1.8 mg/kg)	Dexamethasone (8 Aprepitant (80 mg)		
Granisetron (oral: 2 mg; IV: 1 mg or 0.01 mg/kg)			
Ondansetron (oral: 24 mg; IV: 8 mg or 0.15 mg/kg)			
Palonosetron (IV: 0.25 mg)			
Tropisetron (oral or IV: 5 mg)			
Dexamethasone (12 mg)			
Aprepitant (125 mg)			

Radiation induced (total body)

Prophylaxis with a 5-HT$_3$ serotonin receptor antagonist ± dexamethasone before each fraction and for at least 24 hours after

Chemotherapy induced

Carboplatin, cyclophosphamide <1500 mg/m^2, cytarabine >1 g/m^2, daunorubicin, doxorubicin, epirubicin, idarubicin, ifosfamide, irinotecan, oxaliplatin

Day 1	Day 2	Day 3
5-HT$_3$ serotonin receptor antagonist	5-HT$_3$ serotonin receptor antagonist	5-HT$_3$ serotonin receptor antagonist
Dolasetron (oral: 100 mg) (IV: 100 mg or 1.8 mg/kg)	OR	OR
Granisetron (oral: 2 mg) (IV: 1 mg or 0.01 mg/kg)	Dexamethasone (8 mg)	Dexamethasone (8 mg)
Ondansetron (oral: 16 mg [8 mg twice daily]) (IV: 8 mg or 0.15 mg/kg)		
Palonosetron (IV: 0.25 mg)		
Tropisetron (oral or IV: 5 mg)		
Dexamethasone (8 mg)		

Anthracycline + cyclophosphamide

Day 1	Day 2	Day 3
5-HT$_3$ serotonin receptor antagonist (doses listed above) Dexamethasone (12 mg) Aprepitant (125 mg)	Aprepitant (80 mg) When Apreptitant not given: Dexamethasone (8 mg)	Aprepitant (80 mg) When Apreptitant not given: Dexamethasone (8 mg)

Radiation induced (upper abdomen)

Prophylaxis with 5-HT$_3$ serotonin receptor antagonist before each fraction

Chemotherapy induced

5-Fluorouracil, bortezomib, cetuximab, cytarabine <1000 mg/m^2, docetaxel, etoposide, gemcitabine, methotrexate, mitomycin, mitoxantrone, paclitaxel, pemetrexed, topotecan, trastuzumab

Day 1

Dexamethasone (8 mg)

Radiation induced (lower thorax and pelvis, cranium (radiosurgery) and craniospinal)

Prophylaxis or rescue with 5-HT$_3$ serotonin receptor antagonist before each fraction

Chemotherapy induced

2-Chlorodeoxyadenosine, bevacizumab, bleomycin, busulfan, fludarabine, rituximab, vinblastine, vincristine, vinorelbine

As needed

Prescribe a single dose of dexamethasone 8 mg. Prescribing oral metoclopramide, or a phenothiazine is common.

Radiation induced (head and neck, extremities, cranium, breast)

Rescue with dopamine receptor antagonist or 5-HT$_3$ serotonin receptor antagonist (as needed); continue prophylactically for each remaining radiation treatment day.

Discriminatory immunophenotypes for lymphocytic neoplasms

Table A.5 Discriminatory immunophenotypes for lymphocytic neoplasms

Cells or neoplasm	Positive	Negative
B cells	CD 10,19, 20, 22, 23, 45RA, 79a	
B-lymphoblastic lymphoma	CD 10, 19, 79a [CD 20, 22]; HLA-DR	Tdt
B-cell small lymphocytic lymphoma, chronic lymphocytic leukemia	CD 5,19, 20, 23, 43, [CD 11c]; BCL-2	CD 10; 22/ FMC7
B-cell prolymphocytic leukemia		
Lymphoplasmacytic lymphoma	CD 19, 20, 22	CD 5,10
Follicular lymphomas	CD 10,19, 20 [CD 23]; BCL-2	CD 5,11c, 43
Marginal zone lymphomas (MALT)	CD 19, 20, 22 [CD 11c, 43]	CD 5,10, 23
Hairy cell leukemia	CD 11c, 19, 20, 22/FMC7, 25, 103; TRAP	CD 5,10,23
Mantle cell lymphoma	CD 5,19, 20, 22/ FMC7, 43, [CD 10]; BCL-1	CD 11c, 23
Diffuse large B-cell lymphoma	CD 19, 20, 22 [BCL-2]	CD 5,10
Burkitt lymphoma African-type sporadic type	CD 10, 19, 20, 22; EBV CD 19, 20, 22	CD 5, 23 CD 5, 23
Multiple myeloma	CD 10, 38; PCA-1; BCL-1 Cytoplasmic light and/or heavy chain	[CD45, 79a]
T cells	CD 1, 2, 3, 4, 5, 7, 8, 43, 45RO	
T-lymphoblastic lymphoma	CD 3, 7 [CD 1a, 2, 4, 5, 8]; Tdt	
Adult T-cell leukemia/lymphoma	CD 2, 3, 4, 5, 25; HTLV-1	CD 7,8
T-cell prolymphocytic leukemia	CD 2, 3, 4, 5, 7 [CD 8]	
Large granular lymphocytic leukemia T-cell type NK-cell type	CD 2, 3, 8,16, 57 CD 2, 16, 56, 57	CD 4, 5, 7, 56 CD 3, 4

Table A.5 (Cont.)

Cells or neoplasm	Positive	Negative
Peripheral T-cell lymphoma	CD 4 > CD 8 [CD 2, 3, 5, 7]	
Anaplastic large cell lymphoma	CD 30 [CD 3, 25, 45]; EMA	
Angioimmunoblastic T-cell lymphoma	CD 4 > CD 8 [CD 2, 3, 5, 7]	
NK/T-cell lymphoma	CD 2, 4, 56 [CD 8]	CD 3
Hepatosplenic γ/δ T-cell lymphoma	CD 2, 3, 5, 7; G/d	
Enteropathy-type intestinal T-cell lymphoma	CD 3, 7,103 [CD 8]	CD 4
Subcutaneous panniculitis-like T-cell lymphoma	CD 3, 8	CD 4
Mycosis fungoides	CD 2, 3, 4, 5 [CD 7]	CD 8, 25
Hodgkin lymphoma		
L & H cell of "lymphocyte-predominant" type	CD 19, 20, 22, 45	CD 15, 30; EMA
Reed–Sternberg cells; mononuclear and multinuclear lacunar cells of classic HL	CD 15, 30	CD 20, 45; EMA
Acute lymphoblastic leukemias	See Chapter 41	

[ ], occasionally positive; BCL, breakpoint cluster location [cyclin D]; BCL-1 positive in mantle cell lymphoma and plasma cell malignancies; BCL-2 positive in mantle cell lymphoma, most follicular lymphomas, small lymphocytic lymphoma, chronic lymphocytic leukemia, and some diffuse large cell lymphomas.

CD, clusters of differentiation; CD 22/FMC7, FMC7 epitope of CD 22; CD 45, leukocyte common antigen (LCA); EBV, Epstein–Barr virus; EMA, epithelial membrane antigen; G/d, gamma-delta (γ/δ) T-cell receptor protein; MALT, mucosa-associated lymphoid tissue; PCA-1, plasma cell-associated antigen; Tdt, terminal deoxytransferase (positive in cortical thymic lymphoid cells and lymphoblastic neoplasms); TRAP, tartrate-resistant acid phosphatase.

Casciato, Dennis A. and Barry B. Lowtiz, eds. *Manual of Clinical Oncology*, 4th edition. Lippincott Williams & Wilkins, Philadelphia, 2000. Reprinted with permission.

Table A.6 Common terminology criteria for adverse events v3.0 (CTCAE)

The NCI Common Terminology Criteria for Adverse Events v3.0 is a descriptive terminology that can be used for adverse event (AE) reporting. A grading (severity) scale is provided for each AE term.

Adverse event	Short name	Expected toxicities from chemotherapy treatment				
		Grade 1	Grade 2	Grade 3	Grade 4	Grade 5
Neutrophils/granulocytes (ANC/AGC)	Neutrophils	<LLN–1500/mm^3 <LLN–1.5 × 10^9/L	<1500–1000/mm^3 <1.5–1.0 × 10^9/L	<1000–500/mm^3 <1.0–0.5 × 10^9/L	<500/mm^3 <0.5 × 10^9	Death
Platelets	Platelets	< LLN–75,000/mm^3 <LLN–75.0 × 10^9/L	<75000–50000/mm^3 <75.0–50.0 × 10^9/L	<5000–25000/mm^3 <50.0–25.0 × 10^9/L	<25000/mm^3 <25.0 × 10^9	Death
Fatigue (asthenia, lethargy, malaise)	Fatigue	Mild fatigue over baseline	Moderate or causing difficulty performing some ADL	Severe fatigue interfering with ADL	Disabling	—
Hair loss/alopecia (scalp or body)	Alopecia	Thinning or patchy	Complete	—	—	—

Diarrhea	Diarrhea	Increase of <4 stools per day over baseline; mild increase in ostomy output compared to baseline	Increase of 4–6 stools per day over baseline; IV fluids indicated <24 hr; moderate increase in ostomy output compared to baseline; not interfering with ADL	Increase of >7 stools per day over baseline; incontinence; IV fluids 24 hr; hospitalization; severe increase in ostomy output compared to baseline; interfering with ADL	Life-threatening consequences (e.g., hemodynamic collapse)	Death
Nausea	Nausea	Loss of appetite without alteration in eating habits	Oral intake decreased without significant weight loss, dehydration or malnutrition; IV fluids indicated <24 hrs	Inadequate oral caloric or fluid intake; IV fluids, tube feedings, or TPN indicated ≥ 24 hr	Life-threatening consequences	Death
Vomiting	Vomiting	1 episode in 24 hr	2–5 episodes in 24 hr; IV fluids indicated <24 hr	≥ 6 episodes in 24 hr; IV fluids, or TPN indicated ≥ 24hr	Life-threatening consequences	Death
Neuropathy: sensory	Neuropathy: sensory	Asymptomatic; loss of deep tendon reflexes or paresthesia (including tingling) but not interfering with function	Sensory alteration or paresthesia (including tingling), interfering with function, but not interfering with ADL	Sensory alteration or paresthesia interfering with ADL	Disabling	Death

ADL, activities of daily living; LLN, lower limit of normal. Full listing of CTCAE v3.0 can be found at http://ctep.cancer.gov

Selected oncology web sites

- American Society of Hematology
  http://www.hematology.org/
- American Cancer Society (ACS statistics, other information, links to states)
  http://www.cancer.org/
- American Society of Clinical Oncology (ASCO; physician site)
  http://www.asco.org/
- ASCO—People Living with Cancer (patient site)
  http://www.plwc.org/
- Agency for Healthcare Research and Quality
  http://www.ahrq.gov/
- PubMed, National Library of Medicine (search MEDLINE and get abstracts)
  http://www.ncbi.nlm.nih.gov/entrez/query/
- Health Services/Technology Assessment Text (a helpful collection of HSTAT guidelines, surgeon general reports, technology assessments, and reviews)
  http://hstat.nlm.nih.gov/
- American Pain Society
  http://www.ampainsoc.org
- American Academy of Hospice and Palliative Medicine
  http://www.aahpm.org/
- National Cancer Institute's Cancer Information home page (NCI information, including PDQ, clinical trials information, statistics)
  http://www.cancer.gov
- Cancer Therapy Evaluation Program (CTEP) home page (includes common toxicity criteria)
  http://ctep.cancer.gov/
- Cancer Trials
  http://www.cancer.gov/clinicaltrials; http://www.cancertrialshelp.org
- Centers for Disease Control and Prevention (CDC)
  http://www.cdc.gov
- National Guideline Clearinghouse (guidelines for over 800 diseases and conditions, including many for cancer)
  http://www.guideline.gov/
- National Comprehensive Cancer Network (NCCN) Complete Library of Clinical Practice Guidelines in Oncology, for health professionals (free registration required) and patients
  http://www.nccn.org
- Association of Community Cancer Centers (includes the Compendia-Based Drug Bulletin)
  http://www.accc-cancer.org/
- Rxlist—Internet Drug Index (primarily for patients; includes alternative medicines)
  http://www.rxlist.com

- FDA Oncology Tools Web site (contains information about approved cancer therapies, product labels, approval summaries, what drugs are approved for what diseases, and considerations for making decisions about therapies, including advice on when to contemplate using unapproved drugs and how to obtain access to unapproved drugs)
http://www.fda.gov/Drugs/default.htm
- Drugs@FDA (a catalog of FDA-approved drugs—drug approval letters, labels, and review packages)
http://www.accessdata.fda.gov/scripts/cder/drugsatfda/index.cfm

Index

A

Abiraterone acetate, for prostate cancer, 582
Acanthosis nigricans, 319
Accelerated chemotherapy, 146
Acetaminophen, 257
Acetyl-L-carnitine, 201
Ackerman's tumor, 650
Acquired immunodeficiency syndrome, non-Hodgkin lymphoma with, 786–7
Acral hyperkeratosis, paraneoplastic, 319
Actinomycin D, 116
Acupuncture, 198
Acute graft-versus-host disease (GVHD), post HSCT
  overview, 158
  prophylaxis, 158
  stages and grading, 159t
  treatment, 160
Acute lymphoblastic leukemia (ALL), 724–7
  clinical features, 724
  diagnosis, 724–5
  epidemiology, 724
  mature B-cell, 725
  precursor B-cell, 724
  risk assessment, 725
  supportive care, 726
  T-cell, 725
  treatment, 726–7
    chemotherapy, 727
    consolidation therapy, 726–7
    early response, 726
    induction therapy, 726
    maintenance therapy, 727
    monoclonal antibodies, 727
Acute myeloid leukemia (AML), 718–23
  clinical presentation, 719
  diagnosis and classification, 719–20, 720t
  epidemiology, 718
  etiology, 718
  pathology, 719
  prognosis, 720
  treatment, 721–3
    allogeneic transplantation, 722
    autologous transplantation, 722
    consolidation chemotherapy, 721
    emerging therapies, 723
    general scheme, 722
    induction chemotherapy, 721
    stem cell transplantation, 722
    supportive care, 721
Acute necrotizing myopathy, 311–12
Acute promyelocytic leukemia (APL), 722
Acute renal failure
  with malignant disease, 298
  in tumor lysis syndrome, 300
Addiction, opioid, 263
Adenomatous colon polyps, prophylactic surgery, 37
Adenosine analogs, 127–31
  cladribine, 127–8, 747
  clofarabine, 129–30
  fludarabine, 128–9, 746, 748
  general, 127
  hydroxyurea, 130–1
  pentostatin, 129, 747, 783
Adjunctive radiotherapy, 92
Adoptive therapies, 191
Ado-trastuzumab emtansine, for metastatic breast cancer, 462
Adrenal cancer, 528–31
  epidemiology and etiology, 528
  investigations, 529
  pathology, 528
  presentation and endocrine syndromes, 529, 529t
  prognosis, 531
  treatment
    nonsurgical, 530
    surgical, 530
Adrenal gland anatomy, 528
Adrenal insufficiency (failure)
  late effects of treatment in, 354, 355t
  as metabolic emergency, 294
Adrenocortical tumors, 528–31. See also Adrenal cancer
Adverse events. See also specific agents and cancers
  terminology, 816t–817t
Aflatoxin, 19
Aggressive fibromatosis, 704
Agitation, terminal, 388–9, 390
Air pollution, 24
Alcohol, 19
  head and neck cancers from, 646
Alemtuzumab, 180
  for chronic lymphoid leukemias, 746, 747
Alkane sulfonates, 107
Alkylating agents, 104–11. See also specific agents
  alkane sulfonates: busulfan, 107
  aziridine analogs: thiotepa, 106–7
  mechanism of action, 104
  nitrogen mustards
    chlorambucil, 104
    cyclophosphamide, 104–5
    ifosfamide, 105
    mechlorethamine, 106
    melphalan, 106
  nitrosoureas, 107–9
    carmustine, 108
    lomustine, 108–9
    streptozocin, 109
  nonclassical
    dacarbazine, 109–10
    procarbazine, 110
    temozolomide, 110–11
  resistance, 104
Allodynia, 263
Allogeneic hematopoietic stem cell transplantation, 152
Allopurinol, for tumor lysis syndrome prophylaxis, 300
Alopecia, 816t
Alpharadin, for prostate cancer, 584

α-tocopherol
  supplements, 201
Alternative
  medicine, 195–203
  defined, 196 (See also
    Complementary and
    alternative medicine
    (CAM))
Alveolar rhabdomy-
  osarcoma, 696
Aminoglutethimide, 169
Aminoglycoside antibiotics
  on ears, 358
  on kidneys, 358
Amitriptyline, for
  neuropathic pain, 257
Amplifications, 4
Anal canal, 508
Anal cancer, 508–11
  adenocarcinoma, 511
  clinical presentation, 508
  epidemiology, 508
  etiology, 508
  malignant melanoma, 511
  pathology and natural
    history, 508
  practical points, 511
  staging, 509, 509t
  treatment
    chemoradiation, 149
    initial, 510
    palliative, 510–11
    workup, 510
Analgesic ladder, 256–7,
  256f
Analgesics. See also specific
  agents
  adjuvant, 264
  non-opioid, 257
  opioid, mild-to-moderate
    pain, 257–8
Anal margin, 508
Anaplastic
  astrocytomas, 626–34.
    See also Brain tumors,
    primary
Anaplastic
  (undifferentiated)
  thyroid carcinomas. See
    also Thyroid cancers
  epidemiology and
    etiology, 514
  pathology and
    genetics, 515
  presentation, 517
  prognosis, 526
  staging, 518
  treatment
    external beam
      radiotherapy, 524
    surgery, 521
Anastrozole, 169

Androgen blockade/
  deprivation, for
  prostate cancer, 578,
  581
  combined, 581–2
Anemia, 215–24
  causes, 218
  fatigue from, 216
  hemolytic,
    paraneoplastic, 316
  management, 216
  nutritional, 218
  treatment
    decision
      tree, 222f–223f
    erythropoiesis-
      stimulating
      agents, 218–20
    iron, parenteral, 221
    overview, 218–19
    recommendations, 220
    red blood cell
      transfusions, 218,
      220
Anemia of chronic
  disease, 218
Angiogenesis, 4
  establishment, 13–14
  growth factors in, 14
Angiosarcoma, 704
Anorexia
  defined, 366
  end-of-life care, 366–7
Anthracenedione, 115
Anthracyclines, 112–17
  dactinomycin, 116
  daunorubicin, 113–14
  doxorubicin, 113
  epirubicin, 114–15
  on heart, 358
  idarubicin, 115
  mitomycin C, 116–17
  mitoxantrone, 115–16
  pharmacology, 112
  resistance, 112
  toxicity, 112–13
Antiandrogens, 170. See
  also specific agents
Antiangiogenic therapy, for
  brain tumors, 634
Antibiotic-resistant
  organisms, 237
Antibiotics. See also specific
  types and infections
  antitumor, 112–17 (See
    also Anthracyclines)
  for febrile neutropenia
    empiric, 242–4, 243b,
      244b
  prophylactic, 248
Antibodies. See also specific
  agents

alemtuzumab, 180
bevacizumab, 180
cetuximab, 180
panitumumab, 180
rituximab, 180
trastuzumab, 181
Anticoagulation,
  prophylactic. See also
  specific agents
  clinical practice
    guidelines, 280–2
    American College
      of Chest
      Physicians, 280
    American Society
      of Clinical
      Oncology, 280–2
    National
      Comprehensive
      Cancer
      Network, 280
  for venous
    thromboembolism
    meta-analyses, 278–9
    randomized trials, 278
Antidepressants,
  tricyclic, as adjuvant
    analgesics, 264
Antidiuretic hormone
  (ADH), excess, 294
Antiemetics, 376,
  377t–378t. See also
  Nausea and/or vomiting
  regimens, 812t–813t
Antiestrogens, 169–70
Antifolates, 118–20. See
  also specific agents
  mechanism of
    action, 118
  methotrexate, 118–20
  pemetrexed, 120
Antifungals, for febrile
  neutropenia
  empiric, 242–3
  prophylactic, 248
Antilymphocyte
  globulin (ALG), for
  myelodysplastic
  syndromes, 738
Antimetabolites, 118–31.
  See also specific agents
  adenosine
    analogs, 127–31
    cladribine, 127–8
    clofarabine, 129–30
    fludarabine, 128–9
    general, 127
    hydroxyurea, 130–1
    pentostatin, 129
  antifolates, 118–20
  mechanism of
    action, 118

methotrexate, 118–20
pemetrexed, 120
antipurines, 124–7
cytarabine, 124–5
gemcitabine, 125–6
nelarabine, 126–7
purine analogs, 124
fluoropyrimidines, 121–3
5-fluorouracil, 121–2, 123
5-fluorouracil prodrugs, 122–3
mechanism and sites of action, 118, 119f
thymidylate synthase inhibitors, 121
Antimicrotubule agents, 140, 141t–143t. *See also specific agents*
docetaxel, 143t
estramustine phosphate, 143t
ixabepilone, 140, 143t
mechanism of action, 140
paclitaxel, 143t
vinblastine, 141t
vincristine, 141t
vindesine, 141t
vinorelbine, 141t–142t
Antineoplastons, 202
Antiprogestins, 170
Antipurines, 124–7. *See also specific agents*
cytarabine, 124–5
gemcitabine, 125–6
nelarabine, 126–7
purine analogs, 124
Antitumor antibiotics, 112–17. *See also* Anthracyclines
Anxiolytics, as adjuvant analgesics, 264
APC mutation screening, 56
Apoptosis, 4
defined, 12, 13
evasion, 13
failure to engage, 145
pathways, 13
regulators, 7, 7t
Aromatase inhibitors, 169
for breast cancer, 450
early, 453–5
metastatic, 459–60
+ tamoxifen, 170
Aromatherapy, 201
Art therapy, 200
Ascites treatment, for malignant ascites
palliative surgical, 75
surgical, 80
unsealed radionuclide, 99

Astrocytomas, 626–34. *See also* Brain tumors, primary
ATM, 16
Autologous hematopoietic stem cell transplantation, 152
Axillary lymph node dissection, 449
Ayurveda, 198
Azacitadine, 183
for myelodysplastic syndromes, 738
Aziridine analogs, 106–7

B

Back pain, from spinal cord compression, 332
Bacterial infections, 21
Bacterial vectors, 192, 193t
Barrett's esophagus, prophylactic surgery, 36
Basal cell carcinoma, 680–3
epidemiology and etiology, 680
management, 682–3
presentation, 680, 681f
prevention and future directions, 683
Bathex syndrome, 319
bcl-2, in follicular lymphoma, 14
BCR-ABL kinase inhibitors
dasatinib, 178
imatinib, 178
nilotinib, 178
BCR-ABL translocation, 6
Beam dosimetry, 92
Bellini tumor, 537. *See also* Renal cancer
Benign pigmented nevi, 668, 669f
Benzodiazepines, as adjuvants, 264
β-carotene, 43, 201
Bevacizumab, 180
for brain tumors, 634
for colorectal cancer, metastatic, 504, 505, 505t
for hepatocellular carcinoma, 496
for non–small-cell lung cancer, 408
for pancreatic cancer, 488
for renal cancer, 545t, 546
venous thromboembolism from, 272

Bilharzial bladder disease, 14, 21
Biliary tract cancers, 490–2
bile duct, brachytherapy for, 97
cholangiocarcinoma, 490–1
gallbladder, 491–2
Biofield therapies, 198
Biological therapies. *See also specific types*
for pancreatic cancer, 488
for renal cancer, 543–4
Biological vectors, 192, 193t
Birt-Hogg-Dube syndrome, renal cancer in, 537. *See also* Renal cancer
Bisphosphonates
as adjuvant analgesics, 264
for bone pain, 257
for breast cancer, metastatic, 460
for hypercalcemia, 291
for prostate cancer, 583
for renal cancer, 542
Bladder and ureter cancers, 548–56
epidemiology and etiology, 548
genetics and molecular biology, 549
investigation, 551
pathology, 548–9
presentation, 551
staging, 549, 550t
treatment, 551–6
bladder conservation, 554
chemoradiation, 149
chemotherapy, metastatic cancers, 555–6
chemotherapy, neoadjuvant and adjuvant, 554, 555t
future, 556
muscle-invasive bladder cancer, 552
outcomes, 556
radiation therapy alone, 553
superficial tumors, 551–2
surgery, radical, 552–3
Bladder outlet obstruction, 348–9
Bleomycin, on lungs, 358
Blocking agents, 38, 39t
Body-based methods, 199

Body surface area (BSA) nomogram, 804
Bone metastasis treatment
 surgery, 78
 unsealed radionuclides, 99
Bone pain, analgesia for, 257
Bones, late effects of treatment on, 358
Bone sarcomas, 687–92, 706–14
 chondrosarcoma, 712
 chordoma, 712
 diagnosis and staging studies, 689
 epidemiology, 688
 etiology, 688
 Ewing's sarcoma, 708–10
 giant cell tumor of bone, 713
 osteosarcoma, 706–7
  metastatic, 707–8
 pathology, 689, 689t
 primary malignant spindle cell sarcoma of bone, 712
 staging system, 690, 691t
 surveillance, 714
 treatment
  chemotherapy, 692
  radiotherapy, 690–1
  surgery, 690
Bone-targeted therapy, for prostate cancer, 583–4
Bortezomib, 183
Bosutinib
 for chronic myeloid leukemia, 732
 side effects, 733
Bowel obstruction, 74
Brachial plexus block, 266
Brachytherapy, 96–7
BRAF inhibitors. See also Dabrafenib; Vemurafenib
 for malignant melanoma, 675, 676
Brain metastases, 79, 638–40
 epidemiology, 638
 investigation, 639
 management, 639–40
 outcome, 640, 640t
 pathology, 638
 presentation, 638
Brain tumors,
 primary, 626–34
  epidemiology, 626
  etiology, 626
  hereditary syndromes, 626, 627t

investigations and staging, 628
management, 629–34
 ependymoma, 632
 gliomas, 629–31, 631t, 632t
 medulloblastoma, 632
 meningiomas, 633
 pineal tumors, 633
 pituitary tumors, 633
 recent advancements and future treatments, 633–4
pathology and classification, 626–8
presentation, 628, 629t
BRCA1, 434
 prophylactic surgery, 36
 screening, 54
BRCA2, 434
 screening, 54
Breaking bad news, 382–3
Breakthrough pain, 262–4
 adjuvant analgesics, 264
 dose equivalents, 263t
 general approach, 262
 increasing analgesic requirements and persistent pain, 262–3
Breast cancer, 429–44
 advances, 430
 clinical trials, large, 430
 epidemiology, 432
 etiology and risk factors, 432–3
 follow-up, early-stage patients, 458
 genetics and genetic assessment, 434, 435t
 hereditary, prophylactic surgery for, 36
 male, 433
 pathology
  ductal carcinoma, special types, 436–7
  ductal carcinoma in situ, 436
  histological types, 437t
  invasive ductal carcinoma, 436, 437
  invasive lobular carcinoma, 437
  lobular carcinoma in situ, 436
  Paget's disease of the breast, 437
 presentation and staging, 442–4
  diagnosis, 442
  most common presentations, 442, 443b

 referral to breast clinic, 443b
 TNM staging system, 443, 444t
prognostic factors, 438, 438t
screening, 48, 440–1
spread, 67
survival rates, 72
treatment
 brachytherapy, 97
 palliative resection, 76
Breast cancer management, 446–62
 early cancer, 448–55
  adjuvant, 455t
  chemotherapy, adjuvant, 450–3, 452t–453t
  defined, 448
  endocrine therapy, adjuvant, 450, 453–5
  neoadjuvant, 455, 455t
  overview, 448
  radiotherapy, locoregional, 449–50
  surgery, axillary, 449
  surgery, breast, 448–9
 locally advanced cancer, 456, 457t
 metastatic cancer, 459–62
  bisphosphonates, intravenous, 460
  chemotherapy, 461
  endocrine therapy, 459–60
  incidence, 459
  principles, 459
  radiotherapy, 460
  radiotherapy, reduced fractures, 460
  targeted therapies, 461–2
 multidisciplinary, 447
 noninvasive cancer, 446–7
Breast conservation therapy, 448
Breast/ovarian syndrome, genetic screening, 54
Breast reconstruction, 449
"Breast" syndromes, hereditary, genetic screening, 54
Bronchial obstruction, 338–9
BSA nomogram, 804
Burkitt's lymphoma, 11
 Epstein-Barr virus in, 20, 33
Busulfan, 107

C

Cachexia. See also
  Paraneoplastic
  syndromes (PNS)
  defined, 366
  end-of-life care, 366–7
Calcitonin, salmon, for
  hypercalcemia, 292
Cancer-associated
  retinopathy, 312–13
Cancer biology, 10–14. See
  also specific cancers
  angiogenesis
    establishment, 13–14
  apoptosis evasion, 13
  cell cycle
    deregulation, 10–11
  independence from external
    growth-promoting
    and growth-inhibiting
    signals, 11–12
  invasion and
    metastasis, 14
  limitless
    replication, 12–13
Cancer of bladder and
  ureter, 548–56. See
  also Bladder and ureter
  cancers
Cancer of cervix, 614–17.
  See also Cervical cancer
Cancer of unknown
  primary, 789–99
  clinical presentation, 790,
    796
  etiology and
    pathology, 796
  initial workup, 791, 791t
  malignant pleural
    effusion, 795
  management, 798, 799f
  metastases
    bone, 794
    brain, 794
    liver, 794
    lung, 794
    lymph nodes, 792
    peritoneum, 793
  prognostic factors,
    favorable, 796
Cancer of uterine
  corpus, 610–13
  endometrial
    cancer, 610–12
  sarcoma, 613
Cannabinoids, for end-of-
  life anorexia and
  cachexia, 367
Capecitabine, 122–3
  for metastatic colorectal
    cancer, 504–5

Capsaicin, for neuropathic
  pain, 257
Carboplatin, 133–4
  for non–small-cell lung
    cancer, 406–7
Carboplatin-paclitaxel,
  for non–small-cell lung
    cancer, 407, 408
Carcinoembryonic antigen
  (CEA), 190
Carcinogenesis, 38. See
  also specific cancers
  multistep, 4
Carcinogens,
  genetic (somatic)
    mutations, 17
Carcinoid tumors, 478–81
  diagnosis, 478
  epidemiology and risk
    factors, 478
  future directions, 481
  management, 480–1
  pathology, 478–9
Cardiotoxicity, 358
Carmustine, 108
Carotenoids, 43
Casodex, 170
Caspases, 13
Castration, as hormone
  therapy, 168, 170
Castration-resistant
  prostate cancer, 582
Cataracts,
  treatment-related, 358
Catheter infection, empiric
  antibiotic therapy
  for, 243
Catheter thrombosis,
  central venous
  catheters, 286
Cauda equina
  syndrome, 332
CDH1
  breast cancer, 434
  screening for
    mutations, 55
CD95 ligand, 13
Celiac plexus block, 266
Cell cycle
  in cancer, 11
  checkpoints, 10–11
  deregulation, 10–11
  phases, 10
Cell death. See also
  Apoptosis
  radiation-induced, 84–5
Cell killing, fractional, 102
Central nervous system
  tumors, 625–40. See
  also specific types
  brain tumors,
    primary, 626–34

lymphoma, primary
  CNS, 636–7
metastases,
  brain, 638–40
Central venous catheters,
  thrombosis, 286
Cerebellar degeneration,
  paraneoplastic, 310
Cervical cancer, 614–17
  epidemiology, 614
  etiology and HPV, 20,
    33, 614
  management, 616–17
    brachytherapy, 96, 617
  pathology, 614
  presentation, 615
  prognosis, 615, 616t
  screening, 48
  staging, 615, 616t
Cervical carcinoma in situ,
  prophylactic surgery
  for, 37
Cetuximab, 180
  for colorectal cancer,
    metastatic, 504,
    505, 506
  for head and neck
    cancers, 661
  infusion reactions to, 506
  for pancreatic
    cancer, 488
Checkpoint kinase 2 gene
  screening, 54–5
Checkpoints, cell
  cycle, 10–11
CHEK2
  breast cancer, 434
  screening, 54–5
Chelation therapy, 202
Chemical exposures, 24
Chemoendocrine
  therapy, 173
Chemoprevention. See
  also specific cancers and
  agents
  agents and
    mechanisms, 38–9,
    39t
  clinical trials, 40–1
  defined, 30
  principles, 38
Chemoradiation, 86,
  148–9, 148t
  for anal and bladder
    carcinomas, 149
  concurrent
    combined, 148, 148t
  for esophageal
    cancer, 149
  for head and neck
    cancer, 149
  for lung cancer, 149

Chemoradiation (cont.)
  for rectal cancer, 149
  sequential combined therapy, 148
Chemotherapy, 101–49. *See also specific agents and cancers*
  accelerated, 146
  alkylating agents, 104–11
  antimetabolites, 118–31
  antimicrotubule agents, 140, 141t–143t
  antitumor antibiotics, 112–17 (*See also* Anthracyclines)
  chemoradiation, 148–9, 148t
  cisplatin and derivatives, 132–5
  classification of cytotoxics, 102
  combination therapy rationale, 102
  concurrent with radiation, 86
  dose adjustments
    in hepatic failure, 805t–807t
    in renal failure, 808t–809t
  dose and tumor kill, 102
  dose intensification, 146
  drug resistance, 144–5 (*See also* Resistance, drug)
  topoisomerase inhibitors, 136–8
  venous thromboembolism from, 272
Chemotherapy resistance genes, 188
Chemotherapy sensitization genes, 188
Chewing tobacco, leukoplakia from, 32
Chiropractic, 199
Chlorambucil, 104
  for chronic lymphoid leukemias, 746, 747
Cholangiocarcinoma, 490–1
Chondrosarcoma, 712
Chordoma, 712
Chromophobe, 537. *See also* Renal cancer
Chronic graft-versus-host disease (GVHD), post-HSCT, 160
Chronic lymphoid leukemias (CLL), 742–8
  classification, 742, 743t
  clinical presentation, 744
  diagnostic evaluation, 744, 745b
  epidemiology, 742
  future directions, 748
  management, 744–8
    first-line, 746
    response assessment, 745
    second-line/subsequent, 747–8
    therapeutic criteria, 744–5
  pathogenesis, 742–3
  prognosis, 748
  subtypes, 743
Chronic myeloid leukemia (CML), 730–4
  clinical phases, 730–1
  cytogenetics, 731
  differential diagnosis, 731
  epidemiology, 730
  investigations, 731
  leukocytosis, 731
  management, 732–4
    accelerated phase, 734
    allogeneic stem cell transplant, 734
    blast phase, 734
    chronic phase, 732–4
  pathophysiology, 730
  Philadelphia chromosome, 730
Cigarette smoking, 18, 32
Cirrhosis, alcoholic, 19
Cisplatin, 132–3
  on kidneys, 358
  on nerves, 358
  for non–small-cell lung cancer, 406–7
  renal tubular dysfunction from, 299
Cisplatin derivatives. *See* Carboplatin; Oxaliplatin
Cladribine, 127–8
  for chronic lymphoid leukemias, 747
Class I molecules, 154
Class II molecules, 154
Clinical equipoise, 209
Clinical trials, 205–11. *See also specific agents and cancers*
  cancer prevention, 40–1
  ethics, 208
  fundamentals, 206
  history, 207
  phases, 210–11
  safety and efficacy, 209
Clofarabine, 129–30
Clubbing, digital, 318

Coagulopathy, paraneoplastic, 317
Codeine phosphate, low-dose, 258
Cognitive-behavioral approaches, to pain, 267
Colectomy, prophylactic, 69
Colon cancer
  bowel obstruction, 74
  diet on, 19
  mutations, 4
  survival rates, 72
Colon polyp surgery, prophylactic, 37
Colony-stimulating factors (CSFs). *See also specific types*
  for febrile neutropenia, 246
  prophylactic, 249, 249f, 415, 451, 600, 739
Colorectal cancer, 500–6
  epidemiology and risk factors, 500
  screening, 48
  spread, 67
  staging, 500, 501t
  survival, 500
  treatment, 502–6
    chemoradiation, 149
    chemotherapy, adjuvant, 502–3
    chemotherapy, palliative, metastatic disease, 504–6
      first-line, 504–6, 505t
      second-line, 506
      subsequent, 506
    palliative, metastatic disease, 503–5
    palliative, resection, 76
    prophylactic surgery, hereditary disease, 36
    radiotherapy, 503
    surgery, 500–2
Combination chemotherapy. *See also specific cancers and agents*
  rationale and design, 102
Combined androgen blockade, for prostate cancer, 581–2
Communication
  end-of-life care, 382–3
  last days of life, 391
Complementary and alternative medicine (CAM), 195–203
  alternative medical systems, 198

complex natural products, 202–3
defined, 196
electromagnetic-based therapies, 199
energy therapies, 198–9
exercise therapies, 199
groups, 198
issues, 197
manipulative and body-based methods, 199
mind-body interventions, 200–1
art therapy, 200
meditation, 200
music therapy, 200
yoga, 200
nutritional therapeutics, 201
for pain, 267–8
pharmacologic and biologic treatments, 202
scope, 196
spiritual therapies, 203
Complex natural products, 202–3
Conditioning regimens, hematopoietic stem cell transplantation, 157
Conjugated agents. See also specific agents
denileukin diftitox, 182
ibritumomab, 182
tositumomab, 182
Conservative surgery, 68
Constipation, end-of-life care, 367–9
Correlative science endpoints, 209
Corticosteroids. See also specific types
as adjuvant analgesics, 264
for bone pain, 257
cataracts from, 358
on insulin requirements, 297
osteopenia from, 358
Courvoisier's sign
cholangiocarcinoma, 490
pancreatic cancer, 484
Cowden's syndrome screening, 54
COX-2 inhibitors, for pain, 257
Cushing's syndrome, 306–7
Cutaneous malignancies, 667–84. See also specific types

intraocular melanoma, 678
malignant melanoma, 668–76 (See also Malignant melanoma)
Merkel cell carcinoma, 684
nonmelanoma skin cancer, 680–3
Cyclin-dependent kinases (CDK), activation, 10
Cyclizine, for nausea and vomiting, 341
Cyclophosphamide, 104–5
Cytarabine, 124–5
Cytoreductive surgery, palliative, 76
Cytotoxic chemotherapy. See Chemotherapy

D

Dabrafenib, for malignant melanoma, 675
Dacarbazine, 109–10
for malignant melanoma, 675
Dactinomycin, 116
Dasatinib, 178
for chronic myeloid leukemia, 732
resistance, 733–4
side effects, 733
Daunorubicin, 113–14
Death rattles, 369, 390
Decitabine, 183
for myelodysplastic syndromes, 738
Deep vein thrombosis (DVT), 276, 277t. See also Venous thromboembolism (VTE)
Definitive radiotherapy, 92
Delayed gastric emptying, nausea and vomiting from, 374
Deletions, 4
Delirium, end-of-life care, 370
Demethylation agents
azacitadine, 183
decitabine, 183
Dendritic cells (DCs), 191
Dendritic cell vaccination, 191
Denileukin diftitox, 182
Denosumab, for prostate cancer, 583

Depression, end-of-life care, 384–5
Dermatofibrosarcoma protuberans, 704
Dermatomyositis, 313–14
Desmoid tumors, 704
Dexamethasone
for bone pain, 257
for nausea and vomiting, 341
Diagnosis. See also specific cancers
surgical, 70–1
Diarrhea, 817t
Dichloroacetic acid (DCA), 202
Diet, 19
low-fat, 201
Dietary prevention
carotenoids, 43
fat, 42
fiber, 42
folate, 43
fruits and vegetables, 19, 42
Difluorodeoxy-cytidine, 125–6
Digital clubbing, 318
Disease-free survival, 209
Disodium EDTA chelation, 202
Dissemination. See also specific cancers
principal methods, 67
Distress, end-of-life care
family and caregiver, 386–7
patient, 385–6
DNA methylation, 183
DNA methyltransferase, 183
DNA repair genes, 16
DNA vaccines, 190–1
Docetaxel, 143t
for prostate cancer, 584–5
Donor lymphocyte infusion (DLI), in HSCT, 164
Donors, hematopoietic stem cell, 154–5
haploidentical-related donor-matched transplant, 155
matched unrelated, 154
umbilical cord blood, 154–5
Dose. See also specific agents and cancers
chemotherapy, in tumor kill, 102
radiation therapy, 84
calculation, 93

Dose intensification, 146
Dose response, 146
Dosimetry, beam, 92
Doxorubicin, 113
 on heart, 358
Dronabinol, for end-of-life anorexia and cachexia, 367
Drug resistance, 144–5
Ductal carcinoma in situ (DCIS), 436, 446. See also Breast cancer
Durie-Salmon staging system, 756, 757t
Dying. See End-of-life care
Dysautonomia, nausea and vomiting from, 374
Dysplasia, 650
Dyspnea, end-of-life care, 371–3
 assessment, 371
 causes, 371–2
 management, 372–3

E

Early-responding tissue, radiotherapy, 85
Ears, late effects of treatment on, 358
Efficacy, clinical trial, 209
Efficacy outcomes of interest, 209
EGFR, 12
Electromagnetic-based therapies, 199
Electrons, 88, 89f
Embryonal rhabdomyosarcoma, 696
Embryo storage, 357, 357t
Empiric antibiotic therapy, for febrile neutropenia, 242–4, 243b, 244b
 antifungals, 242–3
 duration, 243–4, 243b
 IDSA guidelines for antimicrobial agents, 242, 243b
 initial, 242
 vancomycin, 242
En bloc surgery, 68
Encephalomyelopathies, 311
Endocrine cancers, 513–33. See also specific types
 adrenal, 528–31
 neuroblastoma, 532, 533t
 thyroid, 514–27
Endocrine dysfunction, as late treatment effect, 354, 355t
Endocrine therapy. See Hormone therapy
End-of-life care, 363–91
 See also specific topics
 definition and scope, 364
 last days of life, 390–1
 multidisciplinary team, 364
 need, 364
 physical symptoms, 366–80
  anorexia and cachexia, 366–7
  constipation, 367–9
  death rattles, 369, 390
  delirium, 370
  dyspnea, 371–3
  lymphedema, 373–4
  nausea and vomiting, 374–8, 375f, 377t–378t
  nutrition and hydration, 379–80
 psychosocial symptoms, 382–9
  communication, 382–3
  depression, 384–5
  distress (family and caregiver), 386–7
  distress (patient), 385–6
  spiritual suffering, 387–8
  terminal agitation, 388–9, 390
 symptom management, whole-person, 365
Endometrial cancer, 610–12
 epidemiology, 610
 etiology and risk factors, 610
 pathology, 610
 presentation, 610
 prognosis, 611, 612t
 treatment
  adjuvant radiation, 612
  brachytherapy, 96
  chemotherapy, 612
  surgery and staging, 611, 611t
Endometrial stromal sarcomas, 613
Endpoints
 correlative science, 209
 surrogate, 209
Energy therapies, 198–9
Enteral nutrition, end-of-life care, 380
Environmental exposure, chemical, 24
Environmental risks, in prevention, 32
Enzalutamide, for prostate cancer, 582–3
Ependymomas, 626–34. See also Brain tumors, primary
Epidermal growth factor receptor (EGFR), 178
Epidermal growth factor receptor (EGFR) inhibitors. See also specific agents
 erlotinib, 178, 488, 496
 lapatinib, 179, 462
 for pancreatic cancer, 488
Epidural anesthesia, 266
Epigenetic changes, 4
Epigenetic molecular alterations, 6
Epirubicin, 114–15
 on heart, 358
Epothilones, 140
Epstein-Barr virus (EBV), 20, 33
 Burkitt's lymphoma, 33
 CNS lymphoma, 636
 head and neck cancers, 646
 Hodgkin lymphoma, 769t
Equipoise, clinical, 209
Erlotinib, 178
 for hepatocellular carcinoma, 496
 for pancreatic cancer, 488
Erythema, necrolytic migratory, 319
Erythema gyratum repens, 319
Erythrocytosis, paraneoplastic, 316
Erythroderma, 319
Erythroplakia, 650
Erythropoiesis-stimulating agents. See also specific agents
 overview, 218–19
 recommendations and dosing, 220
 for renal cancer, 542
 safety considerations, 219, 223f, 224
 venous thromboembolism from, 224, 272
Esophageal cancer
 epidemiology and etiology, 466

Her2Neu testing, 468
staging, 466, 467t
surgical considerations, 468
survival rates, 72
treatment
chemoradiation, 149
localized (resectable) disease, 468-9
recurrent and metastatic disease, 470
Esophageal cancers, 466-70
Essiac, 203
Estramustine phosphate, 143t
Estrogen receptor (ER), 171
Ethics, clinical research, 208
Etiology and epidemiology, 15-24. *See also specific cancers*
alcohol, 19
chemical exposures, 24
diet, 19
gender, 22
genetic factors, 16-17
DNA repair genes, 16-17
proto-oncogenes, 16
tumor suppressor genes, 16
infections, 20-1
radiation exposure, other, 23
smoking, 18, 32
Etoposide, 138
Etoposide plus carboplatin (EC), for small cell lung cancer, 413
Etoposide plus cisplatin (EP), for small cell lung cancer, 413
Ewing's sarcoma, 708-10
Exemestane, 169
Exercise therapies, 199
External beam radiotherapy, 92-5. *See also specific cancers*
adjunctive, 92
definitive, 92
by disease site, 95t
intensity-modulated radiation therapy, 93, 94f
neoadjuvant, 92
palliative, 92
treatment planning, 92-4, 94f

Eyes, late effects of treatment on, 358

F

Familial adenomatous polyposis (FAP)
desmoid tumor, 704
genetic screening, 56
prophylactic surgery, 36
Familial cancer syndromes, 485t
Fat
dietary, 42
low-fat diet, 201
Fatigue, 224-7, 816t
from anemia (See Anemia)
causes, 216
evaluation, 226
treatment
accompanying causes, 226
unexplained fatigue, 227
Febrile neutropenia, 229-50
complications, 234
defined, 230
infectious agents
antibiotic-resistant, 237
bacteria, 236
fungal, 237
parasitic, 237
viral, 237
key point summary, 250
management checklist, 238t-240t
myelosuppression and, 230
patient evaluation
additional, 240t
initial, 236, 238t-239t
sites of infection, common, 236
prophylaxis
antibiotics, 248
colony-stimulating factors, 249, 249f, 415, 451, 600, 739
risk assessment, 245, 245t
risk factors, 232, 233b
in small cell lung cancer, 415
timing, 232
treatment
empiric antibiotic therapy, 242-4, 243b, 244b
initial, 236, 238t-239t

myeloid growth factors, 246
Fentanyl
metabolites and side effects, 259
for step 2 pain relief, 258
Fertility
vs. sexual function, 356
treatment on, 356-7, 357t
Fertility preservation, 356-7, 357t
Fever. *See* Febrile neutropenia; Paraneoplastic syndromes (PNS)
Fiber, 42
Fibromatosis, aggressive, 704
Field design, radiotherapy, 93
Fish, salt, 19
head and neck cancers from, 646
Fistulas
palliative surgery, 75
types, 74
5-Fluorouracil (5-FU), 121-2
adverse events, 121
for anal cancer, 510, 511
for basal cell carcinoma, skin, 682
for biliary tract cancer, 492
for carcinoid tumors, 480
for colorectal cancer, 503, 505t
metastatic, 504, 506
dosing, 122
for esophageal cancer, 468, 469, 470
for gastric cancer, 474, 475
for hepatocellular cancer, 496
modulation, 123
for pancreatic cancer, 487
for penile cancer, 560, 561
pharmacology, 122
sites of action, 119f
for small intestine adenocarcinoma, 480
5-Fluorouracil (5-FU) prodrugs
capecitabine, 122-3
2-fluoro-2'-deoxyuridine (floxuridine), 118, 123

Flavopiridol, for chronic lymphoid leukemias, 748
Floxuridine, 118, 123
Fludarabine, 128–9
 for chronic lymphoid leukemias, 746, 748
2-Fluoro-2'-deoxyuridine (floxuridine), 118, 123
Fluoropyrimidines, 121–3
 5-fluorouracil (See 5-Fluorouracil (5-FU))
 5-fluorouracil prodrugs
  capecitabine, 122–3
  2-fluoro-2'-deoxyuridine (floxuridine), 118, 123
Flutamide, 170
Folate, 43
Follicle-stimulating hormone (FSH), 168
Follicular lymphoma
 bcl-2 gene, 14
 pathophysiology, 14
Follicular thyroid cancer. See also Thyroid cancers
 epidemiology and etiology, 514
 pathology and genetics, 515
Formestane, 169
Fractional cell killing, 102
Fractionation, 84
Fruits, 19, 42

G

Gabapentin
 as adjuvant analgesic, 264
 for neuropathic pain, 257
Gallbladder cancer, 491–2
Ganglion impar block, 266
Gardner's syndrome, desmoid tumor in, 704
Gastric cancer, 472–5
 epidemiology and etiology, 472
 hereditary diffuse genetic screening, 55
 prophylactic surgery, 36
 Her2 testing, 472
 staging, 472, 473t
 surgical considerations, 472–4
 treatment
  localized resectable, 474
  localized unresectable, 474
  recurrent and metastatic, 475

Gastric emptying delay, nausea and vomiting from, 374
Gastrointestinal bleeding, palliative surgery for, 76
Gastrointestinal cancers, 465–511. See also specific types
 anal, 508–11
 biliary tract, 490–2
 colorectal, 500–6
 esophageal, 466–70
 gastric, 472–5
 hepatocellular, 494–6
 pancreatic, 484–8
 small intestine and carcinoid, 478–81
Gastrointestinal stromal tumor (GIST), 694–6, 695t
Gastrointestinal syndromes, hereditary, genetic screening, 56
Gemcitabine, 125–6
 for biliary tract cancer, 492
 for breast cancer, metastatic, 461
 for esophageal cancer, metastatic, 470
 for mesothelioma, 423
 for pancreatic cancer, 487
 for small intestine adenocarcinoma, 480
 for uterine leiomyosarcoma, 705
Gemcitabine-cisplatin
 for bladder cancer, 554, 555, 555t
 for non-small-cell lung cancer, 407
Gemtuzumab ozogamicin
 for acute myeloid leukemia, 723
 hepatic veno-occlusive disease from, 162
Gencidin, 187
Gender, cancer and, 22
Gene delivery, 192, 193t
Genes, 16–17. See also specific genes and cancers
 cancer-associated, 32, 32t
 DNA repair, 16
 proto-oncogenes, 16
 specific, 16–17
 tumor suppressor, 16
Gene therapy, 185–93
 for brain tumors, 633
 categories, 186

chemotherapy sensitization and resistance genes, 188
 evolution and aims, 186
 gene delivery, 192, 193t
 mutant oncogene correction, 187
 regulation, 186
 tumor suppressor gene expression, 187
Genetic-directed enzyme prodrug therapy, 188
Genetic molecular alterations, 6
Genetic prodrug activating therapy, 188
Genetic risk prevention, 32, 32t
Genetic screening, 51–7
 developing issues, 57
 evolution, 52
 general considerations, 53
 purpose, 52
 specific syndromes, 54–6
  checkpoint kinase 2 gene, 54–5
  hereditary "breast" syndromes, 54
  hereditary gastrointestinal syndromes, 56
  serine threonine kinase, 55
Genitourinary cancers, 535–603. See also specific types
 bladder and ureter, 548–56
 penile, 558–61
 prostate, 563–86
 renal, 536–47
 testicular, 589–603
Germ cell tumors, ovarian, 606–9. See also Ovarian cancer
Germ-line molecular alterations, 6
Gerson therapy, 201
Gestational trophoblastic tumor, malignant, 623–4, 624t
Giant cell tumor of bone, 713
Gleason score, prostate cancer, 565, 568, 569
Glioblastomas, 626–34. See also Brain tumors, primary
Gliomas, 626–34. See also Brain tumors, primary

Glucagonoma syndrome, 308
Glucksberg grading system, 159t
Glucocorticoids, adrenal failure from, 354
Glutathione, in drug resistance, 145
Gonadal dysfunction, as late treatment effect, 356
Gonadotropin–releasing hormone (GnRH), 168
Gonadotropin–releasing hormone (GnRH) agonists, 168
Gonzalez regimen, 201
G1 phase, 10
G2 phase, 10
Graft-versus-host disease (GVHD), post-HSCT
 acute
  overview, 158
  prophylaxis, 158
  stages and grading, 159t
  treatment, 160
 chronic, 160
Granulocyte–colony-stimulating factor (G-CSF)
 accelerated chemotherapy, 146
 prophylactic, for febrile neutropenia, 249, 249f, 415, 451, 600, 739
Growth factor receptors, 6, 7t
Growth factors, 6, 7t. See also specific types
 angiogenesis, 14
Growth hormone deficiency, treatment-related, 354
Growth-inhibiting signals, independence from, 11–12
Growth-promoting signals, independence from, 11–12
G1-S transition, 10
Guided imagery, 200
Gynecologic cancer, 605–24. See also specific cancers
 cancer of cervix, 614–17 (See also Cervical cancer)
 cancer of uterine corpus, 610–13
 ovarian, 606–9
 vulvar and vaginal cancer, 618–24

H

Haloperidol
 as adjuvant analgesics, 264
 for end-of-life delirium, 370
 for nausea and vomiting, 341
Haploidentical-related donor-matched transplant, 155
HapMap, 57
Hatha yoga, 200
Head and neck cancers, 643–63
 epidemiology, 644, 648
  cancer of nasal cavity and paranasal sinuses, 648
  cancer of oral cavity, 648
  cancer of pharynx, 648
  laryngeal cancer, 648
  salivary gland cancer, 648
 etiology, 646–7
 intraocular tumors
  melanoma, 664
  retinoblastoma, 664
 investigations, 654–5
 management, 657–61
  chemoradiation, 149
  early stage, 658–60
  locally advanced unresectable, 660–1
  malignant lesions, 657
  metastatic, 661
  premalignant lesions, 657
 overview, 644
 pathology
  other, 650
  salivary gland cancer, 651
  squamous cell carcinoma, 650
 presentation
  cancer of nasal cavity and paranasal sinus, 652
  cancer of oral cavity, 652
  cancer of pharynx, 652–3
  laryngeal cancer, 652
  salivary gland cancer, 653
 prognosis and follow-up
  cancer of nasal cavity and paranasal sinuses, 662
  cancer of oral cavity, 662
  cancer of pharynx, 662
  laryngeal cancer, 662
  salivary gland cancer, 662
 rehabilitation, 663
 screening and prevention, 649
 staging, 656
Heart, late effects of treatment on, 358
Helicobacter pylori infection, 21, 33
Hematogenous metastasis, 14
Hematopoietic stem cell transplantation (HSCT), 151–64
 for acute lymphoblastic leukemia, 727
 allogeneic, 152
 autologous, 152
 conditioning regimens, 157
 donor lymphocyte infusion, 164
 donor selection
  donors, potential, 154–5
  human leukocyte antigen typing, 154
 for multiple myeloma, 762
 post-transplant complications, 158–64
  acute graft-versus-host disease, 158–60, 159t (See also Acute graft-versus-host disease (GVHD), post HSCT)
  chronic graft-versus-host disease, 160
  hepatic veno-occlusive disease, 162
  infection, 161–2
  long-term, 164
  T-cell depletion, 158
 pretransplant evaluation, 156
 umbilical cord blood, 154–5
Hematopoietic support, for high-dose chemotherapy, 146
Hemolysis, 218

Hemolytic anemia, paraneoplastic, 316
Hepatic failure, chemotherapy dose adjustment in, 805t–807t
Hepatic veno-occlusive disease, post-HSCT, 162
Hepatitis B virus, 20, 33
Hepatitis C virus, 20, 33
Hepatocellular carcinoma, 494–6
 diagnosis and prognosis, 494
 epidemiology, 494
 etiology
  aflatoxins, 19
  hepatitis B virus, 20, 33
 management
  best supportive care, 496
  liver-directed approaches, 495
  sorafenib, 496
  surgery, 495
  systemic chemotherapy, 496
 pathology and staging, 495
 symptoms, 494, 495t
Hepatorenal syndrome, 346
Her2, gastric cancer testing for, 472
HER2 amplification/overexpression, breast cancer, 436
 on chemotherapy, 451
Hereditary clear cell carcinoma, 536. See also Renal cancer
Hereditary diffuse gastric cancer
 genetic screening, 55
 prophylactic surgery, 36
Hereditary leiomyoma, 537
Hereditary non-polyposis colorectal cancer (HNPCC)
 genetic screening, 56
 prophylactic surgery for, 36
Hereditary papillary renal carcinoma syndrome (HPRCC), 536. See also Renal cancer
Her2/Neu, 191
 esophageal cancer testing, 468
High-dose rate (HDR) sources, 96

Histone deacetylase (HDAC), 184
Histone deacetylase inhibitors, 184
HLA typing, 154
Hodgkin lymphoma, 768–73
 classification, 768, 769t
 clinical subtypes, 770, 771t
 epidemiology, 768
 etiology, Epstein-Barr virus, 20
 immunophenotypes, discriminatory, 774, 777t–778t, 815t
 management, 772–3
  advanced stage, 772
  early stage (IA and IIA), 772
  late effects, 773
  lymphocyte-predominant HL, 772
  salvage therapy, 773
  secondary malignancies, 359
  thyroid dysfunction from, 354
 pathology, 768
 prognosis, 771–2, 772b
 risk factors, 768, 769t
 staging, 770, 770b
Homeopathy, 198
Hormonal therapy
 for prostate cancer, 582–3
 venous thromboembolism from, 272
Hormone-responsive cancers, 166b
Hormones, 166. See also specific types
Hormone therapy, 165–73. See also specific types
 controversies
  adjuvant therapy duration, 173
  chemoendocrine therapy, 173
 hormone-responsive cancers for, 166b
 principles, 166b
 rationale and aim, 166
 resistance, 172
 response predictors, 171
 types
  agonists and supraphysiological hormone doses, 168–9

  endocrine gland ablation, 168
  single-agent vs. combination, 170
  steroid hormone antagonists, 169–70
  steroid-producing enzyme inhibition, 169
Hoxsey therapy, 203
HTLV-1, 21
HTLV-2, 21
Human immunodeficiency virus (HIV), 21
Human leukocyte antigens (HLAs), 154
 typing, 154
Human papillomavirus (HPV), 20, 33
 anal cancer, 508
 cervical cancer, 614
 head and neck cancers, 646
 immunization, 614
 penile cancer, 558
Hurthle cell carcinomas, 514
Hydatidiform moles, 620–2, 622t
Hydration
 end-of-life care, 379–80
 last days of life, 390
Hydrazine sulfate, 202
Hydromorphone
 metabolites and side effects, 259
 for step 2 pain relief, 258
Hydroxyurea, 130–1
Hyperalgesia
 breakthrough pain, 262
 opioid-induced, 263
Hypercalcemia, 290–2
 acute renal failure from, 298
 in breast cancer, metastatic, 460
 in endocrine paraneoplastic syndromes, 307–8
 in end-of-life care, 366, 367, 374, 376
 in hepatocellular carcinoma, 495t
 in intestinal obstruction, 340
 in multiple myeloma, 752, 754, 755t, 758, 763t
 in non-Hodgkin lymphoma, 781
 in prostate cancer, 569
 in renal cancer, 540, 542

in tumor lysis syndrome, 300
Hyperfractionation, 84
Hyperglycemia, 297
  in Cushing's syndrome, 307
Hypericum perforatum, 203
Hyperkalemia, 296
  in tumor lysis syndrome, 300, 301
  in urinary tract obstruction, 349
Hyperkeratosis, acral, paraneoplastic, 319
Hyperphosphatemia
  in acute leukemia, 726
  in tumor lysis syndrome, 300
Hypertrophic osteoarthropathy, 318
Hyperuricemia
  in acute leukemia, 726
  in acute myeloid leukemia, prevention, 721
  in tumor lysis syndrome, 300
Hypocalcemia
  in acute lymphoblastic leukemia, 726
  from bisphosphonates, 264, 291
  from chelation therapy, 202
  from dactinomycin, 116
  in tumor lysis syndrome, 300
Hypofractionation, 84
Hypogastric plexus block, superior, 266
Hypoglycemia, 297, 308
Hypokalemia
  from cisplatin, 133
  in Cushing's syndrome, 307
  in intestinal obstruction, 340
  in Verner-Morrison pancreatic cholera, 308
Hypomagnesemia
  from cetuximab, 180
  from cisplatin, 133, 600
  from EGFR inhibitors, 506
  from panitumumab, 180
  in tumor lysis syndrome, 300
Hyponatremia, 294–5
  from raised intracranial pressure, 326

Hypophysectomy, as hormone therapy, 168
Hypoxia-induced factor 1α (*HIF1α*), 14
Hypoxia reduction, in radiation oncology, 86

I

Ibritumomab, 182
Ichthyosis, 319
Idarubicin, 115
Ifosfamide, 105
  for desmoid tumors, 704
  for Ewing's sarcoma, 692, 709
  for liposarcoma, 705
  for osteosarcoma, 692, 707, 708
  renal tubular dysfunction from, 299
  for rhabdomyosarcoma, 698
  for soft tissue sarcomas, 691
  for synovial sarcoma, 705
Imatinib, 178
  for acute lymphoblastic leukemia, 726
  for chordoma, 712
  for chronic myeloid leukemia, 732, 734
  for dermatofibrosarcoma protuberans, 704
  for dermoid tumors, 704
  for gastrointestinal stromal tumor, 694, 696
  resistance, 733
  side effects, 733
Immunoaugmentative therapy (IAT), 202
Immunophenotypes, lymphocytic neoplasms
  B cells, 814t
  Hodgkin lymphoma, 774, 777t–778t, 815t
  T cells, 814t–815t
Immunotherapy, 190–1.
  See also specific types
  for malignant melanoma, 674
Infections, 20–1
  bacterial, 21
  in cancer prevention, 33
  parasitic, 21
  post-HSCT, 161–2
  viral, 20–1, 33
Inflammatory breast cancer (IBC), 456
Initiation, 38

Insulin-like growth factors (IGF), from large metastatic tumors, 297
Intensity-modulated radiation therapy (IMRT), 93, 94f
Interferon (IFN), for carcinoid syndrome, 481
Interferon-α (IFN-α)
  for Kaposi sarcoma, 702
  for malignant melanoma, 673
  for osteosarcoma, metastatic, 708
  for renal cancer, 544
Interferon-α2B (IFN-α2B), for malignant melanoma, 674
Interferon-γ (IFN-γ), 190
Interleukin-2 (IL-2)
  high-dose, 190
  for malignant melanoma, 674
  for renal cancer, 543
International Bone Marrow Transplant Registry (IBMRT) grading, 159t
Intestinal
  obstruction, 340–2
  etiology, 340
  investigations, 340
  management
    medical, 341–2
    options, 341
    surgical, 342
  presentation, 340
Intracranial pressure (ICP), raised, 326–8
  anatomy, 326
  clinical presentation, 326
  diagnosis, 327
  management, 327–8
  pathogenesis, 326–7
Intracranial stereotactic radiosurgery (SRS), 98
Intraocular melanoma, 97, 678
Intraocular tumors
  melanoma, 664
  retinoblastoma, 664
Intraoperative radiotherapy, 97
Intrathecal anesthesia, 266–7
Intravenous immunoglobulin (IVIG), for hemolytic anemia, 316
Invasive ductal carcinoma, 436. *See also* Breast cancer

Invasive lobular carcinoma, 437
Ionizing radiation, 23
Ipilimumab, for malignant melanoma, 674
Irinotecan, 136–7
  for brain tumors, 634
  for colorectal cancer, metastatic
    first-line, 504–5
    regimens, 505t
    second-line, 506
  for pancreatic cancer, 487
  for rhabdomyosarcoma, 698
  for small cell lung cancer, 414
  for small intestine tumors, 480
Iron, parenteral, 221
Ixabepilone, 140, 143t

J

Jaundice, obstructive, 344–6
  etiology, 344
  examination, 345
  history, 344
  management, 346
  palliative surgery, 75
Jaw osteonecrosis, from breast cancer radiotherapy, 460

K

Kaposi sarcoma, 700–2
  epidemiology and etiology, 700
  management, 701–2
  pathology, 700
  presentation, 700
  staging, 701, 701t
Karnofsky performance status, 802b
Kattan nomogram, prostate cancer, 572
Ketoconazole
  for adrenocortical tumors, 530
  for Cushing's syndrome, 307
  for prostate cancer, 582
Kidney cancer
  angiogenesis in, 14
  von Hippel-Lindau gene in, 14, 536
Kidney failure, chemotherapy dose adjustment in, 808t–809t

Kidneys, late effects of treatment in, 358
KRAS mutation, in colorectal cancer, 506
k-RAS mutations, 187

L

Lactobacillis, 202
Laetrile, 202
Lambert-Eaton myasthenic syndrome, 313
Lanreotide, for carcinoid syndrome, 481
Lapatinib, 179
  for invasive ductal carcinoma, 436
  for metastatic breast cancer, 462
Large T, 4
Laryngeal cancer, 643–63. See also Head and neck cancers
  epidemiology, 648
  presentation, 652
  prognosis and follow-up, 662
Last days of life care, 390–1. See also End-of-life care
Late-responding tissue, radiotherapy, 85
Late treatment effects, 351–60. See also Treatment effects, late
Lead-time bias, in cancer screening, 47
Leiomyoma, hereditary, 537
Leiomyosarcomas, 613, 705
Lenalidomide
  for chronic lymphoid leukemias, 748
  for multiple myeloma, 758
  for myelodysplastic syndromes, 738
  venous thromboembolism from, 222f, 273, 274t, 753
Length bias, in cancer screening, 47
Leser-Trelat, sign of, 319
Letrozole, 169
Leucovorin, for metastatic colorectal cancer, 504
Leukemias. See also specific types

  acute, 717–27
  acute lymphoblastic, 724–7
  acute myeloid, 718–23
  acute promyelocytic, 722
  chronic
  chronic lymphoid, 742–8
  chronic myeloid, 730–4
Leukocytosis, in chronic myeloid leukemia, 731
Leukoplakia, 650
  chewing tobacco in, 32
Leveen shunts, 75
Levomepromazine, for nausea and vomiting, 341
Li-Fraumeni syndrome, genetic screening, 54
Limb-conserving surgery, 68
Limitless replication, 12–13
Linear accelerator, 88
Liposarcomas, 705
Liver failure, chemotherapy dose adjustment in, 805t–807t
Liver transplantation, 68
Lobular carcinoma in situ, 436, 447. See also Breast cancer
Lomustine, 108–9
Low-dose rate (LDR) sources, 96
Low-fat diet, 201
Low-molecular-weight heparin (LMWH)
  for central venous catheter thrombosis, 286
  for deep vein thrombosis, 276
  for venous thromboembolism, meta-analyses, 278
  for venous thromboembolism prophylaxis
    clinical practice guidelines, 280, 281–2
    regimens and cost, 283t–284t
Lumiliximab, for chronic lymphoid leukemias, 748
Lumpectomy, for early breast cancer, 448

Lung cancer, 396–9. See also specific types
  epidemiology, 396, 397t
  etiology, 396
  genetics, 398
  investigations, 399
  non–small-cell lung cancer, 400–12
  pathology, 397–8
  screening and prevention, 396
  signs and symptoms, presenting, 399
  small-cell lung cancer, 413–18
  smoking in, 18, 32, 34
  superior vena cava syndrome in, 323–4, 415
  survival rates, 72
  treatment
    brachytherapy, 96
    chemoradiation, 149
Lungs, late effects of treatment on, 358
Luteinizing hormone (LH), 168
Luteinizing hormone–releasing hormone (LHRH), 168
Luteinizing hormone–releasing hormone (LHRH) agonists, 168
Lymphedema, end-of-life care for, 373–4
Lymphomas. See also specific types
  CNS primary, 636–7
  hypercalcemia in, 290
  immunophenotypes
    B cells, 814t
    Hodgkin lymphoma, 774, 777t–778t, 815t
    T cells, 814t–815t
  malignant, 767–87
    Hodgkin, 768–73
    non-Hodgkin, 774–84
    non-Hodgkin and AIDS, 786–7
  unsealed radionuclide treatment, 100
Lynch syndrome, genetic screening, 56

M

MAGE-1, 191
Malignant ascites treatment
  surgery, 80
  unsealed radionuclide, 99
Malignant gestational trophoblastic tumor, 623–4, 624t
Malignant lymphomas. See Lymphomas, malignant
Malignant
  melanoma, 668–76
  anal cancer, 511
  anatomy, 668
  benign pigmented nevi, 668, 669f
  clinical presentation, 670
  epidemiology and etiology, 668, 669f
    sun exposure, 22, 32, 668, 670
    ultraviolet light, 32, 668, 670
  investigations, 670
  management, 672–6
    chemotherapy, immunotherapy, and radiotherapy, 673–4
    future directions, 676
    metastatic disease, 674–5
    prognosis and risk of relapse, 673
    surgical and sentinel lymph node biopsy, 672–3, 673t
  pathology, 671
  screening and prevention, 670
  staging, 671
Malignant pericardial effusion, surgery, 80
Malignant pleural effusion
  in cancer of unknown primary, 795
  surgery for, 80
Malignant pleural mesothelioma, 420–4. See also Mesothelioma
Mammalian target of rapamycin (mTOR) inhibitors, 179
Mammography, 440–1
Manipulative methods, 199
Massage, therapeutic, 199
Mastectomy
  for ductal carcinoma in situ, 446
  for early breast cancer, 448
  prophylactic, 69
Matched unrelated donors, 154
Mature B-cell acute lymphoblastic leukemia, 725

MDR1, 188
  in anthracycline resistance, 112
Mechlorethamine, 106
Meditation, 200
Medullary adrenal tumors, 528–31. See also Adrenal cancer
Medullary renal carcinoma, 537. See also Renal cancer
Medullary thyroid carcinoma. See also Thyroid cancers
  epidemiology and etiology, 514–15
  pathology and genetics, 516
  presentation, 517
  prognosis, 527
  screening and prevention, 516
  staging, 518, 518t
  surveillance and follow-up, 526
  treatment
    external beam radiotherapy, 524
    surgery, 521
Medulloblastomas, 626–34. See also Brain tumors, primary
MEK inhibitors, for malignant melanoma, 675, 676
Melanoma
  intraocular, 664, 678
  malignant (See Malignant melanoma)
Melatonin, 202
Melphalan, 106
Meningiomas, 626–34. See also Brain tumors, primary
6-Mercaptopurine (6-MP), 124
Merkel cell carcinoma, 684
Mesothelioma, 420–4
  clinical presentation, 421
  epidemiology, 420
  etiology, 420
  investigations, 421
  management, 423–4
  pathology, 420
  prevention, 420
  staging, 421, 422t, 423t
  treatment outcome, 424
Metabolic dysfunction. See also specific types
  late effects of treatment in, 354–5, 355t

Metabolic
  emergencies, 289–301.
  See also specific types
  acute renal failure,
    malignant
    disease, 298
  hypercalcemia, 290–2
  hyperglycemia, 297
  hyperkalemia, 296
  hypoglycemia, 297
  hyponatremia, 294–5
  renal tubular
    dysfunction, 299
  tumor lysis
    syndrome, 300–1
Metabolic syndrome, late
  effects of treatment
  in, 355, 355t
Metastatic disease, 14,
  78–80. *See also specific
  cancers*
  bone, 78
  brain, 79, 638–40 (See
    also Brain metastases)
  diagnosis, 78
  hematogenous, 14
  indications, 78
  malignant ascites, 80
  malignant pericardial
    effusion, 80
  malignant pleural
    effusion, 80
  positron emission
    tomography,
    preoperative, 67
Methadone
  metabolites and side
    effects, 259
  for neuropathic pain, 259
  for step 2 pain relief, 258
Methicillin-resistant
  Staphylococcus aureus
  (MRSA), 237
Methotrexate, 118–20
Methylprednisolone, for
  bone pain, 257
Metoclopramide,
  for nausea and
  vomiting, 341
MicroRNA genes, 6, 8, 9t
Mind-body
  interventions, 200–1
  art therapy, 200
  meditation, 200
  music therapy, 200
  relaxation and guided
    imagery, 200
  yoga, 200
Mindfulness-based stress
  reduction (MBSR), 200
Minimally invasive surgery
  (MIS), 68

definitive treatment, 73
diagnosis and
  staging, 70–1
Mini-mental test, 631, 632t
Mirtazapine, for end-of-
  life anorexia and
  cachexia, 367
Mismatch repair genes
  screening, 56
Mitomycin C, 116–17
Mitosis (M), 10
Mitoxantrone, 115–16
Mixed mullerian
  tumors, 613
Mixed parotid tumor, 651.
  See also Salivary gland
  tumors
MLH1 screening, 56
Molar pregnancy, 620–2,
  622t
Molecular alterations, 6–9.
  *See also specific cancers
  and types*
  apoptosis regulators, 7,
    7t
  growth factors and
    growth factor
    receptors, 6, 7t
  microRNA genes, 6, 8, 9t
  oncogenes, 6, 7t
  signal transduction
    molecules, 7, 7t
  transcription factors, 6,
    7t
  tumor suppressor
    genes, 8, 9t
  types, 6
Molecular cancer
  biology, 3–14
  cancer biology, 10–14
    angiogenesis
      establishment, 13–14
    apoptosis evasion, 13
    cell cycle
      deregulation, 10–11
    growth-promoting and
      growth-inhibiting
      signals
      independence, 11–12
    invasion and
      metastasis, 14
    limitless
      replication, 12–13
  molecular
    alterations, 6–9
    (See *also* Molecular
    alterations)
  multistep
    carcinogenesis, 4
Monoclonal antibodies. *See
  also specific cancers
  and types*

for acute lymphoblastic
  leukemia, 727
alemtuzumab, 180
bevacizumab, 180
cetuximab, 180
panitumumab, 180
rituximab, 180
trastuzumab, 181
Monoclonal cancers, 16
Morphine
  low-dose, 258
  oral morphine
    equivalents, 258
  for step 2 pain relief, 258
MRP, in anthracycline
  resistance, 112
MSH2 screening, 56
MSH6 screening, 56
Mucinous cystic
  carcinoma, 537–8. *See
  also* Renal cancer
Multidisciplinary
  teams, 62–3
  end-of-life care, 364
Multidrug resistance, 102
  classical, 144
Multidrug resistance–
  associated protein, 145
Multilocular cystic
  carcinoma, 537–8. *See
  also* Renal cancer
Multinational Association
  of Supportive Care
  of Cancer (MASCC)
  scoring index, for febrile
  neutropenia, 245, 245t
Multiple endocrine
  neoplasia, prophylactic
  surgery for, 36
Multiple myeloma
  (MM), 749–64
  classification, 754, 755t
  clinical features, 752–3
  defined, 750
  diagnosis, 754, 754b
  epidemiology and risk
    factors, 750
  hypercalcemia in, 290
  pathogenesis, 751
  staging and
    prognosis, 756, 757t
  treatment, 758–64
    hematopoietic stem cell
      transplant, 762
    indications, 758
    supportive therapy, 762,
      763t–764t
    systemic therapy,
      agents, 758, 759t
    systemic therapy,
      regimens, 758,
      760t–761t

Multistep
  carcinogenesis, 4
Music therapy, 200
Mutant oncogene
  correction, 187
Mutations, 4
MYC, 11
MYC, 11
Myeloablative conditioning
  regimens, HSCT, 157
Myelodysplastic syndromes
  (MDS), 736–9
  classification, 737t
  clinical features, 736–7
  clinical trials, 738
  epidemiology, 736
  management, 738
  pathology, 736
  prognosis, 739, 739t
Myeloid growth
  factors, for febrile
  neutropenia, 246
Myelosuppression, 230
  anemia from, 218
  febrile neutropenia
  and, 230
MYH-associated
  polyposis, 56
MYH screening, 56

N

Naltrexone, low-dose, 202
Nasal cavity cancers,
  643–63. See *also* Head
  and neck cancers
  epidemiology, 648
  presentation, 653
  prognosis and
  follow-up, 662
Nasopharyngeal carcinoma
  etiology
  Epstein-Barr virus, 20, 33
  salt fish, 19
Naturopathy, 198
Nausea and/or vomiting
  management
  antiemetics (See
  Antiemetics)
  end-of-life care, 374–8,
  375f, 377t–378t
  causes, 374–6, 375f
  management, 376,
  377t–378t
  prevalence, 374
  terminology, 817t
Necrolytic migratory
  erythema, 319
Nelarabine, 126–7
Neoadjuvant
  radiotherapy, 92
Nerve blocks, 266

Nerves, late effects of
  treatment on, 358
Neural crest tumors,
  unsealed radionuclide
  diagnosis and treatment
  of, 99
Neuroblastoma, 532, 533t
Neuroleptics. See *also*
  specific agents
  as adjuvant
  analgesics, 264
  for end-of-life
  delirium, 370
Neuronavigation, for brain
  tumor surgery, 633
Neuropathic pain, 255
Neuropathic pain
  management
  analgesia, 257
  methadone, 259
Neuropathy
  peripheral, 310–11
  sensory, 817t
Neuropsychological treatment
  effects, late, 360
Neurotoxicity, 358
Neutrons, 88
Neutrophilic dermatosis,
  paraneoplastic, 318
Neutrophils, 816t
Nevi, benign
  pigmented, 668, 669f
Nicotine addiction, 34
Nilotinib, 732
  for chronic myeloid
  leukemia, 732
  resistance, 733–4
  side effects, 733
Nitrogen mustards. See
  also specific types
  chlorambucil, 104
  cyclophosphamide, 104–5
  ifosfamide, 105
  mechlorethamine, 106
  melphalan, 106
Nitrosamines, head and
  neck cancers from, 646
Nitrosoureas, 107–9. See
  also specific types
  carmustine, 108
  lomustine, 108–9
  streptozocin, 109
Nomograms
  BSA, 804
  prostate cancer, 570–2
Non-Hodgkin
  lymphoma, 774–84
  AIDS and, 786–7
  classification
  immunophenotype and
  cytogenetics, 774,
  777t–778t

WHO, 774, 776b
clinical features, 779,
  780t
gene expression
  profiling, 782–3
incidence, 774
management
  aggressive (diffuse large
  B-cell), 784
  highly aggressive
  (Burkitt,
  lymphoblastic), 784
  initial, 783
  low-grade, 783
  relapsed, 783–4
  unsealed
  radionuclide, 99
prognosis, 781t, 782,
  782t
risk factors, 774, 775f,
  775t
staging, 781, 781t
Nonmelanoma skin
  cancer, 680–3
  epidemiology and
  etiology, 680
  management, 682–3
  presentation, 680, 681f
  prevention and future
  directions, 683
Nonmyeloablative
  conditioning regimens,
  HSCT, 157
Non–small-cell lung cancer
  (NSCLC), 400–12. See
  also Lung cancer
FDG-PET scanning, 400
staging, 400, 401t, 402
superior vena cava
  syndrome in, 324
treatment
  chemotherapy, 400,
  405–8
  chemotherapy,
  preoperative, 402
  modalities, 400
  radiation therapy, 400,
  410–12
  surgery, 400, 402–4,
  404t
Nonsteroidal
  anti-inflammatory drugs
  (NSAIDs), for pain, 257
Nottingham Prognostic
  Index (NPI), 438,
  438t, 450
Nutrition
  end-of-life care, 379–80
  last days of life, 390
Nutritional anemia, 218
Nutritional
  therapeutics, 201

O

Obesity, 19
Oblimersen, 187
Obstructive complications, 337–49. *See also specific types*
  bowel, 74
  bronchial obstruction and stridor, 338–9
  intestinal, 340–2
  obstructive jaundice, 344–6
  urinary tract, 348–9
Obstructive jaundice, 344–6
  etiology, 344
  examination, 345
  history, 344
  management, 346
Octreotide
  for carcinoid syndrome, 481
  for nausea and vomiting, 341
Ocular melanoma, 97, 678
Ocular toxicity, 358
Oltipraz, 38
Omacetaxine, for chronic myeloid leukemia, 732
Oncocytoma, 537. *See also* Renal cancer
Oncogene mutations, 16
  gene therapy correction, 187
Oncogenes, 6, 7t. *See also specific types and cancers*
Oncogenesis, 4
Oocyte storage, 357
Oophorectomy, as hormone therapy, 168
Opioids. *See also* Pain management; *specific agents*
  addiction, 263
  analgesic
    dose equivalents, 263t
    low-dose, 257–8
    more potent, 258–60
  hyperalgesia, 263
  side effect management, 260
  titration, 259, 259f, 262
  tolerance and withdrawal, 262
Oral cavity cancers, 643–63. *See also* Head and neck cancers
  epidemiology, 648
  presentation, 652
  prognosis and follow-up, 662
Oral morphine equivalents (OMEs), 258

Orchidectomy, prophylactic, 69
Orchidopexy, prophylactic, 69
Osteoarthropathy, hypertrophic, 318
Osteonecrosis of jaw, from breast cancer radiotherapy, 460
Osteopenia, from steroids, 358
Osteosarcoma, 706–7. *See also* Bone sarcomas
  metastatic, 707–8
Ototoxicity, 358
Outcomes of interest, efficacy, 209
Ovarian cancer, 606–9
  epidemiology, 606
  etiology and risk factors, 606
  pathology, 606
  presentation, 606–7, 607t
  prognosis, advanced stage disease, 607t
  treatment, 607–9
    bowel obstruction, 74
    chemotherapy, primary, 609
    cytoreductive surgery, 76
    germ cell and sex cord tumors, 609
    new approaches, 609
    recurrent disease, 609
    surgery and staging, 607–8, 608t
Ovarian tissue storage, 357, 357t
Ovarian tissue transposition, 357, 357t
Overall survival, 209
Oxacillin-resistant *Staphylococcus aureus* (ORSA), 237
Oxaliplatin, 134–5
  for metastatic colorectal cancer
    first-line, 504–5
    second-line, 506
Oxycodone
  low-dose, 258
  metabolites and side effects, 259
  for step 2 pain relief, 258

P

p53, 10–11, 16, 145, 187
  screening, 54
Paclitaxel, 143t

Paget's disease of the breast, 437
  osteosarcoma with, 706–7
Pain
  acute *vs.* chronic, 255
  neuropathic, 255
  palliative surgery, 75
  patient interpretation, 255
  somatic, 255
  visceral, 255, 266
  nerve blocks for, 266
Pain management, 251–68. *See also specific agents and therapies*
  basic pillars, 256
  for breakthrough pain, 262–4
    adjuvant analgesics, 264
    dose equivalents, 263t
    general approach, 262
    increasing analgesic requirements and persistent pain, 262–3
  causes
    exacerbating factors, 254
    primary, 254
  general points, 252
  incidence, 252
  oral morphine equivalents, 258
  other
    complementary and alternative medicine, 267–8
    epidural anesthesia, 266
    intrathecal anesthesia, 266–7
    nerve blocks, 266
    palliative radiotherapy, 267
    psychological and cognitive-behavioral, 267
  pain scales assessment, 253
  pharmacologic, 256–60
    analgesic ladder, 256–7, 256f
    side effect management, 2
    step 1: mild-to-moderate pain, nonopioid analgesia, 257
    step 2: mild-to-moderate pain, low-dose opioids, 257–8

step 3: nonresponsive, more potent opioid, 258–60
titration, 259, 259b, 262
understanding in, 255
undertreatment, 254
Pain scales, 253
PALB2, in breast cancer, 434
Palliative radiotherapy, 92, 267
Palliative surgery, 74–6
ascites, 75
bowel obstruction, 74
cytoreductive surgery, 76
fistulas, 74–5
gastrointestinal bleeding, 76
jaundice, 75
pain, 75
primary tumor resection, 76
Pancreatic cancer, 484–8
anatomy, 484
epidemiology, 484
evaluation and staging, 485, 486t
familial syndromes, 485t
future directions, 488
management, 486–8
chemotherapy alone, 487–8
concurrent chemoradiation, 486–7
radiotherapy, 488
recurrence, 486
surgery, 486
symptomatic, 488
targeted biological, 488
pathology, 486
presentation, location in, 484
survival rates, 72
Pancreatic cholera, Verner-Morrison, 308
Pancreaticoduodenectomy, 486
Panitumumab, 180
for metastatic colorectal cancer, 504, 505, 506
Papillary-follicular thyroid carcinoma. See also Thyroid cancers
epidemiology and etiology, 514
pathology and genetics, 515
presentation, 516
staging, 518
surveillance, follow-up, and prognosis, 526

treatment
external beam radiotherapy, 524
radioiodine, 522–3
surgery, 520–1
Papillary renal cell carcinoma, hereditary, 537. See also Renal cancer
Papillary thyroid carcinoma. See also Thyroid cancers
epidemiology and etiology, 514
pathology and genetics, 515
presentation, 516
staging, 518
surveillance, follow-up, and prognosis, 526
treatment
external beam radiotherapy, 524
radioiodine, 522–3
surgery, 520–1
Paracrine signals, 11
Parallel structures, radiotherapy, 85
Paranasal sinus cancers, 643–63. See also Head and neck cancers
epidemiology, 648
presentation, 653
prognosis and follow-up, 662
Paraneoplastic cerebellar degeneration, 310
Paraneoplastic pemphigus, 318
Paraneoplastic retinopathy, 312–13
Paraneoplastic syndromes (PNS), 303–19
cancers with, 304
defined, 304
dermatologic and skeletal acanthosis nigricans, 319
Bathex syndrome, 319
digital clubbing, 318
erythroderma, 319
hypertrophic osteoarthropathy, 318
ichthyosis, 319
necrolytic migratory erythema, 319
pemphigus, 318
pruritus, 319
pyoderma gangrenosum, 318

sign of Leser-Trelat, 319
Sweets syndrome, 318
vitiligo, 319
endocrine, 306–8
Cushing's syndrome, 306–7
glucagonoma syndrome, 308
hypercalcemia, 307–8
hypoglycemia, 308
somatostatin syndrome, 308
syndrome of inappropriate antidiuretic hormone, 306
Verner-Morrison pancreatic cholera, 308
Zollinger-Ellison syndrome, 308
fever and cachexia, 304
hematological coagulopathy, 317
platelet disorders, 316
red cell disorders, 316
white cell disorders, 316
mechanisms, 304
neurological, 310–14
acute necrotizing myopathy, 311–12
dermatomyositis and polymyositis, 313–14
encephalomyelopathies, 311
Lambert-Eaton myasthenic syndrome, 313
paraneoplastic (cancer-associated) retinopathy, 312–13
paraneoplastic cerebellar degeneration, 310
peripheral neuropathy, 310–11
stiff-man syndrome, 312
Parasitic infections, 21
Parenteral nutrition, end-of-life, 380
Pazopanib, for soft tissue sarcoma, 692
Pemetrexed, 118, 120
for mesothelioma, 423, 424
for non–small-cell lung cancer, 407

Pemphigus, 318
Pemphigus vulgaris, paraneoplastic, 318
Penile cancer, 558–61
 epidemiology and etiology, 558
 investigations, 560
 management
  brachytherapy, 97, 560
  primary tumor, 560
  regional lymph nodes, 561
 outcomes, 561
 pathology, 558
 presentation, 560
 staging, 558, 559t
Pentostatin, 129
 for chronic lymphoid leukemias, 747
 for non-Hodgkin lymphoma, 783
Peptide vaccines, 190
Pericardial effusion, malignant, surgery, 80
Peripheral neuropathy, 310–11
Peritoneal-venous shunts, 75
Persistent pain, 262–3
Pertuzumab, for breast cancer, 436
 metastatic, 462
Peutz-Jeghers syndrome, genetic screening, 55
p53 gene therapy, 187
P-glycoprotein, 144
 in drug resistance
  classical multidrug resistance, 144
  vincristine, 141t
P-170 glycoprotein, 112
Pharmacological exposure, chemical, 24
Pharmacological resistance, 144
Pharyngeal cancers, 643–63. See also Head and neck cancers
 epidemiology, 648
 presentation
  hypopharyngeal, 653
  nasopharyngeal, 652
  oropharyngeal, 652
 prognosis and follow-up, 662
Phase 0 clinical trials, 210
Phase I clinical trials, 210
 cancer prevention, 40–1
Phase II clinical trials, 210
 cancer prevention, 40–1
Phase III clinical trials, 210
 cancer prevention, 41

Phase IV clinical trials, 211
Philadelphia chromosome, 178, 730
Photons, 88, 89f
Physical activity, 199
Pineal tumors, 626–34. See also Brain tumors, primary
Pituitary dysfunction, late effects of treatment in, 354, 355t
Pituitary tumors, 626–34. See also Brain tumors, primary
Platelet disorders, paraneoplastic, 316
Platelets, 816t
Pleomorphic adenoma, 651. See also Salivary gland tumors
Pleomorphic rhabdomyosarcoma, 697
Pleural effusion, malignant
 in cancer of unknown primary, 795
 surgery, 80
PMS2 screening, 56
POEMS syndrome, 316
Polymyositis, 313–14
Polyposis syndromes. See also specific types
 genetic screening, 56
Ponatinib
 for chronic myeloid leukemia, 732
 side effects, 733
Portal imaging, 94
Positron emission tomography (PET), preoperative, for metastatic disease, 67
Prayer, spiritual, 203
Precursor B-cell acute lymphoblastic leukemia, 724
Prednisone. See also Corticosteroids
 for bone pain, 257
Pregnancy, molar, 620–2, 622t
Prevention, cancer, 29–43
 chemoprevention
  agents and mechanisms, 38–9, 39t
 defined, 30
 principles, 38
 clinical trials, 40–1
 diet
  carotenoids, 43
  fat, 42
  fiber, 42

 folate, 43
 fruits and vegetables, 19, 42
 environmental risks, 32
 genetic risks, 32, 32t
 infectious causes, 33
 smoking-related cancers, 18, 32, 34
 strategies, 30–1
 surgery, 36–7
Primary central nervous system lymphomas, 636–7
Primary malignant spindle cell sarcoma of bone, 712
Primary tumor resection, palliative, 76
Probiotic supplements, 202
Procarbazine, 110
Progesterone receptor (PR), 171
Programmed cell death. See Apoptosis
Progression, 38
Promotion, 38
Prophylactic cranial irradiation (PCI), for small cell lung cancer, 418
Prophylactic surgery, 36–7, 69. See also specific cancers
Prostate cancer, 563–74
 castration-resistant, 582
 controversies, 564
 epidemiology, 564
 etiology, 564–5
 future directions, 586
 investigations, 568
 nomograms, 570–2
 pathology, 565
 risk categorization, 574
 screening, 48, 566–7
 signs and symptoms, presenting, 569
 staging and prognostic factors, 569, 571t
Prostate cancer treatment, 574–9
 active surveillance, 574, 576t
 brachytherapy, 97, 577–8
 cryotherapy, 578
 external beam radiotherapy, 577
 future directions, 586
 hormone therapy alone, 578
 organ-confined disease, 574–8, 576t
 prostatectomy, radical, 574–5
 PSA failure, 579
 radiotherapy, 575

watchful waiting, 578
Prostate cancer treatment
outcomes, 580–5
early disease, 580
metastatic disease, 580–5
androgen blockade, 581
bone-targeted therapy, 583–4
castration, medical, 581
castration, surgical, 581
castration-resistant, 582
chemotherapy, 584–5
combined androgen blockade, 581–2
fundamentals, 580–1
hormonal therapies, 582–3
Prostate-specific antigen (PSA), 566–7, 569, 572
Proteasome inhibitors, 183
Protons, 88, 89f
Proto-oncogenes, 16
Pruritus, paraneoplastic, 319
PSA failure, 579
Pseudohyponatremia, 294
Psychoeducational approaches, to pain, 267
Psychological approaches, to pain, 267
PTEN
in breast cancer, 434
screening, 54
Pulmonary embolism (PE). See also Venous thromboembolism (VTE)
clinical presentation, 276, 277t
Pulmonary toxicity, 358
Purine analogs, 124
Pyoderma gangrenosum, 318

Q

Quadrantectomy, for early breast cancer, 448
Quality of life, 209
Quinolones, for febrile neutropenia prophylaxis, 248

R

Radiation exposure
ionizing, 23
other, 23
sun, 22, 32, 668, 670
Radiation-induced cell death, 84–5

Radiation
oncology, 81–100
applications, 82
defined, 82
external beam radiotherapy, 92–5
adjunctive, 92
definitive, 92
by disease site, 95t
neoadjuvant, 92
palliative, 92
treatment planning, 92–4, 94f
historical perspective, 82
palliative, 267
radiation physics, 88–90
radiation safety, 90, 90b
sources of radiation, 89, 89t
types of radiation, 88, 89f
radiobiology, 84–7 (See also Radiobiology)
specialized radiation therapy, 96–100
brachytherapy, 96–7
intraoperative radiotherapy, 97
stereotactic radiosurgery, 98
total body irradiation, 98–9
unsealed radionuclides, 99–100
Radiation physics, 88–90
radiation safety, 90, 90b
sources of radiation, 89, 89t
types of radiation, 88, 89f
Radical surgery, 68
Radiobiology, 84–7
dose, 84
fractionation, 84
hypofractionation and hyperfractionation, 84
radiation-induced cell death, 84–5
radiosensitivity, improving, 86, 87t
tumor and organ, 86, 87t
Radioiodine, for thyroid cancer, 522–3
Radioisotopes, 88, 89f
Radionuclides, unsealed, 99–100
Radiosensitivity
improving, strategies, 86, 87t
tumor and organ, 86, 87t
Radiotherapy. See Radiation oncology

Raltitrexed, 121
Ras oncogene, 12
activated, expression, 4
Ras proto-oncogene, 16
Receptor tyrosine kinases (RTKs), 11–12
Reconstructive surgery, 68. See also specific cancers
Rectal cancer. See also Anal cancer; Colorectal cancer
chemoradiation, 149
Red cell disorders, paraneoplastic, 316
Red cell transfusions, 218, 220
Red clover, 203
Reflexology, 199
Regorafenib
for colorectal cancer, metastatic, 506
for gastrointestinal stromal tumor, 694
Regulatory T-cell (Treg) response modulation, 191
Relaxation, 200
Renal cancer, 536–47
epidemiology and etiology, 536
genetics, 536–7
investigations, 538
pathology, 537–8
signs and symptoms, presenting, 540
staging, 538, 539t
treatment, 540–6
adjuvant, 541
biological therapies, 543–4
chemotherapy, 543
future directions, 546–7
molecular targeted therapies, 544–6, 545t
outcomes, 544
radiotherapy, 541
recurrence, prognostic features, 542–3
supportive care, 542
surgery, 540–1
for transitional cell carcinoma, 544
Renal failure, chemotherapy dose adjustment in, 808t–809t
Renal toxicity, 358
Renal tubular dysfunction, 299
Replication, limitless, 12–13

Research ethics, 208
Resection. See Surgical oncology; Surgical resection
Resistance, drug/therapy, 144–5
 alkylating agents, 104
 anthracyclines, 112
 chemotherapy resistance genes, 188
 failure to engage apoptosis, 145
 glutathione, 145
 hormone therapy, 172
 multidrug, 102
  classical, 144
 multidrug resistance-associated protein, 145
 pharmacological, 144
 target or transport mechanism alteration, 144
Response Evaluation Criteria in Solid Tumors (RECIST), 810t
Restriction point, cell cycle, 10
Retinoblastoma, 664
Retinopathy, paraneoplastic, 312–13
Retroviruses, RNA, 21
Rhabdomyosarcomas (RMS), 696–8
 alveolar, 696
 embryonal, 696
 epidemiology and etiology, 696
 management, 697–8
 pleomorphic, 697
 staging, 697, 697t
Rituximab, 180
 for acute lymphoblastic leukemia, 727
 for chronic lymphoid leukemias, 746
 for hemolytic anemia, 316
 for Hodgkin lymphoma, 772
 for non-Hodgkin lymphoma, 781t, 782, 782t, 783, 784, 787
 for small intestine lymphoma, 481
RNA retroviruses, 21
Robotic surgery, 73
R0 resection, 72
R1 resection, 72
R2 resection, 72
RU-486, 170

S

Safety. See also specific agents and therapies
 clinical trials, 209
 radiation, 90, 90b
Salivary gland tumors, 643–63. See also Head and neck cancers
 epidemiology, 648
 pathology, 651
 presentation, 653
 prognosis and follow-up, 662
Salmon calcitonin, for hypercalcemia, 292
Sarcomas. See also specific types
 bone, 687–92, 706–14
 brachytherapy for, 97
 carcinosarcomas, 613
 defined, 688
 endometrial stromal, 613
 Kaposi, 700–2
 leiomyosarcomas, 613, 705
 small intestine, 479–80
 soft tissue, 687–705
 uterine, 613
Schistosoma haematobium infection, 21
Sciatic pain, spinal cord compression, 332
Screening. See also specific cancers
 cancer, 45–8
  limitations, 47
  principles, 46
  tests, 48
 genetic, 51–7 (See also Genetic screening)
Secondary malignancies, treatment-related, 359
Seed and soil hypothesis, 14
Selection bias, in cancer screening, 47
Sentinel node biopsy, 71
Serial structures, radiotherapy, 85
Serine threonine kinase screening, 55
714X, 202
Sex cord-stromal tumors, 606–9. See also Ovarian cancer
Sexual function, post-treatment, 356
Signal transduction molecules, 7, 7t
Sign of Leser-Trelat, 319

Sister Mary Joseph's node, 484
6-Mercaptopurine (6-MP), 124
6-Thioguanine (6-TG), 124
Sjögren's syndrome, radiotherapy-induced, 358
Skin cancer. See also specific types
 etiology
  sun exposure, 22, 32, 668, 670
  ultraviolet light, 32, 668, 670
 malignant melanoma, 668–76
 Merkel cell carcinoma, 684
 nonmelanoma, 680–3
Skull contents, 326
Small cell lung cancer (SCLC), 413–18. See also Lung cancer
 febrile neutropenia in, 415
 fundamentals, 413
 incidence, 413
 staging and prognostic factors, 413
 superior vena cava syndrome in, 323, 324, 415
 treatment
  chemotherapy, 414–16, 416t
  radiotherapy, 418
Small intestine tumors, 478–81
 diagnosis, 478
 epidemiology and risk factors, 478
 future directions, 481
 management, 480–1
 pathology
  adenocarcinoma, 478
  lymphoma, 479
  metastases, 480
  sarcoma, 479–80
Small-molecule inhibitors, 178–9. See also specific agents
 BCR-ABL kinase inhibitors
  dasatinib, 178
  imatinib, 178
  nilotinib, 178
 epidermal growth factor receptor inhibitors
  erlotinib, 178, 488, 496
  lapatinib, 179, 462

mammalian target of
  rapamycin inhibitors
  (temsirolimus), 179
vascular endothelial
  growth factor
  receptor inhibitors
    sorafenib, 179
    sunitinib, 179
Small T, 4
Smoking
  cancer from, 18, 32
    head and neck, 646
    lung (See Lung cancer)
  cessation, 18
  prevention, 34
Soft tissue sarcomas,
  687–705. See also
  specific types
  angiosarcoma, 704
  classification, 694, 695t
  dermatofibrosarcoma
    protuberans, 704
  desmoid tumors, 704
  diagnosis and staging, 689
  etiology, 688
  gastrointestinal stromal
    tumor, 694–6, 695t
  Kaposi sarcoma, 700–2
  leiomyosarcomas, 705
  liposarcomas, 705
  pathology, 689, 689t
  rhabdomyosar-
    comas, 696–8
  staging system, 690, 691t
  surveillance, 714
  synovial sarcomas, 705
  treatment
    chemotherapy, 691–2
    radiotherapy, 690
    surgery, 690
Somatic molecular
  alterations, 6
Somatic pain, 255
Somatostatin analogues. See
  also specific agents
  for carcinoid
    syndrome, 481
Somatostatin
  syndrome, 308
Sorafenib, 179
  for hepatocellular
    carcinoma, 496
  for renal cancer, 545–6,
    545t
Soy phytoestrogens, 201
Sperm storage, 356, 357t
  for testicular cancers, 593
S phase, 10
Spinal cord
  compression, 331–4
  diagnosis, 333
  examination, 333

management, 334
presentation, 332
symptoms, 332
syndromes, 333t
Spindle cell sarcoma of bone,
  primary malignant, 712
Spindle poisons, 140,
  141t–143t
Spiritual care,
  end-of-life, 387–8
Spiritual suffering,
  end-of-life, 387–8
Spiritual therapies, 203
Spread, principal
  methods, 67
Squamous cell carcinoma
  of head and neck, 650
Squamous cell carcinoma
  of skin
  epidemiology and
    etiology, 680
  management, 682
  presentation, 680, 681f
  prevention and future
    directions, 683
St. John's wort, 203
Staging. See also specific
  cancers
  surgical, 70–1
Stem cell transplantation,
  hematopoietic, 151–64.
  See also Hematopoietic
  stem cell transplantation
Stereotactic body
  radiotherapy (SBRT), 98
Stereotactic
  radiosurgery, 98
Steroid hormone
  antagonists, 169–70
Steroids. See also specific
  types
  cataracts from, 358
  osteopenia from, 358
Stiff-man syndrome, 312
STK11
  in breast cancer, 434
  screening for
    mutations, 55
Streptozocin, 109
Stridor, 338–9
Sun exposure, 22, 32,
  668, 670
Sunitinib, 179
  for gastrointestinal
    stromal tumor, 694
  for hepatocellular
    carcinoma, 496
  for renal cancer, 545, 545t
Superior hypogastric plexus
  block, 266
Superior vena cava
  syndrome, 322–4

clinical features, 322
diagnosis, 323
differential diagnosis, 322
etiology, 322
management, 323–4
  in small cell lung
    cancer, 323, 324, 415
Suppressing agents, 38, 39t.
  See also specific agents
Surgical oncology, 65–80.
  See also specific cancers
  diagnosis and
    staging, 70–1
  general principles, 66
  metastatic disease, 78–80
    bone, 78
    brain, 79
    diagnosis and
      indications, 78
    malignant ascites, 80
    malignant pericardial
      effusion, 80
    malignant pleural
      effusion, 80
  outcome, long-term, 72
  palliative surgery, 74–6
    ascites, 75
    bowel obstruction, 74
    cytoreductive surgery, 76
    fistulas, 74–5
    gastrointestinal
      bleeding, 76
    jaundice, 75
    pain, 75
    primary tumor
      resection, 76
  surgical resection, 66
    curative, 72–3
    prophylactic, 69
  techniques
    conservative and radical
      surgery, 68
    en bloc, 68
    minimally invasive
      surgery, 68
    prophylactic, 69
    reconstructive surgery, 68
  tumor biology, 66
Surgical resection, 66. See
  also specific cancers
  curative, 72–3
  excision margins, 72
  prophylactic, 69
  R0, R1, and R2, 72
Surrogate endpoints, 209
Survival. See also specific
  cancers
  disease-free, 209
  overall, 209
  rates, 72
Sweets syndrome, 316,
  318

Syndrome of inappropriate ADH secretion (SIADH), 294, 306
Synovial sarcomas, 705

T

T'ai chi chuan, 199
Tamoxifen
  for breast cancer, 450
    early, 453–5
    metastatic, 459
  cataracts from, 358
  for ductal carcinoma in situ, 446
  prevention with, 40
  treatment with, 169–70
    + aromatase inhibitors, 170
Target definition, radiotherapy, 93
Targeted therapies, 175–84. See also specific types and cancers
  antibodies
    alemtuzumab, 180
    bevacizumab, 180
    cetuximab, 180
    panitumumab, 180
    rituximab, 180
    trastuzumab, 181
  for breast cancer, metastatic, 461–2
  categories, 176
  conjugated agents
    denileukin diftitox, 182
    ibritumomab, 182
    tositumomab, 182
  demethylation agents
    azacitadine, 183
    decitabine, 183
  histone deacetylase inhibitors (vorinostat), 184
  for malignant melanoma, 675–6
  molecular (See also specific agents)
    for renal cancer, 544–6, 545t
  for non–small-cell lung cancer, 408
  pancreatic cancer, 488
  proteasome inhibitors (bortezomib), 183
  rationale and development, 176
  for renal cancer, 544–6, 545t
  small-molecule inhibitors, 178–9 (See also Small-molecule inhibitors; specific types)

Target mutation, in drug resistance, 144
Taxanes, 140. See also specific agents
  on nerves, 358
T-cell acute lymphoblastic leukemia, 725
T-cell depletion, post-HSCT, 158
Teams,
  multidisciplinary, 62–3
  end-of-life care, 364
Telomerase, 4, 12–13
Temozolomide, 110–11
  for glioblastoma, 631
  for gliomas, 630, 631t
  for malignant melanoma, 675
Temsirolimus, 179
  for renal cancer, 545t, 546
Teniposide, 138
Terminal agitation, 388–9, 390
Terminal secretions, 369, 390
Terminology, adverse events, 816t–817t
Testicular cancer, germ cell, 589–603
  epidemiology and etiology, 590
  follow-up, 603
  investigation, 592
  management, 598–602
    carcinoma in situ, 598
    chemotherapy regimens, examples, 603t
    complications of therapy, 602
    intermediate- and poor-prognosis disease, 601
    prophylactic surgery, 36
    relapsed disease, 602
    residual masses postchemotherapy, 600–1
    stage I IA/B seminoma, 599
    stage I IC–III seminoma, 600
    stage I seminoma, 598–9
  pathology, 591
  presentation, 592
  prognostic grouping, 593, 596t
  screening, 590
  sperm storage, 593
  staging, 593, 594t–595t
Testicular cancer, non–germ cell, 603
  epidemiology and etiology, 590
  management
    complications of therapy, 602
    intermediate- and poor-prognosis disease, 601
    relapsed disease, 602
    residual masses postchemotherapy, 600–1
    stage I, 599
  pathology, 591
  presentation, 591, 592
  screening, 590
Testicular tissue freezing, 356, 357t
Thalidomide
  for multiple myeloma, 758
  venous thromboembolism from, 222f, 273, 274t, 753
Therapeutic massage, 199
6-Thioguanine (6-TG), 124
Thiotepa, 106–7
Thoracic cancers, 395–428. See also specific types
  lung, 396–9
  mesothelioma, 420–4
  non–small-cell lung, 400–12
    chemotherapy, 405–8
    radiation therapy, 410–12
    surgery, 402–4
  small-cell lung, 413–18
    chemotherapy, 414–16
    radiotherapy, 418
  thymic tumors, 426–8
Thrombocytopenia, paraneoplastic, 316
Thrombocytosis, paraneoplastic, 316
Thrombosis
  central venous catheter, 286
  venous (See Venous thromboembolism (VTE))
Thymic tumors, 426–8
  clinical presentation, 426–7
  epidemiology, 426
  investigations, 427
  management and staging, 427
  pathology, 426
  treatment outcomes, 428, 428t
Thymidylate synthase inhibitors, 121
Thyroid cancers, 514–27
  epidemiology and etiology, 514–15

investigations, 517
pathology and genetics, 515–16
presentation
 anaplastic, 517
 medullary, 517
 papillary and follicular, 516
prognosis, 526–7
screening and prevention, 516
staging, 518, 518t
surveillance and follow-up, 526
treatment, 520–5
 chemotherapy, 525
 external beam radiotherapy, 524
 radioiodine, 522–3
 surgery, 520–1
 unsealed radionuclide, 99
Thyroid dysfunction, late effects of treatment in, 354, 355t
Thyroidectomy, prophylactic, 69
Tibetan medicine, 198
Titration. *See also specific agents*
 opioid analgesics, 259, 259b, 262
Tobacco
 chewing
  head and neck cancers from, 646
  leukoplakia from, 32
 smoking, 18, 32, 34 (See *also* Lung cancer)
Topoisomerase inhibitors, 136–8. See *also specific agents*
 topoisomerase II inhibitors
  etoposide, 138
  teniposide, 138
 topoisomerase I inhibitors
  irinotecan, 136–7
  topotecan, 137
Topotecan, 137
 for breast cancer, metastatic, 461
 for cervical cancer, 617
 for ovarian cancer, 609
 for small cell lung cancer, 416
Tositumomab, 182
Total body irradiation (TBI), 98–9
Traditional Chinese medicine (TCM), 198
TRAIL, 13

Trametinib, for malignant melanoma, 675
Transcription factors, 6, 7t
Transfusions, red blood cell
 overview, 218
 recommendations, 220
Transitional cell carcinoma. *See also* Renal cancer
 of bladder and ureter, 548–56 (See *also* Bladder and ureter cancers)
 pathology, 538
 treatment, 544
Transport mechanism alteration, 144
Trastuzumab, 181
 for breast cancer
  early, 451
  invasive ductal carcinoma, 436
  locally advanced, 456
  metastatic, 461, 462
  regimens, 452t–453t
 on cardiac function, 358
 for esophageal cancer, 470
 for gastric cancer, 475
Treatment effects, late, 351–60
 endocrine and metabolic dysfunction
  adrenal failure, 354, 355t
  metabolic syndrome, 355, 355t
  pituitary, 354, 355t
  thyroid, primary, 354, 355t
 fertility issues and preservation, 356–7, 357t
 fundamentals, 352
 neuropsychological, 360
 organ-specific
  bones, 358
  ears, 358
  eyes, 358
  heart, 358
  kidneys, 358
  lungs, 358
  nerves, 358
 secondary malignancies, 359
Treatment principles, 61–3
 multidisciplinary teams, 62–3
 multiple clinical disciplines, 62
 range of expertise, 63
Triazole drugs, 169
Tricyclic antidepressants (TCAs), as adjuvant analgesics, 264

Trifolium pratense, 203
Trimethoprim-sulfamethoxazole (TMP-SMX), for febrile neutropenia prophylaxis, 248
Trophoblastic tumors, 620–4
 hydatidiform moles, 620–2, 622t
 malignant gestational trophoblastic tumor, 623–4, 624t
Trousseau syndrome, 317
Tubulin, 140
Tubulin-interactive agents, 140, 141t–143t
Tumor blocking agents, 38, 39t
Tumor cell lysate preparation, 190
Tumor cell mutation, drug resistance, 144
Tumor lysis syndrome, 300–1
Tumor mass, 102
Tumor progression, 38
Tumor resection, primary palliative, 76
Tumor suppressing agents, 38, 39t
Tumor suppressor genes, 8, 9t, 16, 187. See *also* p53
Tumor virus genes, 17
2-Fluoro-2′-deoxyuridine (floxuridine), 118, 123
Tyrosine kinase inhibitors. *See also specific types*
 resistance, 733–4
 side effects, 733

U

Ulcerative colitis, prophylactic surgery for, 36
Ultraviolet light, in skin cancer, 32, 668, 670
Umbilical cord blood transplantation, 154–5
Undescended testis, prophylactic surgery with, 36
Unfractionated heparin (UFH), for venous thromboembolism prophylaxis
 clinical practice guidelines, 280, 281–2
 regimens and cost, 283t

Unsealed radionuclides, 99–100
Ureter cancers, 548–56. See also Bladder and ureter cancers
Ureteric obstruction, 348–9
Urinary tract obstruction
  etiology, 348
  investigations, 348
  management, 348–9
  symptoms, 348
Urothelial tumors, 548–56. See also Bladder and ureter cancers
Uterine cancer, 610–13
  endometrial cancer, 610–12
  sarcoma, 613

V

Vaccines
  dendritic cell, 191
  DNA, 190–1
  peptide, 190
Vaginal cancer, 618–19
Vancomycin, for febrile neutropenia
  empiric, 242
  prophylactic, 248
Vancomycin-resistant coagulase-negative staphylococci, 237
Vancomycin-resistant enterococcus (VRE), 237
Vascular endothelial growth factor receptors (VEGFRs), 179
Vascular endothelial growth factor (VEGF) receptor inhibitors, 179. See also Sorafenib; Sunitinib
  for brain tumors, 634
  for pancreatic cancer, 488
Vectors, gene therapy, 192, 193t
Vegetables, 19, 42
Vemurafenib, for malignant melanoma, 675
Veno-occlusive disease (VOD), hepatic post-HSCT, 162
Venous thromboembolism (VTE), 271–86
  central venous catheters, 286
  clinical practice guidelines, prophylactic anticoagulation, 280–2

American College of Chest Physicians, 280
American Society of Clinical Oncology, 280–2
National Comprehensive Cancer Network, 280
clinical presentation
  deep vein thrombosis, 276, 277t
  pulmonary embolism, 276, 277t
consequences, 275
from erythropoiesis-stimulating agents, 224
key point summary, 285
prevention and treatment, prophylactic anticoagulation
  meta-analyses, 278–9
  randomized trials, 278
regimens and cost, 283t–284t
risk factors, 274t
  biomarkers, 273
  cancer treatment, 272–3
  general, 272
Verner-Morrison pancreatic cholera, 308
Verrucous tumor, 650
VHL, in renal cancer, 14, 536
Vinblastine, 141t
Vincristine, 141t
  on nerves, 358
Vindesine, 141t
Vinorelbine, 141t–142t
Viral infections, 20–1, 33
Viral vectors, 192, 193t
Virchow's node, 484
Virchow's triad, 272
Virus-directed enzyme prodrug therapy (VDEPT), 188
Visceral pain, 255, 266
  nerve blocks for, 266
Vitamin
  A supplements, 201
  Vitamin D + calcium, 201
  Vitamin E, 201
  Vitamin K antagonists
    for venous thromboembolism
      meta-analyses, 278
      regimens and cost, 284t

for venous thromboembolism prophylaxis, 281
Vitiligo, 319
Vomiting, 817c. See also Nausea and/or vomiting
neural mechanisms, 375f
von Hippel-Lindau (VHL) syndrome, 536. See also Renal cancer
von Hipple-Lindau (VHL) gene, in renal cancer, 14, 536
Vorinostat, 184
Vorozole, 169
Vulvar cancer, 619–20, 622t
  epidemiology and etiology, 619
  pathology, 619
  presentation, 619
  prognosis, 620
  staging, 620, 622t
  survival by stage, 622t
  treatment, 620W
Warfarin
  for central venous catheter thrombosis, 286
  for venous thromboembolism
    meta-analyses, 278
    regimens and cost, 284t
  for venous thromboembolism prophylaxis, 281
Web sites,
  oncology, 818t–819t
Wells clinical deep thrombosis model, 276, 277t
Wells clinical pulmonary embolism model, 276, 277t
Whipple procedure, 486
White cell disorders, paraneoplastic, 316
WHO performance criteria, 803b

Y

Yoga (asanas), 199, 200

Z

Zoledronic acid, for prostate cancer, 584
Zollinger-Ellison syndrome, 308